Health Assessment
in Nursing Practice

Health Assessment in Nursing Practice

Fourth Edition

Jorge Grimes, M.S.N., R.N., Ed.D., ANP
Chair of Graduate Nursing
State University of New York
Health Science Center at Syracuse
Syracuse, New York

Elizabeth Burns, R.N., M.S.N., Ed.D.
Dean of Health
Husson College
Bangor, Maine

Little, Brown and Company
Boston New York Toronto London

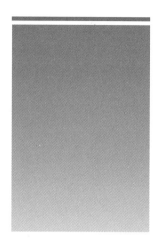

Fourth Edition

Library of Congress Cataloging-in-Publication Data

Grimes, Jorge.
Health assessment in nursing practice / Jorge Grimes, Elizabeth Burns.—4th ed.
p. cm.
Includes bibliographical references and index.
ISBN 0-316-32831-6
1. Nursing assessment. I. Burns, Elizabeth. II. Title.
[DNLM: 1. Nursing Assessment. WY 100.4 G862h 1996]
RT48.G74 1996
616.07'5—dc20
DNLM/DLC
for Library of Congress 95-46922
CIP

Printed in the United States of America
SEM

Editorial: Evan R. Schnittman
Editorial and Production Service: Colophon
Designer: LeGwin Associates
Cover Designer: Hannus Design Associates

Contents

Preface

Professional nurses are in a unique position to meet health care needs comprehensively because they respond to the total needs of the client, emphasizing health, the client's strengths, and the client's involvement in self-care. Professional nurses are committed to client and community education and to the promotion and maintenance of health, as well as to the restoration of health and the detection of illness. Today's nurse provides individuals and families with a humane and continuing point of contact with the health care delivery system.

We believe that maximizing the nurse's ability to provide care requires in-depth knowledge and skill in health assessment. The focus of this book is on providing a systematic approach to the health assessment of individuals of all ages.

The organizing framework of the text integrates four major components of health assessment: social interaction, culture, mental health, and physical health.

Chapter 1 addresses social considerations in health and illness, holistic health, and the interrelationship of nursing and holistic health. It examines the roles of stress, environment, and social class and their relation to an individual's ability to maintain equilibrium for clarity as well as the role that culture plays in an individual's health-promoting activities and response to illness. It is important for nurses to understand culturally relevant approaches in care planning and delivery. In this chapter the nursing process is reviewed and the list of (NANDA) latest nursing diagnoses is included.

Chapter 2 describes aspects of communication essential to comprehensive health assessment. This chapter also emphasizes self-awareness, trust, respect, and empathy, which are factors in the development of a therapeutic milieu.

Chapter 3 provides guidelines for mental health assessment including specific maturational and situational stressors. Much of mental health assessment is accomplished while interviewing the client to obtain a health history.

Obtaining the health history is an important first step in assessing a client's health status. Chapter 4 is designed to provide the nurse with complete information on the client interview and on components of the health history.

Chapters 5 through 16 present steps in the physical assessment of all body systems. Of special assistance to the nurse are the learning objectives, discussion questions, and boxed overviews of the techniques of examination and of appropriate documentation samples provided with every chapter.

Following the systems chapters are three chapters that address assessment of clients at various age levels: Chapter 17, "Assessment of the Newborn"; Chapter 18, "Assessment of the Child and Adolescent"; and Chapter 19, "Assessment of Wellness."

The remaining chapters focus on aggregates: Chapter 20, "Assessment of the Older Adult"; Chapter 21, "Assessment of Women's Health"; and Chapter 22, "Assessment of Men's Health."

We wish to acknowledge the help of Judy Davis Grimes, Ph.D., licensed psychologist. Her contributions to the chapters on communication in health assessment, the health history, and mental health assessment were extensive and helped make these chapters valuable guides for the nurse.

J.G.
E.B.

Acknowledgments

The authors would like to extend a special thank you to the following who have provided photographs and given permission for tables and illustrations.

4: (Fig. 1-1) Adapted from Don Fink, "Holistic Health: Implications for Health Planning," *American Journal of Health Planning,* July 1976.

16 (Fig. 1-6): From John A. Frederich, "Tension Control Techniques," in *Guide to Fitness After Fifty,* Roger Harris and Lawrence W. Frankel, eds. (New York: Plenum Press), 1977.

122 (Figs. 5-4, 5-5, 5-6, 5-7), 123 (Figs. 5-8, 5-9), 145 (Fig. 6-21), 148 (Fig. 6-27), 149 (Fig. 6-29), 150 (Fig. 6-30), 151 (Fig. 6-35), 153 (Fig. 6-37), 157 (Fig. 7-2), 164 (Figs. 7-10, 7-11, 7-12), 166 (Fig. 7-16), 167 (Fig. 7-17B, C), 176 (Fig. 8-7), 177 (Fig. 8-9), 185 (Fig. 8-22), 187 (Fig. 8-26), 211 (Fig. 9-27), 233 (Figs. 10-16, 10-17), 234 (Fig. 10-18), 235 (Fig. 10-20), 298 (Fig. 13-17), 312 (Fig. 14-4), 384 (Figs. 16-25, 16-27), 507 (Fig. 21-3): Used with permission from R. H. Kampmeier and T. M. Blake, *Physical Examination in Health and Disease,* 4th ed. (Philadelphia: F. A. Davis Company), 1970.

124 (Fig. 5-10), 125 (Figs. 5-11, 5-12), 134 (Fig. 6-2), 138 (Figs. 6-3, 6-4), 140 (Fig. 6-9), 143 (Fig. 6-14), 145 (Fig. 6-22), 150 (Figs. 6-31, 6-33), 152 (Fig. 6-36), 165 (Fig. 7-14), 167 (Fig. 7-17A), 186 (Fig. 8-24), 187 (Figs. 8-27, 8-28, 8-29), 184 (Fig. 8-18), 190–192 (all photos), 209 (Figs. 9-21, 9-23), 275 (Fig. 12-5), 292 (Fig. 13-10), 310 (Figs. 14-2, 14-3), 330 (Figs. 14-22, 14-23), 331 (Figs. 14-24, 14-25, 14-26), 387 (Figs. 16-30, 16-31), 377 (Fig. 16-21), color endsheets: Courtesy Erie County Medical Center, Buffalo, New York.

150 (Fig. 6-32): From Abbott Laboratories, *Common Skin Diseases—An Atlas,* 1954. (Fig. 6-34): From Braunwald et al., *Harrison's Principles of Internal Medicine,* 8th ed., © 1977 New York: McGraw-Hill. Reprinted by permission.

144 (Fig. 6-19), 145 (Fig. 6-20), 197 (Fig. 9-6): From Abbott Laboratories, *Some Pathological Conditions of the Eye, Ear and Throat* © 1946.

164 (Figs. 7-10 and 7-12), 185 (Fig. 8-21), 178 (Fig. 8-10), 209 (Figs. 9-19, 9-20, 9-22), 210 (Figs. 2-25, 2-26): From Mahlon H. Delp and Robert Manning, *Majors Physical Diagnosis* (Philadelphia: Saunders), 1981, by permission of the publisher.

164 (Fig. 7-13), 165 (Fig. 7-15), 205 (Fig. 9-17), 241 (Fig. 11-3), 332 (Fig. 14-27): Reprinted from the Revised Clinical Slide Collection on the Rheumatic Disiases, copyright 1981. Used by permission of the American Rheumatism Association.

329 (Fig. 14-20): From John A. Prior and Jack S. Silberstein, *Physical Diagnosis,* 5th ed. (St. Louis: C. V. Mosby), 1977, used by permission of the publisher.

392 (Fig. 17-1): From F. C. Battaglia and L. O. Lubchenco, "A Practical Classification of Newborn Infants by Weight and Gestational Age." *The Journal of Pediatrics,* August 1967, p. 161.

393 (Fig. 17-2): From C. H. Kempe, H. K. Silver, and D. O'Brien, *Current Pediatric Diagnosis and Treatment* (Los Altos, Calif.: Lange Medical Publicaitons), 1980.

397–426: Photos courtesy of Mead Johnson Laboratories.

446–448 (Figs. 18-3–18-6): Courtesy Ross Laboratories.

499, 451, 459: Photos from Daniel Bellack.

454 (Fig. 18-14): Courtesy National Society to Prevent Blindness, New York.

481 (Fig. 20-1): Joan Netherwood.

484 (Fig. 20-2): Courtesy NIH Gerontology Research Center.

506 (Fig. 21-2): Adapted from *Nutrition During Pregnancy and Lactation,* Maternal and Child Health Unit, California Department of Health, 1975, pp. 62–63.

PART I

General Assessment

CHAPTER 1

Holistic Health Assessment

Learning Objectives

1. Identify characteristics of holistic health.
2. Describe the role of nursing in holistic health and wellness.
3. Describe the phases of the nursing process.
4. Explain the concept of data analysis.
5. Define the concepts of health and illness.
6. Discuss the psychosocial and physiologic stages of illness.
7. Give examples of individual reactions to loss of social role.
8. Explain the effect of stress on health.
9. Identify factors in the environment that affect health and illness.
10. Describe the relationship between social class and illness.
11. Define *ethnocentrism.*
12. Identify cultural areas of health assessment.
13. Explain what is meant by "The family is an expression of the culture in which it is found."
14. State examples of religious influence on health care and health status.
15. Recognize that personal space is perceived differently by various cultures.
16. Recognize that attitudes, values, and customs differ among social classes.

Health care and the concept of holistic health are examined in this chapter, with particular attention given to their interface with the nursing process. Common sociologic and cultural factors that affect health are also discussed.

HEALTH CARE

Health professionals and laypeople are becoming increasingly aware that we must go beyond the goal of curing illness. Many illnesses appear to be caused, or at least fostered, by societal demands and conditions and individual lifestyles. Evidence indicates that the shift in emphasis can and should be toward the prevention of illness and the refinement of concepts of wellness and holistic health.

The movement in this direction has been slow for a number of reasons. The health care system has been and continues (to a large extent) to be based on the medical model, in which the focus of health care is on the treatment of illness. Historically, the reason for this emphasis has been society's need to cure communicable disease. This goal has largely been accomplished, and at present the focus of the medical model is on the cure of life-threatening and chronic diseases, such as hypertension, heart disease, stroke, diabetes, and cancer.

An additional and persuasive reason for slowness in the movement toward a wellness orientation is the politics of the illness care system in the United States. The health care industry, focused primarily on illness care, is the third largest industry in the United States and employs 6% of the labor force (Kalisch & Kalisch 1982, p. 93). In addition, most health care insurance is directed toward illness care. Little reimbursement is provided for providers and seekers of preventive health care, health promotion, and health maintenance services. However, the public is beginning to demand care that will increase the level of wellness, reduce the cost of illness care, and enhance quality of life. As a result, medical education is placing increased focus on the preparation of primary physicians, and nursing education continues to emphasize health promotion and disease prevention at both the undergraduate and the graduate levels. Increasingly, graduate nursing programs focus on provision of primary care through the preparation of advanced practice nurses (including nurse practitioners and midwives).

CONCEPTUAL BASES OF HOLISTIC HEALTH

The concept of *holism* must be understood before it can be applied to health and nursing. The philosophical concept of holism defines the whole as greater than the sum of its parts. In 1926, Jan Christian Smuts, in addressing the concepts of holism and evolution, disagreed with the analytical method employed by the life sciences to study organisms. He knew there was more to learn about the human body than could be found by taking each cell part and studying it in isolation. He felt there is an organizing process that pulls everything together in harmony, causing the organism to maintain itself in a fluctuating environment. He referred to this process as "holism."

Philosophically, from the standpoint of holism (which considers the whole to be greater than the sum of its parts), attention should be paid to the interconnectiveness—the relations and the patterns of life and of self—between and within the environment and the universe. Many primitive cultures were "in tune" with the earth and healing. The earth was deemed sacred and a healer by the Native Americans. With an acceptance of the nature of life, illness, suffering, and death become an integral part of living.

Holistic health care is an approach to wellness that is person-oriented rather than disease-oriented. Holistic health assessment recognizes every aspect of the person's interacting with the environment. Holistic health practice encompasses the prevention of illness and maintenance of health as well as the healing process. The average person does not maintain responsibility for health but has relinquished this responsibility to the health care system. Many consumers have come to believe that they can smoke, tolerate obesity, drink to excess, and drive carelessly; they expect that the effects of these excesses can be repaired by the health care system. The holistic perspective requires that the individual become an active participant in maintaining a healthy lifestyle. An additional aspect of holistic health is the view that illness is a creative opportunity for the individual to learn more about himself, to evaluate goals and values, and to engage in self-explanation.

Holistic health care concepts and practices include humanistic medicine, alternative health care, preprimary care, and altered provider-patient relationships (Fink 1976, pp. 23–31).

Humanistic medicine deals with illness but focuses on the presence of health in the person who also happens to be ill. Humanistic medicine attempts to work within the health care system while encouraging it to move toward a more holistic approach. Using this approach, the professional is a technical specialist who supports clients in devising new

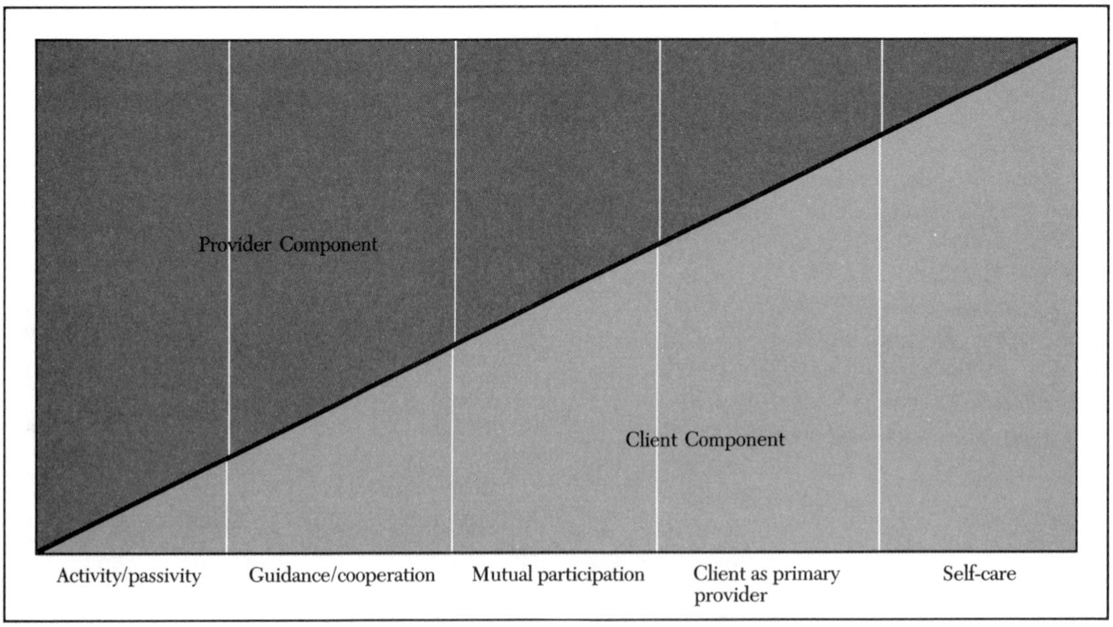

Figure 1-1 Provider-patient relationships.

approaches to health and in assuming responsibility for lifestyle choices.

Alternative health care helps the client to seek several possibilities. Examples of these alternatives are biofeedback, meditation, imaging, massage, rolfing, relaxation techniques, and therapeutic touch. Alternative care can also mean involvement in organized health systems that are not part of Western scientific medicine, such as acupuncture, African and Hispanic healing systems, and homeopathy.

Preprimary care is a health care system in which people manage their own health care problems. This system includes the self-care and self-help movements.

There are five levels to be considered in the *altered provider-patient relationship* (Fig. 1-1).

- *First level:* The patient is passive; the health practitioner relationship resembles the traditional parent-child relationship.
- *Second level:* The patient is ill but aware and capable of following directions and making some choices.
- *Third level:* Mutual participation occurs; the practitioner helps the individual to help herself by sharing information.
- *Fourth level:* The practitioner is a consultant; the individual bears primary responsibility for health or illness.
- *Highest level:* The individual assumes total responsibility for care.

Self-care has captured the imagination and support of many in the United States and is being encouraged by several health insurers as a means of containing health care costs. Currently, however, the majority of health insurers will not financially support physical and psychological health promotion and illness prevention therapies.

NURSING AND HOLISTIC HEALTH

Historically, nursing has had a commitment to holistic health and wellness. From Florence Nightingale in the mid-1800s to the theorists of the past 40 years, nursing has focused on the promotion and maintenance of health. Concepts of health and wellness as related to the individual, family, and community are addressed by nursing assessment and include physical, psychosocial, cultural, spiritual, and environmental factors.

Flynn has purported that the nurse should exhibit "realness, empathetic understanding and unconditioned positive regard for the client" (Flynn 1980, p. 19). She suggests that by gathering the following information, nurses will consciously integrate holistic principles in practice:

- You can attend to the part that your clients' lifestyles play in their levels of wellness. What is the way they live?
- How do their beliefs, values, and needs fit their behavior?
- What are their relationships with others?
- How do they handle stress?
- Do they take care of their bodies?
- Do they recognize their philosophical and spiritual needs, and are they comfortable with that aspect of their life? (Flynn 1980, p. 22)

Holistic nursing practice uses the steps of the nursing process. The following general discussion of the nursing process explains the role of health assessment in the nursing process.

The Nursing Process

The nursing process is a means of problem solving. It is a purposeful process, the ultimate goal of which is to help improve the health status of a client or assist the client in maintaining or returning to his optimum level of functioning and wellness. The phases of the nursing process include

- assessment
- nursing diagnoses
- planning
- implementation
- evaluation

This process is not linear; rather than being sequential, the activities described within each phase are interactive at any point in time. Data evolve as they are critically processed. In other words, as you collect data you are constantly analyzing, validating, and evaluating within each phase.

Assessment

Assessment generally has been described as the foundation of the nursing process. The greater your knowledge and experience, the greater the potential for an accurate and comprehensive assessment. Knowledge aids you in determining when a behavior or response needs to be pursued to collect additional pertinent information. It also helps you to recognize interrelationships of findings and to identify patterns. When the time available for assessment is short, knowledge and experience dictate the priorities for investigation in light of the presenting behavioral responses. During data collection, as well as during the analysis and synthesis of data, knowledge sets the stage by organizing frames of reference.

The process of health assessment is an independent nursing activity. It provides the data necessary for the nurse to make diagnoses and perform tasks and responsibilities within the framework of case finding, health teaching, health counseling, and therapeutic nursing care. In health assessment, models of nursing theorists such as Benner, King, Neuman, Orem, Parse, Peplau, Rogers, Roy, and Watson provide such frames of reference, along with such commonly used nonnursing theories as

- Maslow's hierarchy of needs
- Selye's general adaptation syndrome

- Erikson's psychosocial development theory
- Havighurst's developmental tasks
- Duvall's stages of family development
- Piaget's cognitive developmental theory
- Lewin's field phenomenon

Such theories, plus knowledge of normal ranges and normal variations, provide guidelines for understanding clients and their environments, for decision making in the collection of data about the client's health status, and for analyzing and synthesizing the data base. Assessment establishes the client as a person—as unique—and therefore facilitates the individualization of care.

Data collection is inherent to the assessment phase and is directed toward information relative to health status. Data collection requires

- interpersonal and communication skills
- ability to empathize
- knowledge of nursing and related sciences
- skillful use of the senses

Data collection involves ongoing analysis of interactions, historical aspects, physical findings, and client behaviors. It is performed during all phases of the nursing process.

Generally, data are classified as either objective or subjective. You can measure *objective data;* objective data can be observed and measured similarly by another individual. *Signs* are objective data; you can see, touch, hear, or obtain standardized measurement of it. *Symptoms,* on the other hand, are considered *subjective data.* Subjective data are observable only by the client; therefore, you know these data only if the client communicates them to you. The accompanying lists exemplify objective and subjective data.

Objective data: Examples
Vital signs, deformities, skin lesions, drainage, emesis, edema, feces, urine volume, asymmetry, distention, laboratory results (sonogram, x-ray, ECG, EEG, blood chemistry, urinalysis)

Subjective data: Examples
Pain, nausea, vertigo, palpitations, mood, fear, anger, disappointment, frustration, happiness

You may observe facial expressions or characteristic body positioning or gestures that might be clues that the client is experiencing a particular symptom, but you will never really know what the client is experiencing unless the client tells you during the process of validation. Subjective data are experienced by personal feelings and personal perspectives. They are any data reflected by what the client says or what others (family members, health professionals, even you) say about the client.

Analysis and synthesis of data are paramount to assessment. At times, a given interpretation may prompt further data collection. Accuracy takes precedence. The more thorough and comprehensive the data base, the greater the potential for insight regarding the client or situation. No matter how complete the data base, the data are virtually useless without skillful and knowledgeable analysis.

The analysis of the client's health situation has a different "flavor" when performed by the nurse than when performed by the physician. When the physician screens the client, the goal is to ascertain whether there are existing pathologic conditions that require medical or surgical care. The nurse assesses the client's health status in regard to a pattern of

- risk factors
- health practices
- lifestyle
- culture
- existing health problems
- existing complications related to health problems
- the potential for complications related to health problems
- the potential for health problems
- psychosocial and physical responses to illness
- wellness and assets

In other words, the nurse's focus is on nursing care for the total human being in all phases and life functions.

Regulations governing nursing practice hold the nurse responsible for case finding and for having the client seek medical attention when needed. Recognizing deviations from the norm and seeking consultation or initiating referral are reflective of ethical practice and accountability in nursing practice. These legal obligations require the nurse to have knowledge of norms and differences in norms as influenced by age, race, and gender.

The identification of the client's assets is a key feature of health assessment, because these strengths help the client maintain balance or restore equilibrium when imbalances in health status occur. Examples of client assets are

- a healthy constitution (e.g., decreased vulnerability to illness, minimal disease history)
- decreased exposure to illness-causing variables
- good nutrition
- regular exercise habits
- vital signs and weight within the norm
- temperance in all things
- absence of detrimental habits (e.g., drug abuse, smoking)
- a solid support system
- a love of life
- a thriving spirituality
- stable sexuality
- leisure and hobby interests
- ability to learn quickly
- flexibility (e.g., ability to adapt easily to changing circumstances)

- financial security
- employment
- busy, enjoyable retirement
- good self-esteem
- self-care capabilities
- health insurance

When the client situation is viewed in light of assets, the outlook may not be as dismal as originally thought. For instance, a client who has had a limb amputated as a result of an accident could have a brighter outlook if her many assets are emphasized rather than if the focus is merely on the limb loss and the resulting limitations. In a larger context, analysis of data can lead to the discovery and development of new knowledge and new theoretical frameworks. It can assist in identifying populations at risk. It can aid in the endeavor to develop and perfect assessment tools, to categorize knowledge, and to improve nursing interventions and the implementation and evaluation of nursing care. Analysis determines patterns of client behavior, and nursing diagnoses are the products of analysis and synthesis of the health assessment data base.

Nursing Diagnoses

Most regulations governing nursing practice state that it is the legal responsibility of the licensed registered nurse to make nursing diagnoses. A nursing diagnosis generally has three components:

1. The actual or potential problem
2. The potential or actual factors that may be contributing to the problem—the etiology of the problem
3. The pattern of objective and subjective data (signs and symptoms) that define the health problem

The following is an example of a nursing diagnosis:

Fluid volume deficit
related to persistent diarrhea
as evidenced by dry skin, poor skin turgor, dry lips and buccal mucosa, furrowed tongue, fever, fatigue, weakness, and vertigo

Table 1-1 provides examples of nursing diagnoses and possible etiologies.

The first conference for the purpose of developing a classification system for nursing diagnoses was held in 1973. Table 1-2 lists the diagnostic categories that have accumulated from several subsequent conferences on nursing diagnoses. Once nursing diagnoses have been identified, therapeutic nursing interventions are planned.

Planning

The plans for action must be determined within ethical boundaries and consider the health assessment data, the client's rights, and the nurse's legal responsibilities within

Table 1-1 **Examples of Nursing Diagnoses**

Actual or potential problem		Sample causes
Ineffective breathing pattern	related to	Retained secretions
Alteration in urinary elimination	related to	Incontinence
Sexual dysfunction	related to	Side effects of sedatives
Knowledge deficit	related to	Low-salt diet
Acute anxiety	related to	Impending surgery
Self-care deficit: feeding	related to	Right-side paralysis
Situational low self-esteem	related to	Unemployment
Constipation	related to	Immobility Inadequate fluids Lack of fiber in diet
Noncompliance with diabetic diet	related to	Lack of knowledge Inadequate finances
High risk for trauma	related to	Decreased visual acuity Muscle weakness Throw rugs Absence of handrails
Social isolation	related to	Depression due to death of spouse
Anticipatory grieving	related to	Inability to talk about impending loss of leg

Table 1-2 North American Nursing Diagnosis Association Categories for Nursing Diagnoses

Exchanging

Altered nutrition: more than body requirements
Altered nutrition: less than body requirements
Altered nutrition: high risk for more than body requirements
High risk for infection
High risk for altered body temperature
Hypothermia
Hyperthermia
Ineffective themoregulation
Dysreflexia
Constipation
Perceived constipation
Colonic constipation
Diarrhea
Bowel incontinence
Altered urinary elimination
Stress incontinence
Reflex incontinence
Urge incontinence
Functional incontinence
Total incontinence
Urinary retention
Altered tissue perfusion (specify type) (renal, cerebral, cardiopulmonary, gastrointestinal, peripheral)
Fluid volume excess
Fluid volume deficit
High risk for fluid volume deficit
Decreased cardiac output
Impaired gas exchange
Ineffective airway clearance
Ineffective breathing pattern
Inability to sustain spontaneous ventilation
Dysfunctional ventilatory weaning response
High risk for injury
High risk for suffocation
High risk for poisoning
High risk for trauma
High risk for aspiration
High risk for disuse syndorme
Altered protection
Impaired tissue integrity
Altered oral mucous membrane
Impaired skin integrity
High risk for impaired skin integrity

Communicating

Impaired verbal communication

Relating

Impaired social interaction
Social isolation
Altered role performance
Altered parenting
High risk for altered parenting
Sexual dysfunction
Altered family processes
Caregiver role strain
High risk for caregiver role strain
Parental role conflict
Altered sexuality patterns

Valuing

Spiritual distress (distress of the human spirit)

Choosing

Ineffective individual coping
Impaired adjustment
Defensive coping
Ineffective denial
Ineffective family coping: disabling
Ineffective family coping: compromised
Family coping: potential for growth
Ineffective management of therapeutic regimen (individuals)
Noncomplicance (specify)
Decisional conflict (specify)
Health-seeking behaviors (specify)

Moving

Impaired physical mobility
High risk for peripheral neurovascular dysfunction
Activity intolerance
Fatigue
High risk for activity intolerance
Sleep pattern disturbance
Diversional activity deficit
Impaired home maintenance management
Altered health maintenance
Feeding self-care deficit
Impaired swallowing
Ineffective breastfeeding
Interrupted breastfeeding
Effective breastfeeding
Ineffective infant feeding pattern
Bathing/hygiene self-care deficit
Dressing/grooming self-care deficit
Toileting self-care deficit
Altered growth and development
Relocation stress syndrome

Perceiving

Body image disturbance
Self-esteem disturbance
Chronic low self-esteem
Situational low self-esteem
Personal identity disturbance
Sensory/perceptual alterations (specify) (visual, auditory, kinesthetic, gustatory, tactile, olfactory)
Unilateral neglect
Hopelessness
Powerlessness

Table 1-2 Continued

Knowing	High risk for violence: self-directed or directed at others
Knowledge deficit (specify)	High risk for self-mutilation
Altered thought process	Post-trauma response
	Rape-trauma syndrome
Feeling	Rape-trauma syndrome: compound reaction
Pain	Rape-trauma syyndrome: silent reaction
Chronic pain	Anxiety
Dysfunctional grieving	Fear
Anticipatory grieving	

a nonbiased context of respect and acceptance of the client. The American Hospital Association has published "A Patient's Bill of Rights" (see below) to communicate the rights of clients to all concerned. Professionals must protect and facilitate the client's exercise of ethical and legal rights. The American Nurses' Association has published a "Code for Nurses" (see p. 10) that establishes guidelines to ethical behaviors and responsibilities in nursing practice. A nurse is legally bound to render a certain standard of nursing care contingent on educational level. This expected level of care is judged by what nurses with similar education would do in the client situation. It is assumed that nurses with similar educational backgrounds can make judgments that are reasonably the same.

Outcomes are desired changes in clients' health status. They are defined in response to the nursing goals and according to a time frame. The nursing goal might be to adequately hydrate the client. The nursing diagnosis of "fluid volume deficit related to persistent diarrhea" may have the outcome criteria of "moist lips, good skin turgor, normal temperature, and 3000 mL oral intake in 24 hours." The outcomes can be observed and measured. The therapeutic

A Patient's Bill of Rights

The American Hospital Association presents a Patient's Bill of Rights with the expectation that observance of these rights will contribute to more effective patient care and greater satisfaction for the patient, his physician, and the hospital organization. Further, the Association presents these rights in the expectation that they will be supported by the hospital on behalf of its patients, as an integral part of the healing process. It is recognized that a personal relationship between the physician and the patient is essential for the provision of proper medical care. The traditional physician-patient relationship takes on a new dimension when care is rendered within an organizational structure. Legal precedent has established that the institution itself also has a responsibility to the patient. It is in recognition of these factors that these rights are affirmed.

1. The patient has the right to considerate and respectful care.
2. The patient has the right to obtain from his physician complete current information concerning his diagnosis, treatment, and prognosis in terms the patient can be reasonably expected to understand. When it is not medically advisable to give such information to the patient, the information should be made available to an appropriate person in his behalf. He has the right to know, by name, the physician responsible for coordinating his care.
3. The patient has the right to receive from his physician information necessary to give informed consent prior to the start of any procedure and/or treatment. Except in emergencies, such information for informed consent should include but not necessarily be limited to the specific procedure and/or treatment, the medically significant risks involved, and the probable duration of incapacitation. Where medically significant alternatives for care or treatment exist, or when the patient requests information concerning medical alternatives, the patient has the right to such information. The patient also has the right to know the name of the person responsible for the procedures and/or treatment.
4. The patient has the right to refuse treatment to the extent permitted by law and to be informed of the medical consequences of his action.
5. The patient has the right to every consideration of his privacy concerning his own medical care program. Case discussion, consultation, examination, and treatment are confidential and should be conducted discreetly. Those not directly involved in his care must have the permission of the patient to be present.
6. The patient has the right to expect that all communications and records pertaining to his care should be treated as confidential.
7. The patient has the right to expect that within its capacity a hospital must make reasonable response

to the request of a patient for services. The hospital must provide evaluation, service, and/or referral as indicated by the urgency of the case. When medically permissible a patient may be transferred to another facility only after he has received complete information and explanation concerning the needs for and alternatives to such a transfer. The institution to which the patient is to be transferred must first have accepted the patient for transfer.

8. The patient has the right to obtain information as to any relationship of his hospital to other health care and educational institutions insofar as his care is concerned. The patient has the right to obtain information as to the existence of any professional relationships among individuals, by name, who are treating him.
9. The patient has the right to be advised if the hospital proposes to engage in or perform human experimentation affecting his care or treatment. The patient has the right to refuse to participate in such research projects.
10. The patient has the right to expect reasonable continuity of care. He has the right to know in advance what appointment times and physicians are available and when. The patient has the right that the hospital will provide a mechanism whereby he is informed by his physician or a delegate of the physician of the patient's continuing health care requirements following discharge.
11. The patient has the right to examine and receive an explanation of his bill regardless of source of payment.
12. The patient has a right to know what hospital rules and regulations apply to his conduct as a patient.

No catalogue of rights can guarantee for the patient the kind of treatment he has a right to expect. A hospital has many functions to perform, including the prevention and treatment of disease, the education of both health professionals and patients, and the conduct of clinical research. All these activities must be conducted with an overriding concern for the patient and, above all, the recognition of his dignity as a human being. Success in achieving this recognition assures success in the defense of the rights of the patient.

Courtesy American Hospital Association.

American Nurses' Association Code for Nurses

1. The nurse provides services with respect for human dignity and the uniqueness of the client unrestricted by considerations of social or economic status, personal attributes, or the nature of health problems.
2. The nurse safeguards the client's right to privacy by judiciously protecting information of a confidential nature.
3. The nurse acts to safeguard the client and the public when health care and safety are affected by incompetent, unethical, or illegal practice of any person.
4. The nurse assumes responsibility and accountability for individual nursing judgments and actions.
5. The nurse maintains competence in nursing.
6. The nurse exercises informed judgment and uses individual competence and qualifications as criteria in seeking consultation, accepting responsibilities, and delegating nursing activities to others.
7. The nurse participates in activities that contribute to the ongoing development of the profession's body of knowledge.
8. The nurse participates in the profession's efforts to implement and improve standards of nursing.
9. The nurse participates in the profession's efforts to establish and maintain conditions of employment conducive to high-quality nursing care.
10. The nurse participates in the profession's effort to protect the public from misinformation and misrepresentation and to maintain the integrity of nursing.
11. The nurse collaborates with members of the health professions and other citizens in promoting community and national efforts to meet the health needs of the public.

nursing interventions are the means, planned mutually by the client and the nurse, to help the client achieve the specific outcomes.

Nursing interventions promote and strengthen the client's coping strategies and health resources; they are directed toward the prevention of health problems and complications of illness or healing measures. They are prescribed to eradicate, modify, and control the causes of a health problem; to prevent further debilitation; to promote wellness; and to increase the quality of life.

Client participation in the identification of concerns, the setting of priorities, and the determination of the plans of action is extremely important. A client's concerns, or what he may view as priorities, may go unattended if he is not involved actively in planning. Client participation increases client compliance with nursing and medical treatment. You need to be aware of the client's priorities and work from that basis.

Sometimes the client is unaware of health enhancement priorities. Health teaching provides the client with an opportunity for learning about his health status and alternative means of enhancing it. This additional knowledge gives the client a different perspective and more information with which to evaluate the situation. The added knowledge may affect how the client views his concerns and priorities. Furthermore, the client's perspective may align more with that of the nurse or the physician.

Occasionally, interventions made without the client's participation may prove to be more harsh than necessary. For instance, if bowel elimination complications develop in a client undergoing bed rest, a laxative may be prescribed. The nurse, in planning with the client, may discover a less harsh solution. For this particular client, a glass of prune juice or apple cider in the morning and evening could be as effective as a laxative.

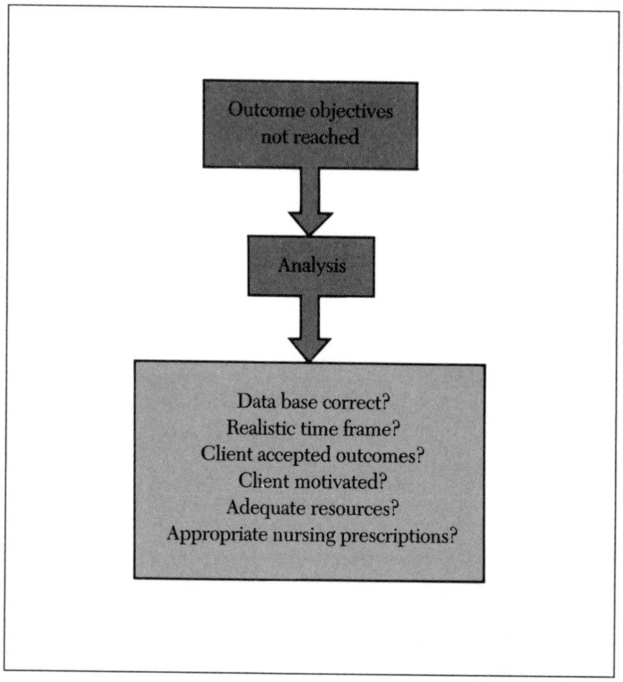

Figure 1-2 Some analytic questions to consider when the desired outcomes are not achieved.

Implementation

Once the nursing interventions have been determined, they must be carried out. This implementation of nursing plans is the action phase of the nursing process. The intervention phase is based on scientific rationale underpinning each purposeful action performed by the nurse or the client. Concomitant assessment, analysis, and evaluation are done with the initiation of each step of the plan. The effectiveness of the intervention in assisting the client to achieve outcome objectives is evaluated.

Evaluation

The evaluation phase judges the degree to which the client's status has progressed toward the established outcomes. Eval-

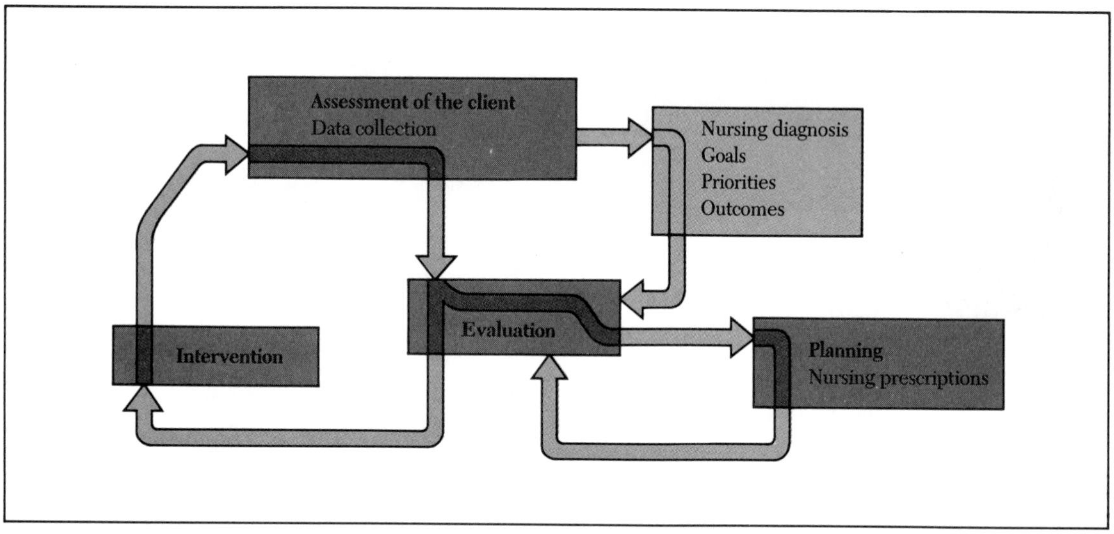

Figure 1-3 The phases of the nursing process are not linear but intertwine. Initial collection of data generates nursing diagnosis; data collection following implementation leads to evaluation of nursing intervention effectiveness or to reformation of the planning phase.

uation determines whether a specific nursing diagnosis has been resolved (or to what degree it is present) and the effectiveness of the nursing interventions.

Care must be taken not to "compare apples and oranges." For example, nursing actions directed toward alleviating stress or pain may be effective despite the client's overall physical deterioration from a debilitating disease. In such a case, the nursing interventions may be promoting wellness, even though the signs of physical illness may be progressive.

If the desired outcomes relative to the specific nursing diagnosis and nursing interventions are not realized, analysis is necessary to determine why. Evaluation may lead to reformulation of nursing diagnoses and nursing interventions (Fig. 1-2). The interrelatedness of the phases of the nursing process is illustrated in Fig. 1-3.

CONCEPTS OF HEALTH AND ILLNESS

According to Dunn (1959, 1977) health and illness are not discrete states of being. They are actually part of a continuum, with optimum health or a high level of wellness at one end and illness and death at the other. Figure 1-4 illustrates this health continuum. Notice that there may be situations in which the body operates with a dysfunction such as diabetes mellitus, yet the overall level of wellness can be maintained through treatment. Therefore, a client who has a chronic illness may, with the proper care, lead a healthy life.

Dunn's concept of health has been criticized as limited because it is an either-or (wellness-illness) phenomenon. Nursing theorists have defined health in a variety of ways (Chinn & Jacobs 1987):

- Orem (1971) conceptualized health as a state of wholeness.
- Levine (1967) and Neuman (1974) talked of health as a holistic balance and a state of homeostasis, respectively.
- Peplau (1952) defined health as a forward-moving process.
- Rogers (1970) explained health as a process of becoming.
- King (1971) and Roy (1976) stated that health was a process of adaptation.
- Parse (1981) described health as a "lived experience"—a continuous, changing process, a way of life that a person co-creates with the environment.

Whether conceptualized as a state or as a process, the common view of health is that it is dynamic, always changing.

Because wellness and illness patterns are reflected in the gestalt of health, their characteristics, along with variables known to influence wellness and illness, are examined to assess health. A person's level of wellness can be changed by stimuli that cause stress. Stressors can be physical, psychological, or social. Regardless of the form of the stressor (see box entitled "Examples of Stressors"), the body responds holistically. Illness arises from the inability to cope with these threats to health.

An individual surrounds herself with protective devices that enable her to maintain health. These devices might be physical, such as clothing and housing; behavioral, such as diet, healthy habits, coping strategies, and hobbies; or psychosocial, such as family ties, love relationships, and a

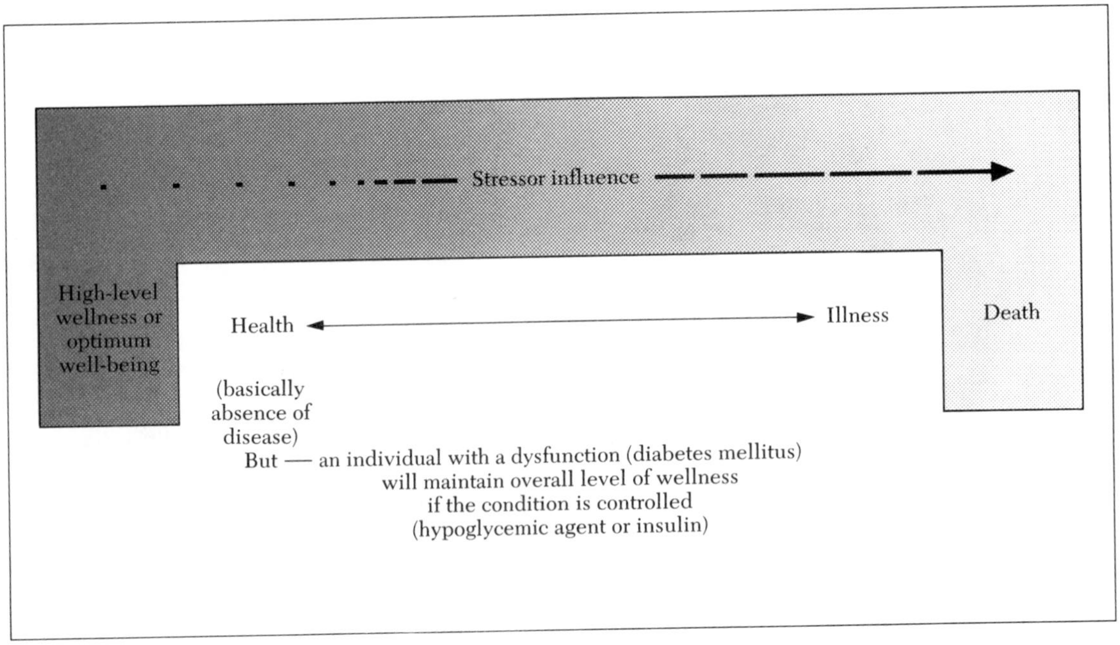

Figure 1-4 Halburt Dunn's health continuum.

Examples of Stressors

Physical:	Viruses, bacteria, trauma (burns, fractures, wounds, surgery)
Psychological:	Separation or death of a loved one; loss; abuse; life demands of family, school, job; illness
Social:	Environmental situation, particular lifestyle, incarceration, divorce, marriage, relocation, poverty

resilient attitude toward life. These protective devices may enable a person to overcome stress easily and regain health. At other times, the stress is too powerful and the individual will become ill.

Figure 1-5 illustrates the physical and psychosocial stages of illness. There are two recognized physical stages of illness: onset and recovery. In addition, Martin and Prange (1962) identified three psychosocial stages of illness that parallel the physical stages but lag behind them:

1. transition to illness
2. acceptance of illness
3. convalescence

Additional time is needed (brown line) before a person can psychologically and socially assimilate the physical changes of illness (gray line).

Two people can have the same illness and respond differently. Some rapidly identify the signs and symptoms of illness and then interrupt their activities. Others may continue to work despite signs such as pain and fever. The latter persons are using the major mental defense mechanism of the transition stage of illness: *denial.* Use of this mechanism may diminish pain or anxiety or alleviate them altogether. It is also common for the mechanism of *rationalization* to occur at this time. The individual attempts to convince himself that he is not ill; he tells himself that he cannot possibly be ill. Otherwise, he could not have continued to unload a ton of cement blocks or play 18 holes of golf. The time lag between physical change and psychosocial assimilation is the period of denial and rationalization (Fig. 1-5, shaded area). Denial can delay necessary health care, but in cases of terminal diagnoses, it also may provide the incentive for the client to live day by day.

As the symptoms become more severe and more specific, the individual enters the second stage of illness: *acceptance.* At this time, she has acknowledged that she is ill and in most cases abandons the mechanisms of denial and rationalization. During this stage, the individual begins to display *regressive* and *passive* behavior; she may lie down and request that someone take her temperature or get her a couple of aspirins or get the nurse or doctor, depending on the severity of the illness. Her dependence on others decreases her anxiety and fear of illness as she reverts to the safe haven of earlier stages of development, in which she was attended to and could physically and psychologically rest. This resting period promotes the healing process. Generally, during this phase most people assume the position of cooperation fostered by the desire for and the social obligation of getting well.

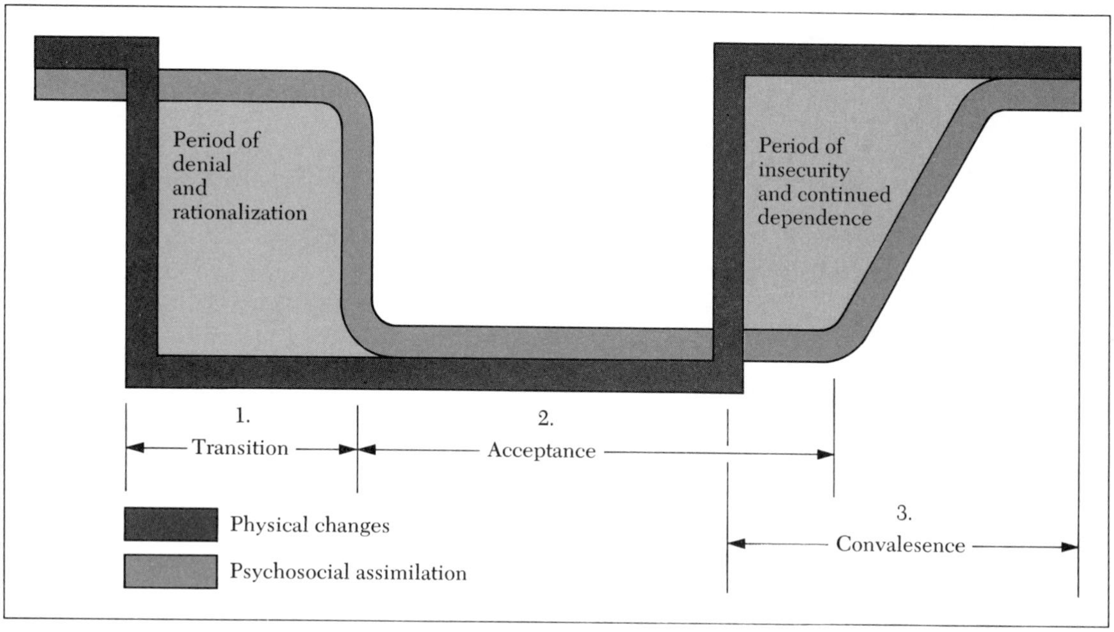

Figure 1-5 Psychosocial lag to physical stages of illness.

In the third stage of illness, *convalescence*, the physical signs of illness are gone; however, this time is characterized by insecurity due to the thought of relinquishing the protective world and its accompanying attentions and kindnesses. In this stage, the nurse must be careful not to reinforce the client's dependent behavior by continuing to feed and bathe her when she is capable of doing so herself. During this phase, the nurse must encourage and support the client in taking steps to resume her independence. The time lag between the physical and psychosocial beginnings of convalescence is the period of insecurity and continued dependence (Fig. 1-5, shaded area).

Not all individuals accept the role of cooperation during illness. Instead, a person may reject this role and become the "difficult" client. With regression, the individual may have childlike temper tantrums and be rebellious. Why a person rejects the desired role requires understanding of the individual and her sociocultural system. There are numerous reasons why a person might choose to reject society's demand for cooperation. The loss of a social role is painful, even as traumatic as the illness itself. The sick mother may fret about not being able to meet her role obligations. The bank president may react angrily at feeling her need to be dependent and being told what to do by others. Disruption of role behavior may cause depression and mental torment: "The most painful thing for me is to see others running around and working. I've worked all my life and now. . . ."

Certain individuals may react angrily or feel worthless when placed in the inactive, dependent role of patient. They may carry this feeling of worthlessness into their affectional relationship, believing they no longer have anything to offer their partners. Mental alienation, sickness, and injury place a heavy strain on life partners. The situation may produce constant friction, or it may increase affection and tighten the interpersonal bond.

For some, illness may be used as an escape from social pressures and responsibilities. All the client has to do is relax and enjoy the dependent position. This type of client will resist returning to the nonsick role. Other clients may use the sick role effectively to control others and therefore be reluctant to relinquish it.

A variety of social, cultural, and biologic factors determine who will become ill and how they will adjust to the sick role.

SOCIOLOGIC FACTORS AFFECTING HEALTH

Health is individually perceived, and in most cases, reaching or maintaining a state of wellness is a goal for all people. However, many people find this task difficult and almost impossible because of numerous factors inherent in their social environments. There are three main sociologic factors that can impede attaining optimum wellness: stress, environment, and socioeconomic level.

Stress

Our fast-paced competitive lifestyle is filled with stress. Our stressful environment, composed of both psychologic and socioecologic factors, creates high levels of nervous tension and anxiety, which influence a person's health.

Stressors may be physical, psychological, or social. Regardless of the form, however, the person will be affected and will respond holistically; both the body and mind will react. For instance, a physical illness produces behavioral changes that are obvious: anger, apathy, withdrawal. A social stressor, such as receiving a jail sentence, may exacerbate a dermatitis. The psychological stress of taking a test can produce such physical symptoms as migraine headache or upset stomach. With extreme psychological shock, physical symptoms can be hysterical blindness, deafness, or muteness.

Regardless of the nature of the stressor, there are three physiologic stages grouped within the General Adaptation syndrome, identified by Hans Selye (1965), that occur throughout the body. They differ only in the degree of the stress response.

The Alarm Reaction Stage

- A short trigger phase sets the mechanism into action—an alert signal for the organism to get prepared.
- Na^+ and Cl^- levels in extracellar fluids fall; K^+ rises.
- Blood pressure falls.

Byrne and Thompson (1978) indicate that explaining treatments to clients will assist them in moving through the alarm stage and into the second stage, at which time the clients are better prepared to tolerate the procedure. The explanation should not be given too far in advance of treatment, as the alarm stage will fade within a short time if the stressor does not materialize. If informed too far in advance, the client may become so apprehensive of the procedure that when it actually does occur, he may be even more vulnerable. To plan the most appropriate time for explanations of this type, you must consider the client's "behavioral stability, his adaptive capacity, as well as the nature of the stressor" (Byrne & Thompson 1978).

The Resistance Stage

- This can be characterized by the statement, "I'm ready; let's get it over with!"
- The organism adjusts to the stressor(s) with the aid of increased ACTH and glucocorticoids.
- Electrolyte blood levels essentially return to normal.
- The body attempts to combat the stress factors and resist further organic damage.

The Exhaustion Stage

- The point at which with prolonged stress, the organism can no longer maintain its adaptive energy resources.
- Cholesterol stores in the adrenals are depleted; ACTH and glucocorticoid secretions dwindle.

Table 1-3 **Life Events and Weighted Values**

Life event	Value	Life event	Value
1. Death of spouse	100	21. Change of responsibility at work	29
2. Divorce	73	22. Son's or daughter's leaving home	29
3. Marital separation	65	23. Trouble with in-laws	29
4. Jail term	63	24. Outstanding personal achievement	28
5. Death of close family member	63	25. Spouse's beginning or stopping job	26
6. Personal injury or illness	53	26. Beginning or ending school	26
7. Marriage	50	27. Revision of habits	24
8. Loss of job because fired	47	28. Trouble with boss	23
9. Marital reconciliation	45	29. Change in work hours	20
10. Retirement	45	30. Change in residence	20
11. Change in health of family member	44	31. Change in schools	20
12. Pregnancy	40	32. Change in recreation	19
13. Sex difficulties	39	33. Change in social activity	18
14. Gain of new family member	39	34. Mortgage less than $10,000	17
15. Change in financial status	38	35. Change in sleeping habits	16
16. Death of close friend	37	36. Change in number of family get-togethers	15
17. Change of work	36	37. Change in eating habits	15
18. Change in number of arguments with spouse	35	38. Vacation	13
19. Mortgage more than $10,000	31	39. Minor violations of law	11
20. Foreclosure of mortgage	30		

Source: Reprinted with permission from T.H. Holmes and R.H. Rahe, "The Social Readjustment Rating Scale," *Journal of Psychosomatic Research,* 11(1967), 213. Elsevier Science Ltd., Pergamon Imprint, Oxford, England.

- Physiologic manifestations that may have originally appeared during the first stage begin to reappear—general malaise, headache, fever, anorexia.
- Reversal may or may not be achieved with external supports such as massive chemotherapy, psychotherapy, blood transfusions, and surgery. (Byrne & Thompson 1978)
- Cellular damage is no longer blocked.
- Increased cellular permeability allows for rapid, extreme electrolyte imbalances.
- Tissue breakdown occurs.
- Massive hemorrhage into the adrenal gland ensues.
- Eventually, the hormones of the gland fail to be secreted.

Selye indicates that death is likely to occur if the stressor(s) continue at the exhaustive stage.

Holmes and Rahe (1967) suggested that significant stress in a person's life, both pleasant and unpleasant, would lower an individual's resistance to disease. Their Social Readjustment Rating Scale (SRRS) lists both positive and negative stressors and may help you ask about specific events that the client may have experienced in the past year or two (Table 1-3). Their study found a positive correlation between the magnitude of the event and the seriousness of the illness. For example, 80% of the study population who had received an SRRS score of over 300 in one year experienced heart attacks or developed other serious illnesses (Table 1-4). One problem in studying stress is that the events may be more or less stressful for individuals, subcultures, or social groups and therefore difficult to measure.

John Friedrich developed a Stress Symptom Checklist self-evaluation tool for monitoring stress (Fig. 1-6). Use of this

Table 1-4 **Scoring the Life-Change Index**

Score range	Interpretation
0–150	No significant problems, low or tolerable life change
150–199	Mild life change (approximately 33% chance of illness)
200–299	Moderate life change (approximately 50% chance of illness)
300 or over	Major life change (approximately 80% chance of illness)

Source: Reprinted with permission from T.H. Holmes and R.H. Rahe, "The Social Readjustment Rating Scale," *Journal of Psychosomatic Research,* 11 (1967), 213. Elsevier Science, Ltd., Pergamon Imprint, Oxford, England.

There are many symptoms of tension which imply a need for relaxation. In order to be able to cope with tension, it is helpful to become aware of some of these symptoms. By completing the following check list, you can gain further insight into your status regarding relaxation.

	Frequently (1)	Quite Often (2)	Seldom (3)	Never (−1)
1. Do you feel insecure?	______	______	______	______
2. Do you often feel over-excited?	______	______	______	______
3. Do you feel anxious?	______	______	______	______
4. Do you worry when you go to bed at night?	______	______	______	______
5. Is it difficult for you to fall asleep at night?	______	______	______	______
6. Do you find it difficult to relax when you want to?	______	______	______	______
7. Do you wake up in the morning feeling tired and loggy?	______	______	______	______
8. Do you find it difficult to concentrate on a problem?	______	______	______	______
9. Do you often feel tired during the day?	______	______	______	______
10. When playing a sport, do you find it hard to concentrate on it?	______	______	______	______
11. Is it hard for you to stay awake at work or in class?	______	______	______	______
12. Do you feel upset and ill-at-ease?	______	______	______	______
13. Do you lack self confidence?	______	______	______	______
14. Do you often worry during the day over possible misfortunes?	______	______	______	______
15. Do you frequently feel bored?	______	______	______	______
16. Do you often feel discouraged?	______	______	______	______
17. Do you have nervous feelings?	______	______	______	______
18. Do you feel depressed?	______	______	______	______
19. Do you have any type of twitch?	______	______	______	______
20. Do you have frequent headaches?	______	______	______	______
21. Do you have frequent colds, earaches, or sore throats?	______	______	______	______
22. Do you have any persistent pains in joints or feet?	______	______	______	______
23. If you feel yourself becoming tense, do you find it difficult to relax?	______	______	______	______
24. Do you notice that you seldom find time to relax or stretch during the day?	______	______	______	______
25. Do you exercise regularly?	______	______	______	______
26. Do you often find that you exhibit tension by scowling, clenching fists, tightening jaws, hunching shoulders or pursing lips?	______	______	______	______
27. Do your shoes, belt or other items of clothing fit too tightly?	______	______	______	______
28. When you notice any of the tension symptoms, do you find it difficult to stop or minimize them?	______	______	______	______
29. Are you unable to "let go" easily when you feel tense?	______	______	______	______

The foregoing was merely designed to bring attention to areas which may reflect tension in your daily life. If you wish to rate yourself, the following scale will reflect, to a degree, your tension potential. Score: Frequently (1), Quite Often (2), Seldom (3), Never (−1).

Score	Rating
0–19	Above average tension control
20–39	Average tension control
40–55	Low tension control
56–84	Poor tension control

Figure 1-6 Stress symptom checklist.

checklist may be helpful to you and the client in identifying symptoms of stress (Friedrich 1977).

At times, clients are unable to recognize early signs of stress in themselves or to identify what situations cause them stress. You can suggest that it would be helpful for the client to record stressful events and the symptoms experienced related to the events. After this has been done for several days or weeks, the client may be able to identify specific areas that need attention to reduce stress. The diary should record time of day, the stressful event, and the symptoms that accompany the event. Additionally, it is helpful to know how the client has dealt with stress in the past, whether it affected his health and/or relationships with others or interfered with his activities of daily living (e.g., self-care, job, family or school responsibilities).

Table 1-5 lists common stressors experienced in illness and hospitalization. Information from this list can be helpful to the nurse assessing the client and, subsequently, in planning care activities to reduce the client's stress.

Although much emphasis has been placed on the role of stress as a cause in the development of certain diseases, you need to realize that stress can serve constructive purposes as

Table 1-5 **Hospital Stress Rating Scale**

Assigned rank	Stress value	Event	
1	13.9	Having strangers sleep in the same room with you	_____
2	15.4	Having to eat at different times than you usually do	_____
3	15.9	Having to sleep in a strange bed	_____
4	16.0	Having to wear a hospital gown	_____
5	16.8	Having strange machines around	_____
6	16.9	Being awakened in the night by the nurse	_____
7	17.0	Having to be assisted with bathing	_____
8	17.7	Not being able to get newspapers, radio, or TV when you want them	_____
9	18.1	Having a roommate who has too many visitors	_____
10	19.1	Having to stay in bed or the same room all day	_____
11	19.4	Being aware of unusual smells around you	_____
12	21.2	Having a roommate who is seriously ill or cannot talk with you	_____
13	21.5	Having to be assisted with a bedpan	_____
14	21.6	Having a roommate who is unfriendly	_____
15	21.7	Not having friends visit you	_____
16	21.7	Being in a room that is too cold or too hot	_____
17	21.1	Thinking your appearance might be changed after your hospitalization	_____
18	22.3	Being in the hospital during holidays or special family occasions	_____
19	22.4	Thinking you might have pain because of surgery or test procedures	_____
20	22.7	Worrying about your spouse being away from you	_____
21	23.2	Having to eat cold or tasteless food	_____
22	23.3	Not being able to call family or friends on the phone	_____
23	23.4	Being cared for by an unfamiliar doctor	_____
24	23.6	Being put in the hospital because of an accident	_____
25	24.2	Not knowing when to expect things will be done for you	_____
26	24.5	Having the staff be in too much of a hurry	_____
27	25.9	Thinking about losing income because of your illness	_____
28	26.0	Having medications cause you discomfort	_____
29	26.4	Having nurses or doctors talk too fast or use words you can't understand	_____
30	26.4	Feeling you are getting dependent on medications	_____
31	26.5	Not having family visit you	_____
32	26.9	Knowing you have to have an operation	_____
33	27.1	Being hospitalized far away from home	_____
34	27.2	Having a sudden hospitalization you weren't planning to have	_____
35	27.3	Not having your call light answered	_____
36	27.4	Not having enough insurance to pay for your hospitalization	_____
37	27.6	Not having your questions answered by the staff	_____
38	28.4	Missing your spouse	_____
39	29.2	Being fed through tubes	_____
40	31.2	Not getting relief from pain medications	_____
41	31.9	Not knowing the results or reasons for your treatments	_____
42	32.4	Not getting pain medication when you need it	_____
43	34.0	Not knowing for sure what illness you have	_____
44	34.1	Not being told what your diagnosis is	_____

Continued

Table 1-5 **Continued**

Assigned rank	Stress value	Event	
45	34.5	Thinking you might lose your hearing	____
46	34.6	Knowing you have a serious illness	____
47	35.6	Thinking you might lose a kidney or some other organ	____
48	39.2	Thinking you might have cancer	____
49	40.6	Thinking you might lose your sight	____
TOTAL			____

Source: Reprinted from B.J. Volicer and M.W. Bohannon, "A Hospital Stress Rating Scale," *Nursing Research,* 24:352–359 (September–October 1975).

well. The stress mechanism is initiated during a rollercoaster ride, a passionate kiss, a jump off the street in response to an automobile horn, or a dash into the house in a rainstorm. It prepares the individual in a crisis situation for fight or flight; by doing so, it reveals itself as a life-saving defense mechanism in league with such other adaptive body mechanisms as the healing process, the clotting mechanism of blood, the inflammatory process, and the immunologic response.

Environment

The concept that environment influences health is not new. In the mid-eighteenth century, the French philosopher Rousseau (1913) espoused the idea that one's style of living is a main source of illness:

> The great inequality of living, the extreme idleness of some, gratifying our sensual appetites, the too exquisite foods of the wealthy . . . the unwholesome food of the poor . . . all these, together with sitting up late, and excesses of every kind, immoderate transports of every passion, fatigue, mental exhaustion, the innumerable pains and anxieties inseparable from every condition of life, by which the mind of man is incessantly tormented; these are too fatal proofs that the greater part of our ills are of our own making, and that we might have avoided them nearly all by adhering to that simple, uniform and solitary manner of life which nature prescribed. . . . What we think of the good constitution of the savages, at least of those whom we have not ruined with our spirituous liquors, and reflect that they are troubled with hardly any disorders, save wounds and old age, we are tempted to believe that, in following the history of civil society, we shall be telling also that of human sickness.

Rousseau spoke of activity. Exercise is a necessity of good health. Thus, it is important to assess the client's work and recreational activities, exercise frequency, and the facilitators and barriers to exercise.

When Rousseau commented on the "too exquisite" foods of the wealthy, he was unknowingly identifying the excessive purine content in such dishes as pheasant under glass, which may cause deposition of urate crystals in and about the joints and tendons, resulting in a pathologic condition known as gout. Additionally, Rousseau noted that diet is socioculturally and economically determined to some extent. In the United States, deficiency-disease malnutrition exists because of poor diets from fast-foods or lack of equal food distribution to all members of society.

The environmental effect on health of which we are most aware is pollution. The urban environment is rife with air pollutants (carbon monoxide, asbestos, iron and steel dust, and the many by-product petrochemicals of industry).

The rural environment has been polluted by chemical dumpsites, unsafe water supplies, improper sewage disposal, unscreened windows, inadequate refrigeration or heating, lack of modern facilities in the kitchen and bathroom, and the scarcity of nursing and modern health facilities. Rural health care is a national concern, and small-scale programs are being established in various regions to provide health personnel and mechanisms of communication and transportation to families living in isolated areas.

Socioeconomic Level

Even though the United States lacks a sense of rigid social class, class consciousness and the striving for upward mobility are clearly present. There are many indicators of social class: wealth, "old" families, education, occupation, background, and neighborhood.

The U.S. government reports usually stratify on the basis of income. Income is not a bad way to gauge someone's health resources, as the amount of money earned determines how much an individual can afford to spend on health care visits, nutritious foods, and medical treatment. However, income is not always a strong predictor of educational background—a university professor and a skilled blue-collar worker can have the same income, yet they differ greatly in prestige and education. Therefore, certain socioeconomic rating scales must consider not only income but also occupation and amount of education.

In the United States, the majority of health professionals come from the middle and upper classes. Therefore, health care tends to be aimed at the client who has the same frame of reference as the health professional and the same expectations of health care. Thus, a health professional may misunderstand the expectations and concerns of clients from a lower social stratum, and they might mistakenly view these clients as irresponsible. Koos (1954) found that the lower-class person identified specific symptoms as needing medical attention to a much lesser extent than did members of the middle and upper classes (Table 1-6).

It is the task of nurses and other health workers to try to understand the circumstances that make some of their clients seem irresponsible. For example, because health care costs are rising much faster than personal income, many people of lower socioeconomic means simply do not have money to pay for health care. Additionally, knowledge deficits, values, and health belief systems could be variables influencing the type and amount of health care sought.

Other problems facing the lower socioeconomic strata are

- substandard housing with poor heating and ventilation systems
- communicable diseases
- rodents
- poor quality and scarcity of food
- poor sanitation services

Within such a social environment, is it any wonder that people in the lower socioeconomic classes are ill more often, more seriously, and for a longer duration than are those of the middle and upper classes?

CULTURAL CONSIDERATIONS IN HEALTH ASSESSMENT

Understanding the concept of values helps you to better assess cultural considerations and their impact on health. Values represent a system of ideas, attitudes, and beliefs about the worth of an entity or concept and are related to customs within specific cultures. They consciously and unconsciously bind together individuals and families in a common culture (Parad & Caplan 1965, p. 58). Values function as general guides to behavior. They help the individual or group understand the nature and meaning of the world and how they fit into that world. Socialization is the process by which values are instilled within individuals. Values, emerging over time, result from personal experience, interpersonal relationships, and the circum-

Table 1-6 **Percentage of Respondents in Each Social Class Recognizing Specified Symptoms as Needing Medical Attention**

Symptom	Upper class (N = 51)	Middle class (N = 335)	Lower class (N = 128)
Loss of appetite	57	50	20
Persistent backache	33	44	19
Continued coughing	77	78	23
Persistent joint and muscle pain	80	47	19
Blood in stool	98	89	60
Blood in urine	100	93	69
Excessive vaginal bleeding	92	83	54
Swelling of ankles	77	76	23
Loss of weight	80	51	21
Bleeding gums	79	51	20
Chronic fatigue	80	53	19
Shortness of breath	77	55	21
Persistent headaches	80	56	22
Fainting spells	80	51	33
Pain in chest	80	51	31
Lump in breast	94	71	44
Lump in abdomen	92	65	34

Source: From *The Health of Regionville* by Earl L. Koos. Copyright © 1954 by Columbia University Press. Reprinted with the permission of the publisher.

stances of the times in which one lives. Individual value systems reflect culture, society, personal needs, and significant reference groups (Rokeach 1973, p. 5). Values are derived from the life that an individual lives, which determines what that person deems important (Kelley 1977, p. 300).

It is vital that you understand the cultural background of the client. This information may not be at your fingertips, so you must review literature pertinent to the particular client. Much can also be learned about the manifest values of the individual's cultural group by observing the verbal and nonverbal communication occurring during the assessment. You can thereby inquire how the client perceives health, illness, wellness, religion, family, friends, and other areas that are often value laden. As health caregivers, we value health, and we can assist the client in the process of valuing health and health-related practices in the following ways:

1. Encourage her to make more choices and to make them freely.
2. Help her to discover alternatives when faced with choices.
3. Help her to weigh alternatives thoughtfully, reflecting on the consequences of each.
4. Encourage her to consider what she prizes and cherishes.
5. Provide opportunities to affirm choices.
6. Encourage her to act and live in accordance with her choices.
7. Help her to be aware of repeated behaviors or patterns in her life. (Raths et al 1978)

Particular beliefs about self, health, and illness are formed largely by one's culture; thus, the nurse in appropriate situations might inquire into the following areas:

- Does the client believe that she has the ability to shape events and that certain behaviors can provide a fuller, happier health?
- Does the client believe that what is happening is an act of God?
- Does the client believe that an evil eye has been cast on her and/or her family?

Individual or family values are a reflection of the community in which individuals live and the subculture(s) with which they identify. Most persons belong to a number of subcultures based on social class, ethnic background, occupational groups, peer groups, and religious affiliations (Friedman 1981, p. 172). These subgroups are influential in the development of values.

Many observers are concerned that the values held by health professionals are not congruent with the values held by a large number of their clients; thus, once the client leaves the health care facility, she is unlikely to follow the prescribed treatment regimen because it is useless to her lifestyle and goals.

If you are aware of the client's cultural values, this awareness becomes an excellent predictive basis for determining behavior and planning the most effective nursing interventions. Most nurses ascribe to Anglo-American middle-class values, which stress individuality, material wealth, physical beauty, democracy, cleanliness, work, education, science, and the legal system. You should be aware of personal value

Checklist for Cultural Assessment

Age
Sex
Race
Developmental stage and tasks of the individual
Ethnic group
Social class
Occupation and education
Financial status
Religious orientation and practices
Communication
- Verbal/language
- Nonverbal behavior
- Time and space

Roles/responsibilities

Family
- Family developmental stage
- Childrearing beliefs and practices
- Kinship
- Decision-making power

Community structure/neighborhood
Occurrence of stressful life events
Health care practices/Healing practices
Restrictions in health care
Explanation of cause (belief) of illness

Table 1-7 Basic Values of Cultures with Selected Cultural Examples

Value	Range of beliefs	Example of cultural/subcultural group adhering to value
Human nature (What is innate nature of man?)	A. The person is basically *evil but capable of achieving goodness* with self-control and effort.	Puritan ancestors; Protestants of Pentecostal or Fundamentalist background; Appalachian subculture
	B. The person is a *combination of good and evil,* with self-control necessary but lapses in behavior understood.	Most people in the United States
	C. The person is basically *good.*	
Man-nature (What is relation of man to nature or supernature?)	A. The person is *subjugated to nature* and cannot change whatever is destined to happen.	Spanish-American culture Appalachian subculture
	B. The person lives in *harmony with nature;* man-nature-supernature exist as a whole entity.	Asian cultures; Navajo Indian culture
	C. The person is to *gain mastery over nature;* all natural forces can be overcome.	Most people in the United States
Time (What is temporal focus on human life?)	A. *Past time* is given preference; most important events to guide life have happened in the past.	Historic China
	B. *Present time* is the main focus; people pay little attention to the past and regard the future as vague.	Spanish-American cultures; Appalachian subcultures
	C. *Future* is the main emphasis, seen as bigger and better; people are not content with the present.	Most people in the United States
Activity (What is the main purpose in life?)	A. *Being orientation.* The person is important just because he is and may spontaneously express impulses and desires.	Appalachian subculture. While no culture allows complete expression of impulses and all cultures must have some work done, the Mexican fiesta and Mardi Gras in New Orleans are manifestations of this value.
	B. *Becoming-in-being orientation.* The person is important for what he is, but he must continue to develop.	Most religious cultures; Native American subcultures
	C. *Doing orientation.* The person is important when he is active or accomplishing something.	Most people in the United States
Relational (What is man's relation to other men?)	A. *Individualistic relations* emphasize autonomy of the person; he does not have to fully submit to authority. Individual goals have primacy over group goals.	Most Gemeinschaft societies, such as folk or rural cultures; Yankee and Appalachian subcultures; middle class America, with emphasis on nuclear family
	B. *Collateral relations* emphasize that the person is part of a social and family order and does not live just for himself. Group or family goals have primacy.	Most European-American ethnic groups, especially Italian-American; Spanish American culture; Native American tribal subcultures; most cultures adhere to somewhat through sibling relations in family
	C. *Lineal relations* emphasize the extended family and biological and cultural relationships through time. Group goals have primacy.	Cultures that emphasize hereditary lines; upper class America; Asian cultures; Middle-East cultures

Source: Beckmann M, Zentner R, Proctor J, *Nursing Concepts for Health Promotion* (3rd ed.). Englewood Cliffs, NJ.: Prentice-Hall, 1985. Pp. 437–438.

orientations as you are assessing the health behavior of clients. Some basic values of cultures with selected cultural examples are shown in Table 1-7. By recognizing the client's values and cultural orientation, you are able to carry out an in-depth and meaningful assessment, which can enhance the helping and caring process.

The concept of culture is essential to nursing practice because the response of an individual to health and illness must be viewed in the *context* of culture. Health professionals are often dismayed to find that their well-intentioned health teaching, guidance, and planning appear to fall on deaf ears. Generally, this "failure to learn" is ascribed to lack of education, ignorance, or indifference. If the situation were to be given further study, however, it might be found that what is considered high-level wellness has no meaning in certain cultures.

Knowledge of cultural differences must come from more than intellectual curiosity. To be truly comprehensive, health assessment and nursing care require active cultivation and use of this knowledge. Ethnocentrism—the tendency to use our own group and our own customs as the standard for all judgments—is counterproductive in intercultural communications. To avoid this narrow perspective, you need to view cultural factors as more than just addendums or last-minute considerations; they must become part of your thinking. This process should not be difficult if you become more aware that health and illness can be determined and influenced by an individual's cultural background.

You are also operating within a cultural context and must understand how it affects your relations with others. One way for you to do so is to examine your own cultural beliefs—how they affect your life and how you may have thought and felt in the past when interacting with someone with beliefs different from your own.

How do we define culture, and how does it relate to and affect health and illness? Culture includes those beliefs, values, attitudes, and customs that shape and color everything in our lives: education, occupation, marriage, family, and the way we experience health and illness. The United States contains many subcultures. As a nurse, you will see many clients from various subcultures as you perform health assessments. A general guide for cultural assessment is presented in Table 1-8.

Family

There are few nurses who do not subscribe to the notion that the family must be included in the planning for the care of the sick individual. How often, however, does the nurse fully investigate the kinship and family roles in specific cultural groups?

- Who makes the decisions in the family?
- Who are considered members of the family?
- During illness, what are the expectations of each family member?
- What does "being healthy" mean to the client?
- What does the client believe caused his illness?
- Who does the client go to see to get better when she is ill?
- Who cares for the children?
- When are the children disciplined, by whom, and how?

To determine answers to these questions for a client in a particular subculture, you may need to consult the literature, observe family interactions, or ask the family or group. Most clients willingly share this information when you display *genuine* acceptance and interest in them as individuals.

Many cultural groups, notably Spanish-Americans, Mexican-Americans, and Native Americans, feel alienated when they are not surrounded by their entire family during illness. This attitude is also evident in Gypsy culture, in which the entire clan comes to the hospital or clinic with the sick member. Such groups often avoid seeking medical attention because they fear separation. The Chinese design their hospitals so that families can remain with the sick person and help care for them.

As a nurse, you must be concerned with the client's perception—and his family's perception—of health and illness. Table 1-9 presents health views of four cultural groups. You need to view wellness and illness not as isolated physiologic or psychological phenomena but as parts of the context of family relationships and religious practice.

The essence of family is living together as a unit—the grouping need not be permanent, conjugal (marriage-bound), or sanguineous (blood-related). In the United States there are a great number of subcultures that share one or more traits and vary on the basis of race, sexual orientation, ethnic origin, social class, religion, lifestyle, and occupation. In this complex society, one must first identify the subculture before attempting to describe a family.

In African-American families, decision-making power is often found to reside with the wife, who is usually dominant (Kephart 1961). This may mean that she will make the health decisions for the family, such as which health services to use and under which circumstances. Another difference in the African-American family structure is the greater role of the grandmother, who may raise her daughter's or son's children and have the responsibility and control of seeing to their health and welfare (Williams 1975).

Another subculture and type of family that you may encounter is Spanish-American or Mexican-American. In her studies of health practices among Spanish-speaking people in northern California, Margaret Clark (1970) found that fathers are the dominant figures in the family. Childbearing is both the privilege and the obligation of the married women. Households are often large and may include not only a large number of offspring but also grandparents.

Table 1-8 Cultural Assessment

Data categories	Guideline questions/instructions
Ethnic origin	Does the family identify with a particular ethnic group (e.g., Puerto Rican, African)?
Race	What is the family's racial background (e.g., African-American, Filipino, Native American)?
Relocations	Where has the family lived (country, city)? How long? Has the family moved recently?
Habits, customs, values, and beliefs	Describe habits, customs, values, and beliefs the family holds or practices that affect its attitudes toward birth, life, death, health, illness, time orientation, the health care system, and health care providers. Does the family have special customs pertaining to the birth and naming of children? Is time in utero incorporated as part of the child's age (for example, is the child considered one year old at birth)? What is the family's degree of belief and adherence to its overall cultural system? Does an older child or adolescent adhere to these customs and beliefs?
Behaviors valued by culture	How does the family value privacy, courtesy, respect for elders, behaviors related to family roles, sex roles, and work ethics?
Cultural sanctions and restrictions	Sanctions—What is accepted behavior by the family's cultural group regarding expression of emotions and feelings, religious expressions, and response to illness and death?
	Restrictions—Does the family have any restrictions related to sexual matters, exposure of body parts, certain types of surgery, discussion of dead relatives, and discussion of fears related to the unknown?
Healing beliefs	Cultural healing system—What cultural healing system does the family predominately adhere to (e.g., Asian healing system, Raza/Latino curanderismo)? What religious healing system does the family predominately adhere to (for example, Seventh-Day Adventist, West African voodoo, Christian Scientist, Fundamentalist sect, Pentacostalist)?
	Cultural health beliefs—Is illness explained by the germ theory or cause-effect relationship, presence of evil spirits, imbalance between "hot" and "cold" or yin and yang, or disequilibrium between nature and human? Is good health related to success, ability to work or fulfill roles, reward from God, or balance with nature?
	Cultural health practices—What types of cultural healing practices does the family use?
	Cultural healers—Does the family rely on cultural healers?
Childrearing	How does the family discipline children? What behaviors are acceptable? What behaviors are unacceptable? How does the child show courtesy and respect for adults?
Childcare	What customs or beliefs influence care of the umbilical cord? What is the family's belief about when newborns should be taken outside the home? What customs or beliefs influence feedings, skin care, hair care, and other areas of personal hygiene?

Source: Adapted from Bloch's assessment guide for ethnic/cultural variations, by B. Bloch. In M. Orque, B. Bloch, and L. Monrroy (eds.), *Ethnic Nursing Care: A Multicultural Approach,* pp. 49–75. Copyright © 1983 by The C. V. Mosby Co. Reprinted by permission.

Family size is another variable that may affect the health of individuals. In large families there are more individuals present to introduce illness. Generally, the living quarters may be small; therefore, transmission and reinfection are the rule among the many family members present in the home.

Religion

Religious beliefs, attitudes, and practices can also be strong cultural forces that affect health status and needs. Questioning in the following areas can aid in assessing spiritual and religious beliefs:

- Would the client like to talk with clergy?
- Does the client participate in any particular religious faith?
- Would the client want you to make arrangements to help her with any particular spiritual ceremonies or practices?
- Who does the client generally turn to for spiritual help?
- From whom or what does the client draw her strength?
- Do any medical or healing approaches conflict with the client's religious beliefs?

Religious Customs

Jewish males are circumcised within a short time after birth. This widespread custom has been linked to the low incidence of cancer of the penis among Jewish men and cancer of

Table 1-9 **Examples of Possible Beliefs and Practices of Some Members of Cultural Groups**

	Native American	Hispanic	Asian	African-American
Views of health	Holistic view: God is seen as the giver of life and health	Holistic view: as a state of equilibrium; children may wear amulets for protection	Seen as a balance of energy, called Yin-Yang	Health means being able to work productively, being in a state of harmony with others in the universe
View of illness	Tied into religion	Has spiritual, social ramifications; good or "natural" diseases due to imbalance; "supernatural" diseases due to satanic forces	Seen as an imbalance of energy	Seen as a state of incapacitation, sense of disharmony, lack of communion
Resource person for treatment	Healing specialists, herbalists, diagnosticians	*Curanderos,* other types of healers	Healers, herbalists	Older woman with experience; the caregiver must develop a healing relationship with the ill person
Treatments	Herbs; sweat baths; a family conference if necessary to decide if a family member enters a hospital (Navajo)	Folk medicine; prayers; herbs; hot-cold foods and fluids to offset specific illnesses classified as derived from "hot" or "cold" causes	Herbs; nutrition; meditation; spiritual healing; massage; acupressure; acupuncture; hot-cold foods and fluids to counteract illnesses; moxibustion	Religious healing; folk remedies; herb teas; poultices
Views of children's health risks	Fear of strangers coming close to infants; fear of "witching" infant (Navajo)	If a stranger lavishes attention on but fails to touch a child, the child may develop "evil eye," i.e., diarrhea, vomiting		A stout child is admired

Source: J. Servonsky and S. Opas, *Nursing Management of Children,* Boston: Little, Brown, 1987. Published by Little, Brown and Company.

the cervix among Jewish women (Damon 1977). Religious groups that do not believe in early circumcision, such as Moslems, or that do not believe in circumcision at all, such as Hindus, have higher rates of these types of cancer. Low rates of cancer of the upper digestive tract and respiratory system among Jewish men are thought to be related to the moderate use of alcohol and tobacco advocated by the Jewish faith (Damon 1977). Total abstinence from tobacco smoking and alcohol drinking are thought to be associated with the low rates of certain types of cancer among Mormons. One group of vegetarian Seventh Day Adventists, whose religion forbids the use of tobacco, alcohol, pork, caffeine-containing beverages, hot condiments and spices, and highly refined foods, was found to have significantly lower systolic and diastolic blood pressures than individuals from the general population (Armstrong et al 1977).

During crises such as severe illness or death, people tend to become more dependent on their religious faith. It is important for you to be aware of the different religious sects in the community in order to facilitate the client's continuing practice of his religion and to recognize when religious beliefs conflict with scientific therapies.

Clients must be able to observe their religious practices during treatment. Such practices might involve talking with religious leaders or following dietary practices or other religious rules. It is essential that you recognize when beliefs and practices run counter to medical treatment or affect a client's perception of a health situation. For example, religious beliefs regarding medicine include the Jehovah's Witnesses' stand against blood transfusion and Christian Scientists' opposition to surgical intervention. In fact, Christian Scientists rely heavily on faith healing and shun various kinds of medical help. The necessity for preventive measures, such as immunizations, may not be recognized by Muslims, as their view is fatalistic in that their lives are in the hands of Allah. It is not your role as a nurse to resolve these conflicts but to assist the client and his family in reaching appropriate decisions.

BIOLOGIC AND CULTURAL VARIATIONS

An Introduction

Specific population groups have higher incidence rates of certain diseases, genetic conditions, and psycho-behavioral disorders. Some well-known examples of genetic disorders associated with certain population groups are Tay-Sachs disease among Ashkenazic Jews and sickle-cell anemia among African-Americans of West African origin. This is not to say that these diseases occur in everyone in the specific population group or that they are restricted to that population group. For example, although the incidence of Tay-Sachs disease is 100 times higher among Ashkenazic Jews than among non-Jews, it still occurs in 1 out of 500,000 non-Jewish births.

Knowledge that there is a higher probability of a certain disease appearing in a particular population group can be useful to diagnosticians and health planners. For example, a diagnostician presented with a case of abdominal pain, fever, and increased white blood cell count would do well to note the population group to which the patient belongs (Damon 1977). In a patient of Mediterranean background, the symptoms might be due to a crisis of familial Mediterranean fever or glucose-6-phosphate dehydrogenase deficiency, both of which are largely found among Syrians, Armenians, Greeks, Italians, and Sephardic Jews. In an African-American or Black African, the same symptoms might be due to a crisis of sickle-cell anemia. In a Native American or person of Western European origin, these may be symptoms of a gallbladder inflammation. Knowledge of disease patterns in different populations aids the clinician in making the diagnoses and, in this case, might prevent unnecessary surgery. Knowing the population in which a disease is likely to occur is also useful to health planners, for it helps them to allocate services and money for health screening and health care. Information on population variation in disease incidence will be found in some of the following chapters under the heading "Biologic and Cultural Variations."

We prefer to use the term *population group* rather than *racial group* or *ethnic group*. Racial group has been used to define a breeding population with distinguishing biologic characteristics and certain genes in common. Ethnic group is used to denote a breeding population sharing cultural characteristics, such as attitudes, religion, and dietary habits. Obviously, there is no such thing as a completely distinct racial or ethnic group, because individuals tend to marry individuals from other groups. Also, although biologic characteristics may be present to a different degree in different racial groups, all biologic traits generally occur to some degree in each group, as we saw in the case of genes for Tay-Sachs disease. Finally, there is variation in the extent to which cultural characteristics are shared by the members of an ethnic group. Thus, we have chosen to use the term *population group* to encompass the meaning of both racial group and ethnic group. A *population group* is an aggregation of individuals who have an increased likelihood of mating with each other and tend to have biologic and/or cultural characteristics in common. Increased probability of disease in a particular population group thus arises from the shared biologic and/or cultural traits.

In some cases, a disease has a strictly biologic transmission and arises from genes found in the population group, such as the gene for producing the deficient enzyme glucose-6-phosphate dehydrogenase in Mediterranean peoples. And sickle-cell anemia is due to a variation in the hemoglobin gene that originally occurred in West African populations and is carried by African-Americans of West African ancestry.

Other diseases result from the interaction of biologic and cultural factors in the population group. African-Americans have higher rates of morbidity and mortality from hypertension. There seems to be an underlying genetic predisposition to develop high blood pressure in this group, but it is probably exacerbated by the lower socioeconomic status, varying dietary patterns, and potentially higher levels of stress among African-Americans. Among other conditions that are probably due to the interaction of biologic and cultural characteristics are lactase deficiency among Asian and African-Americans and atherosclerosis among whites.

In addition, cultural or socioeconomic factors may lead to higher or lower incidences of disease within a population group. For example, the greater incidence of infectious diseases such as pneumonia, tuberculosis, and syphilis among non-whites is related to the greater proportion of low-socioeconomic-status individuals in this group. In some cases, a disease that was formerly thought to be due to biologic factors is now seen to result from cultural or socioeconomic conditions. For example, because Native Americans have high rates of alcoholism, many investigators have researched the possibility that biologic differences in alcohol metabolism might be the cause. However, it now seems that differences in cultural attitudes about alcohol use and drinking behavior may explain the higher Native American alcoholism rates.

These and other examples of biologic and cultural variations in disease patterns will be considered in following chapters.

Ethnic Groups and Ethnomedical Systems

The ethnic group to which one belongs is a variable over which the individual has no control. Within a US community there are often ethnic subcommunities—Italian, Jewish, African-American, Polish, Greek, Mexican-American, and so on. These ethnic groups have their own class structures, styles of living, and entertainment (music and dance), and many may still maintain their own languages, food habits, and different conceptions of familial and personal roles. This maintenance of ethnic and cultural traditions is especially true in first- and second-generation immigrants, but remnants may also be found in beliefs and practices in many succeeding generations.

The following are questions that relate to ethnicity:

- Where was the client born?
- Where were the client's parents born?
- What language is spoken in the home?
- Does the client identify closely with her ethnic group?
- What does the client believe caused her illness?
- Are any foods on the client's diet taboo in regard to religious practices, food intolerance, and personal preferences?

Studies have found that ethnic groups differ in reporting symptoms and in seeking medical aid (Mechanic 1968). They also vary in their willingness to accept psychological interpretations of their complaints (Fink et al. 1969) and in their reactions to pain (Zborowski 1952). Zborowski found, for example, that of the four ethnic groups studied, Irish and Americans (those who had been in the United States for more than two generations) tended to be stoic in their response to pain, while Italians and Jews displayed more overt emotional behavior.

Most cultures have their own health norms and practices. Many groups continue to ascribe their illnesses to an "evil eye," sin, or failure to observe religious practice, while others perceive their conditions as the "will of God" and therefore feel they cannot be treated. For example, the Italian grandmother who believes, even if halfheartedly, that her grandchild's headaches are caused by the evil eye (a curse) will perform the *malocchio,* a ceremony using oil and water, which will validate her suspicion of the presence of the evil eye. The fact that the ceremony is performed provides the cure. Thus, the *malocchio* is a diagnosis as well as a cure.

Leininger (1970) discussed the Spanish-American belief in the evil eye, particularly in relation to children. Spanish-Americans believe that disease occurs because someone has admired the child to an excessive degree. The treatment must then consist of having the person who has cast the *mal-ojo* (evil eye) touch or caress the child. This belief has implications for nursing in that the child should always be touched or caressed when being admired. Many Spanish-Americans believe that illness is the will of God and that preventive measures are therefore of little value. The children are in God's hands, so why should they have to be immunized? They see pregnancy as normal and as something health personnel should not disrupt. Thus, traditional nursing approaches would certainly be ineffective in relating when these beliefs are held.

The African-American folk medicine system has been described as including elements of African beliefs, folk and formal medicines, and modern scientific medicine, interwoven with factors from Christianity, voodoo, and sympathetic magic (Snow 1974). These medical beliefs are strictly followed by many African-Americans. Illnesses are often treated within the community by individuals who try in their own fashion to restore equilibrium. Ministers, adult women, and in rural areas, "root workers" (said to have supernatural powers granted by God) are active in providing health care (Dougherty 1976).

The Navajo places strong credence in the power of spirits. Anthropologist Jeremiah Lyons related an incident that occurred in a tuberculosis hospital in a western state. During a storm one evening, a tree in the hospital courtyard was destroyed by lightning. By morning, every Navajo had left the hospital and would not return until a special ceremony was performed by the medicine man to appease the spirit they believed had destroyed the tree.

You cannot scoff at or disregard the beliefs of others. As a nurse, you must learn to provide health care that incorporates such beliefs, as they are strongly internalized values. Interestingly, medicine men, shamans, and *curanderos* provide a necessary and vital function within the cultural group. Often they are able to "cure" by providing emotional support, as they generally consider the whole person. Further, in many societies these individuals have been taught the basic skills of modern medicine, since they are frequently contacted first by the ill person or family. As a nurse, you must encourage people to seek out so-called standard medical attention, but you must also be aware of the important role cultural healers have in the lives of certain groups. You must learn to provide meaningful health care and still respect—and more importantly, understand—the value system operating within a culture. It may be helpful and necessary to include the client's folk medicine practitioner when providing care.

You also need to consider that many folk remedies are therapeutic. It is important to recognize that herb and plant remedies can be helpful and interfere only to avoid overdoses, or in cases in which incompatibility with prescribed drugs may occur. Such practices as wearing garlic to ward off spirits or wearing copper bracelets to alleviate the symptoms of arthritis should not be ridiculed. Furthermore, you should not ignore clients' fears of spells and hexes.

Communication and Personal Space

Verbal and nonverbal communication are extremely important in health assessment. The ability to communicate effectively is essential. You cannot expect to be fluent in all languages and may need to use an interpreter on occasion; however, if you are actively involved with a specific cultural group, you should be able to communicate in that group's language.

Another problem with language communication may arise from the client's lack of understanding of medical terminology. You need to be quite sure that the client understands directions for medical procedures and prescriptions. The patient may be confused or awed and agree quickly to instructions while not having any real understanding of the information being relayed. To ensure that the client understands what is happening, you may have to spend more time validating his understanding.

Communicating effectively also means listening to what the client brings to the encounter and may necessitate adopting another vocabulary. You need to be aware of such terms as a "risin" (boil), "tizik" (tuberculosis), or "the smothers" (inability to breathe easily) when dealing with low-income clients.

Southern clients may also refer to a class of problems having to do with the state of their blood; "high blood" and "low blood" are terms that have specific meaning for the client (Snow 1976). Table 1-10 lists some folk illnesses in Hispanic and African-American cultures.

Although important, knowing the language does not guarantee effective communication. For example, you should not assume that eye contact and touching are good means of positive reinforcement with a client. Some cultural groups view these behaviors as intrusions on their privacy. Prolonged eye contact is considered disrespectful among Eastern and Asian cultures: "The Indian believes that to touch someone violates his body boundary and takes something away from him as a person" (Fire & Baker 1976). Spanish-

Table 1-10 **Folk Illnesses in Hispanic and African-American Cultures**

Culture	Folk illness	Etiology	Behaviors	Practitioner	Treatment
Hispanic	*Susto* (fright)	An individual experiences a stressful event at some time prior to the onset of symptoms. The stressor may vary from death of a significant person to a child's nightmare to inability to adequately fulfill social-role responsibility. Children are more susceptible to *susto*. It is believed that the soul or spirit leaves the body.	Restlessness during sleep Anorexia Depression Listlessness Disinterest in personal appearance	*Curandero* or *Espiritualista* (*Espiritista*)	A ceremony is performed using branches from a sweet pepper tree and a candle. Motions by the ill person and the curer are performed that form a cross. Three Ave Marias or credos (Apostles' Creed) are said.
	Empacho	Bolus of undigested food adheres to the stomach or wall of intestine. The cause may be the food itself, or it may be due to eating when one is not hungry or when one is stressed.	Stomach pain Diarrhea Vomiting Anorexia	Family member *Sabador* *Curandero*	Massage of the stomach or back until a popping sound is heard. A laxative may be given.
	Caida de la Mollera (fallen fontanel)	Trauma—a fall or blow to the head or the rapid dislodging of a nipple from an infant's mouth causes the fontanel to be sucked into the palate.	Inability to suckle Irritability Vomiting Diarrhea Sunken fontanel	Family member *Curandero*	One or more of these practitioners insert a finger into the child's mouth and push the palate back into place. Hold the child by the ankles with the top of the head just touching a pan of tepid water for a minute or two. Apply a poultice of soap shavings to the fontanel. Administer herb tea.

Continued

Table 1-10 Continued

Culture	Folk illness	Etiology	Behaviors	Practitioner	Treatment
	Mal de ojo (evil eye)	A disease of magical origin cast by a person who is jealous or envious of another person or something the person owns. The evil eye is cast by the envious person's vision upon the subject thereby heating the blood and producing symptoms. Usually a beautiful child is envied or admired but is not touched by the admirer and the evil eye can be inflicted. The admirer may not be aware of the damage done. If the child is admired and then touched by that person, the evil eye is not inflicted.	Fever Diarrhea Vomiting Crying without apparent cause	*Curandero* *Brujo*	Passing an unbroken egg over the body or rubbing the body with an egg to draw the heat (fever) from the body. Prayers such as the Our Father or Hail Mary may be said simultaneously with the passing of the egg. The egg is then broken in a bowl, placed under the head of the bed and left there all night. By morning if the egg is almost cooked from the heat of the body this is a sign that the sick person had *mal de ojo.*
	Mal Puesto (evil)	Illness caused by a hex put on by a *brujo,* witch, or *curandero,* or other person knowledgeable about witchcraft.	Vary considerably Strange behavioral changes Labile emotions Convulsions	*Curandero* *Brujo*	Varies, depending on the hex.
African-American	High blood (too much blood)	Diet very high in red meat and rich food. Belief that high blood causes stroke.	Weakness, paralysis, vertigo, or other behaviors related to stroke	Family member or friend of Spiritualist or self (the latter does this after referring to a Zodiac almanac)	Take internally lemon juice, vinegar, epsom salts, or other astringent food to sweat out the excess blood. Treatment varies depending on what is appropriate for each person according to the Zodiac almanac.
	Low blood (not enough blood—anemia is conceptualized)	Too many astringent foods, too harsh a treatment for high blood. Remaining on high blood-pressure medication for too long.	Fatigue Weakness	Same as for high blood	Eat rich red meat, raw beets. Stop taking treatment for high blood. Consult the Zodiac almanac.
	Thin blood (predisposition to illness)	Occurs in women, children, or old people. Blood is very thin until puberty and remains so until old age, except for women.	Greater susceptibility to illness	Individual	Individual should exercise caution in cold weather by wearing warm clothing or by staying indoors.
	Rash appearing on a child after birth (no specific disease name—the concept is that of body defilement)	Impurities within the body coming out. The body is being defiled and will therefore produce skin rashes.	Rash anywhere on the body; may be accompanied by fever	Family member	Catnip tea as a laxative or other commercial laxative. The quantity and kind depend on the age of the individual.

Continued

Table 1-10 Continued

Culture	Folk illness	Etiology	Behaviors	Practitioner	Treatment
African-American, continued	Diseases of witchcraft, hex, or conjuring	Envy and sexual conflict are the most frequent causes of having someone hex another person.	Unusual behavior not normal for the person Sudden death Symptoms related to poisoning (i.e., foul taste, fall off [weight loss], nausea, vomiting) A crawling sensation on the skin or in the stomach Psychotic behavior	Voodoo Priest(ess) Spiritualist	*Conja* is the help given to the conjured person. Treatment varies depending on the spell cast.

Source: M. A. Hautman, "Folk health and illness beliefs," *Nurse Practitioner: The American Journal of Primary Health Care* 4(4):27 (1979). Reprinted by permission.

Americans, however, feel more comfortable if eye contact is maintained. The Japanese use nonverbal communication effectively, as they place great store in silence. In their culture, laughing or smiling often does not mean happiness, as it might to Westerners. For the Japanese, it may be an indication of anger or grief. Emotions are rarely expressed facially, and direct eye contact often makes the Japanese uncomfortable. The African-American has developed a highly effective means of communicating nonverbally through body movements, expressions, and gestures. Many African-American, Native American, and Appalachian children are taught not to look an adult directly in the eye, as this communicates disrespect.

The use of personal space is an aspect of culture that frequently serves as a means of nonverbal communication (Hall 1960). Different cultural groups perceive personal space differently. For example, Germans are particular about preserving their private sphere; they need to have their own space. The German culture places emphasis on orderliness; it even considers open doors to be sloppy and disorderly. The Polish, on the other hand, appear to like a little disorder, and the private sphere is not defined as rigidly. The English are conditioned to sharing space but have learned to erect behavioral barriers that allow for privacy.

Hospitals, clinics, and nurses rarely consider these spatial differences. Nurses who have a compulsion to keep things neat and orderly may in fact be creating a nontherapeutic environment—orderly, uncrowded rooms are thought by the Navajo to indicate impending death. The neat and orderly look may discourage effective communication.

In Western culture, individuals are more comfortable when they maintain a considerable distance between each other during social contact. They avoid touching, except in special situations. Latin Americans and Arabs, on the other hand, relate to each other in very close proximity, and the Japanese appear to be quite comfortable in crowded situations. "Spatial changes give a tone to a communication, accent it, and at times even override the spoken word" (Hall 1973, p. 180).

Accurate health assessment cannot be made without effective communication. If this important aspect of nursing practice is neglected, valuable knowledge—as well as rapport between the client and nurse—will be lost.

Social Class

Yamamoto and Goin (1966) reported that clients from the lower socioeconomic groups more frequently fail to keep appointments, a behavior that greatly irritates and frustrates most professionals, who tend to view the client's behavior superficially and out of context.

Bello (1976) has wisely pointed out that "attitudes about the poor also interfere with cultural sensitivity. Many health professionals think poor people are hopeless in that they are poorly educated (academically and health-wise)." You must continually ask yourself whether the behaviors you see are representative of the customs of a particular social class or are perhaps occasioned by the circumstances a lower-class client must endure to receive health care. The only way to answer this question is to provide time, interest, and understanding for each client.

Members of each class level have their own sets of values, systems of behavior, and terminology and manner of communicating. Members "culturize" their children, colleagues, students, or neighbors to their beliefs and accepted modes of behavior. Examine, for example, your own socialization

Try For a Moment to Imagine What a Clinic Visit Would Be Like

You have just completed a number of application papers; no one has bothered to ask you how you feel today. They just want to get your address, phone number, and so forth—the same information that you supplied during your previous visit. You wait for hours in a crowded, noisy hall, sitting on a hard wooden chair that has uneven legs. Maybe, you think, they've lost your chart or perhaps the nurse didn't get your name. You try to tell her your name as she runs by . . . "Yes, yes. Just go sit down and wait your turn." You go back and continue to rock on the uneven legs of the miserable chair. Finally, you hear your last name called out, and you get your 3 to 5 minutes with a blasé and impersonal nurse or physician. Your stomach is upset, and you're uncomfortable. It's late afternoon, and you remember how much better you felt when you arrived here at the clinic at 8 AM, shortly after your breakfast. Within your precious 3 to 5 minutes you are reprimanded for not adhering to your prescribed weight-reduction diet. You explain that the dietetic foods you were instructed to buy were too expensive and that you didn't have the money. "We can't help you if you don't want to follow instructions." Then you are dismissed nonchalantly as a hopeless case and a waste of time. The nurse shouts, "Doctor, do you want to see this client next week?" An uninterested reply, "Yeah . . . I guess . . . same day."

into the occupational culture of nursing. Have your value system, behavior, communication style, and jargon changed at all?

Bernard and Thompson (1970) described a number of differences in customs among social classes. They noted that Kinsey reported sexual behavior to be associated with social classes stratified according to education and occupation. Certain sexual behaviors condoned by one class were viewed indifferently or with censure by another, and vice versa. They indicated further that childrearing patterns, attitudes toward cleanliness, and attitudes toward education are quite dissimilar among classes. They noted that some social classes encourage the development of aggressiveness, whereas others discourage it. For example, an elementary school nurse found that her office was constantly filled with students, particularly African-American children, who were referred to her as behavioral problems on the basis of loud, disruptive, or aggressive behavior. When the white middle-class teachers were told that aggressiveness is encouraged and valued as a personal attribute in many African-American families, they were then able to view the behavior in a different light from the generally far-removed perspective of the white middle class.

Health providers who are engaged in private practice or employed in private institutions are most likely to deal with clients from the middle and upper socioeconomic levels—clients who share their emphasis on preventative health measures and medical care. Clients tend to identify better with health workers who share the same social class and common life experiences. Rosenthal and Frank (1958) reported that psychiatrists working in psychiatric outpatient clinics tended to refer those clients for psychotherapy who were most like themselves. Thus, they referred significantly more white than African-American clients, the better educated, and those in the upper rather than the lower income range.

Health professionals find themselves interacting, sometimes not too successfully, with clients having a cultural orientation quite different from their own; they often seem to ignore the sociologic variables that influence the value system of these clients. Although some believe that such health workers simply do not care or try to understand, we feel that perhaps the basic problem stems from the fact that most health workers, including nurses, are not knowledgeable about the social factors and dynamics at work in different social classes.

Although statistics indicate that overall family income and earnings are steadily increasing, this does not apply to all families, nor do increases keep pace with the rise in the cost of living in all cases. Many families that were once economically stable are now treading a fine line between adequate and inadequate income. It is this marginal position that "tends to increase family vulnerability to crisis events. When family expenditures equal or exceed their income, unexpected costs of illness can jeopardize the family's precarious financial balance" (Hill 1968).

Health Teaching

When providing health teaching to persons of varying cultural backgrounds, you need to remember that not all are eager to participate in health care planning and illness prevention. Because some groups may not be future-oriented, your health teaching must appeal to immediate concerns rather than long-range goals. For example, it may be more important to stress the active treatment of obesity than to focus on the long-range effects of being obese. The teaching must appeal to the values held by the individual within the context of her culture. Otherwise, the client may not comply with treatments, and lengthy and expensive health care measures may consequently be ineffective.

The Puerto Rican has a fatalistic attitude toward life, which results in the belief that there is little control over life. Predominant reasons for illness are "God's will" or that someone has done something wrong and must suffer. The illness is outside one's sphere of influence. Because this feeling of powerlessness is part of the Puerto Rican way of life, it has implications for planning educational programs to assist in controlling disease and promoting wellness. The powerlessness has resulted in individuals not seeking help until a disease has progressed to a severe stage.

There are numerous studies in the nursing and anthropologic literature that you can research so that your teaching is meaningful to the specific cultural group, and learning will be facilitated.

SUMMARY

Holistic health assessment is the foundational skill for the nursing process and uses multiple theories as guidelines in collecting and analyzing data. A psychosocial lag to clients' responses to phases of illness were discussed. The sociologic factors of stress, environment, and socioeconomic level were examined in light of their effect on health and the importance of including them in health assessment. The pertinence for the inclusion of cultural components in health assessment was explained. A person's ethnic group and social class affect attitudes toward health and illness, and family groups from various cultures respond in certain culturally specific ways to the illness of a family member. Contributing to these responses are religious beliefs and customs, values, and folk medicine practices. Other factors to be considered are communication and personal space differences when health teaching and providing care for clients of different cultural groups.

DISCUSSION QUESTIONS/ ACTIVITIES

1. Discuss the key words used in the regulations governing nursing practice in your state.
2. Generate nursing diagnoses and contributing factors from a nursing history and compare and discuss them in a group of peers who did the same using the identical nursing history.
3. Choose eight nursing diagnoses and list possible contributory factors and possible signs and symptoms that may occur as a result of each contributory factor.
4. Take the same eight nursing diagnoses and related contributory factors and develop client outcome objectives.
5. Describe the differing responses of two different clients entering the health care system with the same problem, using Martin and Prange's framework of the stages of illness.
6. Use Fig. 1-6 to rate your tension potential.
7. Explore one or several alternative health care modes (e.g., biofeedback, meditation, imaging, massage, relaxation techniques, rolfing, therapeutic touch).
8. Describe the differences between the medical model and the holistic nursing model.
9. In what ways do your ideas, beliefs, practices, and so on, differ from those of your parents? From those of your grandparents? How can you account for the differences?
10. Identify some groups with which you have been associated. How have they influenced you and your lifestyle?
11. Discuss the implications for nursing of the following statements: (1) Cultural behavior is not present at birth but is acquired through learning over a period of years. (2) Cultures are not static but are subject to change.
12. How has your education reflected, influenced, and/or modified your culture?
13. Share examples of folk medicine practices within your own culture and in various other cultures. Identify at least five examples.
14. Identify and discuss at least eight examples of nursing care planning that would incorporate the cultural beliefs and religious practices of various clients.
15. Consider the following nursing situation: Ora Morningstar has been admitted for chest surgery in the morning. She is 62 years old and has lived on the reservation all of her life. This is the first time she has been admitted to a hospital. It is customary to consult a medicine man prior to surgery to ensure a successful operation. A ritual is performed that takes a couple of hours. There are many preoperative measures to be completed this evening prior to the surgery. What would be your approach to Ms. Morningstar? It is now 10 P.M., and visiting hours are over, according to hospital policy. As you see the medicine man leave the corridor, you enter Ms. Morningstar's room to find that there are still nine relatives in the room. The client tells you that they will be staying with her tonight. You realize that it is customary for members of a Native American family to remain with an ill member. How would you handle this situation?
16. Describe your own health values.

REFERENCES

Armstrong, B.; Van Merwyk, A. J.; and Coates, H. 1977. Blood pressure in Seventh Day Adventist vegetarians. *Am. J. Epidemiol.* 105(5):444–449.

Beckman, M.; Zentner, R.; and Proctor, J. 1979. *Nursing concepts for health promotion.* 3rd ed. Englewood Cliffs, N.J.: Prentice-Hall.

Bello, T. A. Feb. 1976. The third dimension: cultural sensitivity in nursing practice. *Imprint* 23:36–38, 45.

Bernard, J., and Thompson, L. F. 1970. *Sociology: Nurses and their patients in a modern society.* St. Louis: C. V. Mosby.

Byrne, M., and Thompson, L. 1978. *Key concepts for the study and practice of nursing.* 2nd ed. St. Louis: C. V. Mosby.

Chinn, P., and Jacobs, M. 1987. *Theory and nursing—a systematic approach.* St. Louis: C. V. Mosby.

Clark, M. 1970. *Health in the Mexican-American culture.* Berkeley: University of California Press.

Damon, A. 1977. *Human biology and ecology.* New York: W. W. Norton.

Dougherty, M. C. 1976. Health agents in a rural black community. *J. Afro-Amer. Issues* 4(1):44.

Dunn, H. L. 1957. High-level wellness for man and society. *J. of Nat. Med. Assoc.* 49:93.

Dunn, H. L. 1959. High-level wellness for man and society. AJPH *American Journal of Public Health* 49(6): 786-792.

Dunn, H. L. 1977. *High-level wellness.* Thorofare, N.J.: Charles B. Slack.

Fink, D. July 1976. Holistic health: Implications for health planning. *Am. J. Hosp. Pract.* 1:23–31.

Fink, R.; Shapiro, S.; and Soldensohn, S. S. 1969. The filter-down process to psychotherapy in a group practice medical care program. *Am. J. Public Health* 59:245–260.

Fire, M., and Baker, C. 1976. A smile and eye contact may insult someone. *J. Nurs. Educ.* 15:15.

Flynn, P. A. R. 1980. *Holistic health: the art and science of care.* Bowie, Md.: Robert J. Brady Company.

Friedrich, J. A. 1977. Tension control techniques. In *Guide to fitness after fifty,* eds. R. Harris and L. W. Frankel. New York: Plenum Press. 337–338.

Friedman, M. M. 1981. *Family nursing: theory and assessment.* New York: Appleton-Century-Crofts.

Hall, E. T. 1960. Language of space. *Landscape* 10:41–42.

Hall, E. T. 1973. *The silent language.* New York: Anchor Press.

Hill, R. 1968. Social stress on the family. In *Sourcebook in marriage and the family,* ed. M. B. Sussman. New York: Houghton Mifflin.

Holmes, T. H., and Rahe, R. H. 1967. The Social Readjustment Rating Scale. *J. Psychosom. Res.* 11:213.

Kalisch, B. J., and Kalisch, P. A. 1982. *Politics of nursing.* Philadelphia: F. A. Davis.

Kelley, E. C. 1977. The fully functioning self. In *Human dynamics in psychology and education,* ed. D. E. Hamacheck. Boston: Allyn & Bacon.

Kephart, W. M. 1961. *Family, society and the individual.* Boston: Houghton Mifflin.

Koos, E. L. 1954. *The health of Regionville.* New York: Columbia University Press.

Leininger, M. 1970. *Nursing and anthropology: two worlds to blend.* New York: Wiley.

Martin, H., and Prange, A. 1962. The stages of illness: psychosocial approach. *Nurs. Outlook* 10(3)168–171.

Mechanic, D. 1968. *Medical sociology: a selective view.* New York: Free Press.

Parad, H., and Caplan, G. 1965. A framework for studying families in crisis. In *Crisis intervention,* ed. H. Parad. New York: Family Service Association of America.

Raths, L. E.; Harmin, M.; and Simon, S. B. 1978. *Values and teaching.* 2nd ed. Columbus, Ohio: Merrill Publishing.

Rokeach, M. M. 1973. *The nature of human values.* New York: Free Press.

Rosenthal, D., and Frank, J. D. 1958. The fate of psychiatric clinic outpatients assigned to psychotherapy. *J. Nerv. Ment. Dis.* 127: 330–343.

Rousseau, J. J. 1913. *The social contract and discourses.* London: J. M. Dent and Sons.

Selye, H. 1965. The stress syndrome. *Am. J. Nurs.* 65:98.

Servonsky, J., and Opas, S. 1987. *Nursing management of children.* Boston: Little, Brown.

Smuts, J. C. 1926. *Holism and evolution.* New York: Macmillan.

Snow, L. L. June 1976. "High blood" is not high blood pressure. *Urban Health* 5:54–56.

Snow, L. L. 1974. Folk medical beliefs and their implications for care of patients: a review based on studies among Black Americans. *Ann. Intern. Med.* 81:82–96.

Yamamoto, J., and Goin, M. K. 1966. Social class factors relevant for psychiatric treatment. *J. Nerv. Ment. Dis.* 142:332–339.

Zborowski, M. 1952. Cultural components in responses to pain. *J. Soc. Issues* 8(14):16–30.

CHAPTER 2

Communication in Health Assessment

Learning Objectives

1. Describe communication from the standpoint of the concept of life field and the context of perceptual psychology.
2. List factors that distort communication.
3. State three general principles of communication.
4. Identify unresolved feelings and needs that may interfere with your interactions with clients.
5. Incorporate trust, empathy, and respect into fostering a therapeutic milieu for clients.
6. Recognize examples of nontherapeutic and therapeutic patterns of communication.
7. Discuss the use of silence as an interview technique.
8. Recognize body language as a form of nonverbal communication.
9. Incorporate a greater variety of responses in your communication with others.
10. Limit the frequency of nontherapeutic communication patterns.

This chapter introduces some aspects of communication that are essential to a successful health assessment. Discussion begins first with a definition of communication and then moves on to three aspects of communication that are important to remember when working with clients. The central part of this chapter is devoted to factors that foster a therapeutic milieu and a detailed examination of nontherapeutic and therapeutic patterns of communication. All of us have unconscious ways of relating to people, some of which are more effective than others. It is important to become aware of the patterns you use and how they affect the person you are encountering. The final part of this chapter discusses kinesics, the study of body language.

WHAT IS COMMUNICATION?

We think that we know what communication is and that we are fairly good at it. We think that if we have "command of the language," we "have it made." Yet if you think back over past days, chances are that you will be able to recall situations in which you or someone else misunderstood what the other meant to communicate. How did this situation affect you? How must the other person have felt? Anxious? Frustrated? Have you ever had the experience of completing a time-consuming assignment only to discover that you did not understand the communiqué and did the wrong assignment? How many times in the past week did you hear the words, "Oh I thought you meant. . . ."?

Communication is commonly defined as the process of transmitting a message or idea. This definition may seem simple and clear, but it is not as simple as you may think. There are many definitions and theories of communication.

The word *communication* comes from the Latin *communis,* meaning to make common to many, to share. Therefore, it could be said that successful verbal or nonverbal communication has taken place when an experience of mutual "meaning" of thoughts, feelings, and ideas has been shared with another. The words or behavior are nothing in themselves; they only "become" when a common understanding has been established. Thus, communication is the process of transmitting meaning. It is this meaning that you must strive to send to another, and to validate when a communication is sent to you.

Chapter 1 revealed how cultural groups provide people with many culturally specific ways of communicating. Therefore, you need to keep in mind that the "meanings" being communicated will vary from person to person, depending on such influencing factors as culture, environment, and life experiences. No two individual experiences are ever alike. Most people would agree that each person's differing experiences are the cause of misunderstandings in communication. However, the true meanings of communication can be more closely reached if you try to see things from the other person's perspective—if you practice empathy along with other communication skills. Two basic concepts in perceptual psychology, as set forth by Combs, fit well with our definition of communication as the transmission of meaning. First, the focus of the perceptual psychologist is on the meaning of the events to the individual. Combs wrote that "the individual's behavior is seen as a direct consequence, not of the fact or stimulus with which he is confronted, but the meaning of events in his perceptual field" (Combs et al 1971, p. 118). Therefore, the aim is to understand the behavior from the person's own viewpoint. Second, the individual's meaning is formed as a result of "how he sees the situation he is in and how he sees himself" (p. 119). It seems, then, that self-concept, as well as events, has great impact on behavior and, indirectly, on communication.

The schema of communication in Fig. 2-1 has been constructed from a particular definition of communication—the concept of *life field*—and from concepts of perceptual psychology. The life field is the molder of meaning of the events an individual experiences. Figure 2-1 shows the primary constructs of the life field: culture (feelings, beliefs, and attitudes; values that are influenced by religion and myths; sexual perceptions reflected in words such as *old maid, gay, bachelor;* relationships such as husband and wife, parent and child, student and teacher, and stranger and stranger; and societal norms), the environment, life experiences, and self-concept (how we value and perceive ourselves and others). These forces not only direct the content of our thought but also create a way of thinking. The results of the process are expressed by the sender in verbalizations or nonverbal behavior. The sender's expression may be further influenced by certain distortion factors before being received cognitively by the receiver. Although several distortion factors (noise, lighting, and so on) are identified in Fig. 2-1, they do not constitute a complete list. The judgment or interpretation aspect of the meaning is in turn influenced by the life field of the receiver. Whether "successful" communication has occurred cannot be established unless the receiver sends feedback to the sender for validation. If the sender responds appropriately to the feedback, it is assumed

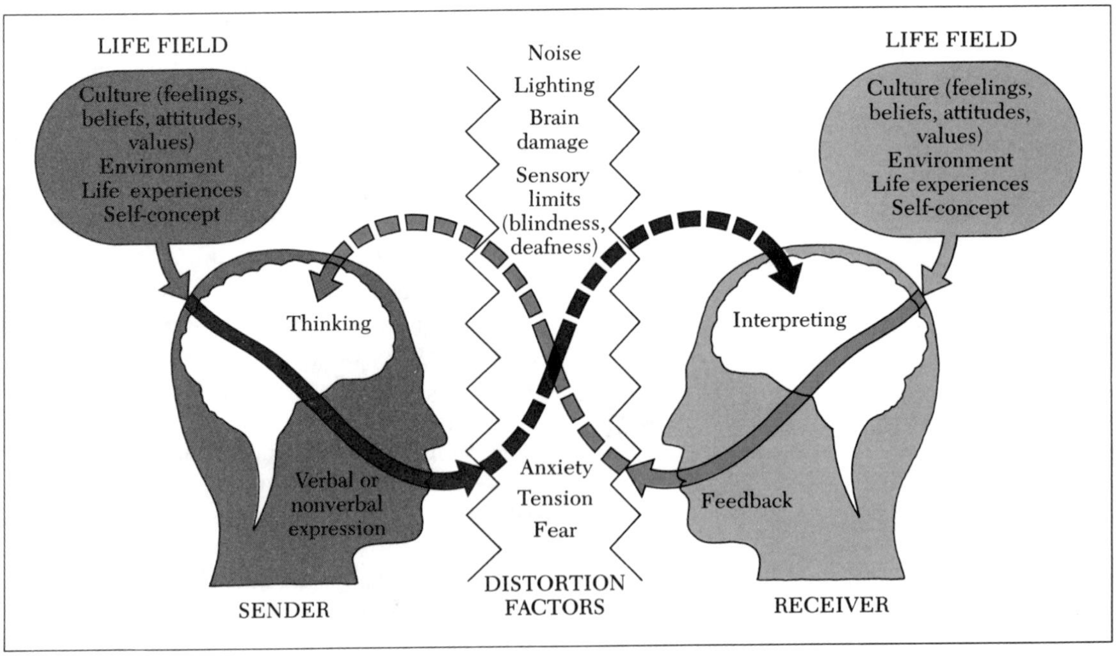

Figure 2-1 A model of communication.

that a close degree of meaning has been shared. Obviously, absolute communication can never be achieved.

PRINCIPLES OF COMMUNICATION

Three basic principles have been selected for discussion to assist improvement of your communication skills.

People communicate in a variety of ways. People communicate via spoken or written symbols. They use body language, such as smiling, covering the face, shrugging the shoulders, or winking an eye. People also communicate by touch, such as a handshake, a pat on the back, a soft caress, a slap on the face. Nonverbal communication is commonly indicated by remarks such as "You could read his expression," "His face was an open book," or "If looks could kill, I'd be dead." All of these methods of communication are expressed and experienced in the context of each individual's life field.

If understanding is absent, communication has not occurred. During health assessment, it is important that you communicate clearly to obtain the needed information. By using words appropriate to the client's level of understanding and avoiding medical/nursing jargon, you will foster understanding. You should not hesitate to question the client to discern whether he understands. Furthermore, using a question such as "What do you mean when you say . . ." may help you understand something the client is attempting to communicate to you. It is wise to remember that the meaning being sent is not always the meaning received. Because nonverbal communication is often a more reliable reflection of an individual's true meaning, your client's meaning may become more clear if you take note of such factors as tone of voice, voice inflections, the loudness and amount of speech, and body positioning and accompanying gestures. In addition, the context (the specific setting, event, or person) may give relevance to the meaning. When a woman says, "I've gotta run!" her exclamation is best interpreted in light of whether she is in a hurry or has a problem with her pantyhose.

Listening is a principal route to awareness and understanding of communication. "A good listener is not only popular everywhere, but after a while he knows something" (Mizner 1955). To be a good listener, you need to exercise your full concentration and listen not only for facts but also for the overall meaning being expressed by the client. Tune in to the main ideas and topics of the client's conversation, along with the choice of words and repetition of key words. Take note of any hesitations and any aggressive expression of words and ideas.

Careful attention is the highest compliment you can pay your client. Basically, you are conveying "I care and want to understand"; this attitude helps to promote a positive and supportive psychological climate in which the client feels free to express herself. Listening, and not talking, is difficult to do. We often cut off communication by quickly jumping to conclusions and offering friendly advice or by giving judgmental comments of approval or disapproval. When you recognize this behavior in yourself, you can often overcome the tendency by consciously substituting a nod of the head, a gesture that usually communicates "I am listening" to the client. As Mark Twain once said, "A good memory and a tongue tied in the middle is a combination which gives immortality to conversation."

FOSTERING A THERAPEUTIC MILIEU

The climate for communication must be viewed as an integral part of the therapeutic milieu. Every day, communication takes place with little thought or genuine response. However, communication, which is at the crux of the interview process and interactions with clients, deserves thoughtfulness and analysis. Attention must be given not only to what transpires between you and the client but also to the creation of a climate for effective communication. You are both an integral part of this climate and a molder of the climate. Understanding yourself places you in a better position to effect a therapeutic milieu.

Self-Awareness

Understanding yourself can greatly enhance your ability to interact effectively with clients. Cormier and Cormier (1979) identified three potential problem areas regarding self-image and have explored how these problems could affect your interactions with clients. These potential problem areas are unresolved feelings and needs in regard to competence, power, and intimacy (Table 2-1, Fig. 2-1).

If you don't feel competent in your professional role, this attitude and self-image may be communicated to your client. This is a common self-image perspective held by beginning health care students. Their interactions with clients often proceed in a manner that meets the needs of the novice rather than the client; that is, these first interactions with clients are more often focused on self than on the client. Problem feelings in the area of competence are incompetence, inadequacy, fear of failure, and fear of success.

A fear of failure can provoke you into ignoring negative and serious topics and keeping the conversation at a superficial or social, conversational level. Fear of success is reflected by a depreciatory self-image accompanied by apologies for self-identified shortcomings, and the interaction is structured to maintain a negative self-image. Also, inadequacies in feelings of masculinity or femininity may cause you to behave in ways that make you feel more secure as a woman or man—for example, seductive behaviors.

Unresolved feelings and needs regarding power are reflected in attitudes of omnipotence and being fearful of control. A power struggle between you and the client is

Table 2-1 Effects of Self-Image on Counseling Interaction

Potential problem area and unresolved feelings and needs	Attitude about self	Possible counseling behaviors
Competence Incompetence Inadequacy Fear of failure Fear of success	1. Pollyanna; overly positive—fearful of failing	Structures counseling to maintain Pollyanna attitude, avoiding conflicts by 1. discounting negative feedback 2. giving "fake" feedback 3. avoiding or smoothing over "heavy stuff"
	2. Negative; overly self-critical—fearful of succeeding	Structures counseling to maintain negative self-image by 1. avoiding positive interactions 2. discounting positive feedback 3. giving self overly negative feedback 4. making goals and expectations too high 5. making self-deprecating or apologetic comments
	3. Not masculine enough or not feminine enough	Structures counseling to make self feel more secure as a male or female by 1. overidentifying with or rejecting very masculine or very feminine clients 2. seducing clients of opposite sex 3. overreacting to or misinterpreting both positive and negative reactions from male and female clients
Power Impotence Control Passivity Dependence Independence Counterdependence	1. Omnipotent—fearful of losing control	Structures counseling to get and stay in control by 1. persuading client to do whatever counselor wants 2. subtly informing client how good or right counselor is 3. dominating content and direction of interview 4. getting upset or irritated if client is resistant or reluctant
	2. Weak and unresourceful—fearful of control	Structures counseling to avoid taking control by 1. being overly silent and nonparticipatory 2. giving client too much direction, as in constant client rambling 3. frequently asking client for permission to do or say something 4. not expressing opinion; always referring back to client 5. avoiding any other risks
	3. Lifestyle converter	Structures counseling to convert client to counselor's beliefs or lifestyle by 1. promoting ideology 2. getting in a power struggle 3. rejecting clients who are too different or who don't respond 4. "preaching"
Intimacy Affection Rejection	1. Needing warmth and acceptance—fearful of being rejected	Structures counseling to make self liked by 1. eliciting positive feelings from client 2. avoiding confronting or offending client 3. ignoring negative client cues 4. doing things for client—favors and so on
	2. Needing distance—fearful of closeness, affection	Structures counseling to maintain distance and avoid emotional intimacy by 1. ignoring client's positive feelings 2. acting overly gruff or distant 3. maintaining professional role as "expert"

Source: Cormier L.S., Cormier W. H. and Weisser R.J.: *Interviewing and Helping Skills for Health Professionals.* © 1986 Boston: Jones and Bartlett Publishers. Reprinted with permission.

Instructions: The following learning activity may help you explore some of your feelings and attitudes about yourself and possible effects on your counseling interactions. The activity consists of a Self-Rating Checklist divided into the three areas of competence, power, and intimacy. We suggest you work through each section separately. As you read the items listed for each section, think about the extent to which the item accurately describes your behavior *most* of the time (there are always exceptions to our consistent behaviors). If an item asks about you in relation to a client and you haven't had much counseling experience, try to project yourself into the counselor's role. Check the items that are most descriptive of you. Try to be as honest with yourself as possible.

Self-Rating Checklist

Check the items that are most descriptive of you.

I. *Competence Assessment*

___ 1. Constructive negative feedback about myself doesn't make me feel incompetent or uncertain of myself.
___ 2. I tend to put myself down frequently.
___ 3. I feel fairly confident about myself as a helper.
___ 4. I often am preoccupied with thinking that I'm not going to be a competent counselor.
___ 5. When I am involved in a conflict, I don't go out of my way to ignore or avoid it.
___ 6. When I get positive feedback about myself, I often don't believe it's true.
___ 7. I set realistic goals for myself as a helper that are within reach.
___ 8. I believe that a confronting, hostile client could make me feel uneasy or incompetent.
___ 9. I often find myself apologizing for myself or my behavior.
___ 10. I'm fairly confident I can or will be a successful counselor.
___ 11. I find myself worrying a lot about "not making it" as a counselor.
___ 12. I'm likely to be a little scared by clients who would idealize me.
___ 13. A lot of times I will set standards or goals for myself that are too tough to attain.
___ 14. I tend to avoid negative feedback when I can.
___ 15. Doing well or being successful does not make me feel uneasy.

II. *Power Assessment*

___ 1. If I'm really honest, I think my counseling methods are a little superior to other people's.
___ 2. A lot of times I try to get people to do what I want. I might get pretty defensive or upset if the client disagreed with what I wanted to do or did not follow my direction in the interview.
___ 3. I believe there is (or will be) a balance in the interviews between my participation and the client's.
___ 4. I could feel angry when working with a resistant or stubborn client.
___ 5. I can see that I might be tempted to get some of my own ideology across to the client.
___ 6. As a counselor, "preaching" is not likely to be a problem for me.
___ 7. Sometimes I feel impatient with clients who have a different way of looking at the world than I do.
___ 8. I know there are times when I would be reluctant to refer my client to someone else, especially if the other counselor's style differed from mine.
___ 9. Sometimes I feel rejecting or intolerant of clients whose values and life-styles are very different from mine.
___ 10. It is hard for me to avoid getting in a power struggle with some clients.

III. *Intimacy Assessment*

___ 1. There are times when I act more gruff than I really feel.
___ 2. It's hard for me to express positive feelings to a client.
___ 3. There are some clients I would really like to be my friends more than my clients.
___ 4. It would upset me if a client didn't like me.
___ 5. If I sense a client has some negative feelings toward me, I try to talk about it rather than avoid it.
___ 6. Many times I go out of my way to avoid offending clients.
___ 7. I feel more comfortable maintaining a professional distance between myself and the client.
___ 8. Being close to people is something that does not make me feel uncomfortable.
___ 9. I am more comfortable when I am a little aloof.
___ 10. I am very sensitive to how clients feel about me, especially if it's negative.
___ 11. I can accept positive feedback from clients fairly easily.
___ 12. It is difficult for me to confront a client.

Figure 2-2 Self-image learning activity.

likely to occur if you are fearful of losing control. On the other hand, if you feel less secure and avoid taking risks, you may find yourself giving the client "free reign" in order to avoid assuming responsibility.

Lastly, problem areas within the realm of intimacy involve feelings and needs for affection and rejection. If you have needs for being valued and liked by the client, you may find yourself subtly seeking positive strokes from the client; selective hearing will tune out any expressions of client dissatisfaction. Taped role play may aid you in identifying this problem area. Fear of intimacy could result in a "strictly business" attitude, wherein you may find yourself behaving aloof and somewhat impersonable. On the other hand, being yourself and using humor when appropriate is therapeutic.

Trust

In a trusting relationship, information shared will be of an honest and often intimate nature. However, a trusting relationship may not be easy to establish because such a relationship is dependent on a variety of factors. Each client will react differently to the sharing of information, depending on past familial/social experiences (beginning with parent bonding and the developmental stage of trust versus mistrust) and past experiences with health professionals. Media also influence attitudes and perceptions. If the client believes the television image of gossiping nurses on soap operas, he is unlikely to divulge private information. The client is also assessing you. He is asking himself, "How much can I tell this nurse? Can I trust this person?" The client may expend considerable energy in testing you. He may be very observant of how you handle information given to you. Therefore, it is extremely important that you specify with whom you will need to share information.

Carelessness in handling information and messages must be avoided. Information given in confidence must be honored, or the client's trust will be broken. When legitimate sharing of information about a client is occurring with another health professional or in a learning setting, privacy must be attended. This type of interchange should not take place in public—in a hallway, nurses' station, restroom, elevator, lounge, public dining area, or even an office, if the door is ajar. Furthermore, talking to a client about staff or another client indiscriminately will cause distrust.

It is often helpful to give a client situation as an example, but the example need not be so explicit as to reveal the individual's identity. For interactions, communication, and history taking to be as meaningful and accurate as possible, the client must feel free to be open and honest and to trust the nurse. Likewise, the nurse must be aware of and adhere to ethical guidelines established by the professional organization (American Nurses' Association Code of Ethics) in regard to confidentiality.

Respect

An essential ingredient in promoting a therapeutic milieu is respect; the client must feel this respect from you. This can be conveyed in ways such as properly addressing the client by title and name—for example, Ms. Jackson, Dr. Harris, and Judge Davis. Respect also entails listening attentively when the client speaks, being nonjudgmental and accepting of the client as he is, placing your own bias and values on the "back shelf," and affording the client common courtesies.

We may not like everyone with whom we come into contact. In light of this, we must admit our feelings and examine them in the context of what they mean to us and our client. If they block the relationship, it may be best for another professional to work closely with the client.

Empathy

Empathy is identification with another's feelings. It means recognizing the other person's perspective or frame of reference, *as if* these feelings were your own—without ever forgetting the "as if." An example of forgetting the "as if" is when you identify so closely with the feelings of a client that you cannot differentiate your own feelings. In this case, you may find it hard to maintain the professional role and provide the guidance and support your client needs. The more the client is like you (in age, sex, and background), and the more the situation is similar to one you have experienced, the more likely it is that you may identify with the client. Even though you may wish to continue working with this client, you may not be able to be objective. In this case, it would be best to refer the client to another professional. Be aware that this is no reflection on your professional capabilities; indeed, it is a reflection of your skill in recognizing your own limitations. This in itself is a mark of a professional. On the other hand, you must be careful not to use this as a "cop-out" whenever you experience uncomfortableness with a client. You need to examine the uncomfortableness. Many times, dealing with the identified cause will allow you to experience personal growth.

To foster understanding, you should attempt to look at life and events from the client's perspective. Obviously, your bias and values exist, but to empathize with a client does not mean that you agree with or hold the same values as the client. The process of empathizing is the sharing of your recognition of the feelings held by the client; it is an additional means of conveying respect. Often, sharing your feelings and experiences with the client can lead to further disclosure. More disclosure can lead to a deeper relationship and understanding.

PATTERNS OF COMMUNICATION

Most of the time, talking occurs without thinking. For instance, the person asking, "How are you?" does not *really* want to know in most cases, and the individual responding, "Fine," may not be fine at all. Such automatic verbalizations are predominant in social conversation but have little value in the health assessment process. A certain degree of communication skill is essential within a relationship model of practice.

- Improve your communication skills by becoming aware of your use of automatic responses and of your personal verbal patterns.
- Learn the principles of various therapeutic communication patterns.
- Plan and evaluate your interactions.
- Make a conscious effort toward replacing nontherapeutic patterns with therapeutic ones.

This last step is perhaps the most difficult, as it takes more energy to unlearn than to learn. However, you will discover that the application and use of therapeutic patterns become easier with practice. In turn, your use of nontherapeutic patterns will slowly diminish. The key is conscious attention and effort.

Nontherapeutic Patterns

Many negative verbal patterns are already a part of most people's communication habits. Therefore, discussion of negative patterns first will help you identify whether you have any of these undesirable habits. These negative patterns are useless for obtaining information, and most actually inhibit communication because of psychological undertones. If any of these patterns characterize your interactions with others, try to "catch" them in the future—it is no crime to stop and think before you respond.

The Value Judgment Pattern

The indiscriminate or constant use of words such as *good, fine,* and *excellent* figuratively places your stamp of approval on the client's actions or ideas. If the client should change her mind and make another decision, she would be in opposition to your sanctioned action or thought. Clients frequently exhibit "nurse-pleaser" behavior. They find it difficult to contradict you because they depend on you in varying degrees and feel they must remain in your good graces should they need you at a future time. Have you ever ceased to create waves to remain on the "right" side of someone at one time or another?

Clients with little self-worth will only suffer more ego deflation if they reject their idea to cling to yours or if they are no longer capable of performing your sanctioned behavior. Even clients with a strong self-concept may avoid telling you they have changed their mind about something. Thus, you unknowingly lose out on sharing, and some communication bonds between you are severed. It is better that you help the client explore her own feelings about her actions and ideas. You can use such prompters as

- "I see you are able to comb your hair (feed yourself, shave) today."
- "How do you *feel* about it?"
- "Are you presently comfortable with. . . ?"

This latter pattern allows the client the freedom to change her mind and feelings should she become uncomfortable with decisions she has made. Conversely, disapproval, expressed in such statements and questions as "That's wrong!" "You shouldn't do that!" "I don't believe you want to say (do) that, do you?" or "You don't have syphilis, do you?" advances your values. If the client's values differ or if she has a disorder of which you disapprove, she infers that she is "bad." Again, the client has been set up either to experience ego deterioration (I'm wrong, I'm bad) or to become defensive. Defensiveness will tend only to strengthen the client's ideas, and she will fight for them all the more. When you impose your values and judgments on the client, you are in essence inhibiting her growth.

You also inhibit the client's growth when you give her advice. This does not mean that it is wrong to offer suggestions, but giving advice is an entirely different matter. By giving advice, you imply that you know best, and you take away the client's opportunity to solve the problem, usurping a responsibility that belongs to her. You may direct the client's thoughts toward other alternatives by asking,

- "Have you considered these possibilities?"
- "Have you weighed the advantages and disadvantages of . . . ?"

Should the client ask you what she should think, do, or feel about a certain situation, rather than jump to conclusions and offer friendly advice, you should help the client to do her own decision making. This process can be initiated by reflecting the request back to the client:

- "What are *your* feelings about . . . ?"
- "What do *you* think?"

This technique not only stimulates the client to rethink the situation but also implies that her thinking has value. One of the therapeutic aims in health assessment and any nurse-client interaction is to free the client, help her grow, and assist her in coming to her own conclusions and decisions.

The Insecure Pattern

Hearing another's anxieties tends to make you uncomfortable. This is what is meant by the expression "Anxiety is contagious." To ease your own discomfort, your first tendency may be to offer a quick shot of what you believe to be "courage-builder" or to give *false reassurance* to the anxious client: "Chin up!" "Keep on smiling!" "Don't worry." "Just listen to the doctors and nurses, and you'll do fine!" "You have a good doctor." "We have the latest and finest equipment." "Things always turn out all right in the end." "You think you're bad off, just think about all the . . . ." Such attempts at solace may ease your anxiety somewhat. You are let off the hook, as these comments have an air of dismissal and will usually cut off any further communication on the subject.

Rather than reject the client and his anxieties by use of these familiar clichés, you can offer your empathy and understanding through the *use of touch,* such as holding the client's hand or placing your arm around his shoulder. With this support, the client can begin to explore and further express his feelings. You can initiate and facilitate this process by such questions or statements as

- "This seems very hard for you."
- "You must feel very bad."
- "What makes you say (do) this?"
- "Would you like to talk about it?"
- "Perhaps if you talk about it, we can discover what it is that makes you feel anxious."

The Defensive Pattern

It is difficult to accept criticism of oneself. Even though you may have groomed the attitude of listening and considering what others say, at times you may find yourself knee deep in rationalization or defensive behavior. When you work closely with other health care workers and with a particular institution, you become identified with them and their cause. In essence, then, an attack on them is an attack on the extension of your self. Because of the frustrations that you may have personally suffered in the bureaucratic system, you may jump to the conclusion that a client's criticism is unfair. It truly may be unjust, but the client needs to express such hurt or angry feelings nonetheless. These feelings exist for the client, regardless of whether they are justified. Some of the common responses you may have used or heard said to a "complaining, ungrateful, hostile" client are "Ms. McKay would never leave you on the bedpan for two hours!" "Dr. Crane is very understanding and a well-known practitioner!" or "Beacon General has an excellent reputation!" If you understand the principles of anxiety and you are a fairly secure individual, you will be able to accept the client's feelings without becoming defensive and help him express them more fully:

- "You sound angry (hurt)."
- "What happened to cause you to feel this way?"
- "Will you try to trace the sequence of events leading up to the point when you began to feel this way?"

Agreeing

A "That's right!" indicates that whatever the client said or decided at the moment is *right.* The client may feel that she cannot change her decision later because then she would be *wrong.* Agreement has pushed the client into a corner in this case. You need to aid the client in gathering as much information as possible so he can arrive at his own conclusions and feel free to change his mind as he continues to ponder the data from various perspectives. When the client asks you to acknowledge a fact, however, this is not vulnerable to a value judgment. You are validating that, for example, "Yes, you are in Beacon Hospital." In no way should you ever agree with a delusion. For example, with a client who believes that he has no stomach, you would not respond to his declaration, "Oh, I now can understand why you are never hungry!" Challenging is no better than agreeing with a delusion; it does not bring reality to the forefront for the client—for example, "If you are dead, then why is your heart still beating?" The same would apply to a client who is experiencing hallucinations. You would not be therapeutic if you responded to a client who said that flies and bugs were crawling all over his body by telling him to "just lie still until I go get a fly swatter to kill them for you." The therapeutic approach in each case is to validate reality for the client.

"Why" Questions

"Why" questions can be or become frustrating. It is not unusual to receive a sarcastic reply to a "why" question such as "If I knew why, I wouldn't be asking you." "Why" questions have an intimidating ring reminiscent of mothers' and teachers' "Why did you do that!" A therapeutic approach would be to focus on the feelings or events.

- "Tell me what has occurred."
- "How do you feel about what is happening?"

Generally the client does not consciously know why, but during the elaboration, data may become clear to him and to you as to the "why."

Therapeutic Patterns

The following therapeutic patterns, when used appropriately, will greatly facilitate the health assessment process. It will be helpful to you and your clients if you become familiar with these patterns and use them consciously in your interactions with others. You will find that with experience you will develop better timing and use of these patterns.

The Open-ended Pattern

Generally, when given the chance, a client will overtly or covertly talk about her concerns. Many clients, however, do not know where and how to begin or progress; they may not be sure of their role in the interaction. An open-ended question or statement not only demonstrates your concern and interest but also points out that it is the client who is the topic of conversation. Examples of open-ended patterns are

- "What brought you to the clinic today?"
- "What do you hope to get from this therapy?"
- "Tell me about yourself."
- "A penny for your thoughts."

At times a client may test your interest to see whether he truly is the focus of conversation. A "needy" nurse will fall prey to such testing and begin to talk about himself. If this happens to you, you are falling short of fulfilling your role as a professional nurse. For example,

Client: "I see you are not wearing a wedding band."
Nurse: "No, I'm not, but we're not here to talk about me, so I would like to continue with the major purpose of the interview, which is . . . ."

You should not ignore the client's comment but simply acknowledge that she has made a correct observation and redirect the focus back to her. If the client persists, you can reiterate your interest in her as a client by saying something like, "I cannot see of what benefit my personal life would be to you, but I do see my role as trying to help you. I feel that to do so I must learn more about you."

The General Lead Pattern

The general lead pattern assures the client that you are listening, interested in, and following him. General leads also encourage the client to continue and elaborate. General leads include

- nodding the head
- raising the eyebrows at appropriate times
- comments such as "Uh huh," "I see," "Continue," "Go on," "And then?" and "Really?"

Did you ever notice the comment made about an individual who uses general leads appropriately? It is said that he is a great conversationalist!

The Reflective Pattern

When you reflect a word, thought, feeling, or idea back to a client, you are doing one or more of the following four things.

1. *You may be stimulating elaboration or more thought on a particular point, behavior, or feeling that the client has expressed:*

- "It's faster?"
- "I see you're biting your nails."
- "You seem to be uncomfortable (anxious, angry, sad, downtrodden, and so on)."

By stimulating elaboration, you keep the conversation flowing and help the client recognize, explore, and begin to deal with her emotions. Do not hesitate to use the word *feelings,* as in

- "What are your *feelings* regarding. . . ?"
- "How do you *feel* about. . . ?"
- "How does this make you *feel?*"

2. *You may be clarifying your understanding of what the client has just said:*

- "Are you saying that. . . ?"
- "In other words. . . ."

If you are not sure what is being communicated or if you have "lost" the progression of thought, you should inform the client that you are not following what she is saying and ask her to repeat what she has just said. Perhaps the client has used a phrase that is unclear to you. For instance, if a client states, "I'm going in circles," what does she mean by this? What is she experiencing? You may begin clarification by reflecting her entire statement: "You're going in circles?" If this approach leads nowhere, perhaps you can help her pinpoint her experience by being more specific: "You're feeling confused (frustrated, dizzy)?"

3. *You may be clarifying the use of dubious pronouns.* Take the following dialogue:

Client: "They told me not to take this medicine."
Nurse: "They?"
Client: "Mr. Pine, the head nurse."

Careless use of pronouns happens with clients and nurses alike. Many clients have difficulty with self-identity, and you may unknowingly compound this problem by careless use of pronouns and by not keeping your identity separate from that of the client. How many times have you heard a nurse say something like, "*We* are going to take our tub bath now." The client could rightly reply, "Who is going to get in first?" or "I doubt if the two of us will fit in that tub!" Clarification of the use of we-us and they-them by either the client or you is always necessary.

4. *You may be summarizing an interaction or requesting a conclusion.* You may reflect what has taken place with such openings as,

- "During the past 15 minutes you and I have been discussing. . . ."
- "What would you say was the main point or focus of what you and I have been talking about?"

Use of the reflective pattern in this way allows you and the client to clearly view the experience and to part with the same idea in mind.

The Silence Pattern

The use of silence following the use of a therapeutic pattern of communication is effective; it gives the client time to think over what has just been expressed and to organize his thoughts for response. It is also a golden opportunity for you to assess the interaction and form alternative plans of response and further communication. In addition, silence coupled with attention can convey acceptance and interest in the client; this attitude will encourage the client to continue his communication.

Most people, particularly Americans, are uncomfortable with silence. U.S. culture is action-oriented. Because silence is not an overt form of action, many people have the impression that nothing is happening, when basically a lot of mental wheels are turning furiously. It is important for you to be aware of this to appreciate the value of silence in communication and to feel more comfortable with using silence therapeutically.

Encouraging Plans

Helping the client think through what would be appropriate actions and coping strategies for future situations is therapeutic. The decisions and plans must be the client's, not yours. You can encourage plans by asking the client such things as

- "What things helped you to handle this situation?"
- "What might you do to handle this the next time it happens?"
- "What activities tend to relax you and that you might use to decrease your tension before it builds up too much?"
- "What could you do to express and release your anger so it doesn't harm you or others?"

Planning in itself doesn't solve future problems. Effective plans need to be implemented. Rehearsing and articulating plans periodically facilitates appropriate behavior through cognitive activity as opposed to impulsiveness.

An awareness of common nontherapeutic and therapeutic patterns of communication will serve as a guide for use in the interviewing process of health assessment. The time and conscious effort you spend to limit the use of nontherapeutic patterns and replace them with more therapeutic ones will be repaid time and time again. Therapeutic communication *is* the hallmark of a relationship model.

KINESICS

Kinesics, the systematic study of body motion and position as a means of communication, is intriguing. What whets the appetite even more is the thought that body language, kinesic behavior, may be an accurate barometer of true feelings and may actually contradict verbal communications. A question of interest is, Does everyone speak the same language when communicating in or by body language? Ekman et al (1969) conducted cross-cultural studies (the United States, Brazil, Japan, New Guinea, and Borneo) and found that facial expressions of emotions are similar regardless of culture. In their studies, the subjects identified sameness of emotion when shown a standard set of facial photographs—for example, they could say that a man expresses happiness, sadness, surprise, and so on. Body language, however, entails more than facial expressions. One speaks with eye and mouth movements, motion in gestures, movement of total body, posture, distance, and position in a room. The narrowed eye or quivering lip must be viewed within the context of the client's idiosyncracy. The narrow eye could be the squinting of happiness or a sinister glance; the quivering lip could be reflective of sadness or anxiety. The waving back and forth (left and right) of the hand with extended index finger tells the receiver, "no, no." Worry, anxiety, impatience—all could be expressed by rocking the total body back and forth in a chair. Slouched shoulders and a bowed head could mean sadness, reverence, or, perhaps, exhaustion. Standing closer than 3 to 5 feet from another person in American culture creates tension and discomfort—the client may feel encroached upon and may become defensive. Sitting in a corner or apart from a group may express shyness or a desire to be left alone.

Interpretation of body language is not simple and clear-cut. The complexity of this interpretation is increased by the fact that body language is a reflection of each individual's experiences; environment (the body language, as verbal expressions, differs in urban and rural communities); socioeconomic group (affluent versus poverty-class body expressions); and cultural group, which includes not only ethnic groups but countercultures such as drug societies and religious cults. Thus, kinesic behaviors cannot be examined in isolation but must be analyzed in conjunction with what occurred before, during, and after the presenting body behavior, as well as in conjunction with accompanying verbal communication. A given culture communicates to its mem-

Table 2-2 **Expressions of Anxiety, Anger, and Sadness**

	Anxiety	Anger	Sadness
Gait	Short steps	Fast, aggressive steps, body leaning forward, arms swinging strongly	Slow steps
Head posture	Head back	Head forward	Head down
Arms	Tightly tucked near body	Crossed tight in front of body	Arms crossed with hands to opposite shoulders
Hands	Fidgeting; tapping	Finger pointing; fist pounding	Limp, dropped at wrist
Feet	One forward ready to walk	Wide stance	Feet loose or crossed at ankles
Respirations	Speaks at height of inspiration	Speaks during inspiration	Speaks at end of expiration

Source: Adapted from Deckert, G. (1974). *Interpreting body language in everyday practice.* (videocassette). Cincinnati, Video Digest.

bers which things to fear—snakes, forbidden areas, communists, and so forth. Most cultures teach its children not to recognize that father is afraid or that father is sad, because these feelings are not to be expressed, let alone experienced by a male member of society. You may therefore feel uncomfortable in reflecting your interpretation of the body language of clients. Facial expression is universal, but one can disguise the mouth. If the mouth is smiling, look at the eyes to see if the "twinkle" of happiness is there. Additionally, you need to recognize that giggling, joking, and laughing may really be a facade for anxiety, nervousness, or fear.

To aid you in increasing your awareness and understanding of body language, Table 2-2 lists expressions of anxiety, anger, and sadness through gait, head posture, arms, hands, feet, respirations, and speech punctuation, according to Dr. Gordon Deckert. Dr. Deckert also identified "respiratory avoidance," a gesture to turn something away, communicated by such behaviors as clearing the throat, coughing, rubbing the nose, or closing the eyes. The message is, " This is something that I would like to get rid of!" He told us to look at former President Nixon's nonverbal message when, speaking with his eyes closed, he said, "I want to make this perfectly clear." Some additional selected behaviors and associated *possible* and *probable* meanings can be seen in Table 2-3. Skill in communication and interpretation of body language is very important in the interview process.

Table 2-3 **Inventory of Nonverbal Communication**

Nonverbal dimensions	Behaviors	Description of counselor-client interaction	Possible effects or meanings
Eyes	Direct eye contact	Client is Anglo-American. Client has just shared concern with counselor. Counselor responds; client maintains eye contact.	Readiness or willingness for interpersonal communication or exchange; attentiveness
	Lack of sustained eye contact	Client is Anglo-American. Each time counselor brings up the topic of client's family, client looks away.	Withdrawal or avoidance of interpersonal exchange; or respect or deference
		Client is a Mexican-American who demonstrates intermittent breaks in eye contact while conversing with counselor.	Respect or deference
		Client mentions sexual concerns, then abruptly looks away. When counselor initiates this topic, client looks away again.	Withdrawal from topic of conversation; discomfort or embarrassment; or preoccupation
	Lowering eyes—looking down or away	Client talks at some length about alternatives to present job situation. Pauses briefly and looks down. Then resumes speaking and eye contact with counselor.	Preoccupation
	Staring or fixation on person or object	Counselor has just asked client to consider consequences of a certain decision. Client is silent and gazes at a picture on the wall.	Preoccupation; possibly rigidness or uptightness
	Darting eyes or blinking rapidly—rapid eye movements; twitching brow	Client indicates desire to discuss a topic yet is hesitant. As counselor probes, client's eyes move around the room rapidly.	Excitation or anxiety; or wearing contact lenses
	Squinting or furrow on brow	Client has just asked counselor for advice. Counselor explains role and client squints, and furrows appear in client's brow.	Thought or perplexity; or avoidance of person or topic
		Counselor suggests possible things for client to explore in difficulties with parents. Client doesn't respond verbally; furrow in brow appears.	Avoidance of person or topic

Continued

Table 2-3 Continued

Nonverbal dimensions	Behaviors	Description of counselor-client interaction	Possible effects or meanings
Eyes, continued	Moisture or tears	Client has just reported recent death of father; tears well up in client's eyes.	Sadness; frustration; sensitive areas of concern
		Client reports real progress during past week in marital communication; eyes get moist.	Happiness
	Eye shifts	Counselor has just asked client to remember significant events in week; client pauses and looks away; then responds and looks back.	Processing or recalling material; or keen interest; satisfaction
	Pupil dilation	Client discusses spouse's sudden disinterest and pupils dilate.	Alarm; or keen interest
		Client leans forward while counselor talks and pupils dilate.	Keen interest; satisfaction
Mouth	Smiles	Counselor has just asked client to report positive events of the week. Client smiles, then recounts some of these instances.	Positive thought, feeling, or action in content of conversation; or greeting
		Client responds with a smile to counselor's verbal greeting at beginning of interview.	Greeting
	Tight lips (pursed together)	Client has just described efforts at sticking to a difficult living arrangement. Pauses and purses lips together.	Stress or determination; anger or hostility
		Client just expressed irritation at counselor's lateness. Client sits with lips pursed together while counselor explains the reasons.	Anger or hostility
	Lower lip quivers or biting lip	Client starts to describe her recent experience of being raped. As client continues to talk, her lower lip quivers; occasionally she bites her lip.	Anxiety or sadness
		Client discusses loss of parental support after a recent divorce. Client bites her lip after discussing this.	Sadness
	Open mouth without speaking	Counselor has just expressed feelings about a block in the relationship. Client's mouth drops open; client says he or she was not aware of it.	Surprise; or suppression of yawn—fatigue
		It has been a long session. As counselor talks, client's mouth parts slightly.	Suppression of yawn—fatigue
Facial expressions	Eye contact with smiles	Client talks very easily and smoothly, occasionally smiling; maintains eye contact for most of session.	Happiness or comfortableness

Table 2-3 Continued

Nonverbal dimensions	Behaviors	Description of counselor-client interaction	Possible effects or meanings
	Eyes strained; furrow on brow; mouth tight	Client has just reported strained situation with a child. Then client sits with lips pursed together and a frown.	Anger; or concern; sadness
	Eyes rigid, mouth rigid (unanimated)	Client states she or he has nothing to say; there is no evident expression or alertness on client's face.	Preoccupation; anxiety; fear
Head	Nodding head up and down	Client just expressed concern over the status of his or her health; counselor reflects client's feelings. Client nods head and says "That's right."	Confirmation; agreement; or listening, attending
		Client nods head during counselor explanation.	Listening; attending
	Shaking head from left to right	Counselor has just suggested that client's continual lateness to sessions may be an issue that needs to be discussed. Client responds with "No" and shakes head from left to right.	Disagreement; or disapproval
	Hanging head down, jaw down toward chest	Counselor initiates topic of termination. Client lowers head toward chest, then says he or she is not ready to stop the counseling sessions.	Sadness; concern
Shoulders	Shrugging	Client reports that spouse just walked out with no explanation. Client shrugs shoulders while describing this.	Uncertainty; or ambivalence
	Leaning forward	Client has been sitting back in the chair. Counselor discloses something about herself or himself; client leans forward and asks counselor a question about the experience.	Eagerness; attentiveness, openness to communication
	Slouched, stooped, rounded or turned away from person	Client reports feeling inadequate and defeated because of poor grades; slouches in chair after saying this.	Sadness or ambivalence; or lack of receptivity to interpersonal exchange
		Client reports difficulty in talking. As counselor pursues this, client slouches in chair and turns shoulders away from counselor.	Lack of receptivity to interpersonal exchange
Arms and hands	Arms folded across chest	Counselor has just initiated conversation. Client doesn't respond verbally; sits back in chair with arms crossed against chest.	Avoidance of interpersonal exchange or dislike
	Trembling and fidgety hands	Client expresses fear of suicide; hands tremble while talking about this.	Anxiety or anger

Continued

Table 2-3 Continued

Nonverbal dimensions	Behaviors	Description of counselor-client interaction	Possible effects or meanings
Arms and hands, continued		In a loud voice, client expresses resentment; client's hands shake while talking.	Anger
	Fist clenching to objects or holding hands tightly	Client has just come in for initial interview. Says that he or she feels uncomfortable; hands are clasped together tightly.	Anxiety or anger
		Client expresses hostility toward boss; clenches fists while talking.	Anger
	Arms unfolded—arms and hands gesturing in conversation	Counselor has just asked a question; client replies and gestures during reply.	Accenting or emphasizing point in conversation; or openness to interpersonal exchange
		Counselor initiates new topic. Client readily responds; arms are unfolded at this time.	Openness to interpersonal exchange
	Rarely gesturing, hands and arms stiff	Client arrives for initial session. Responds to counselor's questions with short answers. Arms are kept down at side.	Tension or anger
		Client has been referred; sits with arms down at side while explaining reasons for referral and irritation at being here.	Anger
Legs and feet	Legs and feet appear comfortable and relaxed	Client's legs and feet are relaxed without excessive movement while client freely discusses personal concerns.	Openness to interpersonal exchange; relaxation
	Crossing and uncrossing legs repeatedly	Client is talking rapidly in spurts about problems; continually crosses and uncrosses legs while doing so.	Anxiety; depression
	Foot-tapping	Client is tapping feet during a lengthy counselor summary; client interrupts counselor to make a point.	Anxiety; impatience—wanting to make a point
	Legs and feet appear stiff and controlled	Client is open and relaxed while talking about job. When counselor introduces topic of marriage, client's legs become more rigid.	Uptightness or anxiety; closed to extensive interpersonal exchange
Total body	Facing other person squarely or leaning forward	Client shares a concern and faces counselor directly while talking; continues to face counselor while counselor responds.	Openness to interpersonal communication and exchange
	Turning of body orientation at an angle, not directly facing person, or slouching in seat	Client indicates some difficulty in "getting into" interview. Counselor probes for reasons; client turns body away.	Less openness to interpersonal exchange
	Rocking back and forth in chair or squirming in seat	Client indicates a lot of nervousness about an approaching conflict situation. Client rocks as this is discussed.	Concern; worry; anxiety

Table 2-3 **Continued**

Nonverbal dimensions	Behaviors	Description of counselor-client interaction	Possible effects or meanings
	Stiff—sitting erect and rigidly on edge of chair	Client indicates some uncertainty about direction of interview; sits very stiff and erect at this time.	Tension; anxiety; concern
Distance	Moves away	Counselor has just confronted client; client moves back before responding verbally.	Signal that space has been invaded; increased arousal, discomfort
	Moves closer	Midway through session, client moves chair toward helper.	Seeking closer interaction, more intimacy
Position in room	Sits behind or next to an object in the room, such as table or desk	A new client comes in and sits in a chair that is distant from counselor.	Seeking protection or more space
	Sits near counselor without any intervening objects	A client who has been in to see counselor before sits in chair closest to counselor.	Expression of adequate comfort level

Source: Cormier L.S., Cormier W.H., Weisser R.J.: *Interviewing and Helping Skills for Health Professionals.* © 1986 Boston: Jones and Bartlett Publishers. Reprinted with permission.

CLIENT INTERVIEW

The interview is the first step in assessing the health status of the client. The health history obtained during the interview is a crucial component in the client's total health assessment. It is also at this point that the nurse-client relationship is initiated. The interview serves as the arena in which rapport is established between nurse and client and from which a trusting relationship can develop. The interview is also a means of mental health assessment and offers insight into possible or existing problems.

The interview provides the principal basis for nursing diagnoses and plan of care in addition to serving as a guide for areas of in-depth focus in the physical examination. For example, if a client complains of headaches, vertigo, and syncope, you would conduct a more highly scrutinizing physical examination of the head and neck and of the cardiovascular and neurologic systems.

To obtain information, you must convey sensitivity toward the client's needs and feelings, creating a climate of warmth and support. Once this climate is established, you will be able to explore more fully the client's beliefs and attitudes about health and illness. These beliefs, attitudes, and feelings will provide further data from which you can determine a client-centered plan of care. Through the interview process, you will be able to elicit information about the client's past and present health status that will be of great value in making subsequent nursing judgments.

To elicit important information, you may want to use open-ended patterns of communication, such as,

- "How do you feel about your family life?"
- "How do you feel about your illness?"

Questions such as these are less limiting than ones that do not encourage the client to express her feelings (e.g., "Do you feel your health is poor?").

At times, it may be necessary for you to ask direct questions about family relationships, financial status, personal habits, and daily life patterns. Allow the client sufficient time to answer these questions. Hurrying to the next question may make the client feel that you are interested only in gathering answers for a form. Be sensitive to the possibility that certain aspects may be uncomfortable and embarrassing to the client. In addition, other aspects of personal life, ethnic background, and religious beliefs may have cultural implications that make it more difficult for the client to be open about addressing them.

If the client demonstrates marked anxiety about any topic, you should not press your inquiries merely to be thorough in completing an established assessment outline, especially if doing so would sacrifice the client's comfort in any way. Sensitive areas may include sexual deviations, secret drinking, family quarrels, or parental attitudes. It might be better if investigation into sensitive areas is left until a time when rapport has been better established, unless it is of extreme import to the client's immediate situation, in which case the client should be made aware of why this information is necessary.

During the interview, you must be supportive of the client by being nonjudgmental and accepting of her feelings and attitudes. The client's nonverbal behavior frequently provides cues for interpreting her verbal messages. You need to listen to what the client says or does not say. Total involvement is necessary for attentive listening. It is also essential that you use words and sentences that the client can comprehend. Many people do not understand such terms as CVA,

MI, or ADL. It is often necessary to rephrase a question or assist the client in returning to the topic. Straying from the question may be an indication that the client is anxious or is trying to avoid disturbing topics. Assure the client that you are not prying, but are attempting to gain information that will be useful in developing a plan of care. Avoid false reassurances and pep talks. Statements such as, "Don't worry about it," "Everything will be just fine," or "Pull yourself together" can create frustration for the client. The client's questions should be answered honestly and directly. Leaving concerns unanswered tends to create anger and anxiety and may destroy the process of interaction. Attention to the client's body language may reveal feelings of anxiety, anger, and hostility.

Confidentiality and privacy are essential and should be maintained for the client. Any transgression could break down or inhibit the establishment of trust in the nurse-client relationship. Trust is important in all interpersonal relationships, but it is especially important when interacting with children. With children, you should be truthful in all things. Perhaps one of the most difficult things to tell a child is that something is going to hurt, but doing so maintains and strengthens the trust between nurse and child. By being honest you also show the child what he can expect of a nurse, and you aid in building the image of the nurse as a "helping" individual.

When you are gathering assessment data, relatives and friends should be asked to leave the room. Once you and the client are alone, you can ask whether the client wishes to have anyone present. In this way, no social or family pressures bear on the client's decision.

Although the client is the best source of information, there are times when the family or a friend must provide the needed information, such as when a child is too young to have adequate verbal skills or is unable to respond because of injury or illness. In such situations you must develop the same trusting relationship with the individuals being interviewed. When you wish to talk to friends and family members about a particular topic regarding an adult client, you should first obtain her permission. For additional suggestions for interviewing the child and adolescent, refer to Chapter 18.

Interview Structure

The interview is not social conversation; it is a goal-directed process of communication. In most cases, it is structured. Basically, the interview structure is composed of three phases: an *introduction,* a *focus,* and *termination.* How and when these phases are initiated depends on such variables as available time, environmental circumstances, and the age, education, and emotional/physical condition of the client.

Introduction

When you first meet someone in a social context, questions usually flow back and forth for the purpose of discovering whether the two of you have anything in common. The mutual interests, values, and experiences that you discover may form the basis for a friendship. Within this type of relationship, each individual generally tries in varying degrees to meet certain needs of the other. In your professional role, however, you are concerned with assisting the client in meeting *his* needs; you must use ways, means, and persons other than the client to meet *your* needs.

In the introduction phase, the information you give the client and your demeanor reflect the expertise you are offering. It is important that you call the client by name and introduce yourself and your status:

- "Hello, Mr. Ralph Ray? *(pause)* I'm Mr. Burns, the head nurse (student nurse, registered nurse, nurse specialist, nurse practitioner)."

It is also necessary to introduce by name and status any health worker who may be accompanying you and to ask the client's permission if others may be present during the interview. You should state the purpose of the interview at the beginning to clarify the client's participation, and, if applicable, you should share your specific role and responsibilities with the client. This latter step informs the client more specifically about what you may be called on to do or on what areas you may be consulted. Depending on the situation, additional contractual information and arrangements may be made, such as regarding time limitations on the interaction(s), fees (the particulars of cost, payment, the client's ability to pay, and available financial assistance), and subsequent interactions (time, place, and expectations of client participation).

In the initial introduction, you must explain the subject of confidentiality, which is vital in maintaining trust and rapport with the client. The client must understand that any information he gives will be shared with other health team members for the purpose of providing the best health care possible. If during the interview the client asks you to keep something to yourself, you need to inform him that you cannot honor such a request if the information negatively affects his well-being or that of another. In all interactions, you need to evaluate what specific information to record. It may be unnecessary to chart certain information that can be kept confidential between you and the client, in which case you need to record only your interpretation of the information.

You need to establish a comfortable climate for the interview, as setting can greatly influence the quality of the interaction. The setting should afford privacy and be free of interruptions and distractions (e.g., radio, television, bright colors, extensive decorations, glaring lights or inadequate lighting, offensive odors, uncomfortable room temperature, poor ventilation and humidity, and a "cluttered" environment). You should make every attempt to promote the client's comfort. If possible, the client should be seated in a comfortable chair so that he can relax. Sitting on a straight chair for prolonged periods can be as uncomfortable as sitting on a cactus.

Most people find communication more difficult if direct eye contact is not maintained; however, there are cultural groups who consider this practice to be disrespectful. It is best for you to be on the same level and face to face with the client during the interview. If it is necessary that the client be interviewed while he is in bed, you should be seated in a chair at the bedside so that you will be at his eye level. In a standing position, you would loom over the client and perhaps appear as an imposing, threatening figure. The standing posture may also imply the attitude of "one foot out the door" to the client. This "too busy" appearance can hamper the interview.

Focus

The focus of an interview is the health assessment of the client. You can learn much by observing the client's behavior—and she can learn much from observing yours. You need to be alert to your own behavior and what it may convey to the client. Gazing out a window may indicate lack of interest to the client; such nervous gestures as finger tapping and leg swinging may be interpreted as impatience.

It is best to encourage the client to initiate the discussion. Once the client begins to voice her concerns, her anxiety level will gradually decline. Then you will be able to focus her energies toward any necessary problem solving. As the client relaxes, she will tend to talk more freely. As the interviewer, you keep your verbal activity to a minimum. A lot of to-and-fro conversation tends to decrease the client's spontaneity and elaboration.

You can help the client relax and begin the discussion by using *open-ended communication patterns* more frequently at the *onset* of the interview. The next step is to keep the ball rolling by interjecting *timely general leads.* The overall communication flow of the interview is optimally free.

Strict adherence to a question-answer format is very mechanical. Consistent use of this format is often symptomatic of a nurse who is uncomfortable when dealing with clients' anxieties, as it can serve as a means of easily circumventing these anxieties. Furthermore, it creates an atmosphere in which the client may find it difficult to seek advice and support for underlying personal problems. Both clients and inexperienced nurses may become preoccupied with the questions and answers of an established interview form as an unconscious escape from facing the truly demanding and threatening problems. In other words, it is the *process* that becomes the main focus, and for the most part, the anxieties go unnoticed. You need to recognize feelings and encourage expression of them. There are times, however, when a modification of this question-answer format is necessary, usually when time is at a premium.

During the interview, you must give guidance to the conversation; you should not allow the client to ramble aimlessly. If you are passive, you may miss pertinent issues, and your passivity may increase rather than reduce the client's anxiety level. Also, the client may interpret passivity as evidence of lack of concern or competence. Rambling is nonproductive and detrimental to the assessment process, particularly when time is limited and there are several pertinent areas to be investigated. A helpful technique for directing the client to specific areas is to use more closed-ended questions that require a yes or no response or short answer. When using this communication pattern, you need to avoid the *common error* of asking more than one question at a time.

If, during the interview, the client does not respond to a specific question, you may try a related question. Should the client state that she would rather not answer or discuss that particular topic, it is generally best to drop the line of inquiry. In this way, you show acceptance of her right to privacy. By having asked the question, you have indicated your interest in the topic, should she care to share information with you at a later time. Marked probing tends to place the client on the defensive and may propel her away from charged areas. Someone once said that probing belongs in surgery.

The more sensitive areas of investigation are best pursued in the latter part of the interview. By this time, a greater degree of rapport has been established with the client, which will facilitate the sharing of more intimate information. Also by this time, you will have collected most of the information relevant to assessing the client's health status, so little information will be lost should the client decrease her communication or become silent in response to the investigation of these demanding areas.

Be on the alert for emotionally charged words or statements spoken emphatically. Take care to identify key words or topics that are repeated frequently. Watch for flushing, facial expressions, and gestures as the client talks about a specific topic or person. Explore the topic or relationship in more depth.

Lastly, part of the interview focus may be on health teaching. In this regard, it is important to remember not to overload the client's circuits; use short learning periods followed by rest (and practice) breaks. When a wealth of information needs to be conveyed, it is sometimes easy for a nurse to become overzealous and "go berserk" with endless, intense explanations and descriptions. Take the client's lead, for example, supplying her with information necessary for the moment, if she seems restless. You may be better informed by asking the client to tell *you* what *she* knows about her health risks, problem, and/or treatment.

Termination

Sadly, termination is a neglected phase of many interviews and nurse-client interactions. Most of us do not enjoy the feeling of hanging at loose ends. The termination phase allows you and the client to reflect on your experience and the work you have accomplished together. It is a time of recapitulation, in which there is some degree of completeness as you and the client evaluate whether your objectives

Checklist for the Interview Structure

- Introduction
  - Give your name and status
  - Give name and status of accompanying health worker(s)
  - State purpose of the interview
  - Clarify your role to the client
  - Clarify the client's role and expectations
  - Discuss contractual arrangement
    - Times
    - Finances
  - Discuss the parameters of confidentiality
  - Setting
    - Privacy
    - Environmental controls
    - Comfort of client
  - Maintain eye contact (when culturally appropriate)
- Focus
  - Body language conducive to the interview process
  - Productive patterns of communication
    - Open-ended
    - General lead
    - Reflection
    - Silence
- Termination
  - Advise client of approaching termination
  - Recapitulate the interview
  - Remind client of the number and times of future sessions (if appropriate)

have been fulfilled. It may be a time of establishing future goals, renegotiating contracts, referring the client to another health worker or agency, or ending the relationship.

Sudden termination without warning may cause difficulty for the client in developing trusting relationships in the future. If you know that there is a time limit to your relationship or that you will be going on vacation or having days off, you should share this with the client as soon as possible. The dependent client—which many "ill" clients are—may be severely distressed at the disappearance of "his" nurse.

In single interview sessions, you should remind the client when the meeting is coming to an end:

- "We are going to have to end our discussion in 10 minutes. Is there anything in particular you would like to talk about, or are there any specific questions you have at this time?"

If you and the client are meeting for a specific number of sessions, the client should be reminded a few sessions from the terminating session:

- "After today, we have three more sessions left in this series."

The chief purpose of the termination phase is to allow people time to adjust and plan for change in order to minimize the stress that is inherent in change.

SUMMARY

This chapter has focused on some concepts of communication essential to effective health assessment. There are three important aspects of communication: (1) People communicate in a variety of ways; (2) if understanding is absent, communication has not occurred; and (3) listening is a principal route to awareness and understanding of communication. Trust, empathy, and respect were described as essential to the creation of a therapeutic milieu. Patterns of communication were discussed and specific examples of nontherapeutic and therapeutic patterns were given. Body language, an important manner of communication, was identified as an index of assessment. The three elements of introduction, focus, and termination within the interview process were discussed.

DISCUSSION QUESTIONS/ ACTIVITIES

1. Describe communication from the standpoint of the concept of life field and the context of perceptual psychology.
2. List factors that distort communication.
3. What is meant by the following statement: "If understanding is absent, communication has not occurred."
4. Role-play an interview session with a colleague. Have another colleague note your communication patterns and interview technique. Role-play or actual interview could be audiotaped or videotaped.
5. Discuss the use of silence as an interview technique. Why is the technique of silence difficult for many people?
6. Describe body behaviors observed in a selected setting and give rationale for interpretation of the kinesics.
7. Keep a communication log of interactions to analyze for the purpose of improving your body language interpretation and use of therapeutic communications techniques and for identifying common nontherapeutic techniques that you tend to use.

REFERENCES

Combs, A. W.; Avila, D. L.; and Purkey, W. W. 1971. *The helping relationship sourcebook.* Boston: Allyn & Bacon.

Cormier, W. H., and Cormier, L. 1979. *Interviewing strategies for helpers: a guide to assessment, treatment, and evaluation.* Monterey, Calif.: Brooks/Cole.

Ekman, P.; Sorenson, E. R.; and Friesen, W. V. April 1969. Pan cultural elements in facial displays of emotion. *Science* 164:3875.

Mizner, W. 1955. In *Speaker's handbook of epigrams and witticisms,* ed. H. V. Prochnow. New York: Harper.

CHAPTER

3 Mental Health Assessment

Learning Objectives

1. List the seven mental functions by which to assess mental functioning.
2. Discuss the characteristics of the ABCs (appearance, behavior, conversation) to be noted during a mental health assessment.
3. Identify the various levels of consciousness.
4. Discuss the techniques used to assess mental functioning.
5. Identify mental dysfunctions characteristic of selected mental illnesses.
6. Describe examples of maturational and situational crises.
7. Describe Kübler-Ross's stages of dying.
8. Recognize signs and symptoms and areas of assessment for situations involving violence, addiction, and loss or impending death.
9. Describe behaviors significant of mild to extreme anxiety states.
10. State the principles important in interactions with depressed and/or suicidal clients.

Everyone has ups and downs and good and bad days. The key to health is a happy medium—a balance. As discussed in Chapter 1, stress has a tremendous impact on this equilibrium. Both body and mind attempt to cope with the impact of stress through their own protective means. The body musters up energy stores, and the mind makes increased use of mental defense mechanisms. The mentally healthy person uses these protective devices to regain homeostasis and is able to function socially; he deals constructively with major tragedies by overcoming misfortunes and using them beneficially. It is when these protective devices fail to recapture homeostasis that illness or an "unhealthy" state exists. In mental illness, these signs and symptoms of dysfunction are part of the client's life and interfere with his ability to function socially.

What is mental health? What constitutes a state of mental well-being? Are there criteria available to assess a client's presence of or lack of mental illness? No concrete definition exists for the term *mental health.* The general consensus, however, is that a mentally healthy individual is one who

- is able to perform the tasks required by his culture.
- has the ability to maintain social relationships.
- is able to establish and maintain intimate relationships.

Mental health does not mean that there is freedom from stressors. The mentally healthy individual is one who actively practices coping strategies and is able to face life's problems.

While many attempts have been made at defining mental health, the surfacing factor in each of these definitions is that *an assessment of mental health of an individual is made in the context of his or her culture or subculture.* For instance, in the eyes of the assessor, folkways and home remedies, such as those of the rural Appalachians, may seem detrimental, and ways of coping with stress or crisis may appear as defeating the purpose or even maladaptive. When taken in the cultural context of the client, however, the behavior and coping mechanisms appear to be adaptive, and the client is deemed to be fully functioning and mentally healthy.

Of course, the presence of signs and symptoms of dysfunction may not necessarily indicate mental illness but in fact may represent a means of coping with a temporary stress situation. The assessment of the client's mental health must encompass

- the signs and symptoms of dysfunction
- preponderance, degree of severity, and duration of symptoms
- extent of interference with social functioning by the symptoms

Additional data from the client's health history will shed light on the mental health assessment. The historical background provides a dynamic perspective for the survey of the nature of the client's current behavior. A review of the client's history in terms of previous personality and characteristic modes of behavior should reveal adaptations that the client has made to life stresses (medical and nonmedical) in the past. The history may indicate the following information, among additional data:

- Does the client have a family history or medical history of mental illness?
- Has the client demonstrated an ability to form close relationships?
- How does the client view himself?
- What has been the nature of the client's interpersonal relationships?
- What is/was the client's degree of dependence-independence?
- What are the client's existing and available support systems?
- What is the client's degree of successful living (jobs, family, friends/scope).

These are aspects that are investigated with every client.

Mental status is evaluated whenever you have multiple interview sessions or subsequent interactions with a client. It is important to remember that because of stress, the client's emotional state may be markedly different from one contact to another. Thus, mental health assessment is an ongoing process—it is never "complete" except for the moment. Method and approach are important. You need to be aware that relentless searching for psychopathology can prove to be a barrier to further assessment and can serve only to anger and alienate the client.

MENTAL FUNCTIONING

The evaluation of mental functioning is part of the mental health assessment. Because mental functioning is an internal process, it is not directly available to observation; therefore, you need to assess it indirectly by analyzing the ABCs of observable data: *appearance, behavior,* and *conversation.* In most cases you will have gathered adequate, observable data on the client's ABCs in the routine course of interviewing, which will serve as a base from which to assess her mental functioning. This assessment is accomplished by viewing the client's ABCs in relation to the following seven mental functions:

1. *Attitude.* What is the client's general overall behavior?
   - How cooperative is she?
   - Does she engage in solitary activity? Parallel activity? Group activity?
   - What is the extent of her participation in interpersonal relationships?
2. *Affect/mood.* Affect is the emotional state of the client—the way she appears to others. Mood is what the client *says* in regard to how she is "feeling"—happy, sad, and so on.
   - Is the client's affect appropriate to the situation? For example, a client who walked about with a constant grin would be displaying inappropriate affect and would not be experiencing her total environment. Appearance may belie feelings. When this happens—as when the client feigns cheerfulness when she actually feels depressed—the affect and mood are in disharmony.
   - Are mood swings present—does the client cry one minute and laugh the next?
3. *Speech characteristics.* These are some of the characteristics of speech that help you detect the presence or absence of difficulties with thought processes. Does the client's speech include
   - circumstantiality?
   - scattering, a loosening of thought associations?
   - a degree of vagueness?
   - a tendency to overgeneralize?
   - the use of global pronouns lacking specific referents (terms such as *they* and *them*)?
   - an inability to describe participation in an experience?
4. *Thought processes*
   - Does the client's conversation flow in a logical sequence?
   - Does the client's conversation make sense?
   - How does the client experience the world around her?
   - Is she in contact with reality?
   - Does she experience hallucinations (sensory impressions that lack external stimuli)?

- Does she experience delusions (false beliefs not based on fact)?

5. *Sensorium and reasoning*
   - Is the client aware of her immediate situation?
   - Is the client alert? Is she oriented to time, place, and person?
   - Do the client's recent and remote memories appear to be intact?
   - Is the client able to perform simple calculations?
   - Is the client able to conceptualize and make appropriate judgments?
   - Does the client understand her condition and the situation in which she finds herself?
   - Does the client know things that would be considered common knowledge?
6. *Potential for danger*
   - Does the client display a positive self-concept?
   - Has the client ever thought about harming or has she actually harmed herself or others?
   - Does the client have a history of uncontrollable temper?
   - Has the client ever been in trouble with the law?
   - Is the client able to cope with situations that are not to her liking?
   - What life stresses has the client experienced?
   - How has the client handled or responded to these life stresses?
7. *Psychological assets.* The outcome of an illness depends as much on the client's assets as on the nature of the pathology.
   - Does the client have a positive self-image?
   - Does the client have a repertoire of coping mechanisms?
   - Does the client have interested and supportive significant others?
   - Does the client have financial stability?
   - Does the client have satisfying interests and hobbies?
   - Does the client have the ability to get along with others?

If, after evaluating your ABC data in light of the seven mental functions, you suspect mental dysfunction, you will need to carefully pursue a more detailed investigation. Signs of disturbances in the client's sensorium, thought processes, or interpersonal relationships would prompt you to further investigate these specific aspects of mental functioning. This investigation requires more extensive techniques that are designed specifically for securing an in-depth evaluation. These special techniques are inherent in the following discussions of each of the ABCs of mental status and functioning.

Appearance

An individual's general appearance can reveal a great deal about him. It must be kept in mind, however, that the description of a client is highly subjective. To exaggerate, a nurse who is as "neat as a pin" may view the "open-collar" client as carelessly dressed; a nurse who is a casual dresser

Checklist for Mental Health Assessment: Appearance

This table presents a *range* of signs and symptoms that *may suggest* dysfunction. They are not in themselves necessarily reflective of mental illness, nor are they all necessarily confined to a specific area of appearance, but may overlap with behavior and conversation.

Mental functions	Appearance	Mental functions	Appearance
1. Attitude a. Cooperativeness b. Interpersonal relationships	Client is aloof, unclean, disheveled, indifferent	4. Thought processes a. Logical b. Coherent c. Perceptual	Client is inattentive, easily distracted, preoccupied
2. Affect/mood a. Appropriate b. Harmony c. Swings	Client has masklike face; is apathetic, flat, rigid, labile, euphoric, depressed, suspicious, hostile; displays inappropriate affect; shows physical signs of anxiety (flushing, sweating, tremors, respirations)	5. Sensorium and reasoning a. Levels of consciousness b. Orientation c. Memory (recent, remote) d. Calculation e. Abstract thinking f. Judgment/insight g. Intelligence	Client displays decreased or absent physiologic reflexes, disinterest, peculiarity of dress, bewilderment
3. Speech characteristics a. Description b. Speed c. Quantity	Client is soft-spoken, loud, boisterous; has monotonous, slow, or rapid speech	6. Potential for danger a. Self-concept b. Harm to self/others	Client is docile, sad, hostile, angry, apathetic
		7. Client's psychological assets	Few or no physical assets

may describe the neat as a pin client as being obsessed with neatness.

- Note the client's body build. Is he short, tall, thin, obese, muscular? Body build may have significant influence on the client's self-esteem and behavior. Body communication is also important to notice.
- Is the client's posture relaxed, tense, erect, or slouched?
- Does the client appear unkempt, careless, and dirty, or is he clean, neat, and tidy?
- Is the client dressed appropriately for the occasion and for his age?
- Is the dress appropriately applied?
- Are the colors bright or subdued?
- Are bizarre outfits or incongruent patterns worn?
- Is the client's facial expression mobile, fixed, bland, furrowed, tense, worried, in pain, sad, angry, sneering, suspicious, frightened, dreamy, laughing, smiling?

The colors of the client's clothing often tell the nurse something about his personality. Self-esteem, stress, mood, and cognitive functioning may be reflected in dress and/or hygiene. Facial expressions reflect affect.

If possible, make observations when the client is unaware of being observed. Under such circumstances, the client may manifest a different appearance. For instance, a client who is normally quite animated and abrasive may be overly docile and polite in an assessment interview when he is under close scrutiny. It is important to recognize that clients often act and appear in a particular manner to please the nurse and significant others.

Behavior

One of the best indicators of the degree of mental functioning is the level of consciousness. There are four basic levels:

1. Conscious and alert
2. Obtundent—has slowed mental processes, lethargy, sleepiness
3. Semicomatose or stupor—is unconscious but can be aroused sufficiently to respond to verbal commands
4. Comatose or unconscious—cannot be aroused; does not respond to painful stimuli; often has accompanying abnormal reflexes and respirations

The client's state of orientation should be determined.

- Is the client oriented in the three spheres—person, place, and time?
- Has there been any recent change in the client's personality or behavior?

Dysfunctional behavior patterns are most likely to be detected or suspected during the routine history-taking process. Difficulties may become apparent when investigating such areas as

- employment (e.g., poor job history, job dissatisfaction)
- school (e.g., discipline problems, poor grades, truancy, inattentiveness, drug abuse)
- family life (e.g., strained or severed relationships, marital difficulties, temper outbursts, trouble with the law, sexual promiscuity/abuse, violence, alcohol abuse or dependency, somatic preoccupation)

Assess whether problems exist in interpersonal relationships by exploring the client's

- ability to work with others
- attitude toward her employer or teachers
- attitude toward rules and regulations
- aspirations
- attitudes toward her parents, siblings, or significant other

In assessing the client's family dynamics, it may be helpful to ask the client to compare herself to her siblings in regard to such aspects as

- role
- responsibilities
- aggressiveness, passivity
- intelligence
- success, failure
- likes, dislikes

Such conditions among family members as jealousy, competitiveness, favoritism, alcoholism, drug dependency, antisocial personality, mental retardation, and psychopathology may be revealed at this time. At this point, you may also want to discuss significant life crises and the client's response to them (adaptation/coping patterns).

- "Tell me about some of the difficult problems you have experienced in your life."
- "How did you deal with those problems?"

If the client reveals sexual problems during the sexual history or if such problems emerge while you are investigating her relationships with others and her lifestyle, you should try to determine their etiology to best direct further exploration.

Conversation

Observing the content, manner, and process of the client's conversation is essential to the assessment of mental functioning. While observing the client's conversation, you should examine his *stream of mental activity*.

Checklist for Mental Health Assessment: Behavior

This table presents a *range* of signs and symptoms that *may suggest* dysfunction. They are not in themselves necessarily reflective of mental illness, nor are they all necessarily confined to a specific area of behavior but may overlap with appearance and conversation.

Mental functions	Behavior	Mental functions	Behavior
1. Attitude a. Cooperativeness b. Interpersonal relationships	Client is negativistic, uncooperative, hostile, belligerent, passive, drooping, withdrawn, impulsive; has slow gait	4. Thought processes a. Logical b. Coherent c. Perceptual	Client avoids anxiety, displays phobic behavior, compulsiveness, echopraxia
2. Affect/mood a. Appropriate b. Harmony c. Swings	Client is overactive, underactive; cries or laughs easily; wrings hands; paces floor; strikes head with hands; holds fixed posture for prolonged periods; has silly smile	5. Sensorium and reasoning a. Levels of consciousness b. Orientation c. Memory (recent, remote) d. Calculation e. Abstract thinking f. Judgment/insight g. Intelligence	Client displays stupor, lethargy, coma, confusion, agitation, delirium panic, twilight state, behavior problems, conduct disorder
3. Speech characteristics a. Description b. Speed c. Quantity	Client grimaces, stammers, stutters; displays uncoordinated or exaggerated movement, mutism, echolalia	6. Potential for danger a. Self-concept b. Harm to self/others	Client has made suicide attempts; is malingering, withdrawn, assaultive, combative, violent; lacks temper control; displays antisocial or criminal behavior (arrests), irritability, explosiveness, excitability, maladaptive coping
		7. Client's psychological assets	Few or no behavioral assets

- Is the client's conversation appropriate?
- Is the client's conversation consistent?
- Does the client ramble?
- Is the client able to proceed logically and to develop a point?
- Is the client's conversation spontaneous and coherent?
- Does the client exaggerate and confabulate (making up for memory gaps by substituting falsehoods)?
- Does the client use circumstantiality ("beating around the bush" before coming to the point)?
- Does the client use tangentiality (going off on a tangent and never reaching the goal, despite refocusing by the interviewer)?
- Is autistic speech present (talking in one's own made-up language)?
- Is the client's speech incoherent?
- Does the client display flight of ideas?
- Are neologisms (made-up, self-coined words) used?

Most of the client's sensorium and reasoning can be evaluated through analysis of conversation. The entire process of history taking affords continuous opportunity for evaluating the client's memory. The reliability of the information received from the client can be checked by follow-up, cross-validation questioning, talking with friends and family, reading past records; and questioning other health personnel who have had contact with the client. These practices will aid in identifying confabulation and memory dysfunction.

The following is the process for a specific test of *recent memory:*

- Tell the client that you are going to show him some items and that you want him to concentrate on them because you will ask him to name them about 5 minutes after you put them away.
- Show the client three or four common items (e.g., pen, keys, watch, coin, toothbrush).
- Have the client repeat the name of the items until he has them memorized.
- Five minutes later, ask him to recall the items.

The average individual is able to remember the items.

Pathology may be reflected in the client's inability to perform *mental calculations.* You can indirectly test the client's ability to do this by asking questions that require the client to calculate his age during a particular year or the

Checklist for Mental Health Assessment: Conversation

This table presents a *range* of signs and symptoms that *may suggest* dysfunction. They are not in themselves necessarily reflective of mental illness, nor are they all necessarily confined to a specific area of conversation but may overlap with appearance and behavior.

Mental functions	Conversation
1. Attitude a. Cooperativeness b. Interpersonal relationships	Client avoids topics; is pessimistic
2. Affect/mood a. Appropriate b. Harmony c. Swings	Client displays disharmony with thought processes; talks of guilt, sin, or unworthiness
3. Speech characteristics a. Description b. Speed c. Quantity	Client displays exaggeration, confabulation, blocking of thought, circumstantiality, tangentiality, autistic speech, incoherence, flight of ideas; is overtalkative; uses neologisms
4. Thought processes a. Logical b. Coherent c. Perceptual	Client displays phobias, obsessions, paranoid ideas, illogical flow; has feelings of strangeness, depersonalization, hallucinations, delusions (somatic, grandeur, persecution, alien control)
5. Sensorium and reasoning a. Levels of consciousness b. Orientation c. Memory (recent, remote) d. Calculation e. Abstract thinking f. Judgment/insight g. Intelligence	Client displays aphasia, memory defect, disorientation, poor judgment, lack of insight, inability of abstract thinking and calculations
6. Potential for danger a. Self-concept b. Harm to self/others	Client has ideas of self-accusation and condemnation, self-depreciation, suicidal ideations
7. Client's psychological assets	Few or no conversational assets

number of years since a particular occasion. In this way, you can avoid placing the client in a testing situation. Failure under a testing-type environment, which in itself usually promotes apprehension, might serve only to increase the anxiety level of the client.

If the client appears to have difficulty with calculation, you can tell him that you would like to test his ability to concentrate. Then ask the client to count forward by adding 3s (1 + 3 = 4, 4 + 3 = 7, 7 + 3 = 10, 10 + 3 = 13, . . .). In most cases, you need not go further than 22 or 25 in order to gauge his ability.

Another commonly used test is to ask the client to start at 100 and subtract 7 from each successive answer (93, 86, 79, 72, 65, . . .). This test is known as serial 7s. Another ability to assess is whether the client is able to "switch" sets. To do this, ask the client a simple arithmetic question wherein you mix addition, subtraction, multiplication, and division exercises. For example, ask the client "2 plus 2 = ? times 3 = ? minus 2 = ? divided by 2 = ?" (the answer is 5). This type of question requires the client to change mind sets.

The ability to *think abstractly* and to conceptualize generally can be assessed during conversation. If the client seems to have difficulty understanding concepts, you could use proverbs to further fine-test his ability for abstract thinking. Ask the client, "What do these sayings mean to you?"

1. People in glass houses shouldn't throw stones.
2. Don't count your chickens before they're hatched.
3. A stitch in time saves nine.
4. No use crying over spilt milk.
5. A rolling stone gathers no moss.
6. You can lead a horse to water, but you can't make it drink.

Each successive set of two proverbs is at a higher level; numbers 5 and 6 require greater abstract thinking ability.

A further test is to ask the client how the following terms are alike: coat/dress, axe/saw, table/chair. If, in the context of conversation, the client seems to display poor *judgment*, you can further test this ability by saying that you would like to have him answer a few questions that you routinely ask all clients. Then ask such questions as

- Why should people pay taxes?
- Why should a promise be kept?
- Why are laws necessary?
- Why do we have child labor laws?
- Why pay bills with checks?

During the history-taking session, you can ease into assessing the client's general *knowledge* (intelligence) by asking him whether he keeps up with the news. Most clients of average intelligence will be able to tell you the name of the president of the United States, the state governor, and the city mayor and will be able to answer such questions as "How many days in a week?" "Where does the sun set?" and "What animal does wool come from?" Because impaired abstract thinking, judgment, and decision making tend to interfere greatly with the client's ability to function at his job and manage his household, examination of his work and home problems may further reveal such impairment.

Finally, you should try to determine whether the client's conversation reveals *suicidal tendencies.* You must be particularly alert for suicide when hyperactivity is coupled with low narcissism or when the client is severely depressed. With all clients you should inquire, tactfully and at an appropriate time, whether they have ever entertained the idea of suicide:

- Is the client sometimes so discouraged that he feels there is no use in going on?
- Is the client ever troubled by thoughts of hurting himself?
- Has the client ever made plans to end it all?

It is also important to investigate avenues that may reveal antisocial behavior:

- What kind of temper does the client have?
- How does the client get along with people?
- Does the client feel he drinks too much for his own good?

In mental assessment, it is quite helpful if you can observe the client interacting with family, with friends, and in other settings and compare your interactions with the client with those of other health team members.

When you record the conclusions of the mental health assessment, including mental functioning, it is desirable to include verbatim wordings and body language samples. With mute clients, you need to keep in mind that they communicate by body language, so the major means you have of evaluating them is nonverbal behavior.

CLINICAL CORRELATES

Appearance

An unkempt appearance often occurs with chronic organic brain disorder and with certain neuroses and psychoses. A severe physical condition or physical handicap could also be responsible for what may appear to be neglect of physical appearance. Clients with chronic organic brain syndrome often have difficulty dressing themselves and may apply their outer garments first and their undergarments on top.

The client's clothing, whether bright or subdued, often tells the nurse something about her personality. Eccentric combinations in dress and inappropriate use of cosmetics are commonly found in clients with schizophrenic or manic personalities.

Behavior

Chapter 2 examined specific body language that may be reflective of mood. Both mental and physical pathology can be communicated via body language. A tense, erect posture accompanied by laughter, fidgeting, or tremors may indicate anxiety; however, you may want to consider the possibility of physiologic dysfunction, such as thyrotoxicosis, when such anxiety symptoms exist. The same can be seen when considering the facies. A flat, mask-like face may be a sign of certain psychoses or of parkinsonism.

Some examples of structural (organic) brain damage that would alter the client's level of consciousness can result from vascular pathology, alcoholic psychoses, toxic psychoses (particularly drug induced), general paresis, meningitis, encephalitis, brain tumors, head injuries, and degenerative disorders (adult hydrocephalus, Pick's disease, Alzheimer's disease, Huntington's chorea). Any situation that alters the normal electrolyte content and pH of the body (acidosis and alkalosis) affects the level of consciousness. Such situations include hypoglycemia, starvation, persistent vomiting, dehydration, cardiorespiratory disease, renal disease, cirrhosis, burns, pyrexia, and use of illicit drugs or improper use of prescribed medications. A cloudy sensorium and confusion are more frequently related to toxic or structural damage than to functional (psychodynamic) factors.

Disorientation in place and person implies cerebral disorder. Such disorientation is commonly observed in elderly clients with circulatory impairments and cerebral degeneration due to the aging process. Coupled with these circulatory and degenerative changes is cerebral hypoxia, observed in elderly clients undergoing general anesthesia. Many an oriented elderly client is sent to surgery only to return postoperatively in a disoriented state of mind caused by hypoxia.

Radical change in environment (from home to hospital room to operating room to recovery room to intensive care unit, and so on) adds to a client's disorientation. Hospitalization and other forms of institutionalization, as well as the separation from one's home and loved ones, upset the client's routine activities. Without the predictability of these daily activities, the client may become bewildered. He is faced with a new set of stimuli that is strange and sometimes frightening.

Disorientation can also result from sensory deprivation, which can occur following ocular surgery (because of the bandages covering the client's eyes), or as a result of isolation, flotation therapy, or immobilization. Again, the elderly individual in our society is more prone to disorientation and other mental disorders because of developmentally related circumstances, such as the loss of spouse and friends by death, social isolation, job retirement, financial deprivation, decreased physical capacity, and decreased resistance, resulting in acute and chronic illnesses.

Sexual problems can result from physical illness, surgery, neuroses, psychoses, and behavioral management problems. Behavioral management problems tend to produce sexual promiscuity, whereas the other etiologies tend to result in a decrease or cessation of sexual activity. For example, the schizophrenic client, who has unstable interpersonal relationships, is actually fearful of getting too close to anyone; even the thought of sexual contact with another may be terrifying to him.

Cadoret and King (1974) have categorized some specific psychiatric syndromes into three groups of behaviors. Following are the three groups and some examples (for further elaboration see their text, *Psychiatry in Primary Care*):

1. *Recent changes in personality or behavior:* (a) Forgetfulness, emotional lability, disorientation, inattentiveness, decreased alertness (organic brain syndrome); (b) inattentiveness, temper outbursts, poor grades, school truancy (drug abuse or dependency).
2. *Lifelong, often chronic, difficulties in behavior:* Home and school discipline problems, sexual promiscuity, poor job history, trouble with the law, drug and alcohol abuse (antisocial personality).
3. *Medical symptoms:* (a) Somatic preoccupation, fatigue, headaches, anorexia, constipation, weight loss, insomnia, decreased libido (depressive syndrome); (b) intermittent attacks of cardiac symptoms and fear, rarely beginning after age 40 and commonly seen in the emergency room setting (anxiety neurosis).

Jenkins (1971) suggests that there may be psychological risk factors for coronary artery disease in addition to the established physical risk factors of age, sex, blood pressure, obesity, and cigarette smoking. Clients with coronary artery disease tend to be serious, shy, and conforming, but self-sufficient. In many cases they are experiencing rejection, marital difficulties, or general dissatisfaction with their jobs. Cassem and Hackett (1971) reported that nearly a third (32.7%) of clients admitted to a coronary care unit were referred for psychiatric consultation because of sexual acting-out, hostile behavior, and noncompliance with the treatment regimen, in addition to anxiety or depressive symptoms.

Conversation

Clinical conditions may be reflected in the content, manner, and process of the client's conversation. For example, the client with a depressive character disorder will have a pessimistic attitude and will avoid certain topics. Because guilt and self-hate are central to depression, the depressed client will tend to talk of guilt, sin, or unworthiness. You may notice disharmony between the client's affect and her thought content. For instance, she may manifest silly behavior when her attitude should be one of concern.

Speech characteristics can be significant. A client with manic psychosis will speak in a rapid, pressured manner, whereas a client who is depressed or has myxedema may speak in a slow monotone. The client with multiple sclerosis will have a staccato pattern of slurred speech.

Difficulty with stream of mental activity can be related to mental dysfunction. Exaggeration and confabulation (making up for memory gaps by substituting falsehoods) are characteristics of clients with Korsakoff's psychosis, amnesia, and other disorders in which clients attempt to hide their memory defects. A blocking or sudden stop in conversation for no apparent reason may result from preoccupation with or interference by delusional thoughts or hallucinations. Circumstantiality and tangentiality are manifestations of either neuroses or psychoses. Autistic speech (talking in one's own made-up language), incoherent speech, flight of ideas, and neologisms are characteristic of schizophrenia. Hallucinations can result not only from psychoses but also from use of various drugs and can occur in delirium tremens, severe myxedema, uremia, and hepatic encephalopathy. A person who is very thirsty, very hungry, severely fatigued, or highly tense may also have hallucinations.

The client with a paranoid psychosis is quite concrete in her thinking and generally exhibits delusions of persecution. She will most likely be suspicious of you in the interview session. Delusions of influence or alien control (by other people or by strange voices) are more characteristic of the client with schizophrenia, as is the delusion that everyone knows what she is thinking. Most of the client's sensorium and reasoning can be evaluated through analysis of conversation.

Loss of memory is an early sign of pathology of the cerebral cortex in general and of the temporal and occipital lobes in particular. Recent memories are those most affected, because remote memory is seldom disturbed and tends to survive disease.

The loss of the ability to perform simple mental arithmetic calculations is a sensitive index of parietal lesions and diffuse cerebral disease. Depression, psychosis, and severe anxiety can also interfere with this cognitive function.

The ability to think abstractly and to conceptualize can be reduced in advanced psychoses and in acute confusional states (inflammatory, metabolic, toxic, or traumatic cerebral disease). Such states also diminish a client's judgment and knowledge base (intelligence). Problems with abstract thinking can also be seen with amnesia, aphasia, schizophrenia, and brain lesions. Clients with such problems may have ideas but can't manipulate them, and their thinking tends to be literal.

Checklist for Assessing Crisis

1. Is the client's chief complaint indicative of internal discomfort?
2. Did the symptoms appear rapidly?
3. Will the situation take time to resolve?
4. Can you identify an event leading up to or contributing to the situation?
5. Does the client show any physical or behavioral signs of disturbance?

If the answers are yes, the client may be facing a crisis. Many times the client may only need support, someone to talk to who will listen and reflect both the content and feeling of the client's statements. In some cases, however, the crisis may become intense and referral for therapy may be warranted.

CRISIS ASSESSMENT

Webster's dictionary defines a crisis as "a turning point for better or worse in an acute disease or fever; an emotionally significant event or radical change of status in a person's life; the decisive moment; an unstable or crucial time or state of affairs." A crisis can be the end of a decade, like turning 40, or a rite of passage, such as the onset of menstruation for the adolescent girl. A crisis can be a marriage or a divorce. It can be a terminal illness diagnosis or an abused spouse or child. Crises range from happiness to violence.

Maturational Crisis

Maturational crises are keyed to the human growth and development process. In some cultures they are celebrated as the rite of passage from childhood to adulthood, and from adulthood to old age. For the early adolescent girl, menarche (first menstrual cycle) signals the beginning of womanhood. For the boy, first ejaculation announces the passage into manhood. Adolescence is the time of physical and emotional growing—of exploring, searching, questioning, and sorting out values to be weighed against those of parents. Adolescence is the time of wondering who am I, where I belong, and how I fit in. It is the time for trying out roles to see which one fits. Likewise, it is a time for decision making and planning one's life. It is a time for doing "my own thing," which may result in rejection by parents and, at times, society. It is a time for recognizing that double standards do exist, and that treatment will not be lenient when a law is violated. The adolescent faces a multitude of crises as he precariously makes his way from the world of the child to that of the adult. Reaching the world of the adult, however, does not signal the end of everyday crises.

Some crises are related more typically to one sex or one age group. Some women, for example, face a crisis or turning point in their lives when their child or children leave home. In what has been labeled the "empty nest syndrome," these women suddenly find themselves with only their spouse to care for. After years of nurturing, parenting, and teaching their children the ways of their culture and society, they discover a void in their lives. Some fill this void by returning to work, seeking volunteer work, or returning to school. Others are engulfed within the void, becoming withdrawn, lonely, or depressed. It is at this point, too, that crises in husband-wife relationships arise. For women, this usually happens after years of cooking, ironing, washing, and cleaning, and perhaps becoming dependent primarily on their children to fulfill their needs.

At about this same time, a man also experiences crises. He may have reached the point in his life where he is taking an assessment of himself. What were his goals when he was young? Where does he stand now in relation to those goals? Can he progress upward? Many times, men feel dissatisfied with their accomplishments in life. They become unhappy with their work and are disenchanted. They feel an urge to take risks, to try new adventures before it is too late. In addition to evaluating themselves relative to their employment and occupational success, they also evaluate other accomplishments. Have they been "good" parents? "Good" spouses? In their eyes, has life been rewarding? And generally, they realize that retirement just around the corner.

Retirement, often associated with aging, brings with it body-image crises. Although body image is important throughout the life span, the sudden realization that body changes have taken place can be a crisis for some. By the natural process of maturing, the body tends to slow down. Gray hairs appear; bald spots become evident; the youthful

Checklist for Assessing Maturational Crisis

1. Are anxiety-arousing or tension-producing events occurring in the client's environment (home, school, workplace)?
2. Have recent changes occurred in the client's lifestyle?
3. Has there been a recent loss of a loved one or significant other through divorce, moving, or death?
4. Does the client have good rapport with family and friends?
5. Is the client satisfied in his/her occupation? If not, how would he/she like it to be?
6. Is the client accepted by his peers?
7. Are there free-flowing lines of communication in the home between husband and wife, parents and child, and between siblings?

figure reflects padding. For some persons, these natural changes are taken in stride. For others, these changes remind them that they are mortal, and the fear of senility and/or death grows out of proportion. The inability to understand and cope with the physical and emotional changes that occur as a result of maturation can present a crisis situation. When assessing the maturational crisis situation, remember that a combination of events, not just one, has usually precipitated the event.

Situational Crisis

Crises of this type arise when the environment in which the client lives is altered dramatically. The homeostasis of the individual is threatened, and bodily responses are usually generated. Three kinds of situational crises are violence, addiction, and loss.

Violence

Victims of violent acts and of continuous physical and/or emotional abuse are present in every community. They include the physically assaulted, rape victims, children who are verbally and physically punished or threatened into submission, spouses who stay in the home and allow beatings to continue out of fear for their safety or the safety of their children, and the elderly who are bullied, pushed, shoved, and sometimes beaten by other members of society, including their own children.

Often, clients who experience physical violence show signs of repeated beatings or shovings. The telltale bruises, black eyes, multiple fractures, or missing teeth are clues that something is amiss. However, verbal assaults and threats are more difficult to detect. Consider the child whose eyes fill with tears of fear or who cowers in the corner when his name is called. Be suspicious when the elderly grandparent begins to tremble or displays other symptoms of anxiety when you ask about his children, grandchildren, or neighbors. You also may encounter a middle-aged woman who insists on going home despite an extreme state of anxiety. These are only a few examples of violence crises and reactions. A screening tool for child abuse is provided as Fig. 3-1.

If you suspect a client is in an abusive relationship, inquire as to what precautions are observed (adopted from Buchalter 1995).

- Does the client know the hotline number and shelter location(s)?
- Does the client have a list of phone numbers to call in an emergency?
- Is the client participating in or possibly interested in participating in a support group?
- Are there firearms in the home? (Keep unloaded.) Ammunition? (Get rid of it, or keep it in a separate place.)
- Does the client have neighbors with whom he can work out a system to signal them to call the police (e.g., shade down in a specific window)?
- Does the client always keep enough money on his person to pay for a cab to quickly get away to a safe place?
- Does the client park his car headed out of the driveway, as well as have adequate gas in the tank at all times?
- Does the client keep an extra key to the house and the car?

Addictions

Addiction and crisis assessment usually address two components: the crisis of the addict and the crisis of the addict's family. For the addict, the realization that she is truly addicted to a substance can be overwhelming. Because of the devastating probabilities, the addict may likely have lost her job, spouse, family, and community support, as well as her self-respect and possibly her identity. In addition to the physical needs of the addict, the psychological needs must be assessed and addressed.

- What does the addict see for herself in the future?
- What does she want?
- Is she willing to begin treatment?
- Is she willing to work toward recovery?

When assessing the needs of the addict, particularly the alcoholic, it is important to keep in mind that the client is sincere in her expressed desire for recovery and fully intends to honor the commitments she is about to make. Realistically, a lot of backsliding generally occurs. Therefore, an assessment of the addict's living environment is important.

- Will moral support and help be available?
- Will backsliding be met with criticisms and put-downs?

Loss

Diagnosis of a terminal illness, advanced aging, accidental death of a family member, or the fear of death itself can initiate a crisis situation in an individual. Kübler-Ross (1975) outlined a model, comprising five stages, that can be used to assess adjustment to death, disability, or loss of something or someone.

Stage 1: Denial

In this stage, the client denies the existence of the loss. "It can't happen to me!" or some other form of disbelief is expressed. One of the dangers in this stage is that by denying, for example, the existence of an illness, the client may neglect treatment until it becomes too late for it to alter the course of the disease. In addition to the client, a family member or close friend may also become involved in denial. This person may refuse to accept the possibility of illness, or in the case of an accidental death, refuse to acknowledge it.

Index of Suspicion: Screening for Child Abusers

Item	Index Score
1. *Attitude in dealing with staff*	
__ Irrationally hostile	3
__ Situationally hostile	1
__ Verbally paranoid (project all blame on others)	3
__ Combative	5
__ Abusive	5
2. *Family structure*	
__ Family together	0
__ Divorce	1
__ Separation exists	4
__ Child/parent role reversal	5
__ Foster home	3
__ One spouse deceased	1
__ Uncontrolled sibling rivalry	3
__ Rigid, compulsive structure	2
__ Loose, ill-defined structure	2
3. *Family problems (parental figures)*	
__ Alcoholism	5
__ Drug abuse	5
__ Frequent visitors to emergency ward	3
__ Evidence of sexual promiscuity	3
__ History of parental figures being abused as children	5
__ Chronic organizational problems in the home because of child	5
__ Psychiatric history	3
__ Unstable job pattern	5
__ Documented assault and/or battery	5
__ Hypertension	2
__ Ulcers	2
__ Past suicide attempt	5
4. *Religious affiliation*	
__ None	5
__ Strong	0
__ Lukewarm	2
5. *Labor and delivery*	
__ High-risk pregnancy	3
__ Low birth weight	5
__ Mental retardation in child, mother, or father figure	5
__ No prenatal care	5
__ Isolation from mother during newborn period	3
__ Born out of wedlock	5
6. *Cultural factors*	
__ Bicultural home	3
__ Interracial marriage	3

Item	Index Score
6. *Cultural factors (continued)*	
__ Patrilineal authority	5
__ Jewish	0
__ Caucasian	3
__ Black	3
__ Hawaiian	1
__ Polynesian	1
__ Chicano	2
__ Puerto Rican	2
__ First generation European immigrant	1
__ Arab	1
__ Matrilineal authority	3
__ Jewish	1
__ Caucasian	3
__ Black	1
__ Hawaiian	0
__ Polynesian	0
__ Chicano	0
__ Puerto Rican	1
__ First generation European immigrant	3
__ Arab	3
__ Metropolitan residency	4
__ Rural residency	2
7. *Child or siblings*	
__ Frequently admitted to hospital	5
__ Diagnosis:	
__ Long bone fractures	5
__ Head injuries	5
__ Hematomas	5
__ Failure to thrive	5
__ Malnourishment	3
__ Bruises (multiple) in various stages of healing	5
__ Multiple scratches	2
__ Burn sites, varying healing stage	5
__ Described by parent figures as discipline problems	5
__ One child or more under 3 years of age	3
__ Parents contradict themselves when describing illnesses and injuries of children	5
__ History of not visiting children when admitted to hospital	5

When the interview for the Index of Suspicion is completed, points assigned the parent for each item are added and the total is ranked: low risk—0 to 40 points, moderate risk—41 to 75 points; high risk—76 to 115; very high risk—116 to 149; and extreme risk—150 points or more.

Figure 3-1 Olson's Index of Suspicion: Identification of parents who are potential child abusers. (Copyright © 1976 The American Journal of Nursing Company. Reprinted from R.S. Olson, Index of Suspicion: Screening for Child Abusers, *American Journal of Nursing,* January 1976, 108–110. Used with permission. All rights reserved.)

Checklist for Assessing Situational Crisis (Violence, Addiction, Loss, or Impending Death)

Assessment for Violence

1. Physical findings suggesting violence/abuse:
   - Bruises
   - Burns (cigarette, rope, hot water, fire)
   - Broken bones
   - Excessively bitten nails
   - Welts on the body
   - Missing hair (excessive hair-pulling)
   - Puffy face
   - Black eye(s)
   - Signs of malnutrition
   - Lumps on the head, trunk, or extremities
   - Concussion
   - Clothing inappropriate for environmental conditions
   - Body twitches when touched
   - Rigid body position, tense muscles
   - Reluctance to go home
   - Unwillingness to disrobe for physical examination
   - Crying uncontrollably
2. Historical findings suggesting violence/abuse:
   - Expression of fear
   - Heightened emotional arousal—e.g., sudden defensiveness or hostility to specific questions
   - Multiple expressions of self-hate
   - Expressions of low self-esteem and insecurity
   - Request that you not report your observations

Assessment for Addiction

1. Physical findings suggesting addiction:
   - Needle marks on arms, legs, trunk, or between fingers and toes
   - Malnourishment
   - Bad breath caused by inability to brush teeth due to extremely sore gums
   - Delerium tremors (DTs) (uncontrollable, heavy shaking)
   - Pupils dilated
   - Evidence of nausea and/or vomiting
   - Slurred speech
   - Unkempt appearance
   - Compulsive alcohol consumption
   - Hallucinatory behavior
   - Memory loss
2. Historical findings suggesting addiction:
   - Inability to maintain employment
   - Loss of family and friends
   - Inability to display socially acceptable behaviors
   - High value given to the addicting substance—e.g., will give up anything for the drug
   - Confused state of alertness
   - Appearance of intoxication but insistence on having "only a couple" drinks
   - Craving for the substance
   - Lies told about drinking patterns; attempts made to minimize the amount consumed; incongruency in answering similar questions
   - Alcohol consumption begun in the morning

Assessment for Denial of Loss or Impending Death

1. Physical findings suggesting loss or impending death:
   - Signs of grieving
   - Signs of advanced, acute, or terminal illness
2. Historical findings suggesting loss or impending death:
   - Refusal to seek medical diagnosis
   - Refusal to follow prescribed treatment plan
   - Avoidance of conversations related to the loss, illness, or individual who is deceased
   - Avoidance of interaction with family members and friends
   - Rejection of suggestions to join support groups
   - In the case of the death of a loved one, behavior continuing as if that significant other is still alive

She, too, may retreat into her own world and pretend that the event never happened. Thus, she continues on as before, but with the unresolved or pending crisis looming over her.

Stage 2: Anger

In this stage, the client expresses anger at life. He is angry because "it" has happened to him, not to others; he can turn the anger inward, cutting off communications necessary for maintaining support, and thus alienate family and friends. In some cases, however, this reaction can work to the client's advantage if you are able to redirect the anger. The client may begin to fight for himself. Hence, in the case of injury or disability, the restoration process can be enhanced.

Stage 3: Bargaining

In this stage, the client or family member tries to strike a bargain with a deity. The client will do anything, such as change her way of living or give more to charity or the church, if only this affliction can be taken away. The family member also makes concessions and promises to be carried out if only her loved one can be saved or if only the pain and agony of the loved one's situation can be spared. When these attempts prove futile, the next stage, depression, is entered.

Stage 4: Depression

At this stage, the client or family member becomes ambivalent and perhaps uncaring. Usually one of two types of depression is demonstrated: reaction or preparatory.

In reaction depression, the client or family member reacts to his environment or life change. In many cases, this type of depression can be maladaptive, locking the individual into this stage and preventing him from resolving his crisis. In preparatory depression, the client or family member can be observed working through the crisis situation—for example, putting his life in order and, primarily for the terminal client, preparing to die. In contrast to reaction depression, preparatory depression can be adaptive in that it allows the client or family member to work toward and possibly accomplish crisis resolution.

Stage 5: Acceptance

In this final stage, the client or family member has worked through the previous stages and accepted her fate. She has resolved the crisis and is ready to continue living. She now appears to become more sociable and content.

When assessing the client and her acceptance of loss or impending death of self or of a significant other, remember that it is not necessary to progress through all of the stages, nor is it necessary to pass through them in any prescribed order. Also, the client may vacillate many times between several of the stages.

ASSESSMENT OF INTERNAL STRESSORS

Anxiety

Although many psychological definitions of anxiety exist, and the construct of anxiety remains obtuse, the consensus is that anxiety results from a stimulation, either physical or emotional, in the environment, which produces a reaction (physical and/or emotional) within the organism. Anxiety ranges from mild to extreme, and various physical and psychological reactions correspond to the various degrees of anxiety.

The degrees of anxiety range on a continuum from adaptive or reactive to maladaptive. There are certain times when anxiety is beneficial and appropriate to the situation, but there are other times when the level of anxiety reaches such proportion that it is detrimental to the person. A common example of this range can occur in the performing arts. Adaptive (mild) anxiety serves as a stimulus to practice, or to perfect the art, but when the stimulus becomes intense, the person may panic or lose confidence in his ability to perform. Thus, the anxiety becomes maladaptive in nature. Another example of reactive anxiety may be seen when persons are forced into situations for which they are unprepared. In these situations, the level or degree of anxiety may reach extreme proportions quickly if the individual lacks competence and coping skills. The client may demonstrate physical symptoms ranging from increased heart rate to incapacitation resulting from fear.

In cases of extreme anxiety, the client may experience anxiety attacks, which may take the form of body tremors, respiratory difficulty, heart palpitations, and a choking sensation. Other degrees of anxiety can produce increased perspiration, clammy palms, gastric distress, diarrhea, loss of appetite, and inability to concentrate.

In the hospital setting, clients who are awaiting tests or surgery generally exhibit symptoms of anxiety. Note whether the client's body tenses or flexes when you touch him. This could be indicative of increased response to stimuli due to fear of the unknown. Unfortunately, heightened anxiety can lead to complications or reactions to drugs. In the surgical area, the client in such a heightened state of anxiety may require more anesthesia than usual to produce the desired effect. Once the desired effect is produced, however, the danger of overdose exists. Anxiety also has the ability to increase blood pressure, pulse, and respiration rates; in some instances, high levels of anxiety can alter test results.

Anger

Anger is a powerful emotion. It is the release of hostilities toward some other object. It is a forceful self-assertion that tends to be destructive in nature. It is a way of venting frustration and confusion associated with a lack of effective coping skills. The behaviors are highly charged and emotionally filled. If these pent-up hostilities are released on others, physical and/or emotional abuses may result. If these hostilities are held within a person, however, physical consequences may result. Blood pressure tends to rise as temper flares. Other physical effects include ulcers, gastric disturbances, sleep disturbances, tension headaches, and increased body tension.

In the clinical setting, you may encounter the client who resists some or all forms of treatment. Instead of countering her hostility with yours, you may be able to defuse the situation and gain her cooperation if you listen to her reasons for the anger. Perhaps she is angry with herself for being ill. She may be feeling guilt or helplessness. Keep in mind

Checklist for Assessing the Degree of Anxiety

Mild Anxiety
1. Client demonstrates an increased sense of alertness and attentiveness.
2. Client is focused more on others than himself.
3. Client displays an interest in the people and objects surrounding him.
4. Client desires to assume responsibility for his own hygiene.
5. Client may become interested in activities.
6. Client may exhibit symptoms such as restlessness, a desire to talk, repeated questions, joking, and procrastination.

Moderate Anxiety
1. Client may demonstrate either an increase in the use of his capacities or demonstrate an unawareness of activities in his immediate environment.
2. Client may indicate a desire to move away from others—to withdraw or isolate himself.
3. Client may display acting-out behavior in the form of complaining constantly, arguing, or excessive teasing.
4. Client may exhibit physical symptoms such as nausea, headache, or low back pain.

Severe Anxiety
1. Client demonstrates inability to make rational decisions; exhibits a state of confusion.
2. Client demonstrates a loss in the body's ability to restore itself.
3. Client appears extremely concerned regarding his condition. This is evidenced through constant questioning, focusing on details, and an impairment in his ability to perceive the situation clearly.
4. Client becomes extremely concerned with routine TPR checks.
5. Client displays automated behaviors such as aimlessly pacing or walking about, picking at clothing and bedding, or conversing without purpose.

Extreme Anxiety
1. Client exhibits a loss of control, and emotions surface.
2. Client can no longer perceive, remember, make decisions, control affect or motor activity, think, or test reality.
3. Client displays relative helplessness.
4. Client may seek escape from life or threats by using rash behaviors.
5. Client may demonstrate the need for comfort from a nonthreatening individual.
6. Client may demonstrate the need for a nonstimulating environment.

Symptoms of Anxiety
- Change in tone of voice
- Increase or decrease in rate of speech
- Change in posture
- Change in pattern of gestures or motions
- Intellectual or emotional preoccupation
- Nonreceptive to communications
- Increased perspiration
- Body tremors
- Lump in throat or choking sensation
- Sinking feeling in abdomen
- Diarrhea
- Vomiting
- Changes in heartbeat, pulse, respirations
- Change in appetite
- Dry mouth
- Sweaty palms
- Increased muscle tension
- Focus on detail
- Physical withdrawal
- Inability to function
- Inability to attend to immediate surroundings
- Immobility or paralysis

Checklist for Assessing Anger

1. Is the client able to control his faculties?
2. Can the client think through the situation?
3. Is the client rational?
4. Is the client becoming physically destructive?

that the client who feels threatened or out of control of the situation may well demonstrate hostility and aggression or anger. For this client, your empathy, caring, and understanding of her needs and concerns may make a difference.

TYPE A, TYPE B, AND TYPE C PERSONALITIES

The type A personality is the emotionally charged, ready-to-go person. He is the first to go when the red light changes to green, he is a half hour early for appointments, and he completes tasks well in advance. Everything must be done ahead of time. He is anxious, impatient, and must always feel in control. When threatened by a stressful situation, he struggles to regain the control he feels he has lost.

Type A personality with underlying feelings of anger is termed type C. The type C personality is highly correlated with coronary disease, angina pectoris, and myocardial infarction. This person tends to work faster, strive harder, and become more aggressive than the type B person.

The type B personality, on the other hand, remains calm when threatened by stressors. He refrains from frantically trying to gain control and maintains energy under prolonged stress. He has been labeled the noncoronary-prone person, who tends to be more relaxed, more accepting of events, and less rushed. While the types of personalities exist, type A falls at one end of a continuum; type B at the other end. The majority of persons fall somewhere in between.

Checklist for Assessing Type A Personality

1. Is the client competitive?
2. Does the client work in a stressful, demanding position?
3. Is the client impatient and always in a hurry?
4. Is the client impulsive?
5. Is the client aggressive?
6. Does the client appear to be a workaholic?

ASSESSMENT OF COPING METHODS

Everyone has her own method of coping with stress; some methods are more adaptive than others (Table 3-1). Defense mechanisms or ego defenses are used to protect the ego from undue stress. The following are commonly used defense mechanisms:

1. *Denial.* Denial is a method of hiding, or burying deeply within oneself, thoughts and feelings. It is a way of pushing these thoughts and feelings into one's unconsciousness. It

Table 3-1 Coping Strategies

Affective-oriented coping strategies	Problem-oriented coping strategies
Hope that things will get better	Try to maintain some control over the situation
Eat; smoke; chew gum	Find out more about the situation
Pray; trust in God	Think through different ways to handle the situation
Get nervous	Look at the problem objectively
Worry	Try out different ways of solving the problem to see which works best
Seek comfort or help from friends or family	Draw on past experience to help you handle the situation
Want to be alone	Try to find meaning in the situation
Laugh it off, figuring that things could be worse	Break the problem down into "smaller pieces"
Try to put the problem out of your mind	Set specific goals to help solve the problem
Daydream, fantasize	Accept the situation as it is
Get prepared to expect the worst	Talk the problem over with someone who has been in the same type of situation
Get mad; curse; swear	Actively try to change the situation
Go to sleep, figuring things will look better in the morning	Settle for the next best thing
Don't worry about it, everything will probably work out fine	Do anything just to do something
Withdraw from the situation	Let someone else solve the problem
Work off tension with physical activity	
Take out your tensions on someone or something else	
Drink alcoholic beverages	
Resign yourself to the situation because things look hopeless	
Do nothing in the hope that the problem will take care of itself	
Resign yourself to the situation because it is your fate	
Blame someone else for your problems	
Meditation, yoga, biofeedback	
Take drugs	

Source: Copyright © 1981 The American Journal of Nursing Company. Reprinted from A. Jalowiec and M.J. Powers, "Stress Coping in Hypertensive and Emergency Room Patients," *Nursing Research*, 30:13 (January–February 1981). Used with permission. All rights reserved.

is a means that can protect against painful memories; once repressed, these memories remain in the unconsciousness despite efforts to retrieve them. With denial, certain aspects of reality are blotted out. An example of denial is the person who, on receiving bad or unwelcomed news, rejects it, pretending it never happened. For instance, the parents who are unable to accept the death of a child may keep the child's room intact for years to come, and they may talk about the child as if she were still alive.

2. *Projection.* Projection is the attributing of your feelings or thoughts to another person. Often, a person unconsciously recognizes some characteristics about herself that make her feel guilty. She then projects, or attributes, these characteristics to someone else, thus releasing herself from guilt and responsibility for them. An example might be an aggressive husband who tells you how hostile his wife is and that he feels he must retaliate in some way. Another example is the mother, married at a very early age, who refuses to allow her daughter to date before mid to late adolescence.

3. *Introjection.* Introjection, which is a way of coping with a threatening situation, involves taking ideas or thoughts incongruent with your own and making them your own. It is a "If you can't beat them, join them" type of behavior. This coping mechanism can come into play in situations in which a threatening issue is in conflict with your set of moral values; to resolve this issue, you make a compromise.

4. *Reaction Formation.* In reaction formation, one expresses the opposite of one's true feelings. This is a means of protection from one's guilt. For instance, when one family member has a deep dislike for another family member, she may go out of her way to express love and caring for this person.

5. *Isolation.* In isolation, the thought and the act connected with the thought are separate, and only the thought is allowed to surface. For example, suppose you have an unpleasant task to do on a beautiful, sunny, summer day. While performing the task, your mind is filled with thoughts of pleasant things that you like to do on these kinds of days. In some cases, the content of the thoughts is socially unacceptable. For instance, suppose someone toward whom you feel animosity is in danger. Suddenly, you are filled with feelings of hostility, and this prevents you from taking swift, appropriate action to help.

6. *Intellectualization.* To intellectualize is to practice exaggerated thinking over feeling. A person using this defense mechanism discusses issues in a very cool, abstract way, without expressing feelings that most persons would express. An adolescent often uses this mechanism when discussing sensitive issues, such as sex. By using this mechanism, she is able to resolve many of the conflicts she must face while growing up.

7. *Undoing.* This is a way of making amends behaviorally for something you wish that you had not done. Shakespeare's Lady MacBeth continuously washed her hands after making arrangements for the death of the king, which was her way of undoing her evil act. Undoing is a way of negating guilt.

Checklist for Assessing Coping

1. Does the client confront situations or withdraw?
2. Does the client deny or accept situations?
3. Does the client have a confidant—someone to talk to?
4. Does the client use defense mechanisms to "get over the rough spots," depend on them for an extended period of time, or use them every time rather than face issues?

There are, however, coping strategies other than the ego defense mechanisms. One way most people cope with difficult situations is to *talk* to someone—a family member or spouse, friend, or religious leader. Some clients seek professional help, but usually after alternative sources have failed. By talking the problem over with someone, the client is able to see the issues from a different perspective, lay the issues out on the table, examine them from all sides, and generate some alternative solutions to the problems at hand.

Another coping strategy is *involvement* in hobbies or volunteer activities. Frequently, people find clubs, church or civic groups, and volunteer agencies helpful and rewarding for providing companionship and filling gaps in their lives. For many, these types of activities provide a change in the daily routine and something to which they can look forward.

Other strategies that are used to release pent-up energies include *physical exercise, long quiet walks,* and *meditation/relaxation techniques.* These help the client relax her body and provide time for rethinking or reexamining her dilemma.

Many people turn to their *religion* as a source of support and a way to cope with daily stressors. They find strength and assurance through their faith in addition to the fellowship and friendships formed with other members. Many times a *sharing of experiences* proves beneficial for all parties involved.

These are only several of the many coping mechanisms used to solve everyday or crisis situations. Remember that facing the problem situation rather than retreating from it or denying its existence is more important than the coping mechanism used to handle the situation.

DEPRESSION

Described as a feeling of sadness, depression ranges from mild to severe. It occurs irrespective of age; however, it tends to occur most often within the adolescent and aging populations. Some depressed clients may appear sad and

Checklist for Assessing Depression

1. Does the client appear withdrawn?
2. Has the client been confronted with a crisis situation in the recent past?
3. Does the client appear excessively active and inappropriately attired (excessive body movements and gaudy attire)?
4. Does the client appear overly talkative and excessively happy for a given set of adverse circumstances?
5. Does the client demonstrate behavior appropriate to the situation?
6. Does the client appear to have difficulty reaching a decision regarding his situation?
7. Does the client complain of changes in weight, appetite, concentration, sleep, or energy level?
8. Does the client express guilt, worthlessness, helplessness, or suicidal ideation?

withdrawn or preoccupied with a serious life event. They appear lethargic and lacking in energy and interest. On the other hand, some depressed clients may appear very active, constantly talking and displaying extensive body movement. They may even appear inappropriately happy.

When assessing the underlying causes and the range of depression, consider several areas:

- loss
- lack of skills
- low self-esteem
- illness
- behaviors

The American Psychiatric Association Diagnostic and Statistical Manual of Mental Disorders identifies the symptoms of major depression as including a depressed or irritable mood and the loss of interest or pleasure in usual activities, plus at least four of the following symptoms over a 2-week period:

- changes in appetite and weight
- disturbed sleep
- motor retardation or agitation
- fatigue and loss of energy
- feelings of worthlessness, self-reproach, excessive guilt
- suicidal ideation or attempts
- difficulty thinking or concentrating

Loss

Depression due to loss can result from many things: loss of a spouse or significant other through separation, divorce, or death; loss of a limb or limbs; total or partial body paralysis; and loss of job, home, or prestige within a community. When assessing the client suffering from loss and depression, remember that, given a sufficient amount of time, most clients will be able to work through the grieving process described earlier in this chapter and resolve their crisis. Be a good listener and try not to offer platitudes. Above all, do not tell the client that he should not feel depressed, that he has no good reason to feel depressed, or that things always work out for the best. From the client's perspective, he has every reason to feel sad and depressed. For many clients, depression may result from a combination of issues.

Lack of Skills

Another contributor to depression is lack of skills, including such common skills as those of communication, problem solving, and sociability. Begin by investigating the client's support system.

- Does the client have someone with whom to talk?
- Does the client have the skill and vocabulary to express herself?

The depressed client may withdraw from family and friends, because she may feel that if she opens up to a family member, she will be rejected.

For adolescents, the lines of communication between parent and child are often tense, if not severed. A special effort needs to be made to help the adolescent understand that you are listening without judging or moralizing and that you are trying to understand. Frequently, when the client is assisted in verbalizing the problem or area of concern, she is able to examine the situation and formulate some viable alternatives.

For the older adult, particularly men, support networks may have been established only with the spouse or with the spouse and one or two significant others (Preston & Grimes 1987). When death of one of these support figures occurs, the network weakens or vanishes altogether; the survivor may not have the skills to establish a new network. In this case, your listening, empathy, understanding, and encouragement may help to raise the client's level of self-confidence and enable the risk taking needed for meeting new friends. If a lack of problem-solving skills exists, this may add to the state of depression. The more the client ruminates over the problem, the more intense the depressed state may become, and, in efforts to solve or resolve a conflict, the client may easily succumb. Helping the client identify the problem or face the issue and generate some realistic, concrete solutions may begin to lead her out of her depression.

Low Self-Esteem

The feelings of uselessness, helplessness, and worthlessness may be overwhelming to a client; he may have depended on a significant other for reinforcement and a feeling of self-worth. Now he may have to face life without a substitute reinforcer. He may easily fall into a trap of self-pity, or, because he has low self-esteem, he may feel incapable of making decisions or coping with the situation. He may feel helpless to change his environment, or he may feel that the situation is out of his control. This would be especially true in the case of an older adult who is suddenly told that he is incapable of making critical decisions in his life with regard to finances, living arrangements, lifestyle, and food.

Illness

Illness, especially one that may require modifying or changing one's lifestyle, may contribute to depression. Questions regarding the prognosis and long-term effects or duration of the illness, plus a lack of understanding of the disease, can contribute to excessive dwelling on the issue by the client. Unexpressed fear can also be a contributor. While assessing the client for depression, make an attempt to encourage the client to discuss the issue(s), express her concerns and fears, and ask any questions she may have.

Checklist for Assessing Suicide

1. Does the client talk of suicide? He might say things like, "I won't be here to bother you," or "You won't have to put up with me much longer," or "I wish I were dead," or "No one cares whether I live or die." He may ask how you would feel if he were dead.
2. Does the client appear extremely depressed; does he want to talk but is reluctant to do so?
3. Is he beginning to give away his most cherished possessions? This is a big clue.
4. Does he appear to have made a big decision and is now at peace with himself? Is his turmoil or crisis over? It is at this point that the danger of successful suicide exists. Up to this point, family and friends have been keeping a close watch on the client, but they relax their vigil because they mistakenly think nothing will happen. But the decision to make the attempt has now been made, the method chosen, and the time and place picked out.
5. Has the client attempted suicide and failed? He will most likely try again . . . and succeed.

Behaviors

In the traditional sense, the depressed client is thought to be solemn and withdrawn, very quiet, and preoccupied with himself; he appears to be anxious and yet sad, fearful of the unknown, and lacking in self-confidence. Keep in mind, however, that other behaviors also are indicative of depression. For example, a client experiencing depression may be dressed quite gaudily, act bubbly and talkative, and display a lot of body movement as he tells you about the situation in which his wife just ran off with another man. He says that he is left with no job and no skills, and he tells you that he feels depressed. The surface value seems to tell you not to believe his assessment, but, in truth, the effervescence is only a charade—an act that allows the client to hide the difficulty of exposing his true feelings.

Indecisiveness also may be a reflection of a depressed state. The client is aware of his situation or his reason for feeling depressed, but is unable to make a decision regarding what kind of action, if any, he wishes to take. Other behaviors observed with depression are over- or undereating, insomnia, a prolonged sleeping pattern, headache, confusion, or preoccupation.

SUICIDE

When depression becomes severe, the client may not be able to think rationally. She wants the situation to end. She is tired, frustrated, and confused. Suicide seems to be the only choice. Suicide is an individual act and, like depression, is no respecter of age. The methods used in suicide attempts vary according to sex, and this accounts for the fact that although women attempt suicide more than men, men are more successful in their attempts. Men use methods that have the potential for being more lethal, such as guns, hanging, and jumping out of high windows. Women use drug overdose more often. (With the women's liberation movement, however, there has been an increase in the use of more lethal methods of suicide by women.)

A suicide attempt is a cry for help, and the actual attempt is a last resort. Prior to the attempt, the client usually has been giving out signals or hints. For assessment, you need to be aware of these cues.

Culture and ethnic background are reflected in suicide rates. Native Americans have a suicide rate above the national average; in some traditional Asian cultures, if you have been disgraced, you are expected to take your own life. In Western society, however, suicide is viewed as a tragedy and, in some cases, a disgrace to the family.

The client who attempts suicide will most likely be found to have a history of long-standing problems, which had escalated and eventually reached a point at which they were unbearable; this latter point in time generally will occur 2 to 3 days prior to the suicide attempt. The approach for assessment is to establish a nonjudgmental relationship in which you listen and reflect the client's feelings. *Confrontation* is an important part of the assessment.

BIOLOGIC AND CULTURAL VARIATIONS

Populations More Prone to Suicide

Urban dwellers more than rural

Protestants more than Catholics

Singles more than family group members

Divorced persons

Unemployed persons

Ill persons

Men, who are five times more successful at suicide than women

Psychotic clients, some of whom have voices telling them to kill themselves

Clients with a history of the following:
- Early loss of family member (especially father)
- Parent-child conflict
- Sibling conflict
- Substance abuse including alcoholism
- Socioeconomic concerns
- Death of another family member or significant other by suicide

- Ask the client if she is thinking about committing suicide.
- Assess the lethality of the situation. For example, ask the client if she has a plan, and what that plan might be.
- Promote catharsis; allow and encourage the client to explore and express her feelings.
- Try to get the client to reach a decision and to express an interest in and commitment to living.

If you feel that the client may attempt suicide, ensure that someone is with her at all times and refer her for treatment. If necessary, make the appointment and take the client.

Table 3-2 is a brief analysis of disease conditions delineating the characteristics of common psychopathologies. Table 3-3 provides an overview of the definition, dynamics, symptomatology, and bases of nursing care for psychoneurotic reactions.

SUMMARY

This chapter presented several factors necessary for completion of a mental health assessment. Mental functioning is an internal process and is not directly available to observation. Such aspects as attitude, affect/mood, speech, thought processes, sensorium and reasoning, potential for danger, and the psychological assets of the client are reflectors of mental functioning. Manifestations of mental dysfunctions are revealed in the client's appearance, behavior, and conversation. Some examples of appearance and behavioral and conversational manifestations of organic pathology and psychopathology were given in the section on clinical correlates. Situational and maturational crises were presented. In particular, the situational crises of violence and addiction were examined. Sources of internal stress, such as anxiety, anger, and personality, were discussed along with ego defense mechanisms and other coping strategies. The symptoms of depression and cues for suicide were highlighted. A brief descriptive analysis of disease states that may be reflected in mental dysfunctioning was presented in table format. One last note: The pathologic conditions and medical diagnoses mentioned in this chapter were not presented for the purpose of providing you with knowledge to establish etiologies or medical diagnoses of mental dysfunctions; rather, they were used to emphasize the fact that ABC data need to be carefully evaluated in terms of need for nursing intervention and/or referral.

DISCUSSION QUESTIONS/ ACTIVITIES

1. Discuss the importance of noting the client's appearance in relation to altered mental states.
2. Identify factors that can affect level of consciousness.
3. Name ten findings in mental health assessment that require the client to be referred to a specialist in that area. Compare these findings with those of your peers, and discuss them.
4. Discuss examples of situational and/or maturational crises that you have experienced personally or peripherally (e.g., those of a relative, friend, or client). Do not reveal another person's identity.
5. Identify your personal ways of coping with stress. Compare these with those of your peers, and discuss them.
6. Role-play a crisis situation and have an observer note your interpersonal and communication techniques. Critique the role-play.

Table 3-2 **Descriptive Analysis of Disease Conditions**

	Psychoneurosis	Psychophysiologic, autonomic, and visceral disorders (psychosomatic)	Personality disorders	Psychosis	Acute and chronic brain disorders
Definition	A psychological disability resulting from an individual's inability to cope with emotional conflicts or stressful environmental problems	A maladaptive emotional reaction in which the symptoms are expressed in organs innervated by the autonomic nervous system, producing physiologic change concurrent with psychological disequilibrium	Entrenched, chronic, maladaptive characterologic patterns in which an individual experiences little or no anxiety or guilt	Psychogenic reactions in which the individual experiences severe personality disorganization and disintegration along with marked distortions of reality	A disorder in which the individual sustains psychological and physiologic dysfunction as a consequence of damaged brain tissue
Types	Anxiety neurosis Phobic neurosis Conversion neurosis Dissociative neurosis Depressive neurosis Obsessive-compulsive neurosis	Gastrointestinal reactions a. Peptic ulcer b. Ulcerative colitis Cardiovascular reactions a. Essential hypertension b. Migraine Respiratory reactions a. Bronchial asthma b. Hyperventilation syndrome Genitourinary reactions a. Impotence or frigidity b. Amenorrhea Musculoskeletal reactions a. Functional backache b. Rheumatoid arthritis Skin reactions a. Psoriasis b. Neurodermatitis Endocrine reactions a. Diabetes mellitus b. Hyperthyroidism	Personality disorders a. Schizoid b. Paranoid c. Inadequate d. Passive-aggressive e. Antisocial Sexual deviation Alcoholism Drug dependence Maladjustment reactions to living	Schizophrenia a. Simple b. Hebephrenic c. Catatonic d. Paranoid e. Schizoaffective f. Chronic undifferentiated g. Childhood schizophrenia Major affective disorders a. Manic-depressive: manic b. Manic-depressive: depressed Involutional melancholia Paranoid states	Delirium tremens Korsakoff's syndrome Cerebral arteriosclerosis Intercranial neoplasms Brain trauma Encephalitis Systemic intoxication or poisoning and others
Etiology	Disruption in the developmental pattern or in interpersonal experiences Multiple, intrapsychic conflicts resulting from unresolved guilt, fear, prolonged stress or crisis Conflict between what patient believes society expects and the bipersonal self	Internalization of feelings Internalization of negative emotions Internal discharge of negative emotions Constitutional organ susceptibility	Faulty or arrested emotional development which interferes with adequate social control or superego formation. Constitutional pre-disposition Deprivation of basic needs in early childhood Physical and/or emotional trauma in childhood or adolescence	Multiple causality, most likely a combination of biochemical, social, and psychological factors	Any condition or agent that produces central nervous system pathology and cerebral tissue impairment

	Underlying and sustained conflict arising from the dichotomy of bicultures and subcultures				
Characteristics	A strong sense of personal discomfort; heightened levels of anxiety Major personality organization remains intact Maintains contact with reality Maintains usual roles, activities, or employment Decreased productivity and creativity Fixed attitudes, affections and/or mannerisms Excessive dependency or domination Correlation between thought and feeling content	Organ pathology Physical illness is the expression of prolonged or intense emotional stress. Physical rather than emotional symptoms dominate the clinical picture. Excellent ability to overtly mask stress and conflict If unchecked and unresolved, physical symptoms may be fatal.	Lifelong, repetitive, maladaptive, and often self-defeating behavior Anxiety is not apparent. Seldom seeks help on own initiative Tolerance to frustration and stress is low. Occasional intellectual insight Pathology is directed outward toward and against others Frequent confrontation with society's mores, norms, and laws	Major personality disorganization Marked interference with ability to function, personally and interpersonally Significant discrepancies between thoughts, feelings, and behavior Substitution of fantasy for reality Presence of delusional and hallucinatory systems Disorientation in the three spheres Regression	Reversible or irreversible Deficits in intellectual functioning Impaired orientation Lability of affect Primary and secondary personality changes Alterations in the levels of consciousness Memory and/or speech impairment
Dynamics	Unresolved emotional conflict is complicated with underlying feelings of guilt resulting in overwhelming anxiety Unsatisfactory relationships with parents, siblings, or peers in the developmental process The resultant symptomatology offers the individual an external means of expressing repressed material thereby allowing both primary and secondary gains for the ego	Psychological stress is converted into anxiety, which is directed internally through the nervous system. The individual experiences pathophysiologic, functional, or structural changes of the organs. Sustained or prolonged conflict causes internalization of fear, hostility, and/or guilt.	The individual operates from an egocentric viewpoint and remains narcissistic. Interpersonal relationships are not important unless they can be used to achieve specific need gratification. A concealed "taking" relationship predominates as opposed to a mutual "give and take" relationship. Avoidance of expectations, discomfort and/or stress-producing situations Disproportionate projection and accusations toward persons, places, and objects in the environment.	Loss of ego boundaries Denial of reality Severe regression Security and identity are threatened. Interpersonal relationships are superficial. Failure or inability to trust self or others	Interference with or destruction of cerebral tissue Libidinal energy is released as a result of organic changes Loss of ability to control libidinal drives Interruption of learning and coping potential

Continued

Table 3-2 Continued

	Psychoneurosis	Psychophysiologic, autonomic, and visceral disorders (psychosomatic)	Personality disorders	Psychosis	Acute and chronic brain disorders
Concepts and principles for nursing care	The presence of anxiety is a universal phenomenon. Knowledge and understanding of "normal anxiety" will provide the nurse with a base to assess the level of patient dysfunction. The symptom picture is usually indicative of the underlying conflict. Rituals are accompanied by profound dread and apprehension. All behavior is meaningful. Nursing care is directed toward the relief of physical and psychological symptoms. The patient's self-esteem is enhanced by the nurse's demonstration of acceptance, respect, and concern for his well-being. Positive, satisfying experiences are introduced to correct developmental and maturational deficits.	Any attitude, behavior, or situation that produces a sense of insecurity arouses anxiety. The overt expression of feelings alleviates internal stress. Disturbed family relationships play an important role in the development and outcome of the patient's illness. In psychosomatic illness interpersonal factors and physical disease are woven together into a single process. Effective treatment depends on a dual emphasis, physical and psychological. A planned schedule of social and recreational activities provides release from tension. Diversion deflects mental preoccupation with self and disability. Know the source or cause of the stresses, tensions, or problems creating the physical reactions. Give priority to the exploration of the primary causes of repressed feelings with the patient.	A firm, calm, consistent, quiet approach is most effective and will produce the least amount of manipulative or explosive response behavior. The nurse must protect other patients from being manipulated or exploited by an individual with a personality disorder. Give clear, concise explanations and directions to avoid verbal entanglements with the patient. Uniform scheduling and consistent application of firm limit setting offers positive guidance toward establishing self-control. Consistency in decision making enables the nurse to maintain an objective viewpoint.	The attitude of personnel makes or breaks the possibility of recovery for the psychotic patient. Care must be directed toward the maintenance of reality relationships. Genuine interest, honesty, warmth, and optimism are essential for establishing contact with psychotic persons. Physical and psychological needs merit equal attention. Familiar routines and persons contribute to security. As a social being, human psychological equilibrium needs to be maintained through satisfying relationships with others, both individually and in groups.	Cerebral damage produces physiologic and psychological malfunctioning. Organic conditions produce mental dysfunction, alteration in mood, physical manifestations and disrupted interpersonal relationships. Acute conditions require immediate interventive techniques to maintain life. Chronic conditions require supportive care coupled with an attitudinal approach of hopefulness. Patients with impaired judgment are unable to function independently and therefore require close observation and protective supervision. Familiarity with the environment promotes feelings of security while change produces frustration. Loss or impairment of physical functioning contributes to increasing the level of fear, anxiety, and confusion.

Source: H. Kreigh and J. E. Perko, *Psychiatric and Mental Health Nursing: A Commitment to Care.* Englewood Cliffs, N.J.: Reston Publishing Co., 1979.

Table 3-3 An Overview of Psychoneurotic Reactions

Condition	Definition	Dynamics	Symptom picture	Concepts and principles for nursing care
Anxiety neurosis	A reaction in response to no apparent or insufficient environmental stimulus	Persistent overuse of *repression* to control emotionally charged thoughts and feelings The presence of socially unacceptable thoughts, feelings, wants, or desires that if actualized would cause loss of approval, acceptance, or love from others Fear of censure, disapproval, or rejection threatens the self-concept.	Free floating and recurrent acute anxiety Dramatic increase in the level and diffusion of anxiety Somatic symptoms are associated with the autonomic nervous system. Decreased ability to focus on the situation at hand Interruption of judgment Sudden onset of panic	Intervention is imperative before anxiety mounts and becomes uncontrollable. Remaining with the patient and providing a warm, concerned human environment enhances the patient's security and reduces the level of anxiety. The nurse listens carefully to the expression of somatic concerns and does not challenge or cast doubt on their validity.
Phobic neurosis	A reaction of intense recurrent, unreasonable fear attached to a specific object or situation	Incomplete repression with *displacement* of anxiety onto an external focus which the individual can then avoid. Particular phobias assume a *symbolic* significance with respect to underlying emotional conflicts or unacceptable desires.	Intense, prolonged, irrational, and disabling fear Common phobias include fear of the dark; open and closed spaces; heights; animals and birds; and dirt or germs. Avoidance of socializing behavior and frequent reclusiveness results in eccentricities.	Phobias are *real* to the individual. The nurse demonstrates acceptance of the patient's avoidance patterns as being necessary for his survival. The nurse assumes initiative in seeking out the patient and provides opportunities for the verbal expression of feelings. Assisting the patient in exploring the "source" or primary painful life experience or trauma that eventuated in displacement
Conversion neurosis	A reaction in which the individual unconsciously transforms his underlying conflict into specific kinds of motor or sensory dysfunction	*Conversion* of anxiety into somatic symptoms, *symbolic* of the underlying conflict Primary gain is relief from emotional tension. Secondary gain is the advantage the symptom provides in meeting the need for dependency. Outcome is the avoidance of responsible, independent functioning. Avoidance of an anticipated, emotionally, and/or physically painful experience. *Denial* of an unpleasant and/or uncomfortable reality in one's life.	Physical manifestations in the form of blindness, deafness, aphonia, laryngitis, and convulsions Displays a lack of concern or indifference toward the existing symptom Minimal observable anxiety	The individual does not consciously invent or choose the condition. Conversion involves the voluntary and sensory systems. The physical symptoms serve to lessen any consciously felt anxiety. Nursing care is focused on the individual and his feelings, not on his symptoms.

Continued

Table 3-3 **Continued**

Condition	Definition	Dynamics	Symptom picture	Concepts and principles for nursing care
Dissociative neurosis	A reaction in which certain aspects of the individual's personality are split off, separated, or detached from his conscious awareness	Employs mechanisms of *dissociation, conversion,* and *symbolism.* Ego attempts to protect itself from critical and/or dangerous pain. *Denial* is used to escape from reality.	Alterations in the state of consciousness, in the person's identity or memory Depersonalization Overwhelming anxiety Manifested through amnesia, fugues, and twilight states.	The nurse must view the patient's emotional functioning as the outcome of his growth and developmental process. It is necessary for the nurse to understand the patient's feelings and behavior and not pass judgment on his actions. Understand the dynamics of this problem to maximize interventive techniques.
Obsessive-compulsive neurosis	A reaction in which the individual experiences persistent, distressing thoughts or impulses resulting in irresistible acting-out behavior	Unsuccessful repression is reinforced through the use of such defensive responses as: *displacement, reaction formation, undoing,* and *symbolism.*	Ambivalence Doubt Vacillation Persistent, recurring ideation Repetitive, stereotyped motor activity	The patient recognizes the unreasonableness of his obsessions and compulsions. Rituals release tension, and temporarily reduce the level of anxiety. Interruption of ritualistic behavior increases the patient's anxiety and guilt. Protect patient from ridicule. Assist the patient to develop new interests outside self.
Depressive neurosis	A reaction in which the individual experiences a state of sadness due to disappointment, an upsetting life event, or a loss of a significant person, possession, or position	Damage to self-esteem with associated repressed anger Disparity between the superego value system and the ego activity, which results in guilt Feelings of inadequacy and inferiority are more pronounced due to exaggerated ego ideal. Depressive features existent throughout the life experience	Marked ambivalence Diffused anger and hostility Fluctuations in mood Difficulty in concentration Reduction in psychomotor activity Reality oriented Appetite and sleep disturbances Somatic complaints Pessimism Vacillation between ability to function and immobility Numerous suicidal threats Accidental death	Provide external structure and milieu that gradually allow the patient to assume responsibility for his life experiences. Verbal or behavioral expression of anger or hostility provides a release for internalized emotion. Persuasion is a useful tool for meeting the needs for acceptance and attention. Reassurance is conveyed through the setting of realistic limits. Feelings of adequacy can be promoted by opportunities for achieving small goals. Allow patient to experience success and accomplishment via a short-term project.

Source: H. Kreigh and J. E. Perko, *Psychiatric and Mental Health Nursing: A Commitment to Care.* Englewood Cliffs, N.J.: Reston Publishing Co., 1979.

REFERENCES

Buchalter, G. 1995. What you can do if you are battered. *Parade Magazine* March 26, 1995.

Cadoret, R. J., and King, L. J. 1974. *Psychiatry in primary care.* St. Louis: C. V. Mosby.

Cassem, N. H., and Hackett, T. P. 1971. Psychiatric consultation in a coronary care unit. *Ann. Intern. Med.* 75:9–14.

Jenkins, C. D. 1971. Psychologic and social precursors of coronary disease. *N. Engl. J. Med.* 284(5):244–255.

Kreigh, H. Z., and Perko, J. E. 1979. *Psychiatric and mental health nursing: commitment to care and concern.* Reston, Va.: Reston Publishing.

Kübler-Ross, E. 1975. *Death: the final stage of growth.* Englewood Cliffs, N.J.: Prentice-Hall.

Preston, D., and Grimes, J. 1987. Study in differences in social support. *J. Gerontol. Nursing* 13(2):36–40.

CHAPTER

4 The Health History

Learning Objectives

1. Recognize the importance of the health history as a component of the assessment of health beliefs, practices, experiences, and status.
2. Describe the components of the health history.
3. Identify guidelines designed to elicit information about the client's current health status or history of present illness.
4. Describe the areas of the client's lifestyle that are investigated during health history taking.
5. Differentiate lifestyle factors that enhance health status from those that are a risk to health status.
6. Identify the purpose of the review of systems used in health history taking.

The health history is a chronologic and detailed health record of the client. Its purpose is to elicit information regarding all of the variables that may affect the client's health experiences and status. These data are then used to develop nursing diagnoses and subsequent plans for individualized care. For the ill client, the health history serves as background material related to the development of present symptoms and associated difficulties. For the well client, such as a student who is having a routine physical assessment and health history update, it supplies data by which you can provide health preventive, maintenance, and promotion counseling and establish a need for immunizations and eye or dental care. With the well client, your time is usually limited, and there is a great deal of information to gather to complete the record. Thus, you need to be skilled in the interview technique in order to best guide the client through the process in a logical order. Increasingly, many aspects of the health history are being tabulated through health history forms or checklists that the client completes and that are then quickly validated at the beginning of the interview. Further, computer technology is enhancing the collection and recording of accumulated health history records.

The interview does not necessarily follow the format for documentation of health history data. The client usually will follow general leads and open-ended questions by discussing primary concerns or areas that are comfortable for him to address. As data are shared by the client, you are continuously evaluating what additional data are necessary and what the client is telling you in ways such as avoidance, omission of topics, recurring themes, or body language. You conduct the interview with purposeful communication skills to gather adequate data for accurate decision making. Certain data in the health history will change from time to time.

Health status, practices, beliefs, and attitudes are not static; there is a need for continuous review and reassessment of these variables in light of a client's individual experiences related to health. This review is necessary not only to detect changes and possible problems but also to update the record on both interim illnesses and health promotion activities, such as incorporating jogging into the daily pattern of living. Baseline laboratory data are also part of the client's health history record and are carefully reviewed or compared with recent laboratory tests.

COMPONENTS OF THE HEALTH HISTORY

In documenting a health history, most forms follow a relatively standardized content format. Although history forms may vary slightly, they contain essentially the same basic information. Generally, there are specific forms or sections to document the health history of an infant or a child (containing questions related to growth and development patterns and to school and social history) and for documenting an obstetric history.

As a general rule, the following information is obtained during the health history interview or on a self-completed checklist:

1. biographical data
2. reason for seeking health evaluation or chief complaint
3. current health status or history of present illness
4. personal history and patterns of living
5. previous experience with illness
6. review of systems
7. client profile

Biographical Data

The client's biographical data are helpful to you in anticipating the special needs of the client and in comparing her background with epidemiologic studies. See the Checklist for Biographical Data for what information generally is documented.

Cultural traditions, ethnic background, and religion are important because these factors can influence the client's health and her belief and attitudes toward health care. The client interprets her current situation on the basis of values and norms that exist within a social and cultural structure. Knowing these parameters of your client will assist you in understanding why the client responds as she does toward health, illness, hospitalization, and those professionals responsible for providing her health care.

The gender and age of your client will alert you to direct history taking and counseling toward sex-specific and age-related morbidity and mortality health problems. Gender would direct your investigation away from opposite-gender-specific health problems and, for example, toward the possibility of tubal pregnancy or ovarian cysts in women and testicular or prostatic cancer in men.

Checklist for Biographical Data

- Name
- Address
- Sex
- Age/birth date
- Marital status/compatibility and adjustment
- Current occupation
- Religion/practice and attitude toward religion
- Race
- Ethnic origin
- Level of education/ability to read and write
- Health history informant and reliability

Although the four leading causes of death in the United States are heart disease, cancer, cerebrovascular disorders (stroke), and accidents, the leading causes are quite different in specific age groups. By knowing the client's age, you can anticipate general disease/injury preventive, promotional, and maintenance health care guidance and health teaching needs. For instance, in children ages 1 to 14, the leading cause of death is accidents; this would require assessment of potential hazards and anticipatory safety counseling. If the community population is composed largely of teenagers, you may expect to find an increased incidence of venereal disease, drug abuse, smoking, accidents, suicide, and juvenile crime. As persons age, the risk for developing heart disease and cancer increases. Because such age-specific health problems occur, your awareness of these differences can assist you in conducting a more thorough health assessment.

Marital status also can be viewed in light of epidemiology. For example, more single men attempt suicide than married men. Marital status also has important bearing on possible economic problems, rehabilitation potential, and future health needs of the family.

Current occupation is traditionally noted in biographical data. Further investigation of occupational history is documented in a later section. Occupations have epidemiologic and economic significance.

Mortality and morbidity rates may vary by racial population groups. Although both African-American and white middle-aged men tend to die of problems involving the circulatory system and the heart, the cause of death tends to be different in these two population groups. African-American middle-aged men tend to die of the secondary effects of hypertension, such as stroke, kidney failure, or myocardial infarctions (Mausner & Bahn 1974). White middle-aged men, however, tend to die of coronary failure associated with chronic heart disease and atherosclerosis. This difference in mortality patterns is probably due to a combination of factors, including population genetic differences, socioeconomic differences, and such subcultural differences as lifestyle and dietary habits.

Childhood morbidity and mortality also vary by subculture. Children whose families are poorer and tend to live in areas with poor sanitation and housing are most likely to die from accidents, pneumonia, congenital malformations, gastroenteritis, and other infective and parasitic diseases. It is obvious that poverty and differences in lifestyle result in high rates of infectious disease.

Knowledge of education and academic abilities are necessary so that communication can be tailored for clarity at the client's level of understanding. Many times the client's ability to read and write are not assessed; more than once a client has been given written instructions, only to reveal on subsequent contact that she did not understand or follow the instructions because she was unable to read them.

Biographical data note the reliability of the health history informant. Should someone other than the client provide the health history information, her name and relationship to the client must be identified on the record. In most cases, this person will be a parent, spouse, friend, or relative. In the case of accident, it may be a total stranger who has witnessed what happened to the client. Whatever the case, you should make a statement about your perceived reliability of the informant, describing her mental status (e.g., alert, well oriented, confused, or anxious). Confusion or anxiety, for example, may alter the accuracy of the record.

Reason for Seeking Health Evaluation or Chief Complaint

Identify the reason for which the client is seeking health care attention. It may, for example, indicate his attitude toward health and health practices, as when a client wants an annual physical checkup or employment health clearance. Some clients often experience symptoms for some time before they seek attention. This information may be important to you in evaluating the client's perception of the situation as well as in establishing guidelines for further investigation.

Checklist for the Reason for Seeking Health Evaluation or Chief Complaint
Annual check-up
Employment health clearance
Follow-up care and evaluation
Signs and symptoms that led client to seek health care
Monitoring of existing health problem(s)

It is vital that the client be allowed to describe the reason or complaint in his own words. To facilitate a description of the chief complaint from the client, use open-ended questions or statements at this point in the gathering process, allowing the client to talk freely without interruption. Ask the client to tell you why he is here today. At the end of his explanation,

- you will have obtained most of what the client views as important complaints or reasons for seeking health evaluation
- generally, you will have a basic feeling for his attitude toward health care services and personnel
- you will most likely be able to evaluate his ability to organize his thoughts and ideas

Record the chief complaint in the client's own words. Occasionally, the client will say something like, "I have heart trouble," "I have cancer," or "I have multiple sclerosis." When the client uses such terms or diagnoses, ask him to elaborate. Ask him what symptoms led to his conclusion or what he means by *multiple sclerosis.* Many times, a client will self-diagnose if he manifests a sign or symptom similar to something he has read or that his neighbor, relative, or friend has been medically diagnosed as having. Further investigation will usually produce a chief complaint such as, "I've had chest pains for the past 2 hours," "I've lost 60 pounds in the past month," or "I've had muscle cramps and weakness in my legs for 4 months." From these examples you can see that the chief complaint is a brief statement of only one or two signs or symptoms and their durations. (A *sign,* such as weight loss or weakness, is objective—you can weigh the client or test muscle strength; a *symptom,* such as pain or cramps, is subjective—you are unable to observe it.)

If the client uses vague terms such as *bowel trouble* or *not feeling well,* ask him to clarify what he means:

- What is it that makes the client say he has bowel trouble (is not feeling well)?
- What is happening that causes the client to say this?

These questions may produce such concrete responses as "vomiting and diarrhea for the past 4 days," or "headache and general weakness for the past 2 days."

In recording, *do not* alter the client's chief complaint into medical terminology, such as "occipital lobe headache—intermittent for 2 months' duration."

Current Health Status or History of Present Illness

Ask the client how she would describe her health up until this time. The client who has described numerous past illnesses and then describes her state of health as "good" may be trying to minimize or deny certain problems. Whether the client describes her health as "terrible" or "good," you should ask for some clarification (e.g., "What do you mean by terrible?"). How individuals perceive their general health has bearing on how well they are able to participate in their health care planning.

If the client has a major complaint, you should encourage the client to provide a factual account of the illness. Take care not to jump to conclusions or to bias the account by adding professional judgments or opinions. Questions should be phrased so that the client will not give a simple yes or no answer. Many clients are suggestible. If you use questions like, "You have more pain when you sit up?" or "Your illness began just a short time ago?" they might agree even if the answer is not exactly true. It is better to ask the client about what brings on the pain or how long she has been ill. This gives the client the opportunity to qualify the information.

A thorough investigation of a particular sign or symptom is accomplished by using guidelines designed to elicit essential information. One effective guideline is the "Seven Variables of Investigation," suggested by Morgan and Engel (1969):

1. bodily location
2. quality
3. quantity
4. chronology
5. setting
6. aggravating and alleviating factors
7. associated manifestations

Bodily Location

- Where is the sign or symptom located?
- Is it a small, well-defined area or a larger, more diffuse one?
- Ask the client to indicate the location and outline it, if possible, with a finger or hand.

Checklist for Current Health Status or History of Present Illness
Location
Quality
Quantity
Chronology
Setting
Aggravating and alleviating factors
Associated manifestations
Effect on ADLs and other life areas
Review of relevant body system(s)

- If the symptom radiates, ask the client to indicate the path of radiation.

Quality

Ask the client to describe the quality of the symptom. For example, pain may be described as dull, sharp, aching, gnawing, churning, or throbbing.

- Is this the worst pain the client has experienced?
- What kind of pain has the client experienced in the past?
- How does this pain compare with past pain? Is it like having a baby, or an abscessed tooth, or a broken bone?

Additionally, the client's posture and facial expression can often give you a clue to the type of pain. For example, the client may grimace or bend over during the interview.

For the client who complains of being nervous, you might reflect, "Nervous?" or ask, "What makes you say this?" If the client has difficulty describing the nervousness, you might ask

- Do the client's hands shake?
- Is the client unable to sleep?
- Is it difficult for the client to sit still or concentrate?

If you can see possible manifestations of his statement in his behavior, you might reflect such observations: "I see you have been tapping your fingers since we began talking."

With a complaint of dizziness, you should determine the degree.

- Does the client feel faint?
- Does the client feel like he is spinning, or does the room seem to spin about him?
- Is the client's vision blurred?
- Is there ringing in the client's ears?
- Does the dizziness cause the client to lose his balance?
- Is the dizziness accompanied by nausea or vomiting?

Quantity

Terms such as *frequency, volume, number, size,* and *extent* can be used to quantify the severity or intensity of the symptom.

- Is the symptom continuous? Intermittent?
- How long has/does the client experience(d) the symptom?
- How has the symptom affected patterns of living?
- Is there anything the client cannot do now that she was able to do prior to the onset of the symptom?
- Has the symptom affected the client's everyday bodily functions, such as eating, walking, lifting?
- Has the symptom altered the client's activities, such as job performance, family relationships, sexual activity, recreation?

Chronology

- When did the symptom first appear?
- Can the client pinpoint the date and/or time?
- Was the onset gradual or abrupt?
- How long has the symptom persisted (duration)?
- Is it constant or intermittent?
- Did it occur abruptly and last for several weeks, or does it occur periodically (exacerbations and remissions)?

If the complaint is an exacerbation of previously established medical condition, the client's knowledge and understanding of his condition should be assessed.

Setting

Setting refers to the precipitating factors and circumstances under which the symptom occurs; it could be a particular place, activity, or person. Setting can be determined by asking the client the following questions.

- Where was the client when this occurred?
- Where was the client prior to this?
- What was the client doing (prior to) at the time?
- Who was with the client?
- Was the client with anyone else prior to this happening?
- Does the symptom occur when the client is lying down, sitting, exercising?
- Is the symptom related to tension at work or in the home?
- Does the symptom follow the ingestion of a meal?

Certain gastrointestinal complaints might occur after a meal; a tension headache might follow an argument or upsetting home or business situation. It is thus important to investigate the circumstances that surrounded the client before and during the onset of a sign or symptom.

Aggravating and Alleviating Factors

What, if anything, causes the complaint to become better or worse? Aggravating factors might include physical exertion, position, ingestion of spicy foods or cold liquids, cold weather, or loud noises. Ask about alleviating factors, such as home remedies and medical treatment:

- "What have you tried to relieve the problem?"
- "Has it worked?"

Associated Manifestations

With the exception of generalized symptoms such as chills, fever, weakness, or fatigue, it is most unusual for a symptom to occur without other related manifestations.

- What other symptoms does the client experience?

Most symptoms suggest disturbances in one or more body systems. As you are listening and guiding the client in describing her illness, you should cluster symptoms together and begin thinking of possible causes of the problem. When you have identified possible involvement of a certain body system, you can proceed to reviewing the entire system at this time instead of waiting until the review of symptoms (ROS) portion of the health history interview. (Some examples are seen in the corresponding box.) At this time, laboratory data can be enlightening.

Knowing which systems to review in relation to the present illness requires not only a thorough knowledge of pathophysiology and pathopsychology but also a great deal of experience. However, any apprehensions you may have should be somewhat relieved by realizing that the routine ROS will identify disorders in systems other than those you considered significant and reviewed during the investigation of the present illness. Thorough documentation of your

Examples of Symptoms and Possible Related Systems

Swelling of the ankles and feet	Ask questions related to both cardiac and renal function.
Shortness of breath following activity	Determine the amount of activity necessary to cause dyspnea. Ask whether the client experiences orthopnea or paroxysmal nocturnal dyspnea, or has a history of respiratory problems or symptoms.
Abdominal upset	Ask specifically whether the client has experienced episodes of pain, nausea, vomiting, diarrhea, changes in bowel habits, melena, clay-colored stools. Ask questions related to both the integumentary and the urinary systems as many gastrointestinal dysfunctions have related skin manifestations (for example, cirrhosis is often accompanied by pruritus, spider angiomas, and palmar erythema); thus, the ROS for the integumentary system may be completed at this time. As well, the urinary system may also be reviewed here, as gastrointestinal signs and symptoms sometimes reflect renal problems; nausea, vomiting, and diarrhea commonly accompany such kidney conditions as nephritis and uremia.

findings is vital to the further analysis of the client's data base by the advance practice nurse or physician.

Personal History and Patterns of Living

Information relating to occupational history, financial status, family history of illness, geographic exposure, and lifestyle is documented in this section of the health history. These data aid you in determining environmental factors that influence the client's health. Specifically, analyze how the client's personal habits, daily activities, and financial status impact on health. The data gathered are of great importance in determining a plan of care, because the conditions and the way in which people live often contribute to disease and illness.

Occupational History

Have the client describe her current or most recent job—what she actually does, what are her work hours, does she like her job, is there anything she doesn't like about her job? Has the client missed a lot of work days? A poor work history showing any of the following symptoms could be an indication of beginning illnesses, or it could be an indication of problem drinking.

- What is the client's work history?
- Are days of work missed because of illness, inability to "get going" on Monday mornings, or a variety of reasons for not being able to get to work on time?
- Does the client have a history of accidents while on the job?
- Is the client presently employed or unemployed?

If unemployed, it may be beneficial to determine which type of unemployment situation the client is facing. For example, if the unemployment is due to seasonal fluctuation, such as is common in the construction industry, her mental health status and stress levels may be more adaptive to the situation than that of the client facing chronic or long-term unemployment. Some clients may be unemployed due to the economy or supply and demand of the job market. A client also may be facing the issue of whether to remain in the present geographic location or relocate, and complicating the issue will be the age of the client. For the worker over age 50, the possibility of employment or career change may appear bleak. These factors, either in combination or singly, can alter the client's stress levels, thus lowering her resistance to illness, both physical and psychological.

Checklist for Personal History and Patterns of Living

Occupational history

Financial status

Family history of illness/past and present

Pertinent negatives of specific illness in family

Example: No history of hypertension, strokes, TB, ulcers, mental illness, alcoholism, epilepsy, gout, bleeding disorders

Significant for diabetes, heart disease, cancer, arthritis, ulcerative colitis

Geographic exposure
- Places
- Date and length of time

Lifestyle
- Personal habits
  - Smoking—type and pack years
  - Alcohol—type and amount
  - Drugs—type, amount, and pattern of use
- Diet
  - Mealtimes
  - Prepared by
  - Special diet/type and when started
  - Vitamins and/or diet pills
  - Specific difficulties

Sleep and rest patterns
- Hours of sleep and awakening
- Naps
- Difficulties/remedies tried

Activities of daily living

Home and neighborhood
- Living arrangements/resources
- Quality of interpersonal relationships

Recreation/hobbies

Sexuality
- Values
- Self-image
- Sexual function
- Sexual difficulties

- Is the client retired or soon to be retired?
- Determine if the client is or was retired voluntarily (worker chose to retire) or involuntarily due to health problems or age.

The worker who voluntarily chooses to retire is usually more prepared for the retirement life than the worker who was involuntarily retired, and thus may have more coping skills. The client's ability to work, despite an impending or existing state of retirement, has implications for an individual's feeling of well-being. Another factor that may contribute to the worker's mental and physical well-being is the opportunity to participate in preretirement workshops.

- What are the occupational hazards of the client's job?
- Where is the geographic location of the work site?
- What kind of stress does the individual perceive in her work role?
- What is the level of the client's job satisfaction?
- Does the client have friends and a support system at work?

A client who is complaining of pain in the chest and coughing and who has worked with industrial solvents for some years may help pinpoint a contributing factor to the illness. If the employment area is outside, environmental pollutants such as dust, soot, coal dust, and other airborne particles may aggravate a previously existing condition. Additionally, financial stressors can have major consequences for health.

- What debts or monetary concerns does the client have?
- Is the client's insurance adequate?
- Will the client be able to pay for treatment, medications, and medical care?

There are a multitude of important avenues the nurse can explore in relation to the client's occupation.

Financial Status

Financial status is closely related to occupation. The ability to meet financial obligations relative to personal needs, family, food, and housing is often a major cause for concern. The best way to determine financial status is to use open-ended questions, such as,

- "How would you describe your financial status?"

Information regarding salary is often considered personal; asking the client to quote his salary may create blocks to communication.

Other specific aspects to explore are whether

- the client is employed in a job paying minimum wage
- the client is holding down more than one job
- the client's income falls just above the cut-off for social supports such as food stamps, access to well-baby clinics, or other low-cost health care facilities

A young divorced mother with dependent children may postpone health care for herself because of the inability to pay for it. Other victims of difficulties with financial status are people living on low fixed incomes; this may include both the young and the elderly. Food and shelter are basic necessities of life, but for these people, shelter often takes priority over food. Because they are unable to eat properly, they are often weak and anemic or obese and malnourished. For persons in the lower income areas, clothing is many times a luxury, and the lack of proper or adequate clothing decreases protection and opens the individual to recurring illnesses. Another result of lower financial status may be the inability to afford proper or adequate sanitation, heat, or utilities such as electricity and gas.

Family History of Illness

General background and familial tendencies are related to the development of many illnesses. Information about the family can provide important evidence about the client's complaints. As Fig. 4-1 demonstrates, this information should include the ages of siblings, parents, and grandparents; their current state of health; and if they are deceased, the cause of death. Special attention should be paid to such disorders as heart disease, hypertension, cancer, diabetes, obesity, allergies, jaundice, bleeding, ulcers, migraine headaches, alcoholism, arthritis, and tuberculosis. If absent, these items are recorded as pertinent negatives (i.e., no history of heart disease, hypertension, cancer, diabetes, and so on).

Geographic Exposure

With the ease of worldwide travel, there is increased exposure to diseases that are indigenous to foreign lands. Therefore, you should ask the client about any travel to those areas. Inquiring about military service may reveal a tour of overseas duty. Occasionally, the birthplace of an individual provides additional clues.

Checklist for Previous Experience with Illness

Childhood illnesses
Immunizations
Allergies—type, response, treatment
Past illnesses
Surgery
Blood transfusions
Trauma

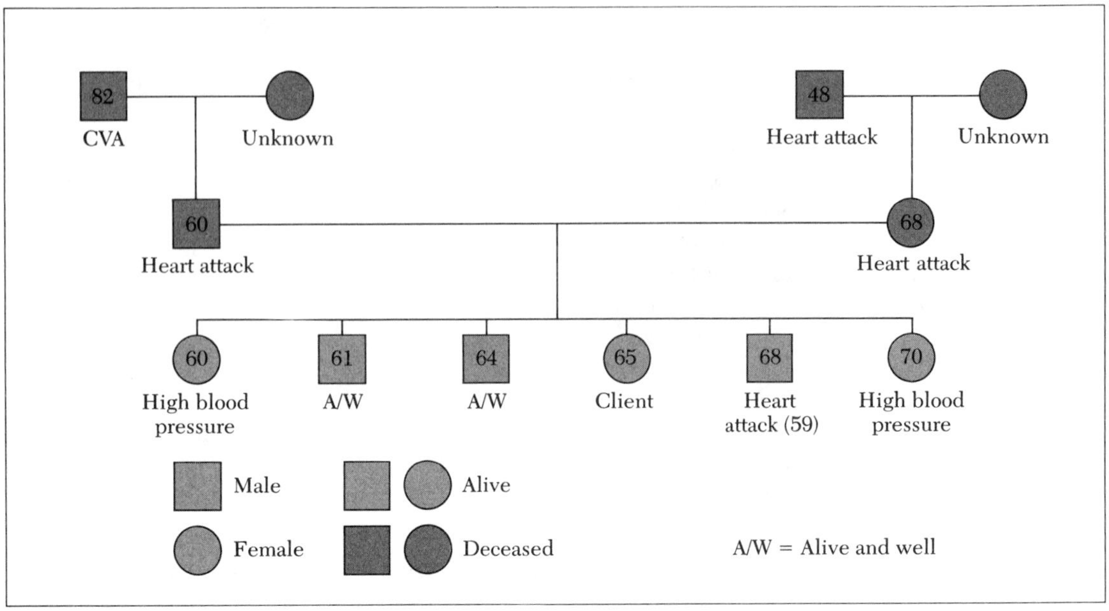

Figure 4-1 Family genogram.

Lifestyle

The investigation of an individual's lifestyle will give you some idea of factors that can be used for health maintenance or restoration. The sample questions in Table 4-1 aid in the assessment of some cultural values and practices related to health care.

Personal Habits

Information should be obtained regarding use of

- tobacco
- alcohol
- over-the-counter (OTC) drugs (including caffeine)
- past and current prescription drugs
- recreational or illicit drugs

Smoking must be described in "pack years," which is calculated by multiplying the number of packs the client has smoked each day by the number of years the client has smoked. For example, the client who smokes one and a half packs a day and has smoked for 20 years, is said to have smoked 30 pack years. Irreversible lung tissue damage is said to occur with the amount of 40 pack years.

Studies have found evidence that second-hand smoke is more detrimental to health than actually smoking tobacco. The American Cancer Society (1994) published the changes in the body beginning from 20 minutes to 15 years after a person quits smoking cigarettes (Fig. 4-2).

People vary greatly in the amount of alcohol they consume and in the body's ability to process this consumption. The rate of metabolism of alcohol is influenced by a variety of factors, including total body weight, sex, age, multiple drug use, and physical condition. The tolerance level of the individual also needs to be considered when trying to determine the degree of a drinking problem. An individual with a low tolerance level for alcohol, meaning he may be able to handle only one drink every hour or two, is an indication of low alcohol consumption. On the other hand, the person who can "handle" three or four drinks per hour is indicative of an experienced drinker. As previously stated, tolerance levels relate to body weight, sex, and experience. As alcohol consumption accelerates, however, the tolerance level does not rise uniformly. First, as consumption increases, the tolerance level also rises, but only until it peaks. Then the tolerance level decreases as the consumption increases. This explains why the novice drinker and the alcoholic become drunk quicker than the more experienced drinker.

Social drinking is usually described as a few drinks now and then, but the distinction between the problem drinker and the alcoholic is less clearly defined. To pinpoint the extent of your client's social drinking or drinking problem, you must go beyond asking the number of cans of beer consumed per week or the number of cocktails consumed on a weekend. The following questions will help you elicit indicators that the client may be experiencing drinking problems as opposed to social drinking.

- What time of day does the client begin drinking?
- Does the client have a hidden supply of alcohol?
- Does the client drink alone?
- Has the client switched from a popular alcoholic drink or beverage to a less popular drink or beverage in order to protect the supply?
- Does the client drive when drinking?

Table 4-1 Assessment of Cultural Values and Practices Related to Health Care

Cultural factor	Assessment questions
Language	What is the first language of the family?
	If English is not spoken, is there a family member or friend who can speak for the others?
	Is an interpreter necessary? Should language cards be used? (These cards are pictures with appropriate statements or questions in a specified foreign language.)
Diet	Does the family have cultural food preferences?
	Are any foods forbidden by the family's cultural or religious beliefs?
	Is there special etiquette surrounding eating practices (for example, a practice that eating is done only in privacy)?
	Is special preparation of foods required?
	Are there special foods for certain occasions?
	What are the customary mealtimes in the family's culture?
Health and illness beliefs	How are health and illness described in the family's culture? Do all family members hold these beliefs?
	What are the family's beliefs about the causes of illness (e.g., punishment for sin, an imbalance of the body system)?
	Whom does the family respect as a health practitioner (e.g., a physician, public health nurse, grandmother, *curandero,* spiritualist, herbalist, acupuncturist)?
	What are the usual remedies used by the family for illness (e.g., home remedies, over-the-counter medications, herbs, prayers, prescription drugs)?
	What are the family's customs and beliefs related to death?
Child-family relationships	Are there religious practices surrounding birth, illness, and death? What are they?
	How is the birth of a child received in the family?
	What are the family's goals for the child? What approach does the family take to help the child reach those goals?
	What health care practices for the child's welfare does the family value? Are there cultural objections to any practices (e.g., immunizations, dental care, teaching of hygiene and other self-care practices)?
	From what source does the family derive its greatest support (e.g., extended family, religion, friends)?
	What role does the extended family play?
	What are the major values of the family (e.g., education, wealth, spiritual life, sports)?

Source: J.P. Bellack and P.A. Bamford. *Nursing Assessment: A Multidimensional Approach.* Boston: Little, Brown, 1987.

- Has the client ever had any problems with the law related to drinking alcohol?
- Are there family problems due to drinking?
- Has the client lost a job or work time due to drinking?
- Does the client gulp down drinks? Chug-a-lug?
- Has the client experienced blackouts? (Blackouts are loss of memory, not loss of consciousness.)
- Does the client have sore gums?
- Is the client malnourished?

Questions about alcohol are often omitted with the young client, yet teenage alcoholism is a very real problem. Alcohol-related highway fatalities are the number-one killer of America's youth; to discount adolescent drinking is foolhardy. In addition, the number of women experiencing drinking problems and alcoholism is on the rise, opening up another new area of concern—fetal alcohol syndrome. A full understanding of the effects of alcohol on the fetus is not yet known, but studies show that as few as two drinks of alcohol per day (not an average of two drinks per day) can cause damage to the fetus. This damage is mainly in the form of abnormalities and mental retardation or learning disabilities. Many of your pregnant clients may be unaware of this potential problem.

WHEN SMOKERS QUIT

Within 20 minutes of smoking that last cigarette, the body begins a series of changes that continues for years.

20 MINUTES
- Blood pressure drops to normal
- Pulse rate drops to normal
- Body temperature of hands and feet increases to normal

8 HOURS
- Carbon monoxide level in blood drops to normal
- Oxygen level in blood increases to normal

24 HOURS
- Chance of heart attack decreases

48 HOURS
- Nerve endings start regrowing
- Ability to smell and taste is enhanced

2 WEEKS to 3 MONTHS
- Circulation improves
- Walking becomes easier
- Lung function increases up to 30 percent

1 to 9 MONTHS
- Coughing, sinus congestion, fatigue, shortness of breath decrease
- Cilia regrow in lungs, increasing ability to handle mucus, clean the lungs, reduce infection
- Body's overall energy increases

1 YEAR
- Excess risk of coronary heart disease is half that of a smoker

5 YEARS
- Lung cancer death rate for average former smoker (one pack a day) decreases by almost half
- Stroke risk is reduced to that of a nonsmoker 5-15 years after quitting
- Risk of cancer of the mouth, throat and esophagus is half that of a smoker's

10 YEARS
- Lung cancer death rate similar to that of nonsmokers
- Precancerous cells are replaced
- Risk of cancer of the mouth, throat, esophagus, bladder, kidney and pancreas decreases

15 YEARS
- Risk of coronary heart disease is that of a nonsmoker.

Source: American Cancer Society; Centers for Disease Control and Prevention

AMERICAN CANCER SOCIETY®

THERE'S NOTHING MIGHTIER THAN THE SWORD

Figure 4-2 Bodily changes occurring subsequent to cessation of smoking. (Courtesy of the American Cancer Society, November 1994.)

It is essential to determine how many and what kinds of OTC drugs the client buys and uses regularly, as well as whether he uses street drugs.

- What kind of drugs does the client use?
- What is the route of drug administration?
- How does the client feel when he takes the drug?
- How often does the client use drugs?
- How old was the client when he first used drugs?
- Does the client share needles?

For characteristics of psychoactive chemical abuse, see Table 4-2.

Many clients who take OTC drugs do not think they are important enough to mention in a health interview. However, *aspirin* accounts for the largest percentage of drug overdoses. Women are particularly prone to taking nonprescriptive *diet pills* and OTC *diuretics.*

Another abused drug is *caffeine,* which is a stimulant. Because using stimulants provides longer periods of intellectual functioning, many students drink excessive amounts of coffee or take caffeine-containing drugs. They may not consider such practices dangerous and therefore may not mention them unless questioned directly. As a drug, caffeine can become addictive, and withdrawal symptoms such as tremors and headache may be experienced 18 to 24 hours after the last ingestion of the drug. Caffeine is a diuretic and can cause insomnia, restlessness, dizziness, irritability, chronic headache, agitation, anxiety, and psychophysiologic disorders. It has been shown that there is a high correlation between drinking more than five cups of coffee a day and heart disease. Moreover, caffeine also has been linked to other disorders, such as peptic ulcer, hiatal hernia, bladder cancer, birth defects, noncancerous fibrocystic breast disorders, and menstrual cramps. Caffeine is present in a variety of products, ranging from coffee and tea to colas and OTC preparations for headache, allergy, and cold symptoms. It can even be obtained from a chocolate bar.

- Caffeine consumers come from all socioeconomic levels, but the greatest consumers are also high users of minor tranquilizers, sedative-hypnotics, alcohol, and tobacco (cigarettes).

Diet

At first glance, questions about diet may seem straightforward and directed mainly at determining whether the client's diet is well balanced. In Fig. 4-3, the food guide pyramid shows the food groups and the U.S. dietary goals for percentage of calories that are to come from each food group. In general, one needs to eat less fat and sugar and more carbohydrates. One method of calculating daily caloric needs uses basal metabolism and activity level (Table 4-3). Basal metabolism rate is the amount of energy needed for basic life functions. Table 4-4 lists some examples of determinants

Table 4-2 **Characteristics of Psychoactive Chemical Abuse**

Psychoactive substance[a]	Common terms[b]	Usual route of administration	Abuse: signs/symptoms	Overdose: signs/symptoms	General comments
Narcotics					
Opium derivatives					
Heroin	H, Harry, horse, brother, scag, smack, junk	Intravenous Intranasal	Pupil constriction, euphoria followed by CNS depression (impaired coordination, lethargy, cyanosis, coma)	Respiratory arrest, death	Relatively small proportion of youth abuse this Schedule I–controlled substance. Tolerance and a strong physical and psychological dependence usually develop rapidly. Potential for perinatal/neonatal addiction and/or effects exists.[c]
Morphine	M, white stuff	Intravenous Oral Intranasal	Euphoria, pupil constriction, constipation, nausea, skin flushing, sweating, respiratory depression, cyanosis, coma	Coma, respiratory arrest, death	Schedule II–controlled substance with high physical and psychological dependence capability. Tolerance develops rapidly, and naloxone hydrochloride (morphine antagonist) will precipitate *withdrawal symptoms* (muscle cramps, stomach cramps, diarrhea, rhinitis, restlessness, and convulsions). Potential for perinatal/neonatal addiction and/or effects exists.[c]
Codeine	Schoolboy	Oral	Mild euphoria, constipation, nausea	Depressed blood pressure and respirations	Schedule II–controlled substance, less likely to produce physical dependence. Large doses produce paradoxical stimulation. Less frequently abused drug by youth except in combination with other substances—e.g., a *Load* is 3 Doriden and 3 codeine.
Synthetic opiates					
Methadone (Dolophine)	Meth, dollies	Oral (preferred) Intravenous	Euphoria, nodding-dozing state, restlessness	Respiratory depression, convulsions, or death	Schedule II–controlled substance causing *severe withdrawal symptoms* including diarrhea, stomach pain, hot and cold flashes, insomnia, and sweating. Tolerance develops slowly, but all components of addiction occur. Potential for perinatal/neonatal addiction and/or effects exists.[c]
Meperidine (Demerol)		Intravenous	Pupil constriction, sweating, respiratory depression, cyanosis	Cold, clammy skin; depressed respirations; decreased blood pressure; shock; coma; death	Schedule II–controlled substance available in hospitals; therefore, abuse potential for medical personnel. Tolerance and physical and psychological dependence develop. Potential for perinatal effects (depressed infant) and perinatal addiction exists.[c]

Continued

Table 4-2 Continued

Psychoactive substance[a]	Common terms[b]	Usual route of administration	Abuse: signs/symptoms	Overdose: signs/symptoms	General comments
Pentazocine (Talwin)	Ts	Oral Intravenous		Similar to opiate overdose, particularly respiratory depression May be lethal if combined with barbiturates or alcohol	Schedule IV–controlled substance for which tolerance and psychological dependence develop after prolonged use.
Depressants					
Alcohol (ethanol)	Booze, hootch, suds, juice	Oral	Progressive stages of intoxication: euphoria, loss of inhibition, emotional lability, impaired judgment, aggressiveness, hostility, incoordination, lethargy, and stupor Blackouts (drug-related memory failure without loss of consciousness, i.e., amnesia)	Coma, death (especially when combined with barbiturates and some tranquilizers—e.g., diazepam)	Alcohol-induced judgment impairment and incoordination are highly correlated with moving vehicle accidents during adolescence. Alcohol dependence is a progressive disease. Psychological dependence precedes physical dependence. Tolerance develops at varying rates, and high tolerance is suggestive of alcoholism. Blackouts are indicative of alcoholism. Some adolescent ethanol deaths have been reported due to a single large intake episode. *Withdrawal:* Anxiety, tremors, hallucinations, hyperreflexia, convulsions, and death Brain damage (subtle to pronounced), liver damage Transmitted through placenta, fetal alcohol effects may occur as well as fetal alcohol syndrome.[c]
Barbiturate Sedative-hypnotics	Barbs, downers	Oral Intravenous	Slurred speech, ataxia, slowed reflexes, constricted pupils, short attention span, impaired judgment, combativeness, violence, paranoid delusions	Respiratory depression, coma, death	Schedule II–controlled substance. Tolerance and physical and psychological dependence develop. High potential for homicide or other violence with intravenous use. Combined with alcohol can cause extreme violence or coma or death. *Withdrawal:* hyperreflexia, irritability, convulsions, death. Transmitted through placenta: perinatal barbiturate effects include inattentiveness and permanent neurological sequelae with excessive amounts.[c]
Secobarbital (Seconal)	Reds, red devils, red birds				
Pentobarbital (Nembutal)	Nembies, yellow jackets				
Amobarbital (Amytal)	Blues, blue heavens				

Nonbarbiturate Sedative-hypnotics					Schedule II–controlled substance with high abuse potential. Tolerance and physical and psychic dependence develop.
Methaqualone (Quaalude)	Quads, Sopers, ludes	Oral	Euphoria, irritability, sleeplessness, delirium tremors	Convulsions, cutaneous and pulmonary edema, shock, respiratory arrest	*Withdrawal:* Similar to barbiturates; often fatal if detoxified without medical supervision. (If convulsions are not treated, status epilepticus usually develops.)
Glutethimide (Doriden)		Oral	Dilated pupils	Prolonged coma, absence of reflexes, fever, and death	Schedule III–controlled substance. Tolerance and physical dependence develop fairly rapidly. Psychic dependence occurs. Potentiated effect with alcohol or other sedatives (e.g., Loads) can cause fatal respiratory and circulatory failure.
Minor tranquilizers					Schedule IV–controlled substance. Prolonged use can result in tolerance and physical dependence. Moderate to high potential for psychological dependence.
Chlordiazepoxide (Librium) Diazepam (Valium) Meprobamate (Equanil)	Tranks	Oral Intravenous	Occasional disinhibition, various nonspecific symptoms	Similar to barbiturate or alcohol intoxication Depressants, including alcohol, potentiate effects and may cause coma and death.	*Withdrawal:* Tremor, abdominal and/or muscle cramping, sweating, and convulsions may occur as late as 14 days following discontinuation of the drug. Sometimes used following stimulant abuse to counteract the effects; rarely used alone by youths. *Special pediatric concerns:* Accidental and nonaccidental tranquilizer poisonings of young children have been reported. Potential for perinatal/neonatal effects and/or addiction exists.[d]
Stimulants					
Amphetamines Amphetamine Sulfate (Benzedrine) Dextroamphetamine (Dexedrine) Methamphetamine (Methedrine)	Uppers, bennies, dexies, pep pills, speed, crystal	Oral Subcutaneous Intravenous	Hypertension, weight loss, dilated pupils, sweating (if injected), psychological and motor stimulation, insomnia, pronounced euphoric state	Cardiac failure, convulsions, coma, cerebral hemorrhage	Schedule II–controlled substance. Tolerance and psychic dependence develop. *Prolonged use:* impaired judgment, pronounced euphoric state, paranoid psychosis. *Withdrawal:* severe depression with suicidal tendency. Potential for perinatal/neonatal effects exists.[d]

Continued

Table 4-2 **Continued**

Psychoactive substance[a]	Common terms[b]	Usual route of administration	Abuse: signs/symptoms	Overdose: signs/symptoms	General comments
Cocaine	Coke, snow, crack, rock	Intranasal Intravenous Intrapulmonary (smoking)	Hypertension, tachycardia, hyperreflexia, hyperactivity, intense euphoria	Tachycardia, hallucinations, nausea, vomiting, muscle spasms Respiratory failure, convulsions, coma, and circulatory collapse	Schedule II–controlled substance. Powerful psychological dependence usually develops. Stimulation is more pronounced than with amphetamines, accompanied with illusion of great physical strength and mental capacity. Expense factor is decreasing as cocaine is being made into a smokable form. Probability of abuse increases with greater financial resources and availability. *Withdrawal:* severe depression. Potential for perinatal/neonatal effects exists.[d]
Hallucinogens					
Cannabis (marijuana, hashish)	Joint, grass, pot, weed, reefer, Mary Janes, stick, hash	Intrapulmonary (smoking) Oral	Mild euphoria, intoxication, heightened sensory awareness, drowsiness, tachycardia, delayed response time, poor coordination, occasional depressed or anxiety reactions Large doses produce hallucinatory effects	Physical exhaustion, convulsions, anxiety, and paranoia (bad trip)	Schedule I–controlled substance. Classified as hallucinogen but closer to an intoxicant in effect. Physical dependence does not occur, but psychological dependence may. Marijuana as a substance of abuse for adolescents and children is on the increase. A major problem is that use of this or other psychoactives may retard individual and group social development—i.e., the substance becomes the recreational focus. Moderate to heavy use is correlated with amotivational syndrome in adolescents and is hazardous to normal personality development. *Withdrawal:* irritability, sleep disturbances, sweating, anorexia, gastrointestinal upset, weight loss

Phencyclidine	PCP, angel dust	Intrapulmonary (smoking)	Dilated pupils, reddened eyes, occasionally hypertension, hyperthermia, piloerection, euphoria, heightened sensory awareness, hallucinations, confusion, paranoia	Hypotensive crisis, intracerebral hemorrhage, convulsions, death	Schedule I–controlled substances. Physical dependence does not occur, but tolerance probably does.
Lysergic acid	LSD, acid	Oral			PCP, STP, DMT, and LSD are major street drugs; LSD may be a deliberate contaminant as a substitute for other substances.
N-N-dimethyltryptamine	DMT, cohoba				*Psychiatric complications:* drugs intensify latent psychotic tendencies, panic, suicide potential, flashbacks (particularly with LSD).
2,5-dimethoxy-4-methyamphetamine	STP, DOM				Potential for perinatal/neonatal effects exists.[d]
Inhalants and organic solvents Hydrocarbons and fluorocarbons (glue, cleaning fluid, aerosol sprays, nail polish remover, gasoline)		Intranasal	Some degree of short-term intoxication, euphoria, impaired perception and coordination, loss of consciousness	Moderate overdosage: unconscious, in no immediate danger of death High overdosage: adrenergic crisis, status epilepticus, respiratory failure	Some degree of psychological dependence in the broad sense—i.e., abuser becomes dependent on the euphoric state. Most often seen with younger substance abusers. Users have an increased probability of alcohol or other substance abuse. Medical complications: asphyxia from plastic bags used to inhale fumes, ventricular fibrillation or other arrhythmias, secondary trauma Lead poisoning Possible irreversible damage to central nervous system, kidneys, liver, and bone marrow Psychosis similar to that evoked by hallucinogenic drugs may occur.

[a]The list covers only the major chemicals or drugs abused.

[b]Common terms vary from area to area across the country.

[c]This is conclusive evidence of the effect on the neonate.

[d]A potential risk of neonatal effects exists. These may be subtle neurologic effects, such as hyperactivity or learning problems, that are not detected until later childhood.

Source: J. Servonsky and S. Opas, *Nursing Management of Children,* Boston: Little, Brown, 1987.

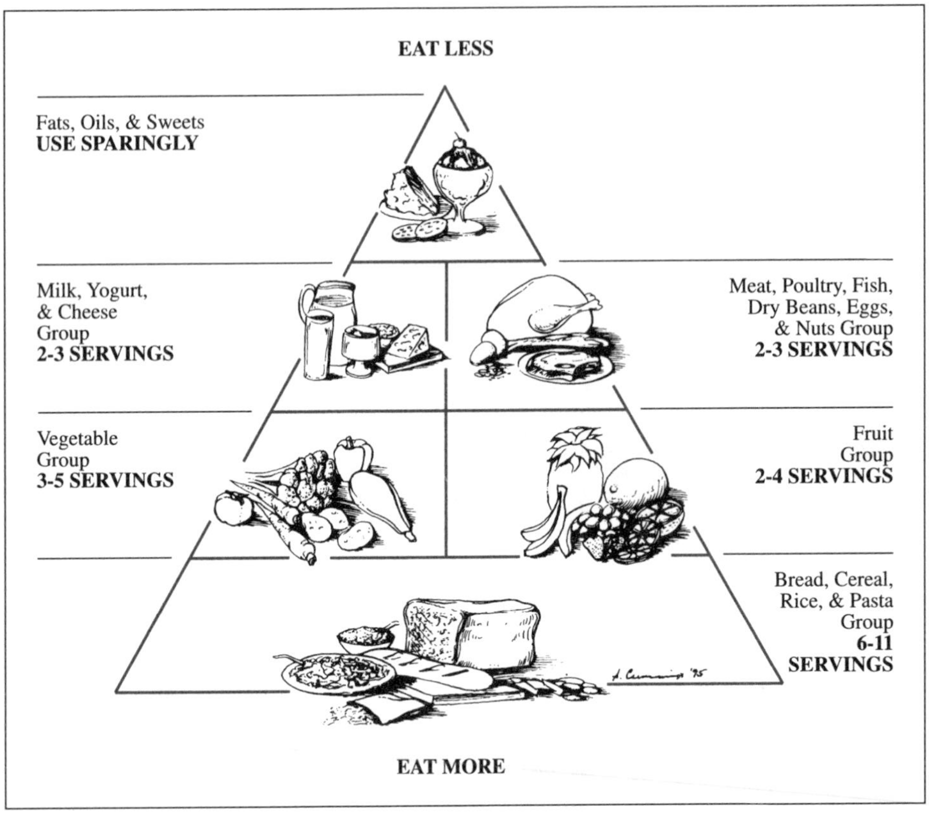

Figure 4-3 Food guide pyramid. (From: U.S. Department of Agriculture and the U.S. Department of Health and Human Services.)

Table 4-3 One Method of Calculating Daily Caloric Needs According to Basal Metabolism and Activity Level

Physical activity	Total calories needed daily
Sedentary to light	$\frac{130}{100} \times$ basal caloric need
Moderate	$\frac{150}{100} \times$ basal caloric need
Strenuous	$\frac{(175 - 200) \times \text{basal caloric need}}{100}$

Source: H.Y. Hui: *Human Nutrition and Diet Therapy.* © 1983 Boston: Jones and Bartlett Publishers. Reprinted with permission.

of caloric needs. Another method for calculating daily caloric needs is provided in Table 4-5.

Knowing a person's diet, eating habits, and eating patterns provides additional invaluable information. Food preferences reflect cultural background, age, financial status, self-image, body image, and a number of other significant factors (Table 4-6). A client's eating patterns may be the clue to a problem of obesity or may be the signal that the malnourished or underweight client may be suffering from psychological problems leading to anorexia or bulimia. In either case, further investigation into the eating patterns of the client and the client's self-image or body image would be warranted. In addition to eating patterns, the client's eating habits may also direct you to areas for further assessment; for example, the adolescent who exists on fad foods may develop skin problems, obesity, or anemia, while the elderly person subsisting on tea and toast may be in fluid and electrolyte imbalance and malnourished. Table 4-7 lists physical signs and symptoms of undernutrition that may be readily observed during the interview and the physical examination. You need to have the client keep a log of what and when he eats for at least 3 days to get a trend of his eating habits.

Sleep and Rest Patterns

The most common sleep disorder is insomnia. Clients with psychoses and neuroses suffer from insomnia. As psychological states (e.g., distress, obsessive behavior, depression, or anxiety) lessen, the client will sleep for longer periods. Initial insomnia occurs when the client has difficulty falling asleep. Emotional factors such as excitement or anxiety may be the cause. At one time or another, all of us have tossed and turned and been unable to fall asleep quickly before a trip or celebration day, such as the night before a holiday. Sudden and diverse stimuli, such as strange noises, also may interfere

Table 4-4 Examples of Determinants of Caloric Needs

Climate/temperature	Warm (Africa) climate requires fewer calories.
	Cold (Yukon) areas require more calories.
Exercise	Requires more calories
Stress/illness/surgery	Requires more calories
Muscle mass	Women require fewer calories than men because women have less muscle mass.
	With aging muscle mass is lost and thus fewer calories are needed.
Growth	Increased calories per body size are necessary in the fast-growing years; there is a big drop in the BMR between 1 and 2 years of age; it levels out at 11–12 years of age, peaks at 23 years of age, and then begins a gradual decline.

Table 4-5 USDA Rule of Thumb for Calculating Daily Caloric Needs

Physical activity	Total calories needed daily*	
	Women	Men
Sedentary	Ideal body weight × 14	Ideal body weight × 16
Moderate	Ideal body weight × 18	Ideal body weight × 21
Strenuous	Ideal body weight × 22	Ideal body weight × 26

*All ideal body weights expressed in pounds.

Source: H. Y. Hui: *Human Nutrition and Diet Therapy.* © 1983 Boston: Jones and Bartlett Publishers. Reprinted with permission.

Table 4-6 Why Do People Eat What They Eat?

Culture	Malaysian source of protein is from insects, e.g., grasshoppers.
	Slaves were forced to eat what others discarded, e.g., chitlins.
	Cows are sacred in India; therefore, milk and beef are not consumed.
Religion	Mormon Practice: no stimulants (caffeinated coffee, tea, colas).
	Seventh Day Adventist does not eat red meat.
	Jewish Laws (depends on degree of orthodoxy) deny pork and shellfish; no meat eaten with dairy products.
Age	Sweet taste buds are the last to degenerate; 2% of taste sensitivity tends to be lost each decade. The elderly generally have a preference for sweets.
Economics	Less money equals more starch in diet; as food money increases, starch decreases in the diet and generally sugar and meat increases.
Convenience	Busy people tend to eat fast foods (high in fat, salt, and sugar).
Psychological	Advertisement/media influences; peer pressure (especially adolescents); rewarding self with comfort foods (ice cream).
Availability	Seasonal foods of the geographic area; no transportation

with falling asleep. Nutritional disorders and excessive alcohol or caffeine intake also can affect sleep. Initial insomnia tends to occur in clients when they are first admitted to the hospital.

Intermittent insomnia is indicated when the client awakes frequently throughout the night; it may result from noise (clanging bedpans, loud voices, slamming doors) as well as from physical causes such as poor ventilation and illness symptoms. The more prevalent physical predisposers to insomnia are chronic pain, diabetes mellitus, hyperthyroidism,

Table 4-7 **Physical Signs and Symptoms of Undernutrition**

Organ/tissue	Undernutrition	Good nutrition
Hair	Dry, wirelike Stiff, often brittle May exhibit some bleaching of normal color Easily pluckable (pediatric form)	Shiny, lustrous Healthy scalp
Eyes	Thickened, opaque bulbar conjunctivae with angular lesions Increase in vascularity, conjunctival injection Xerosis conjunctivae (the conjunctivae, on exposure by holding the lids open and having the subject rotate the eyes, appear dull and lusterless and exhibit a striated or roughened surface) Bitot's spots—small circumscribed grayish or yellowish dull, dry, foamy superficial lesions of the conjunctiva; seen most often on lateral aspect of conjunctiva and in children; not to be confused with pterygium Xerophthalmia—recorded when bulbar conjunctiva and cornea are dry and lusterless with a decrease in lacrimation; often associated with evidence of infection or, in extreme cases, keratomalacia Keratomalacia (pediatric form shows corneal softening with deformity, either localized, usually central part of lower half of cornea, or total)	Bright, clear, moist
Mouth and tongue Mucous membranes	Lips—angular lesions and scars, indicating cheilosis Tongue—Filiform papillary atrophy (smooth slick), hypertrophy/hyperemia, geographic tongue, fissure/serrations or swelling, red, scarlet, beefy (glossitis), magenta colored (color of alkaline phenolphthalein)	Reddish-pink color to lips, tongue, and mucous membrane Absence of lesions Adequately moist Surface papillae present on tongue
Teeth and gums	Teeth—visible caries Gums—atrophy, recession, inflammation; marginal redness or swelling (marginal redness is a definite red border along dental margin of gum, marginal swelling in a swollen border of gum, which may be spongy or firm); swollen red papillae; bleeding gums, which either bleed spontaneously or bleed on slight pressure with a swab stick	Teeth straight, bright without crowding, no evidence of caries Gums firm, reddish pink with no evidence of swelling or bleeding
Skin	Follicular hyperkeratosis—rough, dry Xerosis—dry or scaling Hyperpigmentation—seen most frequently on dorsa of hands and lower forearms, particularly where skin hygiene is poor; skin is rough and dry, and often has a grayish cyanotic base. Thickened pressure points (other than elbows and knees); look especially at belt area, ischial tuberositis, sacrum, over greater trochanters.	Smooth, slightly moist, good color
Abdomen and lower extremities	Potbelly (pediatric form only), hepatomegaly Pretibial edema (bilateral) Calf tenderness (adult form only) Absent knee/ankle jerk (adult form) Absent vibratory sense (adult form): test with tuning fork over lateral malleoli; record as positive only if absent bilaterally	Abdomen flat No tenderness, weakness, or swelling of feet and legs

Table 4-7 Continued

Organ/tissue	Undernutrition	Good nutrition
Skeletal (pediatric form only)	Beading of ribs	Good posture
	Bossing of skull	No malformations
Face and neck	Malar pigmentation (adult form)—areas of dark brown pigmentation over malar eminences	Skin of face and neck clear, smooth
	Nasolabial seborrhea—a definite greasy, yellowish scaling or filiform excrescenses on nasolabial area, which become more pronounced on slight scratching with a fingernail or tongue blade	No thyroid enlargement
	Parotid glands visibly enlarged	
	Thyroid enlarged	
Muscles	Flaccid underdeveloped, or wasted in appearance, tender	Well developed, firm

Specific Questions Related to Diet Assessment

1. Is the client subject to food fads?
2. How much does the client eat?
3. Does the client think he is too fat?
4. Does the client binge eat and then vomit?
5. What is the typical diet on a normal day?
6. How many meals does the client have per day?
7. Does the client eat snacks? If so, how many a day and of what kind?
8. Does the client have free access to snacks?
9. Who prepares the client's meals?
10. Is the client on a special diet? If so, for how long? Does he understand and feel comfortable with the diet?
11. Does the client take vitamins, minerals, or diet pills? If so, what is the variety of pills taken and the number of each variety?
12. Has the client had any disturbances in digestion, chewing, or swallowing?

angina pectoris, gastric ulcer, and respiratory disorders. Terminal insomnia occurs when the client awakes in the early morning and cannot return to sleep. Excitement, anxiety, and change in sleeping habit may be causes of terminal insomnia. An example of the latter would be the client who is wide awake at 4 A.M. Since being hospitalized, however, she has been going to sleep earlier in the evening or napping during the day and, therefore, has had a good night's sleep by that time. If the client does not display sleep deprivation symptoms or exhaustion, her need for sleep has most likely been met.

Some physical characteristics that may indicate troubled sleeping patterns are

- dark circles under the eyes
- puffy eyelids
- bloodshot eyes
- irritability, headache
- fatigue, decreased attention span

Sleep and rest clearly affect the total well-being of the client. The following types of questions will aid you in assessing the sleep and rest patterns of your clients:

1. "When you wake up, do you feel rested?"
2. "When do you usually retire and awake each day?"
3. "How many hours, generally, do you sleep?"
4. "Have you experienced any difficulty in sleeping?"
5. "If you have experienced difficulty, what remedies have you tried?"
6. "Has anything happened recently to which you might attribute your sleeping difficulty?"
7. "What comfort measures do you usually employ that help you sleep well?" Examples might include reading before retiring, watching TV, setting the radio on automatic "off," opening the window, drinking a warm beverage, having a glass of wine, taking a sleeping medication, and so forth.
8. "Do you have trouble falling asleep?"
9. "Do you wake up often during the night? If so, can you easily fall back to sleep?"
10. "Do you wake early in the morning feeling fatigued?"
11. "Do you nap during the day?"
12. "Do you experience nightmares? Sleepwalking? Bedwetting?"

Sleep patterns specific to age are discussed in the appropriate age-related chapters of the text.

Activities of Daily Living

When assessing daily activities, you are actually gathering the client's perception of any difficulties he may be experiencing in the basic activities of eating, grooming, dressing, elimination, and locomotion. At this time, you may want to discuss the effects of handicaps on the client's abilities, or he may reveal any covert handicaps.

You also determine whether the client is independent in performing daily activities or whether he needs supervision or assistance.

1. Is he unable to carry out certain activities?
2. How much assistance does he need?
3. Does he require adaptive devices or prostheses to perform certain activities?
4. Can the client feed himself? Does he need help cutting meat and opening containers? Does he need to be fed? Does he eat at the table? In a dining room? In bed?
5. Is the client independent in grooming himself? Can he bathe (bed, tub, shower)? Can he brush his teeth? Can he comb and wash his hair?
6. Can he care for his nails? Shave? Is he able to apply cologne or deodorant?
7. Does dressing present any difficulties?
8. Is the client able to go to the bathroom by himself?
9. Is he able to care for altered routes of elimination if they are necessary (colostomy, ureterostomy)?
10. Can he get out of bed (transfer)?
11. Can he get into and out of a chair?
12. Does he have any difficulty with standing? Walking? Ascending or descending stairs?
13. If wheelchair bound, is he able to propel the chair by himself?

Home and Neighborhood

The client's physical and emotional environment may create problems, or it may provide an atmosphere conducive to well-being.

- Determine the conditions of the home and neighborhood and the services available.
- Do the drugstores accept Medicare and Medicaid?
- Do the grocery stores accept food stamps?
- Are there community services available to meet the needs of the disabled—food services, modified access routes, transportation?

Investigation of the client's housing conditions and facilities may reveal surprises. Many economically deprived elderly persons live in unheated apartments or rooms with few comforts and little food. If there are children in the home, it is important to evaluate safety measures regarding such things as poisons, bare electrical wires, and other home accident factors.

Your investigation of the client's homelife may be opened by asking the client whether he lives alone or other persons live with him.

- How does the client feel about this arrangement?
- How much time does the client spend at home and away?
- Does the client share values and goals with those living with him?
- Is the client involved in the planning of family activities?
- What support systems—family, friends—are available to the client?
- What is the quality of these support relationships?
- Is a relationship characterized by trust, distrust, mutual support, competition, dominance, submission?
- Has the relationship been harmonious, strained, or interrupted?

To understand specific relationships you might ask the client,

- "How would you describe your mother?"
- "How would your mother describe you?"

A client who expresses concern about a family member might be encouraged to elaborate if you offer a general lead such as, "Tell me more about it."

Recreation/Hobbies

Recreation is generally considered a part of an individual's lifestyle. Discussion might include such things as exercise activity and tolerance, hobbies and other interests, vacations, and even the amount of time spent with family and friends. In the case of a child, you would also be interested in whether her play is generally isolated, parallel, or interactive. The play style should then be assessed according to developmental criteria based on the child's age.

Because lifestyles are so varied in the United States, you need to be open, imaginative, and tactful in your collection of data and to sort out the information necessary for a health history that is truly in the interest of the client's health status. Table 4-8 is a self-test for wellness lifestyle.

Sexuality

Assessment of sexuality is done about as frequently as rectal examinations. In fact, it is probably the most neglected area of health assessment; it is not even addressed in most instances, whereas the existence of the rectal examination as part of health assessment is at least acknowledged, if only by the words "referred" or "not done." Some nurses believe that sexual matters are personal and should not be explored. Others ignore assessment of sexuality because of their own discomfort with the topic. Furthermore, young nurses may find it difficult to discuss sexuality with persons who are older. They may also find it difficult to think of elderly men and women as having sexual feelings, needs, and relationships.

Well-being and sexual functioning are interrelated. If the client is sick or in poor shape, energy, enthusiasm, and interest for sexual activity are generally decreased. Including the assessment of sexual functioning near the end of history taking allows you and the client to feel more comfortable in the roles of nurse and client—that is, in exploring sexuality in relation to health status and in divulging the information.

Table 4-8 Self-Test for Wellness Lifestyle

Behavior		Scoring	Almost always	Sometimes	Almost never
Cigarette smoking	If you never smoke, enter a score of 10 for this section and go to the next section "Alcohol and Drugs."				
	1. I avoid smoking cigarettes.		2	1	0
	2. I smoke only low-tar-and-nicotine cigarettes OR I smoke a pipe or cigars.		2	1	0
		Smoking Score:	____	____	____
Alcohol and Drugs	1. I avoid drinking alcoholic beverages OR I drink no more than 1 or 2 drinks a day.		4	1	0
	2. I avoid using alcohol or other drugs (especially illegal drugs) as a way of handling stressful situations or the problems in my life.		2	1	0
	3. I am careful not to drink alcohol when taking certain medicines (for example, medicine for sleeping, pain, colds, and allergies) or when pregnant.		2	1	0
	4. I read and follow the label directions when using prescribed and over-the-counter drugs.		2	1	0
		Alcohol and Drugs Score:	____	____	____
Eating Habits	1. I eat a variety of foods each day, such as fruits and vegetables, whole-grain breads and cereals, lean meats, dairy products, dry peas and beans, and nuts and seeds.		4	1	0
	2. I limit the amount of fat, saturated fat, and cholesterol I eat (including eggs, butter, cream, shortenings, fat on meats, and organ meats such as liver).		2	1	0
	3. I limit the amount of salt I eat by cooking with only small amounts, not adding salt at the table, and avoiding salty snacks.		2	1	0
	4. I avoid eating too much sugar (especially frequent snacks of sticky candy or soft drinks).		2	1	0
		Eating Habits Score:	____	____	____
Exercise and Fitness	1. I maintain a desired weight, avoiding overweight and underweight.		3	1	0
	2. I do vigorous exercises for 15 to 30 minutes at least 3 times a week (examples including running, swimming, brisk walking).		3	1	0
	3. I do exercises that enhance my muscle tone for 15 to 30 minutes at least 3 times a week (examples include yoga and calisthenics).		2	1	0
	4. I use part of my leisure time participating in individual, family, or team activities that increase my level of fitness (such as gardening, bowling, golf, and baseball).		2	1	0
		Exercise and Fitness Score:	____	____	____
Stress Control	1. I have a job or do other work that I enjoy.		2	1	0
	2. I find it easy to relax and express my feelings freely.		2	1	0
	3. I recognize early, and prepare for, events or situations likely to be stressful for me.		2	1	0

Continued

Table 4-8 Continued

Behavior		Scoring	Almost always	Sometimes	Almost never
	4. I have close friends, relatives, or others whom I can talk to about personal matters and call on for help when needed.		2	1	0
	5. I participate in group activities (such as church and community organizations) or hobbies that I enjoy.		2	1	0
		Stress Control Score:	____	____	____
Safety	1. I wear a seat belt while riding in a car.		2	1	0
	2. I avoid driving while under the influence of alcohol and other drugs.		2	1	0
	3. I obey traffic rules and the speed limit when driving.		2	1	0
	4. I am careful when using potentially harmful products or substances (such as household cleaners, poisons, and electrical devices).		2	1	0
	5. I avoid smoking in bed.		2	1	0
		Safety Score:	____	____	____
		Total Scores:	Cigarette Smoking		____
			Alcohol and Drugs		____
			Eating Habits		____
			Exercise/Fitness		____
			Stress Control		____
			Safety		____
			Total:		____

Interpretation of scores for each category:

Scores of 9 and 10: Excellent! Your answers show that you are aware of the importance of this area to your health. More important, you are putting your knowledge to work for you by practicing good health habits. As long as you continue to do so, this area should not pose a serious health risk. It's likely that you are setting an example for your family and friends to follow. Since you get a very high test score on this part of the test, you may want to consider other areas where your scores indicate room for improvement.

Scores of 6 to 8: Your health practices in this area are good, but there is room for improvement. Look again at the items you answered with a "Sometimes" or "Almost Never." What changes can you make to improve your score? Even a small change can often help you achieve better health.

Scores of 3 to 5: Your health risks are showing! Would you like more information about the risks you are facing and why it is important for you to change these behaviors? Perhaps you need help in deciding how to successfully make the changes you desire. In either case, help is available.

Scores of 0 to 2: Obviously, you were concerned enough about your health to take the test, but your answers show that you may be taking serious and unnecessary risks with your health. Perhaps you are not aware of the risks and what to do about them. You can easily get the information and help you need to improve—if you wish. The next step is up to you.

Source: Test developed by United States Public Health Service. National Health Information Clearinghouse, Washington, D.C.

Sexuality is an identity fashioned greatly by morality, which in turn is developed by the direct influence of the guidance and values of parents and significant others (e.g., peers, other adults, and teachers) generally in concordance with accepted roles and formal laws of religion and society. Thus, there exists a wide cross-cultural variation in attitudes toward sexuality and in sexual behavior (Table 4-9).

Ebersole and Hess (1981, p. 329) define sexuality as "love, warmth, sharing, touching between people, not just the physical act of coitus." Intercourse is only a part of sexuality. Sexuality is being a woman. It is being a man. It is being sensual. It is the total personality (Griggs 1978).

The use of Maslow's well-known model of hierarchy allows the nurse to see that sexuality is a part of the person's total being, as shown in Fig. 4-4. Maslow (1954) postulated that human behavior is motivated by certain categories of basic needs, which are arranged in a hierarchic fashion. In a gestalt mode, all needs and levels of need exist simultaneously; in most circumstances, however, the primary or lower level needs take priority over seeking satisfaction of the higher level needs. The primary physiologic needs include oxygen, food, water, shelter, elimination, activity, rest, pain avoidance, and sexual activity. The emphases of sexuality at the primary level can be viewed as procreation and sexual

Table 4-9 Some Cultural Aspects Affecting Sexuality Assessment

Culture/subculture	Religious/family orientation	Privacy/modesty needs	Other
Mexican-Americans	Family and religion important. Few decisions made without husband. May utilize only a Catholic obstetrician.	Very modest: Man unlikely to undress, provide urine specimens, or allow examination by woman; Man likely to remain with woman during obstetric or urologic exams. Body in general is considered private, even sacred, and is not to be exposed.	Believe males should have higher education and more privileges than females.
Puerto Ricans	Often matriarchal, large, with strong home orientation. Religion often important.		
Native Americans	Religion and medicine are intertwined. Decisions often made by the family as a unit.	Privacy important for their medicine ceremonies. Very modest: may require permission to touch body, e.g., to bathe, brush hair: unlikely to undress with someone in room.	Avoid eye contact because believe one sees into the soul through the eyes and may take soul away. Heavy labor often part of female life; so must consider when providing instructions regarding limitations of activities.
Asians	Often patriarchal; husband may speak for wife.	Very modest	Schools are sex segregated from childhood on.
African-Americans	Not necessarily matriarchal as often believed. Husband and wife work together. Children valued. Often a strong religious orientation.		
Appalachians	Strong family orientation; often bring whole family to hospital or clinic.		Upper and middle classes are similar to general U.S. upper and middle classes. Poor and working classes may differ: "neutrality" ethic prevails; nonassertive, nonaggressive, avoid eye contact, "mind own business" attitudes are valued.

Source: Adapted from *Human Sexuality: A Nursing Perspective,* by R. Hogan (ed.). Copyright © 1980 by Appleton-Century-Crofts. Reprinted by permission.

activity, including sexual exploration, arousal, novelty, and sexual release. Safety and security needs in light of sexuality are the desire for trusting sexual relationships and acquisition of knowledge regarding contraception and the means to prevent and recognize sexually transmitted diseases. Sexually, the needs for love and belonging are reflected in behaviors of sexual intimacy, wherein closeness, loving, and sharing abound, and the need to be accepted as a sexual being regardless of age. Having a sexual identity and feeling that one is sensual satisfy the need for self-esteem in regard to sexuality; this includes the recognition of sexual, physical changes. The pinnacle of Maslow's hierarchy is self-actualization; this encompasses aesthetic needs and, in the sphere of sexuality, is represented by feelings of sexual completeness and an appreciation of the beauty of sexuality.

Alterations in sexual functioning may occur because of social barriers, myths, or effects of illness. Table 4-10 lists diseases and medical therapies that may interfere with sexual health. For example, diabetes can have a significant effect on sexual functioning. Men with diabetes may experience absence of emission (a "dry orgasm") caused by diabetic neuropathy wherein the semen is forced back into the bladder (retrograde ejaculation). Surgical penile implants are used for maintaining erection. For the diabetic woman, the most common problem affecting sexual functioning is fungal infections of the vagina. Treatment of the infection ends painful intercourse. Medications may also affect sexual functioning (Table 4-11). The client should be educated about the possible side effects of decreased or increased libido. If this is distressing to the client, perhaps the possibility of

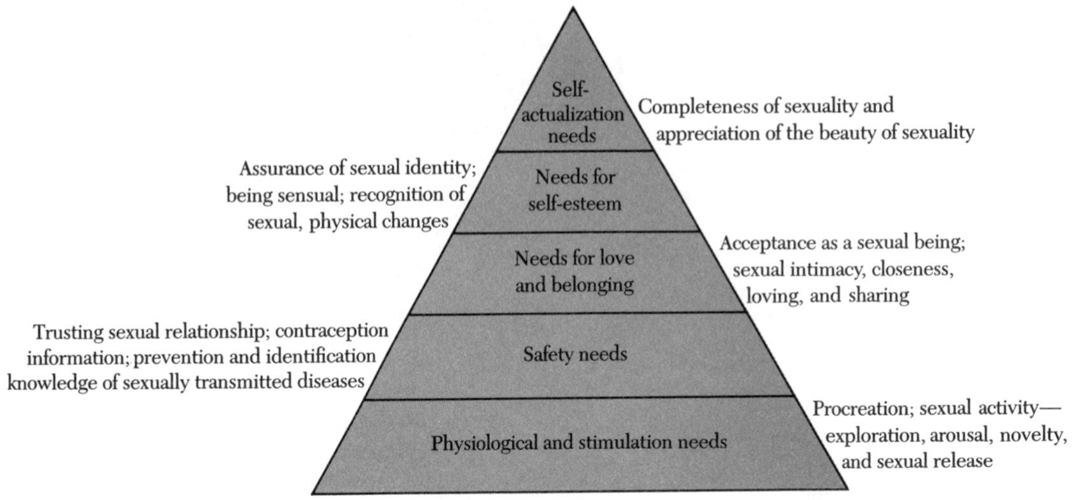

Figure 4-4 Schema of Maslow's hierarchy of needs, with identification of sexuality emphases throughout.

Table 4-10 Physiologic Interferences with Sexual Health

Interferences	Hypothesized mechanism of action
Systemic diseases Pulmonary disease Renal disease Malignancies Infections Degenerative diseases Some cardiovascular diseases	Debility, pain, and depression probably interfere with libido as well as sexual expression.
Metabolic disruptions Cirrhosis Mononucleosis Hepatitis Hypothyroidism Addison's disease Hypogonadism Hypopituitarism Acromegaly Feminizing tumors Cushing's disease Diabetes mellitus	Hepatic problems in the man result in estrogen buildup related to inability of the liver to conjugate estrogens; similar processes occur in the woman along with general debility. By depression of the CNS function, general debilitation, and depression, libido may be decreased, and impaired arousal in the woman and impaired erectile abilities in the man may result. With diabetes there is a hypothesized relationship between neuropathic and vascular damage and retrograde ejaculation and impotence or secondary orgasmic dysfunction, dyspareunia, or adolescent amenorrhea.
Genital interferences Priapism Peyronie's disease Balantitis Phimosis Genital herpes Trauma to the penis Vaginal infections Senile vaginitis Vulvitis	Each of these problems involves damage to the genital organs, which may result in painful intercourse.

Table 4-10 Continued

Interferences	Hypothesized mechanism of action
Leukoplakia Bartholin cyst Allergic response to vaginal sprays, deodorants Vaginitis following radiation therapy Pelvic inflammatory disease Fibroadenomas Endometriosis Uterine prolapse Anal fissures, hemorrhoids Pelvic masses Ovarian cysts Reduced vaginal lubrication, postpartum or with aging Prostatitis Urethritis	Local irritability, damage to genitals, and consequent interference with reflex mechanisms involved in erection and ejaculation
Medical or surgical castration Orchiectomy Radiation therapy Ovariectomy, adrenalectomy	Lowered androgen levels depress libido and lead to impotence, retarded ejaculation, and/or impaired sexual responsiveness.

Source: Adapted from Kaplan, H. S. *The New Sex Therapy.* New York: Brunner/Mazel, Inc. 1974; and Phipps, W.; Long, B.; Woods, N. F.; and Cassmeyer, V. *Medical Surgical Nursing: Concepts and Clinical Practice,* 4th ed. St. Louis: C. V. Mosby, 1991, p. 1520.

Table 4-11 Potential Effects of Drugs on Sexual Function

		Probable mechanism of action	
Drug or drug category	Effect	Physiologic	Psychological
Recreational drugs			
Alcohol	Small amounts transiently positive		Reduced inhibitions
	Large amounts or prolonged use negative	CNS depressant Impotence Premature ejaculation Associated with fetal alcohol syndrome in pregnancy	
Amphetamines and cocaine	Transiently positive	CNS stimulant Rapid and long-lasting erection Intensification of orgasm Decreased fatigue	Mood enhancement Increased mental alertness
	Enduring—negative	Impotence Decreased vaginal secretions resulting in painful intercourse	Decreased libido
Amyl nitrite*	Questionable	Peripheral vasodilation may enhance orgasm but can also produce dizziness, headache, and syncope.	

Continued

Table 4-11 **Continued**

Drug or drug category	Effect	Probable mechanism of action: Physiologic	Probable mechanism of action: Psychological
Caffeine	Transiently positive	CNS stimulant—may reduce fatigue	
	Large amounts or prolonged use—negative	May produce a "nervous reaction"	
Canthoris (Spanish fly)	Negative	Irritation and inflammation of GU tract, systemic poisoning	
Hallucinogens	Questionable		Alters perceptions with either heightened sexual sensations or inability to focus on sexual activity
Nicotine	Negative transient effects	Vasoconstriction with decreased oxygen level and decreased blood flow to sex organs	
	Negative enduring effects	Decreased spermatogenesis	
		Decreased sperm motility	
		Increased incidence of abortion, stillbirths and small-for-gestational age babies	
Opiates*	Transiently positive	CNS depression	Reduced inhibitions
Codeine Heroin Methadone Morphine	Negative—enduring effects	Impotence	Decreased sexual enjoyment
		Decreased ejaculate volume	Decreased libido
		Decreased sperm motility	
Opium		Amenorrhea, dysmenorrhea, infertility, increased incidence of abortion	
Potassium nitrate (saltpeter)	Questionable	Diuresis	
Sedative-hypnotics* Compazine Librium Marijuana	Transiently positive	CNS depressant	Reduced inhibitions
		Tranquilization	
		Relaxation	
Mellaril Thorazine Valium	Large doses negative	Lethargy	Decreased libido
		Decreased coordination	
Therapeutic drugs			
Antidepressants	Negative and positive	CNS depression	Increased libido if depression is reduced
		Impotence	
		Inhibited ejaculation	
		Orgasmic difficulties	
Antihistamines	Transiently negative	CNS depression	Decreased libido
		Decreased vaginal secretion	
Antihypertensives	Negative	Peripheral blockage of innervation of sex organs	Decreased libido
		Decrease or absence of ejaculate; retrograde ejaculation; impotence; orgasmic difficulties; breast tenderness; menstrual irregularities; gynecomastia	

Table 4-11 **Continued**

Drug or drug category	Effect	Probable mechanism of action	
		Physiologic	Psychological
Antipsychotics	Transiently negative	Dry ejaculation Erectile difficulties Gynecomastia Decreased vaginal lubrication Spontaneous flow of milk from breasts Amenorrhea	Decreased responsiveness
Antispasmodics	Negative	Vasoconstriction Ganglionic blockage of innervation of sex organs Impotence Decreased vaginal lubrication	
Corticosteroids	Negative—enduring	Decreased spermatogenesis Can precipitate latent diabetes mellitus	
Cytotoxins	Negative, usually only transient	Decreased spermatogenesis Amenorrhea	Decreased libido and potency
Diuretics	Transiently negative	Impotence Gynecomastia Amenorrhea Breast tenderness	
Hormones			
Sex hormone preparations	Negative	Antiandrogenic effects	Decreased libido Decreased potency
Oral contraceptives	Usually positive	Anovulation Amenorrhea	Concern regarding conception separated from sexual activity
Clomid	Usually positive	Increased testosterone in male Stimulation of ovulation	Decreased libido Decreased potency
L-Dopa and P-chorophenylalanine	Questionable		Improvement of well-being
Selenium	Questionable	Supports fertility in laboratory animals	
Strychnine	Questionable	Stimulation of neuraxis Priapism	
Vitamin E	Questionable	Supports fertility in laboratory animals	
Yohimbine	Questionable	Stimulation of lower spinal nerve centers	

*Also considered a therapeutic drug.

Source: Adapted from Wood, J.S. "Drug Effects on Human Sexual Behavior." *In:* Woods, N. F. (ed.). *Human Sexuality in Health and Illness,* 2nd ed. St. Louis: C. V. Mosby, 1979, pp. 378–379; Ball, W.D. "Drugs That Affect Sexuality." *In:* Hogan, R. (ed.). *Human Sexuality: A Nursing Perspective.* New York: Appleton-Century-Crofts, 1980, pp. 712–726; and Partridge, R. V. "Sexuality and Drugs." *In:* Lion, E. M. (ed.). *Human Sexuality in Nursing Process.* New York: John Wiley & Sons, 1982, pp. 331–339.

alternative treatment could be discussed with the advance practice nurse or physician. Often, the client is relieved to know that sexual dysfunction is caused by the medication and that sexual powers have not been lost. The knowledge that increased or decreased libido is due to a medication may be sufficient. For additional information on sexual dysfunction in men, see Chapter 21.

Keeping in mind the nursing goals of promoting and maintaining health status and having background knowledge of sexuality will enable you to pursue this pertinent area of health assessment with your clients. Assessment of the client's knowledge, assets, needs, and losses in the area of sexuality will help you provide measures for expression of sexuality—for example, use of cosmetics; attractive clothing; opportunities for closeness, touching, kissing, and holding. When sexual activity is not desired or available, suitable substitute activities are listening to music, dancing, relaxing in a rocking chair, and stroking a pet. Alternative choices or options are masturbation, sexual fantasies, oral stimulation, and same-sex relationships. If sexual intercourse is fatiguing to the client, due to a chronic illness or handicap, use of a vibrator may be of benefit. Your suggestions will depend on the client's values, medical condition, psychological health, and social situation. An important role will be to assist the client in accepting normal changes in sexuality and appreciating alternative practices of maintaining sexuality and sexual functioning.

Questions of relevance to sexual health include the following:

- Has the client had any contact with a person who has AIDS or illnesses related to AIDS?
- Does the client use a condom when having sexual intercourse?
- Who are her sexual partners?
- Is the client satisfied with her sexual performance?
- Is she satisfied with the performance of her partner?
- Does the client engage in oral or anal sexual activities?
- Do the client and her sexual partner use contraceptives? If so, what types; how long have they been used; have there been any complications or side effects; is she satisfied with the method(s)?
- Does the client have any questions or concerns about sexual functioning that she would like to discuss?

Previous Experience with Illness

Knowledge of previous illnesses can often be useful in interpreting the significance of the client's present status and his reactions to illness and therapy. Direct questioning may be necessary to obtain information in the areas of childhood illnesses, immunizations, allergies, and medical history.

Childhood Illnesses and Immunizations

It is not sufficient to ask whether the client has had the "common" childhood illnesses, because what is common to one age group is not to another. She should be asked specifically about measles, mumps, chickenpox, diphtheria, and smallpox. The dates or the age of the client when she had any of these diseases must be documented carefully. (For more information on childhood infectious diseases see Appendix D.) Many older people have difficulty remembering a specific disease but can recall having had a high fever with their skin peeling off or an uncomfortable rash that left scars.

The dates and types of all immunizations should be recorded. This information is difficult for many to recall; at least, try to pinpoint at what age the client received the immunization(s). Record information about such immunizations as diphtheria, tetanus, pertussis (whooping cough), rubella (German measles), rubeola (regular measles), mumps, and poliomyelitis. If you work with children, you will need to secure the most recent recommendations for first vaccinations developed by the American Medical Association and the American Academy of Pediatrics, as these are updated periodically.

Individuals over 65 years of age and clients with chronic illness (heart disease, lung disease, diabetes) are generally advised, for temporary protection, to have an influenza vaccination in the fall. Because the medium used for the production of the flu vaccine is eggs, vaccination against influenza is not recommended for those individuals who are allergic to eggs. It is recommended that adults receive a tetanus-diphtheria booster shot every 10 years. Students, health workers, and military personnel are most likely to have had recent immunizations. People who have traveled abroad also are likely to have received immunizations, the types dependent on where they have traveled.

Allergies

Allergic responses to any substance, including drugs, food, pollen, clothing, and chemicals, should be explored.

- What type of allergic reactions did the client experience?
- Where and when did the allergic reaction occur?
- What was the number of allergic reactions?
- What was the treatment used? The results? What does the client do for relief of these allergies?

Information about allergies can be important in diagnosis and treatment of other disorders. For example, the client who has severe "hay fever" may be more susceptible to upper respiratory infections. Allergies to drugs (e.g., penicillin) or to preparations containing iodine or eggs are significant, as the client may be unable to be treated or tested with these substances.

Medical History, Surgical History, and Traumatic Injuries

All statements regarding past illnesses should be investigated thoroughly. These include symptoms, course of treatment, complications, and hospitalization. Many diseases have an acute phase earlier in life and then reappear at a later time. For example, an individual who had rheumatic fever as a child may now demonstrate such symptoms as shortness of breath, weakness, and swelling of ankles and feet.

- What were the major illnesses that the client experienced in his life?
- For what illnesses has the client gone to a physician or clinic?
- Has the client ever been hospitalized?

Inquiry regarding mental illness and emotional stress may be difficult. Often, clients will not volunteer such information, because mental illness is still considered by some to have a social stigma.

- Has the client ever had a nervous breakdown?
- Does the client have frequent crying spells?
- Has the client ever been depressed?
- Has the client had to deal with intense stress at any time in his lifetime?
- How does the client generally resolve stressful situations?
- Has the client received professional support in coping with emotional problems?

Information related to all past surgical procedures is an important part of the history.

- What kind of surgery has the client had?
- When (year or age) was each surgery done and where (in what institution)?
- How long was the recovery period after each surgery? Any complications?

Frequently, clients who have had surgery know little about the exact nature of the operation or the findings. Transcripts of the client's chart can be sought if more information is needed. This same kind of inquiry should be made regarding all major injuries.

- Has the client ever had any traumatic injuries, or has he been involved in any accidents?
- Was he ever seen or treated in an emergency room?
- Has the client ever had a blood transfusion? If so, when, why, how many, and were there any adverse reactions?

Inquire about any incidences of violence.

- Has the client ever been assaulted? Raped?
- Is he in a violent relationship?
- Has he had any counseling or treatment related to violence?

Every bit of information that the client is able to offer may have a bearing on the diagnosis and subsequent planning for the current problem. This information often is essential in evaluating the client's current situation.

Review of Systems

The purpose of the ROS is to ensure that no important clues have been overlooked by the client or nurse. If, in the history of current illness, you have already reviewed one or more systems, do not review them again. Some of the questions will seem repetitive and annoying to clients, so make sure you explain the purpose of the review. If the client identifies one or more symptoms that have not previously come to light, they should be explored in depth. The review should eventually be memorized, but the beginning nurse interviewer might use 3 × 5 cards for some assistance. The absence as well as the presence of symptoms should be recorded. In the example that follows, the review is stated in terms understandable to the general population. In the recording of these data, medical terminology is used, however, so medical terms are included within parentheses.

1. *General health.* Has the client currently or lately experienced any fever, chills, weight loss, tendency to fatigue easily, weakness, mood changes, night sweats, profuse perspiration (diaphoresis), intolerance to heat or cold, excessive thirst (polydipsia), increased appetite (polyphagia), or increased urination (polyuria)? A change in hat, glove, or shoe size? A tendency to easily bruise or bleeds? Transfusions?

2. *Skin, hair, and nails.* Has she had a history of skin diseases, changes in skin color (pigmentation), jaundice, excessive dryness or moisture, eczema, psoriasis, dandruff (seborrhea), lumps, hives, acne, rashes, bruising (ecchymosis), itching (pruritus), or moles (nevi) that have changed in color or size, open sores that are slow to heal, itchy scalp, frequent loss of hair, hirsutism, changes in hair texture or nail appearance, nail biting? Hygienic or cosmetic care

Checklist for Review of Systems

General health
Integument
Head and neck
Breasts
Respiratory
Cardiovascular
Gastrointestinal
Genitourinary
Gynecologic/obstetric
Musculoskeletal
Neurologic

patterns of skin, hair, and nails? Any necessary protective devices, such as sunscreen, protective clothing, gloves?

3. *Head.* Does the client experience unusually frequent or severe headaches, pain, convulsions, dizziness (vertigo), fainting (syncope), head injury (treatment, sequelae)? Use seatbelts, helmets, any other necessary protective devices?

4. *Eyes.* Is there a history of infections, discharge, injuries, visual changes, eye pain, double vision (diplopia), blurring, excessive tearing (lacrimation), pain when looking at light (photophobia), itching, spots in front of eyes, blind spots, flashing lights or halo-rainbows around objects? History of glaucoma or cataracts? Does she wear glasses? For near or far vision? Bifocals? When was her last eye examination? How often does she get her eyes examined? Any activity requiring safety glasses?

5. *Ears.* Is there a history of infections, loss of hearing, pain, discharge, ringing in the ears (tinnitus), hearing noises, dizziness (vertigo)? Care of ears and use of aids for hearing? Exposure to loud noise? Protective ear muffs/plugs needed?

6. *Nose, nasopharynx, and paranasal sinuses.* Is there a history of discharge, frequent colds, sneezing, nosebleeds (epistaxis), allergies, frequency of colds, sinus infections, hay fever, injury, loss or poor sense of smell, obstruction, postnasal drip, pain, tenderness?

7. *Mouth and throat.* Has the client experienced bleeding gums; frequent sore throat; soreness or lesion of the mouth, lips, or tongue; persistent white spots in the mouth; difficulty with taste, chewing, or swallowing (dysphagia); voice changes; hoarseness; toothaches; cavities (dental caries)? Does she wear dentures? When was her last dental appointment? What are her dental hygiene practices? How often does she go to the dentist?

8. *Neck.* Does the client experience pain, stiffness, lumps, swelling (edema), limitation of movement? Have a history of swollen glands, thyroid problems?

9. *Breasts.* Is there nipple discharge, scaling and cracks (fissures) around nipples, dimpling of skin, lumps, tenderness, pain (mastodynia), skin discoloration, or lesions? When was the last examination performed by an advance nurse practitioner or a physician? Does the client practice self breast examination? Mammography? Is there a history of breast-feeding, fibrocystic breast disease, breast cancer?

10. *Respiratory.* Has the client experienced persistent cough, frequent pneumonia, sputum (amount, color, consistency), shortness of breath (differentiate between dyspnea at rest and/or on exertion [how much exertion before becoming dyspneic?], orthopnea, and paroxysmal nocturnal dyspnea), pain in the chest, palpitation, fainting (syncope), wheezing, coughing up blood (hemoptysis)? Is there a history of asthma, pleurisy, bronchitis, TB? Does she know anyone with TB? Has she ever had a test for TB? Chest x-ray? When? Results? Smoking and exposure to secondhand smoke? Exposure to air pollutants? Any need or use of respiratory safety (e.g., mask)?

11. *Cardiovascular.* Has the client had chest pain, palpitations, high blood pressure, anemia, heart attack, Rheumatic fever, murmur, varicosities, an ECG? When? Results? Coolness or change of color of extremity? Cyanosis? Pain in lower extremities when walking? Varicose veins? History of sores that are slow to heal, leg ulcers, thrombophlebitis? Hair loss on legs? Results of cholesterol and lipid tests? When done?

12. *Gastrointestinal.* Has there been nausea, vomiting, loss of appetite (anorexia), indigestion (dyspepsia), heartburn (pyrosis), food intolerance, bright blood in stools, tarry black stools (melena or iron supplements)? When was the last hemoccult test? Results? Has there been rectal gas (flatulence), excessive belching of gas (eructation), change in abdominal size or shape, abdominal hernias, abdominal pain, diarrhea, constipation, piles (hemorrhoids), rectal pain? What are her bowel habits (every day, every third day, etc.), color of stool, consistency of stool (hard, soft, formed, liquid)? Any change in shape of stool (ball-, ribbon-shaped)? Laxative and antacid use? History of hepatitis, liver disease, gall bladder disease, ulcers, colitis?

13. *Genitourinary.* Does the client have frequency or urgency of urination, urination at night (nocturia), difficulty in starting stream, blood in urine (hematuria), dribbling, unable to control bladder (incontinent), flank pain or burning upon urination, excessive amounts of each urination (polyuria)? What is the color of urine? Urine odor? Is there a history of bladder/urinary infection, stones, bed wetting? Has she had a venereal disease (may need to be said in lay terms, i.e., "clap" or "morning drip" instead of gonorrhea, "bad blood" instead of syphillis)? If so, any treatment? Is she sexually active? Are condoms used? For male clients, any penile discharge? Able to have erection, ejaculation? Any lesions or discharge from penis? Scrotal enlargement, masses, hernias?

14. *Gynecologic and obstetric.* Obtain information concerning menarche (onset age of menstruation), last menstrual period, regularity of cycle, duration of menstrual flow, volume (amount) of daily flow, use of tampons or pads, painful menstruation (dysmenorrhea), bleeding between periods (metrorrhagia), excessive bleeding (menorrhagia), bleeding following intercourse, pain during intercourse (dyspareunia), vaginal discharge (color, amount, consistency), vaginal pruritus, number of pregnancies (para), live births (gravida), term deliveries, any labor or delivery or postdelivery (puerperium) complications, abortions (spontaneous or induced; gestation), stillbirths, method of birth control, menopause (symptoms, treatment), postmenopausal bleeding. When was the last pap smear? Results? Frequency of pap smears? Diethylstilbestrol exposure? Fertility problems? Able to enjoy sexual relations? Protective measures taken during coitus?

15. *Musculoskeletal.* Does the client experience muscular pain, stiffness, swelling, weakness, muscle twitching (fasciculations), soreness in joints, limitation of movement, leg

cramps? Have flat feet, back problems? Is there a history of arthritis, gout, broken bones (fractures), dislocations, sprains, deformities, congenital defects? Corrections? Is there use of proper body mechanics when bending over and lifting?

16. *Neurologic.* Has the client experienced unconsciousness, difficulty walking, nervousness, anxiety, convulsions/seizures, blackouts, dizziness (vertigo), fainting (syncope), pain in the arms or legs, paralysis, numbness, tingling, burning, "crawling" sensations (anywhere in body), decreased strength in arms or legs, weakness on one side of the body, unclear thinking, forgetfulness, disorientation, nightmares, tremors, mood changes, sleep disturbances, speech problems? Has there been exposure to toxic substances?

Client Profile

The client profile is a brief summary of your impression of the client based on the information obtained during the process of gathering the health history. It serves to personalize the data and to communicate a concise picture of the total person. Examples of client profiles are given in Fig. 4-5.

Client profile: Ms. J. is a 29-year-old Caucasian woman who appeared anxious during the interview. This was noted in her inability to maintain eye contact and constant wringing of her hands. She expressed concern because she has no health insurance.

Client profile: Mr. G. is a 38-year-old Black male who appeared calm and comfortable during the interview. He has a good understanding of his current health status. His reason for seeking health assessment is for health maintenance.

Figure 4-5 Examples of client profiles.

Checklist for Health History

1. Biographical Data
   - Name
   - Address
   - Sex
   - Age/birth date
   - Marital status/compatibility and adjustment
   - Current occupation
   - Religion/practice and attitude toward religion
   - Race
   - Ethnic origin
   - Level of education/ability to read and write
   - Health history informant and reliability
2. Reason for Seeking Health Evaluation or Chief Complaint
   - Annual check-up
   - Employment health clearance
   - Follow-up care and evaluation
   - Signs and symptoms that led client to seek health care
   - Monitoring of existing health problem(s)
3. Current Health Status or History of Present Illness
   - Location
   - Quality
   - Quantity
   - Chronology
   - Setting
   - Aggravating and alleviating factors
   - Associated manifestations
   - Effect on ADLs and other life areas
   - Review of relevant body system(s)
4. Personal History and Patterns of Living
   - Occupational history
   - Financial status
   - Family history of illness/past and present
   - Pertinent negatives of specific illness in family
   - Example: No history of hypertension, strokes, TB, ulcers, mental illness, alcoholism, epilepsy, gout, bleeding disorders

Significant for diabetes, heart disease, cancer, arthritis, ulcerative colitis

Geographic exposure
- Places
- Date and length of time

Lifestyle
- Personal habits
  - Smoking—type and pack years
  - Alcohol—type and amount
  - Drugs—type, amount, and pattern of use
- Diet
  - Mealtimes
  - Prepared by
  - Special diet/type and when started
  - Vitamins and/or diet pills
  - Specific difficulties
- Sleep and rest patterns
  - Hours of sleep and awakening
  - Naps
  - Difficulties/remedies tried
- Activities of daily living
- Home and neighborhood
  - Living arrangements/resources
  - Quality of interpersonal relationships
- Recreation/hobbies
- Sexuality
  - Values
  - Self-image
  - Sexual functioning
  - Sexual problems

5. Previous Experience with Illness
   - Childhood illnesses
   - Immunizations
   - Allergies—type, response, treatment
   - Past illnesses
   - Surgery
   - Blood transfusions
   - Trauma
6. Review of Systems
   - General health
   - Integument
   - Head and neck
   - Breasts
   - Respiratory
   - Cardiovascular
   - Gastrointestinal
   - Genitourinary
   - Gynecologic/obstetric
   - Musculoskeletal
   - Neurologic
7. Client Profile

Name: Mary Jones

Address: 234 Any Street, Anytown, Anystate

Sex: Female

Age: 35

Birthday: 7/17/63

Marital status: Married—states "happily married"

Occupation: Part-time clerk in variety store

Religion: Protestant (attends church on irregular basis)

Race: Caucasian

Ethnic origin: Polish

Education: High school graduate (plans to take college courses when children get in high school)

Informant: Client; reliable historian

Chief concern: Lump in left breast of 2 days' duration

History of present illness: Client first noticed lump in left breast 2 days ago while bathing. Denies pain or tenderness. No history of trauma to the area. Describes lump as being soft and about the size of peach pit. States there has been no change in the size of her breasts and no skin discoloration. Denies nipple drainage. Very anxious concerning the lump as mother died of breast cancer in 1975. Client feels she is in good health except for the lump. Knowledgeable of SBE procedure but does it sporadically. Sees physician or nurse practitioner at the HMO only when she has a health problem.

Personal history and patterns of living: Has worked part-time as a clerk in a variety store for 4 years (yard goods dept.). Prior to this time remained home caring for family since birth of first child in 1984. Two children: boy 14 yrs and girl 11 yrs. Husband employed at steel company (salary: $39,500). Her salary: $8,000. Describes financial status as adequate for personal and family needs. Two-car family with $56,000 house mortgage. No other large debts. Blue Cross and Blue Shield health insurance.

Family health history: Denies family history of diabetes, arthritis, TB, alcoholism, bleeding disorders, mental illness, stomach problems, liver disorders, kidney

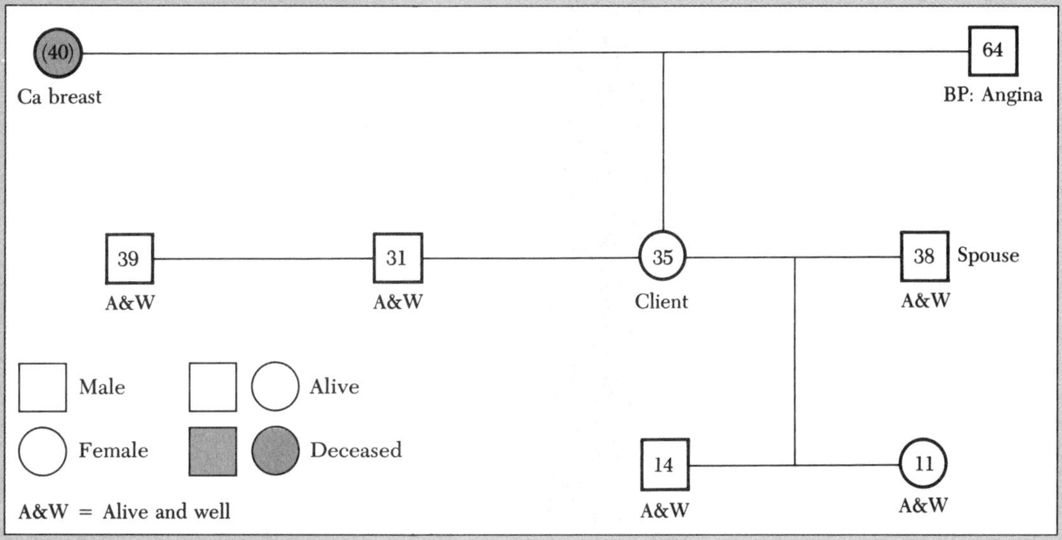

diseases. Family history significant for cancer, heart disease, hypertension.

Geographic exposure: Has never traveled out of state.

Lifestyle:

1. Personal habits—Smokes 1½ ppd (25½ pk yrs). Beer or whiskey 2–4 × /mo—no more than 3 drinks at the most. Takes OTC cold pills (2 × /yr) when necessary. ASA for headache 2–4 × /yr; Caffeine: coffee—4 cups/day; coke—2 bottles/day. Has never experimented with recreational drugs. Is not on any prescription drugs.

2. Diet—Client does most of cooking. Family eats three meals/day. Breakfast—fruit, coffee, toast. Lunch—(brown bag) sandwich, cookies; buys ice cream and coke in vending machine. Dinner—red meat 2–3 × /wk; poultry, fish 4–5 × /wk; potatoes or noodles, bread, vegetable (beans, peas), dessert (cookies, cake) almost every night. Family usually snacks at bedtime (crackers, chips). Denies dieting or use of diet pills. Can eat almost anything and doesn't gain weight. Occasionally takes multi-vits during cold weather. No apparent difficulty with diet, i.e., no indigestion or swallowing difficulties.

3. Sleep and rest patterns—Denies any sleeping difficulties in general but since discovery of lump in breast has awakened several times in the past night and had difficulty falling back asleep. Usually sleeps 7½–8 hrs/day and feels rested upon awakening.

4. Activities of daily living—No difficulties caring for self and carrying out her responsibilities of living.

5. Home and neighborhood—Home in middle-class neighborhood. Living arrangements more than sufficient for family needs (2 bathrooms; each child has own bedroom).

6. Interpersonal relationships—Describes family relationships as close and very good. No family tensions. Keeps close to extended family members on both sides of the family. Annual family reunions.

7. Recreation—No regular active recreation. Watches TV most evenings. Picnics on Sunday afternoons during the summer months. Likes to knit.

8. Sexuality—Traditional values of monogamy. Husband has been sole sexual partner since their marriage 15 yrs ago. Satisfactory sexual activity—no expressed difficulties; however, now worried about image as woman as she states, "I am worried how my husband will react if I must have a mastectomy." States "loving relationship" and considers husband her best friend.

Previous experience with illness:

Childhood illnesses: Measles, chickenpox, scarlet fever, rheumatic fever (not sure of exact age—10?).

Immunizations: Smallpox (age 6); polio vaccine (1969).

Allergies: Denies any known allergies.

Past illness, injuries, surgery: No significant illnesses or injuries until car accident (1988) in which she sustained concussion, broken nose, and multiple bruises to both legs. Was hospitalized 2 days at Community General Hospital (CGH). Appendectomy (1985), discharged in 3 days from CGH. No complications. Never had any blood transfusions.

Review of systems:

1. General health—Denies fever, chills, weight loss, fatigue, weakness, changes in mood, night sweats, diaphoresis, intolerance to cold, polydipsia, polyphagia,

Example of a Health History (continued)

polyuria, being easily bruised, bleeding tendencies, and change in size of hat, gloves, or shoes.

2. Integument—No hx of skin diseases. Denies any changes in skin pigmentation, excessive dryness or moisture, jaundice, eczema, psoriasis or seborrhea, hives, acne, rashes, ecchymosis, pruritus, nevi that have changed in color or size, open sores that are slow to heal, itchy scalp, frequent loss of hair, and nail biting. Uses moisturizing body lotion after A.M. shower. Washes hair qd and uses hair conditioner. Keeps hair short and rarely has permanents—none for the last 6–8 yrs. "Treats" self to nail manicure q 2–3 mo at local department store. Fair skin—uses sunscreen, long sleeves, and hat protection. Hx of severe sunburns of shoulders as a child and teenager.

3. Head—Denies unusually frequent or severe headaches, vertigo, syncope, and seizures. Concussion (1988)—see past injuries (car accident).

4. Eyes—No hx of infections or pain. Wears eyeglasses for close work. Last eye exam 1995. Denies diplopia, blurring, excessive lacrimation, photophobia, pruritus, and spots before eyes or halo-rainbows about lights. Has eye exam q 2 yrs. No hx of glaucoma or cataracts.

5. Ears—No hx of infections. Denies loss of hearing, pain, discharge, tinnitus, auditory hallucinations, and vertigo. Uses OTC medication for effectively cleaning out ear wax q 2–3 yrs—when she notices her hearing is decreased.

6. Nose, nasopharynx, and paranasal sinuses—No discharge, colds 1–2×/yr. Denies sneezing, epistaxis, allergies, loss of smell, obstruction, postnasal drip, pain, and tenderness.

7. Mouth and throat—Denies bleeding gums; frequent sore throat; soreness or persistent white spots in or around mouth, lips, or tongue; dysphagia; voice change; hoarseness; toothaches; dentures. Last dentist appointment—can't remember: "long ago." Visits dentist only when experiencing dental "problems." Uses antiplaque solution and brushes and flosses every A.M.

8. Neck—Denies pain, masses, edema, stiffness, limitation of movement. No hx of swollen glands or thyroid problems.

9. Breasts—(see HPI).

10. Respiratory system—Nonproductive morning cough since 1987. Last chest x-ray in 1988 (neg.). Denies sputum, shortness of breath, wheezing, hemoptysis, or contact with anyone having TB. No hx of pneumonia or bronchitis. No exposure to air pollutants. Workplace has no smoking, and husband doesn't smoke—very little exposure to second-hand smoke. Does not smoke around her children.

11. Cardiovascular system—Denies chest pain, palpitation, syncope, dyspnea, orthopnea, and PND. Never had anemia, heart attack, high blood pressure, clots, phlebitis, or varicosities. Was told she had slight murmur when given physical examination in high school; no follow-up on this was ever done. Never had an ECG.

12. Gastrointestinal system—Denies nausea and vomiting, anorexia, dyspepsia, pyrosis, food intolerance, bright blood in stools, melena, flatulence, excessive eructation, pain, hemorrhoids, and rectal pain. Soft, formed brown stool q AM after hot coffee. Never uses laxatives or antacids. Has not had gall bladder or liver disease, ulcers, or colitis.

13. Genitourinary system—Denies frequency, urgency, nocturia, difficulty in starting stream, hematuria, dribbling, incontinence, pain or burning upon urination, polyuria, and VD. Does not have a hx of bladder/urinary infections or kidney stones. Urine is light yellow with no noticeable odor. Sexually active 2×/wk and is satisfied with sex life. No known exposure to anyone HIV+.

14. Gynecologic and obstetric—Menarche age 12. LMP 2122187. Reg. 28-day cycle. Flow duration of 5 days—1st day heavy flow (4 pads) (avg. 3 tampons other days). Denies dysmenorrhea, metrorrhagia, menorrhagia, dyspareunia, bleeding following intercourse, vaginal discharge, or pruritus. Para 2, gravida 2. Term deliveries—No labor or puerperal complications. No abortions. No exposure to DES. Birth control—uses diaphragm.

15. Musculoskeletal system—Denies muscular pain, stiffness, edema, weakness, faciculations, joint soreness or pain, leg cramps, flat feet, back problems, arthritis, gout, fractures (other than nose in 1988 car accident), dislocation, sprains, and congenital defects.

16. Neurologic system—No hx of unconsciousness. Denies difficulty walking, convulsions, vertigo, pain in arms or legs, numbness, paralysis, tingling or burning anywhere in body, decreased strength in arms or legs, weakness in one part of the body, nightmares, tremors, changes in emotional states, and speech problems. Has felt nervous and anxious past 2 days since discovered lump in breast. Some forgetfulness attributed to anxiety manifested during these past 2 days. No known exposure to toxic substances.

Client profile: Ms. Mary Jones, 35-year-old woman, appears apprehensive. Speech is rapid; logical thought processes. Tears in eyes. Very concerned about breast lump due to mother's cancer of breast and subsequent death at age 40. Otherwise appears in good health generally. Seems anxious for help.

SUMMARY

In this chapter, the health history was discussed in detail. Elements of the client interview and the components of the health history were presented, as well as the rationale and techniques for careful recording of biographical data and the chief complaint. Guidelines to enhance the investigation of signs and symptoms were discussed. Emphasis was placed on the sensitivity needed in exploring the personal history and the specific areas within this portion of the history. This chapter concluded with discussion of the investigation of previous experiences with illness and a detailed description of the ROS. The information gathered in each of the component areas of the health history is useful for interpreting the client's present status, making nursing diagnoses, and planning individualized nursing care. An example of a completed health history was presented.

DISCUSSION QUESTIONS/ ACTIVITIES

1. What is the purpose of the health history?
2. Give examples to demonstrate the use and purpose of the specific information included in the biographical data section of the health history.
3. Describe how the chief complaint is recorded.
4. List and discuss each of Morgan and Engel's seven variables of investigating present illness.
5. Document the following chief complaints, using hypothetical information that reflects the inclusion of the variables of investigation: headache, vomiting, diarrhea, shortness of breath, and rash.
6. What information would you obtain relating to the client's personal history and patterns of living?
7. What is the rationale for the ROS?
8. Why is it important to identify pertinent negatives in the recording of health history, particularly with the ROS and the family health history?
9. Role-play (and videotape, if possible) portions of a history-taking interaction with a client; then critique it. This exercise could be done on an individual basis or in a class session.

REFERENCES

Bellack, J. P., and Bamford, P. A. 1984. *Nursing assessment: a multidimensional approach.* Boston: Jones and Bartlett.

Ebersole, P., and Hess, P. 1981. *Toward healthy aging.* St. Louis: C. V. Mosby.

Griggs, W. 1978. Sex and the elderly. *Am. J. Nurs.* 77:1352–1354.

Hui, Y. H. 1983. *Human nutrition and diet therapy.* Boston: Jones and Bartlett.

Maslow, A. H. 1954. *Motivation and personality.* New York: Harper & Row.

Morgan, W. L., and Engel, G. I. 1969. *The clinical approach to the patient.* Philadelphia: W. B. Saunders.

Servonsky, J., and Opas, S. 1987. *Nursing management of children.* Boston: Jones and Bartlett.

PART II

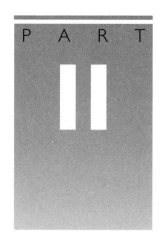

Systems Assessment

CHAPTER

5 Introduction to Physical Assessment

Learning Objectives

1. Recognize that senses can be sharpened to enhance the physical assessment process.
2. Identify general principles of the physical assessment modes of inspection, palpation, percussion, and auscultation.
3. State the areas of the hand best used for the assessment of skin temperature, vibration, and the characteristics of texture, moisture, shape, and consistency.
4. Describe the correct technique used to percuss.
5. Name the various notes produced by percussion.
6. List the components of a general impression.
7. Describe general principles used in the approach to a client to perform a physical assessment.

A complete physical assessment serves as a screening device for detecting abnormalities that are unknown to the client and for identifying signs that may suggest illness or deformity. The findings may serve as support to validate problems suspected from the client's history. The historical information helps you zero in on relevant observations of physical assessment when time is limited for examination.

CULTIVATING THE SENSES

Every minute of every day you are gathering data via your sensory system. You see, touch, hear, smell, and taste. It is these senses that are used in the data-gathering process of physical assessment. The sense of taste was skillfully applied in ancient times—to detect glycosuria, for example. A glass catheter was used to obtain a sterile urine specimen, which was then tasted to detect whether a sweetness was present. Today this means of data gathering has been replaced by laboratory tests.

You must recognize that each of your senses can be cultivated. You need only look about you for evidence—the wine taster who has groomed his ability to taste and smell, the musician who has refined his tone and pitch consciousness. The findings gathered by each sense are made meaningful by association to background knowledge; thus, it is practice and experience, coupled with background knowledge, that will lead to the cultivation of your senses for more effective use in physical assessment.

Throughout the process of physical assessment, your senses of smell, sight, hearing, and touch are concentrated on the client. Most of the nursing literature overlooks the sense of smell, perhaps because the use of this sense requires some sophistication. There is only one ground rule in using smell in assessment: If you detect a peculiar odor that is out of the limits of the normal, you should investigate it further and seek consultation if in doubt.

Although the whys and the wherefores of specific odors are beyond the scope of this text, a few examples are helpful:

1. *Skin odors.* The sense of smell can give you clues about the client's hygiene or body functioning. The client may emit a strong body odor or scents of urine or feces. Immediate conclusions might be that the client does not bathe too frequently or too efficiently or, in the case of the odors of urine or feces, that the client is incontinent. It is necessary to investigate further and to validate any assumptions with the client or with a significant other. It may well be that the client practices good hygiene but that he does not use an effective deodorant or that it is the client's clothing that contains the odor. Clothing, especially wool sweaters and suit jackets, become permeated with body odor, and you may need to recommend more frequent cleaning of clothes. Incontinence is not the only cause of urine or fecal odors—the individual may have been holding an infant whose diaper proved insufficient. And, of course, these odors may be quite normal from a younger child who is still learning to control his normal physiologic functioning. More seriously, though, an ammoniacal skin odor may indicate severe renal dysfunction (uremia).
2. *Mouth odors.* Halitosis (bad breath) can result from dental caries or from dyspepsia. Alcohol may be detected on the breath. A sweet, juicy-fruit breath odor may result from the ketoacidosis of diabetic coma or from prolonged use of starvation diets. Foul-smelling sputum may indicate a pharyngeal or lung abscess or bronchiectasis.
3. *Body secretion odors.* Feces that have a foul-smelling, penetrating, pungent odor are commonly found with biliary tract problems (gallbladder or pancreatic dysfunction) and with malabsorption syndrome. A strong ammoniacal odor of the urine may indicate fermentation within the bladder.
4. *Vomitus and pus odors.* Sour-smelling, fermented emesis may indicate food retained in the stomach for a prolonged period or increased gastric acidity. Fecal-smelling vomitus is observed with prolonged vomiting in peritonitis and in intestinal obstruction. The odor of alcohol as well as phenol and other poisons and irritants may be present in vomitus. Purulent material with an odor similar to strong-smelling cheese may be found in abscesses or cysts containing proteolytic bacteria. A nauseating, sweet smell of pus occurs with pseudomonas infections, and a pungent, sweet odor (similar to the smell of rotting apples) occurs with gas gangrene.

TECHNIQUES OF ASSESSMENT

Four basic methods are used to systematically guide the uses of the remaining senses of sight, touch, and hearing in physical assessment. They are *inspection, palpation, percussion,* and *auscultation.*

Inspection

Inspection is the visual scrutiny of the client that begins at the first moment of contact. All observations must be conducted with adequate lighting, and as the physical assessment proceeds, each bodily area examined must be adequately exposed. To effectively use the method of inspection, you must train your sense of sight to focus on detail. The more knowledge and clinical practice you accrue, the more you will improve your ability of inspection.

As you examine the client, you should compare the two sides of her body. Normally, there are slight deviations between the left and right sides of the body, but general symmetry should prevail upon inspection.

With its variety of lenses, the use of the ophthalmoscope enhances the examination performed by the naked eye. Additional facilitating instruments include speculums (nasal, vaginal), mirrors (head reflector, pharyngeal), and additional sources of light (penlight). Also, the use of x-rays, ECG, and other laboratory tests is a common means of extending the process of inspection.

Palpation

Palpation employs your sense of touch. The roughness, smoothness, hardness, softness, moistness, dryness, motility, and configuration of a body surface or of a nodule or mass can be determined by touch. The tactile sense also reveals the temperature of a given part (such as the coolness of an area of arterial insufficiency). Palpation can also inform you of vibrations (such as the presence of a cardiac thrill or of fremitus) and of position.

Because prolonged heavy pressure on the fingertips can dull your tactile sensitivity, light palpation is used for the majority of the examination. It is through light palpation that areas of tenderness may be elicited; these areas should be carefully examined last, in order not to aggravate pain and interfere with the further gathering of pertinent data. The most sensitive area of your hand is the fingertips, but the dorsum of the hand is more sensitive to temperature because the skin is much thinner there. The palmar aspects of the fingers best detect the presence of vibration (Fig. 5-1). Other palpation techniques are deep palpation and bimanual palpation. These techniques are described in appropriate portions of the text where their use in the assessment process is necessary.

Percussion

Percussion is the striking of a body surface area, noting the "feel" and sounds produced. An evaluation of the underlying structures can be made by interpreting the quality of such

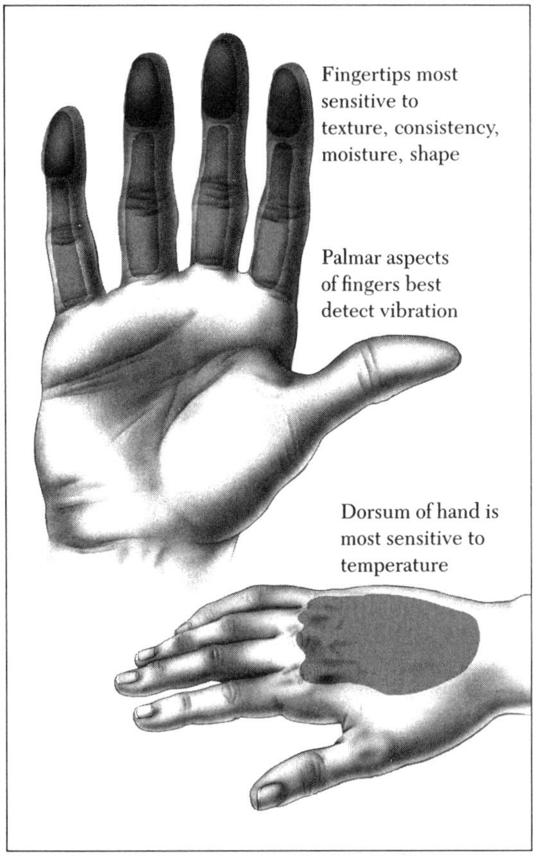
Fingertips most sensitive to texture, consistency, moisture, shape
Palmar aspects of fingers best detect vibration
Dorsum of hand is most sensitive to temperature

Figure 5-1 Sensitive areas of the hand.

stimuli, which vary according to density. There are two basic types of percussion: direct and indirect.

In the direct technique, the body is lightly tapped directly with the fingers or hand. This technique is usually employed when seeking areas of tenderness. Light percussion may aid not only in identifying areas of tenderness but also in differentiating superficial from deep pain. Tapping over an infected sinus will produce pain, as will a blunt but light blow over an infected kidney. A sharp quick blow with a percussion hammer over a tendon will elicit a reflex (the evaluation of reflexes is an essential part of neurologic assessment).

The indirect method is done bimanually. For indirect percussion to be performed properly, the fingernail of the *plexor* should be trimmed short. This protects the *pleximeter* from injury and produces a much better sound quality than using a pad for percussion. Generally, the pleximeter of the left hand (vice versa for those who are left-handed) is placed firmly on the surface to be percussed. The remaining fingers and the palm of the hand are raised off the area. If the hand or other fingers are allowed to rest on the surface, the sound vibrations will be dampened, much like a drumroll is muffled when a hand is placed on the drumhead. The bull's-eye area of the pleximeter (the distal phalanx) is struck by the tip of the plexor of the right hand. A light tap is best. Some individuals find that using the index and middle fingers together as plexors or striking the pleximeter with the narrow point of a percussion hammer proves to be the best method for them. Wrist action is the salient feature of any technique for producing good quality percussion notes. The elbow and shoulder should not move during the delivery of the necessary brisk, staccato blow—only the wrist should move. Action is much like the wrist action used in spinning a yo-yo.

To reach a point at which you can easily and comfortably perform this technique, and to grasp the concept of the changing vibrations and tones that reflect the underlying density of structure, you may want to initially practice percussion techniques on the wall of a room. As you proceed along the wall, you can hear the difference in vibrations and sound as you meet a studboard behind the wall. The more solid the underlying structure, the lesser the vibrations and the shorter the duration of the percussion note. A more solid structure will also have a higher-pitched note on percussion. Thus, percussion notes can be arranged according to the density that produces them (Fig. 5-2). The classifications of the percussion notes in Table 5-1 are arranged from the most dense to the least dense underlying body structures. Such classification of percussion notes and vibrations will not take on any real significance until you couple this knowledge with actual practice.

The technique of percussion can be used to detect painful body areas, to map out the size of areas of greater density (liver, spleen, tumors, fluid), and to identify the location of the lung bases as well as ascertain diaphragmatic excursion (an indirect measurement of lung inflation). You will need

Most dense tissue				Least dense tissue
Flat	Dull	Resonant	Hyperresonant	Tympanic

Figure 5-2 The continuum of percussion notes.

Table 5-1 Classification of Percussion Notes

	Intensity	Pitch	Duration	Area or organ where percussion sound may occur
Flat	Soft	High	Short	Muscle, bone, thigh
Dull	Medium	Medium	Medium	Liver, spleen
Resonant	Loud	Low	Long	Lung
Hyperresonant	Very loud	Very low	Very long	Emphysematous lung
Tympanic	Loud	High	Medium	Gastric air bubble

a flexible plastic ruler or a tape measure in centimeters to describe the size of masses and to measure organ sizes percussed. It is also important to realize that the percussion technique is not as helpful with obese individuals, as most general organ structures or masses over a depth of 5 cm go undetected.

Auscultation

Auscultation is the process of listening to sounds produced within the body. Before the advent of the stethoscope, auscultation was done by applying the examiner's ear directly against the client's body; important information went undetected with this method. An adequate stethoscope about 30 to 35 cm long and about 0.3 cm internal lumen diameter, with both *diaphragm* and *bell* (Fig. 5-3), will enable you to appreciate the method of clinical auscultation. A stethoscope without these qualities will be good for listening only to blood pressure readings. In general, the diaphragm best transmits high-pitched sounds, whereas the bell best transmits low-pitched sounds. Thus, breath sounds, friction rubs, heart sounds, bowel sounds, and crepitus are best heard with the diaphragm, while bruits (pronounced "bru-ees") of stenotic arteries, heart murmurs, and venous hums are best detected with the bell.

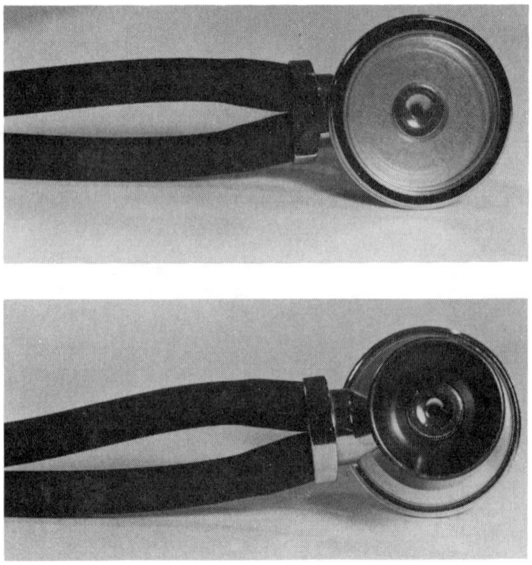

Figure 5-3 Stethoscope with diaphragm *(top)* and bell *(bottom)*.

A comfortable and properly fitting stethoscope is paramount. A poorly fitting stethoscope will be as good as a poorly fitting pair of shoes. Because stethoscope earplugs are interchangeable, you should try various sizes to identify your correct size. The soft rubber earplugs are usually considered the most comfortable because of their flexibility, but this is an individual preference. The two metal tubular portions of the stethoscope should be bent slightly with a pair of pliers so that they comfortably fit the angle of your external auditory canals. The metal span tension should be adjusted by manually bending the earpieces closer together or farther apart until the earplugs fit snugly and comfortably. Such fitting of the stethoscope to the individual is necessary for comfortable and efficient use.

APPROACHING THE CLIENT

The practice of washing one's hands before and after performing an assessment should be strictly followed and should preferably take place in the client's presence, thus conveying an attitude of cleanliness and protection. You can express thoughtfulness for the client's comfort by using warm water and by making appropriate remarks suggesting your recognition of the discomfort derived from the "cold hands" of an examiner. It may be necessary that you wear gloves, masks, gowns, and caps and that you take necessary precautions for the use and care of equipment used in the examination. Their use is dependent on whether contact with blood and bodily fluids is a potential and on the specific condition of the client. The same consideration is shown by warming the stethoscope with your hands before applying it to the client's body. A proper physical environment and appropriately applied clothing (examination gown, drapes, and so on) are necessary to provide privacy for the client. The room should be decently soundproof, quiet, warm, properly screened, and well-lighted. Natural light is superior to artificial light for examination and should be used whenever possible.

An unhurried atmosphere accompanied by a warm, personable client-centered approach is best. The examination should not be prolonged, nor should it be performed in such a rush as to sacrifice effectiveness. If a client is seriously ill, attend to the most pertinent portions of the physical assessment first. Provide rest periods if the client becomes fatigued.

Position of the client is important to the performance of the physical examination. A very ill client may not be able to be in a tiring or uncomfortable position for a prolonged period or to be able to switch back and forth from lying to sitting positions. Therefore, as you perform the examination, you will need to organize portions that can be done with the client in one position before having the client change positions. This decreases the frequency with which the client needs to be changing positions and will be less tiring. Summaries of your position as the examiner and the client's position, whether the client is ambulatory or bed-bound, are provided in Tables 5-2 and 5-3.

At the beginning of the examination, you should explain generally what is to be done. Periodically throughout the examination, instruct the client on how to cooperate, and give a step-by-step explanation of your actions. You need to be careful to use language that is understandable to the client and to avoid ill-founded comments of reassurance. Instruct the client at the onset to inform you if he should become tired or experience any pain. In addition, forewarn the client if a specific procedure may be uncomfortable or hurt. Honesty is the best policy for establishing and maintaining a trustful nurse-client relationship. If it is necessary for a client to undergo an uncomfortable or painful procedure, it is helpful to defer it until the end of the physical assessment process.

An effective physical assessment requires that the portion of the client's body being examined be adequately exposed. At the same time, the client must be protected from drafts and overexposure. It is of prime importance that the client's comfort level, physically and psychologically, be monitored carefully throughout the entire health assessment, as well as during the physical examination.

Table 5-2 A Summary of the Examiner's and Patient's Positions during the Physical Examination

	The ambulatory patient	
Region	The examiner's position	The patient's position
1. General inspection and vital signs	Standing before the patient and moving as needed	Sitting, or lying on the bed or examining table
2. The head	Standing, facing the patient	Sitting on the side of the bed or examining table
3. The neck	Standing, facing the patient, then moving behind him	Sitting on the side of the bed or examining table
4. The back; posterior thorax and lungs	Standing behind the patient	Sitting on the side of the bed or examining table
5. The anterior thorax and lungs	Standing, facing the patient	Sitting on the side of the bed or examining table
6. The breasts and axillary regions	Initially facing the patient, then examining from the patient's right side	Sitting, facing the examiner, then lying supine
7. The heart	Standing at the patient's right	In three positions: sitting, lying on his back, and on his left side
8. The abdomen	Standing at the patient's right	Lying on his back
9. The extremities	Standing, facing the patient, and moving to the patient's right	Lying flat, then sitting on the side of the bed, and finally standing
10. The male external genitalia	Standing before the patient and slightly to his right	Standing, facing the examiner
11. The female genital tract	Sitting on a stool facing the perineum, and standing for part of the examination	Lying on her back on an examining table with both knees flexed and her feet in stirrups
12. The rectum	Standing, facing the buttocks	Bending at the hips over the bed or examining table. The woman retains the same position used in the examination of the genital tract

Source: W. Morgan and G. Engel, *The Clinical Approach to the Patient,* Philadelphia: W.B. Saunders Company, 1969.

Table 5-3 A Summary of the Examiner's and Patient's Positions during the Physical Examination

Region	The bed-bound patient	
	The examiner's position	The patient's position
1. General inspection and vital signs	Standing at the foot of the bed	Lying on his back with the head of the bed slightly elevated
2. The head	Standing at the right side of the bed, then moving to the left side	Lying on his back with the head of the bed slightly elevated
3. The neck	Standing at the right side of the bed	Lying on his back with the head of the bed slightly elevated
4. The back; posterior thorax and lungs	Standing at the right side of the bed, examining across the bed, or from the right posterior oblique side of the chest	Sitting on the left side of the bed with his back to the examiner or sitting up in bed with assistance
5. The anterior thorax and lungs	Standing at the right side of the bed	Lying on his back
6. The breasts and axillary regions	Standing at the right side of the bed	Lying on his back
7. The heart	Standing at the right side of the bed	In three positions: lying on his back, on his left side, and sitting
8. The abdomen	Standing at the right side of the bed	Lying on his back
9. The extremities	Standing at the right side of the bed	Lying flat on his back, then on his abdomen: if able, sitting on the side of the bed facing the examiner
10. The male external genitalia	Standing at the right side of the bed	Lying on his back
11. The female genital tract	Sitting on a stool facing the perineum, and standing for part of the examination	Lying on her back obliquely across the bed, with both legs flexed
12. The rectum	Standing at the right side of the bed	Lying on his left side with both legs flexed at the hip

Source: W. Morgan and G. Engel, *The Clinical Approach to the Patient,* Philadelphia: W.B. Saunders Company, 1969.

These techniques for securing an effective physical assessment and for providing client comfort during the process are presented for a specific purpose—improving the delivery of health care services provided by nurses. It is not unusual to hear clients speak of past experiences in which they were treated impersonally or were made either psychologically or physiologically uncomfortable. Clients complain that their bodies and their care are fragmented—that health personnel are interested only in body "parts," not in them as a person, as a "whole." Is it any wonder that in order to get attention a psychosomatic individual will complain of body dysfunction or a lonely institutionalized client will use the ploy of pain or illness to get the nurse to his bedside?

Clients reveal that they have often felt like a "number" or one of a group of herded cattle. Some say they have received the impression that they are bothersome and have been hurried through on that account. Others tell of frightening experiences as a child, such as "surprise attacks" with painful procedures or an aggressive, rough-handling examiner. Many clients describe experiences of uncomfortableness, running the gamut from "cold hands" to lack of privacy to no explanations. Do you need to be reminded that an explanation couched in technical terms is as good as no explanation?

Purposeful planning is imperative in order to avoid reinforcement of such negative feelings and to eliminate such impersonal or uncomfortable experiences for clients in the future. It is trusted that all nurses appreciate the importance of physical and psychological comfort for the client during health assessment and to place emphasis on its provision.

DEVELOPING A GENERAL IMPRESSION

Your general impression of the client begins to form during the initial observation. It is representative of your opinion of the client's overall appearance. Despite the inclusion of objective data, the general impression is nevertheless your interpretation of the client as a whole and therefore somewhat subjective. Much of the information discussed in Chapter 3 is recorded in the general impression, especially if it is within normal range. If the mental health assessment reveals problems requiring nursing interventions, the general impression may be of considerable length, or a separate report, under the title "mental health or psychological assessment," may be warranted. This latter approach is used particularly when a standardized record form limits the space provided for the recording of the general impression (although some standardized record forms have a specific heading and space provided for psychological assessment). The basic elements usually included in the recording of a general impression are state of consciousness, age, race, sex, development, nutritional state, general state of health, gross abnormalities, striking features, height, weight, and vital signs.

The following discussion of the basic elements provides the rationale for their inclusion and gives examples to aid you in constructing a general impression. By no means are the examples comprehensive, nor is it necessary that all the elements be included in every case. The general impression usually consists of from one to five sentences, so the elements must be stated briefly and succinctly.

State of Consciousness

Terms used to describe the client's conscious state include *alert; lethargic; dull; slow or quick to respond; disoriented to person, place, or time; responsive only to pain;* and *comatose.* Evaluation of the state of consciousness is an important determinant of the approach to be taken with the particular client and of other specific nursing interventions.

Age

Chronologic age is given, if known. Some pathologies are predominant in certain age categories. Obvious examples would be the diseases of childhood (measles, mumps, chickenpox); Perthes' disease, anorexia nervosa, and acne of adolescence; myocardial infarction and gallbladder dysfunction of middle age; and arthritis, diabetes, peripheral vascular diseases, and depression of old age. Knowing the connections between age and disease not only facilitates diagnostic conclusions but also enables you to anticipate possible difficulties and to conduct appropriate preventive health teaching.

You should note whether the client appears to be her stated age or whether she appears older or younger than her chronologic age. Frequently, clients who are alcoholics, who are severely debilitated, or who may be harboring a chronic illness appear to be much older than their actual age.

Race

Knowledge of race directs your attention toward investigating possible racial customs—an important constituent of client data that is necessary to considering the client as an individual when planning nursing care. As with age, there are pathologies that are predominantly found in particular races. For example, there is a higher incidence of skin cancer among whites and a higher incidence of sickle-cell anemia among individuals of African ancestry.

Sex

A client's sex may make her more prone to develop certain diseases. For example, men are more prone to develop gastric ulcers and myocardial infarctions, whereas women are more prone to develop breast carcinoma. Young women are more prone to develop anorexia nervosa, whereas young men are more prone to develop Perthes' disease. Certain pathologies of the gonads are sex-specific, such as epididymitis, prostatitis, and priapism in men, and salpingitis, ovarian cysts, and fibroid uterus in women. Some conditions are genetically sex-linked, such as hemophilia and color blindness, both of which result from a recessive gene carried only on the X chromosome. Such conditions occur primarily in males and are transmitted by normal heterozygous women who carry the recessive gene.

Development

To assess the development of a child, you need to have background knowledge of the normal growth and development phases of the early years of life, because marked changes in both mental and physical abilities occur over a short period. A condensed table of age-related developmental abilities and stages is provided in Appendix C. One of the most common screening tools, used with children up to the age of 7, is the Denver Developmental Screening Test (included in Chapter 18). The developmental testing of the child is usually done at the conclusion of the interview and prior to the physical examination. This sequence often aids in establishing a working relationship with the child prior to the physical examination and results in subsequent cooperation. If a sibling is present for health assessment, begin with the older child, who is more likely to cooperate. The older child will generally set a good example for the younger to follow.

For adults, development generally means physical maturation or normal body growth (height, symmetry) and the presence of secondary sex characteristics.

Many developmental abnormalities are results of dysfunction of or damage to the adenohypophysis (anterior lobe of the pituitary gland). The adenohypophysis releases four hormones that stimulate target areas of the body (the target area of each is within parentheses): thyrotropin (thyroid), gonadotropin (sex organs), adrenocorticotropin (adrenal cortex), and somatotropin (general growth). Developmental anomalies can also occur secondary to chronic diseases in childhood, whether nutritional, infectious, cardiac, renal, or metabolic in origin. Some developmental abnormalities in adults are shown in Figs. 5-4 through 5-8.

Nutritional State

You may want to note whether the client is well nourished or is either overweight or underweight. Extremes may be

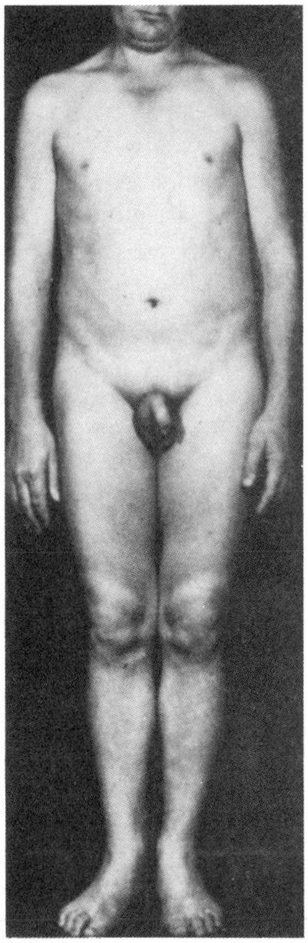

Figure 5-4 Hypopituitarism (chromophobe adenoma). This 33-year-old man lacks a beard and axillary and pubic hair and has lost his libido.

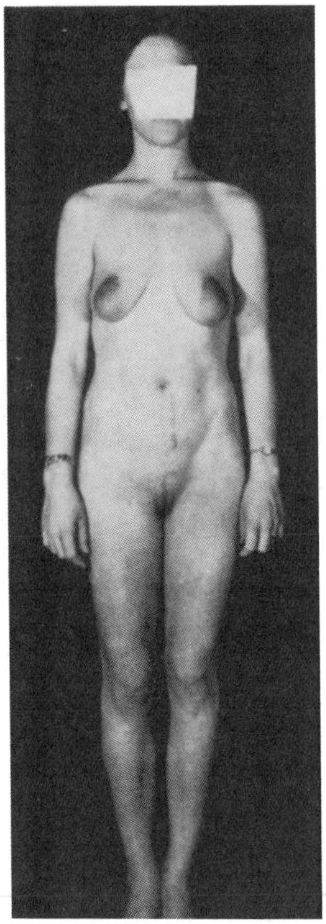

Figure 5-5 Hypopituitarism typical of Sheehan's disease. It is characterized by absence of pubic hair and weight loss.

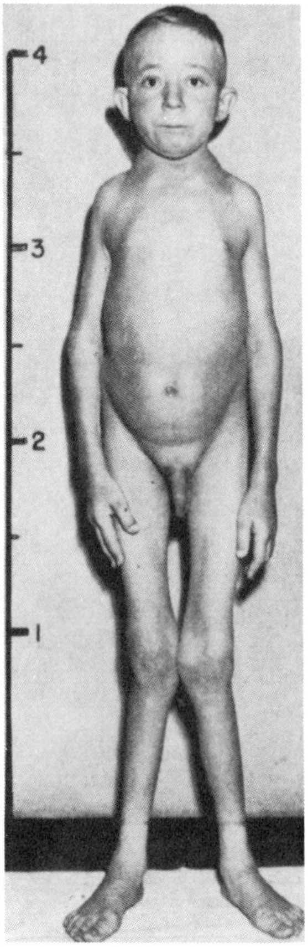

Figure 5-6 Renal dwarfism. This 21-year-old man with chronic renal disease since childhood has stunted growth as a result of severe disturbances in mineral and amino acid metabolism.

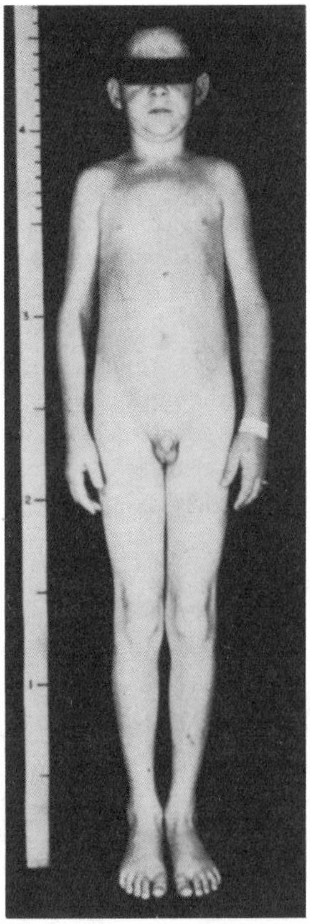

Figure 5-7 Pituitary dwarfism. This 18-year-old man is 54″ tall and weighs 67 pounds. He has no body hair and immature testes.

described using such terms as *malnourished, cachectic* (Fig. 5-9), and *obese.* Often, with a rapid weight loss, the skin will be loose and sagging, but this phenomenon is also common in the elderly as the result of a lifetime of gravitational pull on the loose tissues of the body.

General State of Health

You should note whether the client appears to be in excellent health; shows any signs of distress; appears chronically, acutely, or gravely ill; or is in no apparent distress.

Gross Abnormalities

Note any gross congenital or acquired defects, such as missing limbs, webbed digits, torticollis, or abnormal curvature of the spine. Describe abnormal positions, such as opisthotonos (seen in severe cases of meningitis and tetanus) or a curled fetal-like position (observed in cases of severe withdrawal and sometimes with abdominal pain). Record marked aberrations of body movements, such as athetosis or tics. If the client displays an obvious abnormal gait or speech defect, you may record it here, but such signs would warrant further consideration during the portion of the physical examination that focuses on neurologic function.

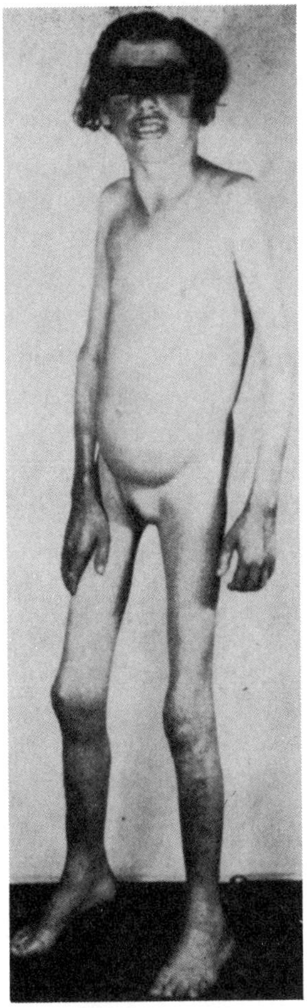

Figure 5-8 Cretinism, which results from hypofunction of the thyroid gland during gestation or infancy, is associated with various degrees of mental retardation. Note the dull expression, thick lips and tongue, potbelly and umbilical hernia, and shortened extremities in relation to trunk from retarded bone growth.

Striking Features

Striking features run the gamut from physical features to personality characteristics to behavior—whatever seems to "jump out" at you. Endocrine disorders, in particular, produce striking physical changes, as seen in Figs. 5-10 through 5-12.

It is often difficult to decide which observations to list under which category. Many of the signs, symptoms, and behaviors discussed so far could be discussed under several; therefore, such categorization is somewhat arbitrary. The important point is that these aspects must be documented somewhere in the general impression.

Height and Weight

The client's height and weight are recorded, and his usual weight is also recorded if he has undergone a marked loss or gain. To assess whether the client's weight is in the normal range, consult height, weight, and body frame tables. Weight

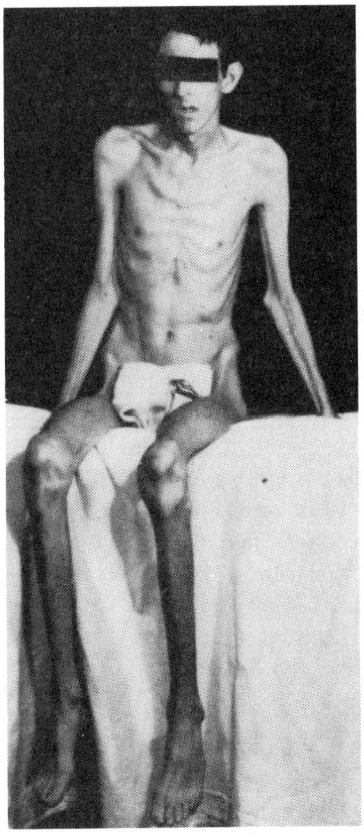

Figure 5-9 Cachexia in a 26-year-old man due to fibrosis of the pituitary.

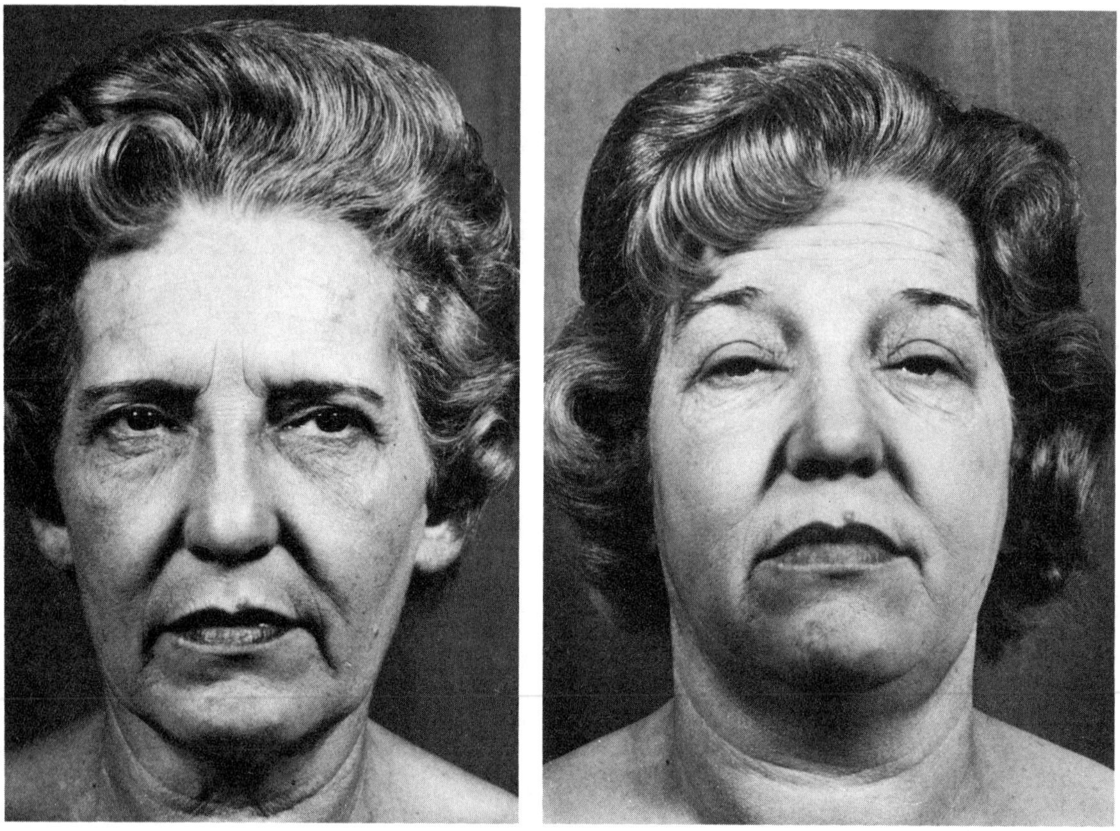

A B

Figure 5-10 **(A)** Client prior to onset of myxedema. **(B)** Facies with onset of myxedema (hypothyroidism in adulthood). Note the coarseness of skin, puffy face, and apathetic expression.

standards for men and women are shown in Tables 5-4 and 5-5. A gross estimate of ideal body weight (IBW) can be calculated using a rule of thumb, as illustrated in Table 5-6.

Vital Signs

Vital signs for adults include temperature, pulse, and respirations (TPR), and blood pressure (BP). For infants, they would also include head circumference and crown-rump height. In special situations, central venous pressure would be considered a vital sign.

Vital signs are initially recorded to establish a baseline against which changes can be compared and to identify trends; subsequent recordings should be made as often as you deem necessary. There is no need to wait for a scheduled time to take vital signs if you suspect a change from other observations. It is important that you know the normal range of vital signs according to developmental aspects and that you identify the client's personal variations.

Temperature

The normal range of body temperature in the resting person is 98.6 ± 1°F orally. Axillary temperature registers approximately 1° lower than the average oral temperature (97.6°F), whereas rectal temperature is about 1° higher than the oral body temperature (99.6°F). Rectal readings are most often taken with children and with adult clients who are mouth-breathers, who are confused, or who are receiving oxygen therapy. It is also necessary to use this method with clients who are unconscious, who have experienced severe trauma (lacerations of the mouth), or who have undergone facial-mandibular surgery (wired fractured jaw, glossectomy).

Each individual has a personal temperature variation. Most commonly, a client's early-morning temperature will register 2+ degrees lower than her average temperature, and her temperature in the late afternoon or early evening will register 0.5° to 1° higher.

The menstruating female exhibits a well-known temperature pattern. Her body temperature usually drops about 24 to 36 hours before ovulation. Then, as ovulation occurs, her morning temperature will rise and remain at this high level until just prior to the onset of her menstrual period.

Infants and young children do not have body temperature as well-controlled as adults. The toddler's average rectal temperature is usually 99° to 100°F (37.2–37.8°C) or higher. Even with minor infections, the infant or young child's temperature may rise to 103° to 105°F. Yet with a severe infection, the infant's temperature may actually be normal or even subnormal.

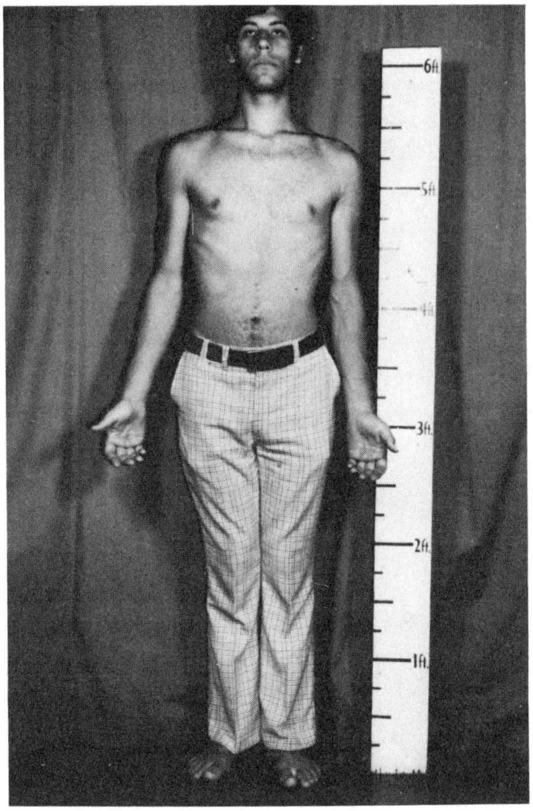

Figure 5-11 Acromegaly. Note the elongation and enlargement of bones, especially of the extremities and jaw, and the soft tissue enlargement of the face, especially of the nose and lips.

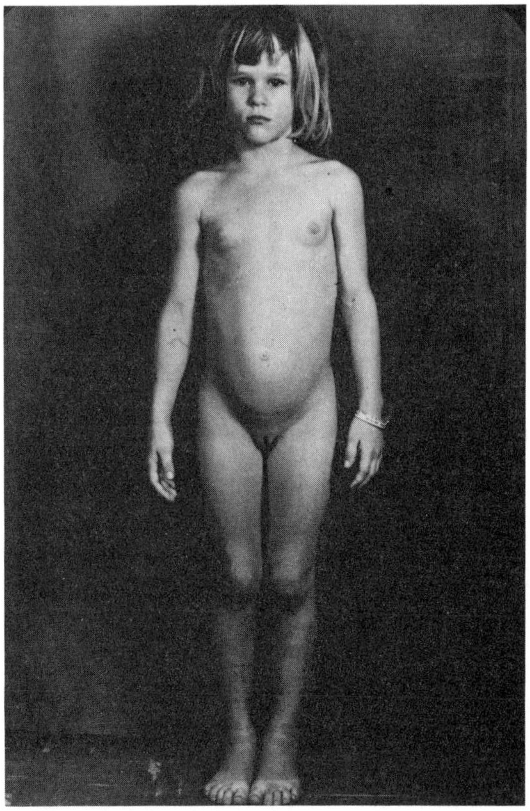

Figure 5-12 Adrenocortical hyperfunction in a preschool girl. Note the breast enlargement.

Table 5-4 Weight According to Frame (Indoor Clothing), Women of Ages 25 and Over*

Height†			Small frame		Medium frame		Large frame	
Feet	Inches	cm	Pounds	Kilograms	Pounds	Kilograms	Pounds	Kilograms
4	10	147.3	92–98	41.7–44.5	96–107	43.5–48.5	104–119	47.2–54.0
4	11	149.9	94–101	42.6–45.8	98–110	44.5–49.9	106–122	48.1–55.3
5	0	152.4	96–104	43.5–47.2	101–113	45.8–51.3	109–125	49.4–56.7
5	1	154.9	99–107	44.9–48.5	104–116	47.2–52.6	112–128	50.8–58.1
5	2	157.5	102–110	46.3–50.0	107–119	48.5–54.0	115–131	52.2–59.4
5	3	160.0	105–113	47.6–51.3	110–122	49.9–55.3	118–134	53.5–60.8
5	4	162.6	108–116	49.0–52.6	113–126	51.3–57.2	121–138	54.9–62.6
5	5	165.1	111–119	50.3–54.0	116–130	52.6–59.0	125–142	56.7–64.4
5	6	167.6	114–123	51.7–55.8	120–135	54.4–61.2	129–146	58.5–66.2
5	7	170.2	118–127	53.5–57.6	124–139	56.2–63.0	133–150	60.3–68.0
5	8	172.7	122–131	55.3–59.4	128–143	58.1–64.9	137–154	62.1–69.9
5	9	175.3	126–135	57.2–61.2	132–147	59.9–66.7	141–158	64.0–71.7
5	10	177.8	130–140	59.0–63.5	136–151	61.7–68.5	145–163	65.8–73.9
5	11	180.3	134–144	60.8–65.3	140–155	63.5–70.3	149–168	67.6–76.2
6	0	182.9	138–148	62.6–67.1	144–159	65.3–72.1	153–173	69.4–78.5

*For women between 18 and 25, subtract 0.5 kg (1 pound) for each year under 25.

†With shoes on—5.1 cm (2-inch) heels

Courtesy of the Metropolitan Life Insurance Company.

Table 5-5 Weight According to Frame (Indoor Clothing), Men of Ages 25 and Over

Height*			Small frame		Medium frame		Large frame	
Feet	Inches	cm	Pounds	Kilograms	Pounds	Kilograms	Pounds	Kilograms
5	2	157.5	112–120	50.8–54.4	118–129	53.5–58.5	126–141	57.2–64.0
5	3	160.0	115–123	52.2–55.8	121–133	54.9–60.3	129–144	58.5–65.3
5	4	162.6	118–126	53.5–57.2	124–136	56.2–61.7	132–148	59.9–67.1
5	5	165.1	121–129	54.9–58.5	127–139	57.6–63.0	135–152	61.2–68.9
5	6	167.6	124–133	56.2–60.3	130–143	59.0–64.9	138–156	62.6–70.8
5	7	170.2	128–137	58.1–62.1	134–147	60.8–66.7	142–161	64.4–73.0
5	8	172.7	132–141	59.9–64.0	138–152	62.6–68.9	147–166	66.7–75.3
5	9	175.3	136–145	61.7–65.8	142–156	64.4–70.8	151–170	68.5–77.1
5	10	177.8	140–150	63.5–68.0	146–160	66.2–72.6	155–174	70.3–78.9
5	11	180.3	144–154	65.3–69.9	150–165	68.0–74.8	159–179	72.1–81.2
6	0	182.9	148–158	67.1–71.7	154–170	69.9–77.1	164–184	74.4–83.4
6	1	185.4	152–162	68.9–73.5	158–175	71.7–79.4	168–189	76.2–85.7
6	2	188.0	156–167	70.8–75.8	162–180	73.5–81.6	173–194	78.5–88.0
6	3	190.5	160–171	72.6–77.6	167–185	75.8–83.9	178–199	80.7–90.3
6	4	193.0	164–175	74.4–79.4	172–190	78.0–86.2	182–204	82.6–92.5

*With shoes on—2.5 cm (1-inch) heels.

Courtesy of Metropolitan Life Insurance Company.

Table 5-6 Calculation of a Gross Estimation of Ideal Body Weight

1. For a **woman** with a **medium-frame** body:

   Allow 100 pounds for the first 5 feet of height.

   Allow 5 pounds per inch over 5 feet of height.

   For example, calculation for a woman 5′5″ tall is

   100 lbs (for the first 5′ of height)

   +25 lbs (inches over 5′ = 5″ × 5 lbs = 25 lbs)

   125 lbs is an estimate of IBW for a woman 5′5″ tall, of medium build.

2. For a **man** with a **medium-frame** body:

   Allow 106 pounds for the first five feet of height.

   Allow 6 pounds per inch over five feet tall.

   For example, calculation for a man 6′2″ is

   106 lbs (for the first 5′ of height)

   +84 lbs (inches over 5′ = 14″ × 6 lbs = 84 lbs)

   190 lbs is an estimate of IBW for a man 6′2″ tall, of medium build.

3. **To determine body frame,** encircle the client's dominant wrist with your thumb and index finger.

   Small frame = index finger touches the first knuckle (distal joint) of the thumb.

   Medium frame = tips of index finger and thumb touch.

   Large frame = unable to touch tips of index finger and thumb.

4. The IBW of an individual with a small body frame is **minus 10%** of the IBW of a medium-framed woman or man as calculated in items 1 and 2.

   For example, the IBW of the medium-framed woman in the example is 125 lbs (10% of 125 = 0.10 × 125 = 12.50). Thus, the IBW of a small-framed woman 5′5″ tall would be 112.5 lbs (125 − 12.5 = 112.5).

5. The IBW of an individual with a large body frame is **plus 10%** of the IBW of a medium-framed woman or man, as calculated in items 1 and 2.

   For example, the IBW of the medium-framed man in the example is 190 lbs (10% of 190 = 0.10 × 190 = 19.5). Thus, the IBW of a large-framed man 6′2″ tall would be 209.5 lbs (190 + 19.5 = 209.5).

It is common to witness slight fever a day or two following surgery; pyrexia is also characteristic of vascular, respiratory, and urologic infections and of wound infection. Pyrexia, as well as subnormal temperatures, can also occur from a direct influence on the thermoregulatory centers in the hypothalamus, such as occurs with head injury, cerebrovascular accident, and cerebral edema or tumor. It is important to remember that anxiety, as well as physical stress, may elevate body temperature.

Clinical thermometers do not record temperatures below 95°F (35°C), so whenever a temperature is recorded in this range, the true temperature should be checked with more sensitive devices. Hypothermia is a particular threat to the elderly, many of whom live in cold conditions and cannot afford the high cost of fuel.

Pulse

The pulse recorded with the TPR is the radial pulse in the child and adult and the temporal or apical pulse in the newborn and infant. Pulse is assessed according to rate, rhythm, and quality. The apical pulse is routinely examined in the adult and child during the cardiac portion of the physical assessment. With cardiac arrest, the carotid or femoral pulse is used to determine perfusion.

The pulse rate varies with age, sex, physical exertion, and emotional status. In children, it is best to take the pulse for a full minute because there is a greater variation in the pulse rates of infants and children (Table 5-7). In the adult, you can take the pulse for 30 seconds and multiply the result by 2. If you note any irregularity, take the pulse for the entire minute. The normal pulse rate in the resting adult ranges from 60 to 100 beats/min and is slightly faster in women than in men. Because of arteriosclerotic tendencies with age, the pulse in the elderly client may feel hard and cordlike and may be of a faster rate.

Stimulation of the sympathetic nervous system will increase the heart rate; thus, tachycardia is present in clients experiencing pain, anxiety, anger, or fear. Clients who require greater cardiac output because of situations that have a greater demand for oxygen also display tachycardia. Such situations include exercise, toxic states with high fever, severe anemia, thyrotoxicosis, shock, hypoxia, congenital heart disease, and congestive heart failure. Bradycardia is not unusual in the physically fit athlete, but it can also be indicative of parasympathetic stimulation in digitalis poisoning, syncope, increased intracranial pressure, myxedema, obstructive jaundice, heart block, and septal defect.

Table 5-7 **Pulse Rates per Minute at Rest for Boys and Girls up to 18 Years**

	Boys			Girls		
Age in years	No. of tests	Mean $\pm$ σ_m	SD	No. of tests	Mean $\pm$ σ_m	SD
0–1	33	135 ± 3.1	18	56	126 ± 2.8	21
1–2	82	105 ± 1.8	16	93	104 ± 1.8	17
2–3	150	93 ± 1.0	12	177	93 ± 0.7	9
3–4	157	87 ± 0.7	9	145	89 ± 0.7	9
4–5	157	84 ± 0.7	8	137	84 ± 0.7	8
5–6	150	79 ± 0.6	7	129	79 ± 0.6	7
6–7	146	76 ± 0.6	8	122	77 ± 0.7	8
7–8	140	75 ± 0.7	8	117	76 ± 0.8	8
8–9	142	73 ± 0.7	9	114	73 ± 0.6	7
9–10	168	70 ± 0.6	7	106	70 ± 0.7	8
10–11	164	67 ± 0.6	7	98	69 ± 0.8	8
11–12	129	67 ± 0.6	7	84	69 ± 0.8	7
12–13	131	66 ± 0.6	7	72	69 ± 0.9	8
13–14	110	65 ± 0.8	8	68	68 ± 0.9	8
14–15	106	62 ± 0.7	7	57	66 ± 1.1	8
15–16	76	61 ± 0.9	8	47	65 ± 1.1	8
16–17	45	61 ± 0.9	6	30	66 ± 1.4	8
17–18	38	60 ± 1.4	8	20	65 ± 1.7	7

Source: Adapted from A. Iliff and V. A. Lee. "Pulse Rate, Respiratory Rate, and Body Temperature of Children Between 2 Months and 18 Years," *Child Development*, 23 (1952): 237. By permission of the Society for Research in Child Development, Inc.

The normal pulse rate is of regular rhythm. However, a state of sinus arrhythmia, in which the pulse rate increases at the peak of respiratory inspiration and decreases on expiration, is a common nonpathologic phenomenon observed in children and young adults. In such cases, the pulse will beat in regular rhythm when the client holds his breath. Cardiac arrhythmias may be indicated by an irregular pulse rhythm and by a pulse deficit, which occurs when the radial pulse rate is less than the apical pulse rate. Occasionally, a person may experience a premature beat, often described as the heart's "skipping a beat." In this case, some other pacemaker fires ahead of the sinoatrial node. Frequent premature ventricular contractions (PVCs) can indicate cardiac irritability from such things as digitalis toxicity, potassium imbalance, or hypoxia, or they may represent more serious cardiac arrhythmias. Pairs of beats or triplets aggregated and followed by a pause are termed *bigeminal* and *trigeminal* pulses, respectively. Premature contractions are the most common cause of bigeminal or trigeminal pulse irregularities. However, they may be symptomatic of overdigitalization or of partial or 2° heart block.

The quality of the pulse is an important factor. A thready, weak pulse is present in shock and in heart failure. A weak pulse is found distal to a partial occlusion of an artery and may also occur with cardiac valvular stenosis, myocardial infarction or myocarditis, and pericardial effusion or constrictive pericarditis. These are conditions in which cardiac output is reduced. A full, strong, bounding pulse (pulsus magnus) accompanies systolic hypertension and may occasionally occur in the normal client during anxiety, excessive physical exertion, or fever. Pulsus alterans, with alternating strong and weak beats, is observed in left ventricular failure, coronary artery disease, and severe arterial hypertension.

Respiration

Normal respirations are effortless, regular, and smooth. Average respirations per minute varies with age. Infants to 2 years of age average 24 to 34 respirations per minute; children to puberty range from 20 to 26 per minute; and normal adults average 12 to 18 per minute. Clients with an increased need for oxygenation of the blood, as with exercise or fever, will show an increased rate of respirations. Changes in respirations can also be caused by interference with the respiratory center of the medulla oblongata.

The depth of respirations determines the volume of air moving in and out of the lungs. Extremes of depth vary from shallow breathing to the deep respirations of Kussmaul's breathing. Exact measurement of the depth of respirations requires a spirometer. A decrease in both respiratory rate and depth is seen with metabolic alkalosis, in which the body is attempting to retain carbon dioxide. Conversely, the increase in the rate and depth of respirations seen in metabolic acidosis is the compensatory mechanism that blows off the excess carbon dioxide and neutralizes the excess amounts of hydrogen ions.

When dyspnea is present, it is important to determine how much exertion is necessary to cause it or whether it occurs at rest. You should look for signs of respiratory obstruction as you note the rate and depth of respirations. You should carefully note whether the chest movement is symmetrical with respirations, whether intercostal or sternal retraction is present, and whether there is nasal flaring. Particularly in chronic obstructive pulmonary disease (COPD), there is obvious use of the accessory muscles in the neck for breathing. The client with COPD assumes a characteristic forward position with her hands on her knees or her elbows on the table. This position compresses the abdomen and increases the intrathoracic pressure, thus facilitating expiration. In clients with asthma or emphysema, you may observe a bulging of the interspaces caused by trapped air during forced expiration.

Blood Pressure

BP tests measure vascular pressures. During cardiac systole (contraction of the ventricles of the heart), the maximum pressure of the blood is exerted against the arterial walls by the left ventricle. This is called the *systolic pressure.* The *diastolic pressure* on the walls of the arteries is continually present and reflects blood vessel resistance.

BP is lowest in the newborn and increases with age. It also increases with exercise and emotional stress and with a gain in weight. Ordinarily, it is at its lowest in the early morning after a night's sleep. A client's BP is also lower when measured in a supine position as compared with a sitting or standing position. The cuff used should cover at least half of the portion of extremity used and not more than two thirds of the area. Methods for taking BP readings are summarized in Table 5-8.

BP is taken in all four extremities in clients suspected of having cardiac problems, in those with weak or absent femoral or popliteal pulses, and in children or young adults with hypertension. This last situation could mean coarctation of the aorta (a congenital narrowing). With coarctation, the systolic pressure of both arms is surprisingly high, and the systolic pressure of the lower extremities is lower than that of the upper extremities because the femoral arteries are at the lower portion of the aorta and thus below the stenosed segment. Normally, the BP reading for the legs is slightly higher than that for the arms because the larger muscle mass exerts more resistance to arterial compression by the BP cuff. Figure 5-13 illustrates that the cuff should be placed at the lower third of the leg with the stethoscope over the popliteal artery. There

Table 5-8 **Blood Pressure Reading Methods**

Palpatory systolic pressure	Auscultatory method	Flush method (for newborns or infants)
1. Place client's arm at heart level. 2. Avoid clothing constriction. 3. Cuff evenly over brachial artery. 4. Palpate radial pulse. 5. Inflate cuff until radial pulse disappears. 6. Inflate cuff 30 mm Hg more. 7. Release pressure of cuff slowly. 8. Read systolic BP at return point of radial pulse.	1. Place client's arm at heart level. 2. Avoid clothing constriction. 3. Cuff evenly over brachial artery. 4. Palpate radial pulse. 5. Inflate cuff until radial pulse disappears. 6. Inflate cuff 30 mm Hg more. 7. Place stethoscope over brachial artery in anticubital space. 8. Release cuff pressure. 9. The point at which you hear the first sound is systolic pressure. Damping or muffling is diastolic pressure. 10. Also record the final sound. Example: 116/80/76.	1. Put cuff around ankle or wrist. 2. Elevate leg or arm. 3. Squeeze or wrap leg or arm with elastic bandage to occlude blood from the part. 4. Inflate to 120–140 mm Hg. 5. Release squeeze or bandage. 6. Release cuff. 7. The point of flush return is the mean diastolic-systolic pressure.

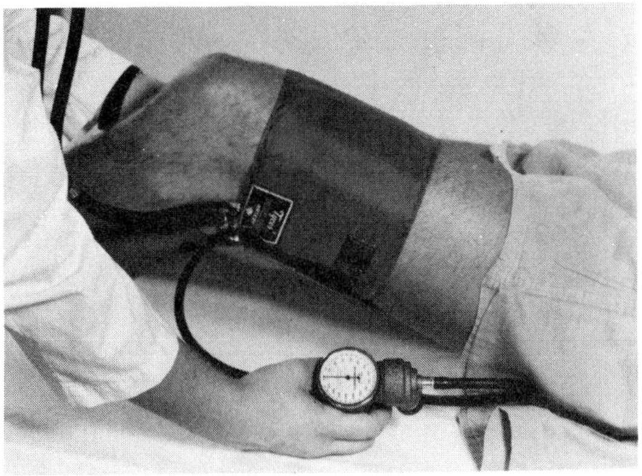
Figure 5-13 Technique for taking BP on the leg.

is usually very little if any difference in BP between the two upper extremities; a significant discrepancy could be a result of aortic aneurysm.

Pulse pressure is the difference between systolic and diastolic pressure readings. Normally, it is 25 to 50 mm Hg. A decrease in pulse pressure may be a sign of heart failure, massive pericardial effusion, aortic stenosis, or mitral stenosis. A widening pulse pressure can be caused by vigorous exercise, fever, increased intracranial pressure, thyrotoxicosis, severe anemia, or severe atherosclerosis of the aorta and large arteries.

Hypertension, as defined by the World Health Organization, is a persistent elevation of BP above 140 mm systolically and 90 mm diastolically (140/90). A pressure below 95/60 is generally considered to be hypotension. However, a hypertensive client may be hypotensive at 150/90.

Essential hypertension is of an unknown etiology. Hypertension can be caused by kidney disease and is usually accompanied by headaches, blurred vision, and renal failure symptomatology. Other causes are coarctation of the aorta, pheochromocytoma, and polycythemia. Associated manifestations of hypertension include epistaxis, headaches, and irritability. There is a familial tendency for hypertension.

An increased systolic pressure as the result of an increase in cardiac output with a stable diastolic pressure can be found in older clients with atherosclerosis and in clients with anemia, arteriovenous fistula, aortic regurgitation, or hyperthyroidism.

A BP decrease occurs following an acute myocardial infarction, as a result of the diminished cardiac output. Hypotension is also seen with hypovolemia, which can occur in shock from hemorrhage, in burns, in dehydration, and in hypoadrenalism. Oliguria or anuria is an early sign of hypovolemia.

BIOLOGIC AND CULTURAL VARIATIONS

Hypertension Among African-Americans

The National Health Survey has determined that 20 to 25 million Americans have either a casual systolic BP of 150 mm Hg or higher or a diastolic BP of 95 mm Hg or higher. However, these high BP levels are twice as frequent among African-Americans as among whites at all ages up to 80 years; hypertension affects 30% of all African-American adults, compared with 16% of all white adults. Hypertension is the disease or physiologic disorder diagnosed when an individual consistently has BP readings above 140 mm Hg systolic/90 mm Hg diastolic. African-Americans are also more likely to suffer from severe hypertension, the relative rate being 3.3 times higher for African-American males than for white males. Mortality rates for African-Americans from hypertension and disorders stemming from hypertension (such as cardiac complications, cerebrovascular disease, and uremia) are similarly higher.

The most significant epidemiologic finding concerning hypertension in the United States is the high morbidity and mortality rates of African-Americans. There has been a limited attempt to explain these higher rates. One or several of the factors involved in hypertension might occur to a greater extent among African-Americans. Alternatively, it might be that they are more sensitive to one or more of the agents. For example, overweight and obesity are two nutritional conditions that have been found to be highly associated with hypertension. Could this be a factor? As a group, African-Americans are leaner than whites; however, it may be that there are more obese African-Americans than whites. Still, this slight difference in the incidence of obesity would not be enough to explain the great difference in high BP rates. Also, one study has shown that weight is less correlated with BP in African-Americans than in whites (Tyroler et al 1975). Thus, more evidence concerning overweight is needed.

Short-term stress can elevate BP markedly. It has been proposed that chronic stress might lead to elevated BP. It is possible that African-Americans and whites are subjected to different amounts of life stress and that the higher BP of African-Americans arises from greater life stress. Although this proposition has intuitive appeal, it would be extremely difficult to investigate. For one thing, it is extremely hard to define stress as a variable and measure it. Thus, investigations along these lines have had inconclusive results.

A review of the literature on socioeconomic status and hypertension in the United States shows that the higher the social class, the lower the prevalence, morbidity, and mortality rates (Howard & Holman 1970). Since African-Americans as a group are more disadvantaged than whites, this suggests that the higher African-American rates might be due to social class differences. However, studies that have compared African-American and white rates in each social class have shown that African-Americans still have much higher mortality rates in every class (Howard & Holman 1970). Thus, although social class seems to be an important determinant of BP, the additive effect of race and social class seems to be an even stronger determinant.

There may be certain traits in the genetic composition of the African-American population that determine the higher prevalence of hypertension. These traits could involve the metabolism of certain etiologic agents, such as sodium or cadmium, or the mechanisms of certain systems, such as the autonomic nervous system. Few studies have investigated these possibilities. Thus, genetic differences and environmental factors interacting with this genetic component may explain the high BP differences.

Obviously, the reasons for the higher rate of hypertension among African-Americans remain unclear. This is a question in need of further investigation.

Checklist for Developing a General Impression

State of consciousness
Age
Race
Sex
Development
Nutritional state
General state of health
Gross abnormalities
Striking features
Height and weight
Vital signs

General impression: Mr. J., an apprehensive 18-year-old white male, college freshman, well developed and well nourished. In acute distress — pale, dyspneic, diaphoretic, leaning forward in a sitting position braced by extended arms, and receiving nasal O_2 (4L/min). No apparent speech defects, but his voice is weak and breathless. Mental processes are slowed. TPR 102-110-36. BP sitting left arm: 100/56. Ht: 5'11" Wt: 160 lbs. (normal wt: 175 lbs).

Figure 5-14 Example of a general impression evaluation.

SUMMARY

This chapter introduced you to the basic techniques of physical assessment. It described the four classical methods: inspection, palpation, percussion, and auscultation. Inspection relies primarily on the visual sense, while palpation employs the sense of touch for evaluating such aspects as temperature, contour, surface texture, consistency, and vibration. Percussion requires considerable practice to perfect and is useful in determining density and size of organs and tumors as well as the presence of pain. The sense of hearing is used in auscultation, a technique central in assessing the cardiovascular, respiratory, and gastrointestinal systems.

Also, the approach to the client in performing physical assessment was described as taking into consideration the client's comfort, safety, and age. Then, each of the components within the general impression (state of consciousness, age, race, sex, development, nutritional state, general state of health, gross abnormalities, striking features, height, weight, and vital signs) was discussed. Vital signs (TPR and BP) were described carefully and clearly to assist you in understanding their significance in a complete physical assessment.

DISCUSSION QUESTIONS/ ACTIVITIES

1. Discuss how you use each of your senses in physical assessment.
2. Of what benefit is your general impression of the client to you or to other health professionals?
3. Why does the initiation of taking vital signs fall into the category of a nursing diagnosis?
4. What would prompt you to take the vital signs of a client and why?
5. Write a general impression of yourself, a classmate, and a client (see Fig. 5-14 for an example).

REFERENCES

Howard, J., and Holman, B. L. 1970. The effects of race and occupation on hypertension mortality. *Millbank Memorial Fund Quarterly* 48:263–296.

Tyroler, H. A.; Heyden, S.; and Hames, C. G. 1975. Weight and hypertension—Evans County studies of blacks and whites. In *Epidemiology and the control of hypertension*, ed. P. Oglesby. New York: Stratton International.

CHAPTER

6 Assessment of the Integument

Learning Objectives

1. Review the structure and function of the skin.
2. Describe the techniques and characteristics of the skin used for inspection and palpation.
3. Describe the techniques and characteristics of the hair used for inspection and palpation.
4. Describe the techniques and characteristics of the nails used for inspection and palpation.
5. Recognize biologic and cultural variations in assessment of the integument.
6. List the characteristics used to describe skin lesions.
7. Identify primary and secondary skin lesions.
8. Recognize physical findings of the integumentary system that are not within the norms.

The integument, or covering, of the body is the skin, the body's first line of defense. It protects the body from trauma and infection and aids in temperature regulation. The appendages of the skin are part of the integumentary system: the sweat glands, sebaceous glands, hair, and nails. Inspection and palpation of the client's hands and fingernails is a nonthreatening beginning to physical assessment. At this time, you can not only notice abnormalities in appearance of these bodily parts, but you can also assess the client's grasp and the existence of stiffness or bony enlargement of the interphalangeal, metacarpophalangeal, and wrist joints.

STRUCTURE AND FUNCTION OF THE SKIN

Figure 6-1 illustrates the three basic layers of the skin: the *epidermis,* the *dermis,* and the *subcutaneous* tissue.

Epidermis

The epidermis is avascular. Devoid of blood vessels, the uppermost layer of the epidermis lacks nutrition and consists of dead keratinized cells. This outermost layer, referred to as the horny layer (stratum cornium), is continuously being shed, a process called desquamation. Excessive desquamation may be observed in severe dehydration and in dermatologic conditions such as psoriasis and contact dermatitis. The dead keratinized cells may accumulate into plaque formations or into horny, wartlike structures (keratosis). Keratosis is commonly observed in the elderly (Fig. 6-2). Hyperkeratosis at the hair follicles is characteristic of vitamin A deficiency. The keratinized cells pile up around the

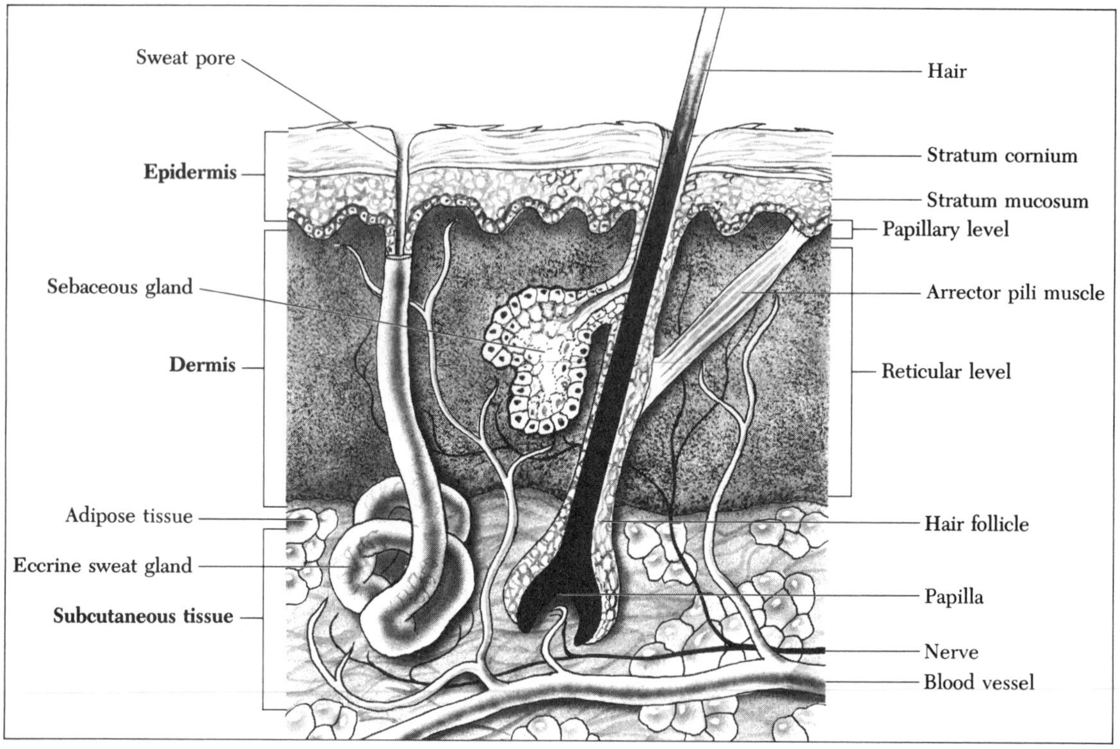

Figure 6-1 Anatomy of the skin.

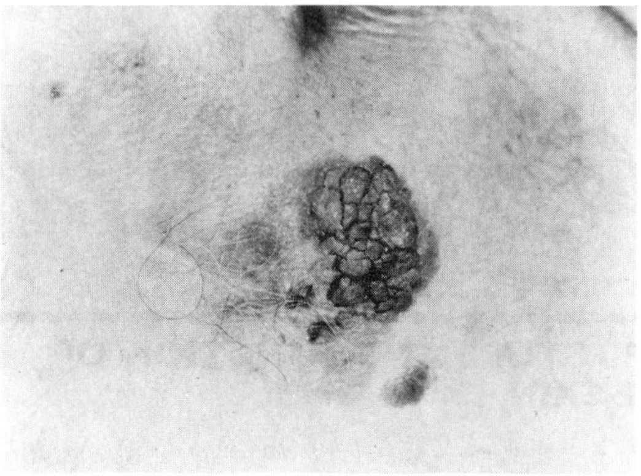

Figure 6-2 Keratosis. These horny plaque formations are commonly observed in the elderly.

external hair shaft, producing a sandpaper-like skin, usually on the upper arms and thighs.

The second layer of the epidermis, the stratum mucosum, derives nutrition for its keratinocyte and melanocyte cells from the underlying vascular tissues. Both keratin and melanin are formed in the stratum mucosum.

Dermis

The dermis acts as a water and electrolyte storage compartment. The uppermost layer of the dermis, the papillary level, consists of dense connective tissue that is molded into the epidermis and that also provides the dermal lining of the hair follicles. The lower reticular level, also composed of many connective cells, contains blood vessels, lymphatics, the sensory nerve endings for the skin, the sweat glands, the sebaceous glands, and the hair follicles. The eccrine sweat glands are coiled tubules leading to an opening (pore) on the skin surface; their primary function is heat regulation via evaporation. The apocrine sweat glands, found primarily in the axillary and genital areas, produce secretions that usually find their way to the skin surface via hair follicles. Body odor is the result of bacterial decomposition of apocrine secretions. The sebum-secreting cells of the sebaceous glands are contained in the dermal lining of hair follicles.

Technique of Inspection of the Skin

1. Adequate lighting and room temperature
2. Adequate exposure of area being inspected
3. Equipment: centimeter ruler or tape
4. Alternate processes: (a) Inspect entire skin surface of body with client disrobed; or (b) as you proceed with the examination of the various anatomical parts, first examine the skin of the particular area being assessed.
5. Characteristics: color, type, pattern, bodily area, size, abnormalities

Sebum, a fatty substance that acts as a protective agent for the skin, enters the distal end of the hair follicle via a connecting duct.

Subcutaneous Tissue

The subcutaneous tissue layer of the skin is the depot for fat storage. Some of the sweat glands and the roots of some hair follicles may extend down into this layer.

CHARACTERISTICS AND TECHNIQUES OF EXAMINATION

Skin

The inspection of the integumentary system begins during the general survey. In fact, a skin disorder may be the most striking feature noted at this time. The integumentary system is often overlooked, and thereby valuable information may be lost about the client's health status. If you consciously place priority on assessment of the integumentary components during each phase of the physical assessment procedure, helpful clues to the state of health of the client will not go unheeded.

- As each anatomical portion of the body is exposed for inspection during the physical assessment process, you should assess the size, shape, and symmetry and then the characteristics of the skin.
- Assessment of each bodily area should begin on the outside surface with the skin and then inward, to the muscles, bones, and underlying organs.
- Inspection and palpation are the chief methods of assessing the integument.

Inspection

Melanin, hemoglobin, and carotene are the basic pigments in the human body. Racial groups have varied degrees of melanin, which account for the differences in skin color (Table 6-1). The body responds to the irritation of physical agents by increasing pigment deposits. The protective mechanism of increased melanin and the subsequent browning of exposed skin areas is well known and readily apparent in individuals who have repeated and prolonged exposure to the sun or sun lamps; to the heat waves of a stove, boiler, or open grate fire; to hot water bottles or heating pads; and to x-ray therapy.

- Be alert for behaviors that may suggest skin problems, such as scratching, rubbing, and picking at the skin.

Color

The color of the skin is inspected to detect any changes in the generalized fleshy color of the individual.

- Inspect for color changes of generalized or localized areas of hyperpigmentation, yellowing of the skin, paleness, cyanosis, erythema, rashes, and lesions (see Box on page 134).
- In dark-skinned clients, observe for color changes in the sclera, palpebral conjunctiva, lips, buccal mucosa, hard palate, tongue and under the tongue, palms, soles, and nails.

Table 6-1 Racial or Ethnic Variations of the Integumentary System

Racial or ethnic group	Predominant skin color	Predominant hair color and texture
African-American	Light brown to deep brown tones	Black; curly and wooly
Raza and Latino (Mexican or Chicano, Puerto Rican, Cuban, Spanish, Central and South American)	Tan, olive, to dark brown tones	Black or dark brown; wavy, curly, or straight
Filipino	Brown tones	Black; coarse, straight or wavy
Chinese	Yellow tones	Black; coarse, straight or wavy
Japanese	Yellow tones	Black or brown-black; coarse, straight or wavy
Vietnamese	Brown tones	Black; coarse, straight or wavy
Eskimo and Aleut	Yellow tones	Black; straight
Native American	Brown-red tones	Black; straight
Caucasian	Pale pink, tan, olive tones	Black, brown, red, or blond; straight to curly, coarse to very fine

Source: Compiled from *Ethnic nursing care: a multicultural approach,* by M. Orque, B. Bloch, and L. Monrroy (St. Louis: The C. V. Mosby Company, 1983), pp. 102, 139, 169, 197, 263, and 290.

BIOLOGIC AND CULTURAL VARIATIONS

Skin Cancer and Skin Color

Differences in body constitution among population groups are linked to varying rates of cancer mortality. One interesting association is that between skin cancer and skin color. Population groups with dark skins, such as African-Americans, have rather low rates of skin cancer, whereas population groups with lighter skin color have significantly elevated rates. It has been hypothesized that darker skin, with its greater pigmentation, offers protection against the sun's radiation. One study concluded that skin cancer is 45 times as common among whites as among non-whites in Hawaii (Allison & Wong 1968). The non-white group comprised population groups with somewhat darker skin color, such as Koreans, Chinese, Japanese, Hawaiians, and Filipinos. Their darker skin colors presumably offered some protection against the damaging effects of the ultraviolet rays of the sun.

- The buccal mucosa and gums of the dark-skinned client may have darker pigmented or dark blue blotchy macules or patches.
- Pallor is manifested in the brown-skinned client as a yellowish brown tinge, and as an ashen-gray skin color in the black-skinned client.

Petechiae, ecchymoses, and a fine macular rash can be differentiated from erythema by stretching the skin gently with your thumb and index finger. The red hue of erythema will diminish in color, whereas the color of the others will be accentuated. Blanching will not occur with petechiae.

Common vascular lesions of the skin are listed and described in Table 6-2. Spider angiomas (Fig. 6-3) are arterial in origin. They appear as a fiery red center with radiating legs, most often surrounded by an area of erythema. They are generally found on the face, neck, shoulders, and upper chest. If a glass slide is placed over the spider angioma, a pulsation of the central body may be detected; however, a definite blanching will occur. Blanching can also be demonstrated by using the point of a pencil to apply pressure to the spider body. At times, spider angiomas may be observed during pregnancy or with vitamin B deficiency. They may also occur in some normal people.

A venous star (Fig. 6-4) is a bluish area that occasionally may be found on the anterior chest but is most often observed on the legs. It results from increased pressure in a superficial vein (varicose veins). Blanching does not take place with applied pressure.

Table 6-2 **Common Vascular Lesions**

Terminology	Characteristics	Comments
Petechiae	Tiny reddish purple spots	Will not blanch. Assess for other signs of bleeding, hepatic dysfunction, subacute bacterial endocarditis.
Spider angioma	Bright red center with radiating legs generally on face, neck, shoulders, upper chest	Will blanch. Assess for liver dysfunction, vitamin B deficiency, and pregnancy.
Venous star	Bluish area most often on legs but may occur on anterior chest	Will not blanch. Assess for sources of increased pressure in superficial veins, e.g., distention, activity, and occupation.
Cherry angioma	Bright red, round lesion, may turn brown with age; usually on torso and extremities; usually papular and surrounded by pale halo	Nonpathologic, increase in size and number as aging proceeds in the adult.
Telangiectasia	Dilation of capillaries and thinning of vascular walls. Frequently on face and thighs as erythemic to bluish lines	Check history of alcoholism, polycythemia, and family (Osler-Weber-Rendu disease is hereditary, can affect nose, skin, GI and GU tract; has hemorrhagic tendency). Will blanch with pressure. Check for signs of bleeding—e.g., Hqb, Hct, urinalysis.

Skin Color Changes

HYPERPIGMENTATION

A diffuse or localized melanin hyperpigmentation may be observed during pregnancy. The face, nipples, areolae, and vulva are affected. A dark line extending from above the umbilicus to the pubic region may appear during the last trimester. This brown line, called the linea nigra, is of no concern; it will gradually fade away after parturition. Mongolian spots, blackish blue areas of the lower back and buttocks, are nonpathologic and are seen particularly in African, Native American, and Asian newborns. The spots disappear in early childhood.

YELLOWING OF THE SKIN

Jaundice

Jaundice is a yellowing pigmentation that appears first in the posterior portion of the hard palate and the sclerae (when the serum bilirubin is only 24 mg/100 ml). As the bilirubin level rises, jaundice can be observed in the mucous membranes and generally throughout the skin of the rest of the body. Its presence is best detected in natural non-glare daylight rather than in artificial light. A normal physiologic jaundice appears the third or fourth day of life in about half of all newborns. It may persist from a week to a month. Jaundice that develops within the first 24 hours after birth or after 2 weeks of age should be regarded with suspicion of pathology.

Carotenemia

Carotenemia produces yellowing of the skin but does not involve the sclerae or mucous membranes. It may occur with an excessive intake of food containing carotinoids (carrots, sweet potatoes, corn, squash), or it may be present in myxedema, hypopituitarism, and diabetes mellitus. Occasionally, carotenemia may be observed during pregnancy. It is typically found on the palms, soles, and face.

PALLOR

In dark skinned individuals, pallor is best detected in the nail beds, palpebral conjunctivae, oral mucosa, and tongue.

CYANOSIS

Cyanosis is most readily detected around the lips, on the earlobes, in the nail beds, and under the tongue. A similar bluish gray skin color occurs from prolonged use of medications containing certain metal salts, such as silver, gold, and bismuth.

ERYTHEMA

Redness of the skin can be caused by dilatation of the superficial capillaries as a result of irritation, inflammation, heat, chilblain, fever, or a sympathetic nervous reaction, such as is seen in embarrassment. Transient heat rashes occur in the diaper area of infants.

ECCHYMOSIS

Black and blue marks are called ecchymoses, and are most commonly caused by physical trauma. The underlying mechanism is the extravasation of blood into the tissues. At first, a deep purple-blue color appears; with time, the color begins to fade to a green-brown and then yellow as the blood is reabsorbed into the vascular system.

PETECHIAE

Petechiae are purpuric lesions of the skin.

Cherry angioma is a nonpathologic lesion that increases in size and number as the individual grows older. It is a bright or ruby-red color, may turn brown with age, and is found on the torso and extremities. It is usually papular (raised), round, and may be surrounded by a pale halo (Fig. 6-5).

Telangiectasia (essential) is nonpathologic other than in an effect it may have on body image. It presents as a small network of dilated superficial venous plexi generally on the face or thighs. However, a rare hereditary hemorrhagic form (Osler-Weber-Rendu), which becomes progressively severe with age, may cause anemia from continuous bleeding from nose, mouth, stomach, bowel, and urinary lesions. Bleeding can occur with trauma or spontaneously.

Pattern

Lesions of the skin at times assume characteristic patterns that may aid in the diagnosis of particular skin diseases. Common patterns include generalized, annular, arciform, iris cluster, zosteriform, polycyclic, and linear (Fig. 6-6). Annular and/or arciform lesions are arranged in circles, arcs, or irregular combinations of the two.

Location

Specific lesions may occur on a particular portion of the body. For instance, acne is commonly present on the face, shoulders, and upper trunk (Figs. 6-7 and 6-8). The pattern for herpes zoster lesions (Fig. 6-9) and the body areas for

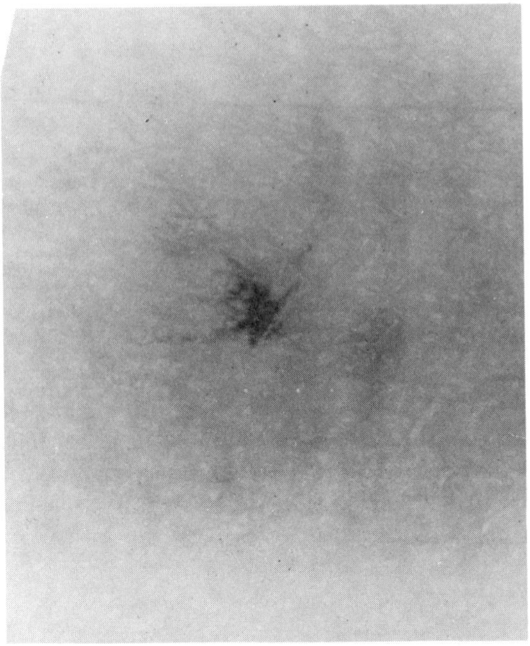

Figure 6-3 Spider angioma, a type of vascular lesion of the skin.

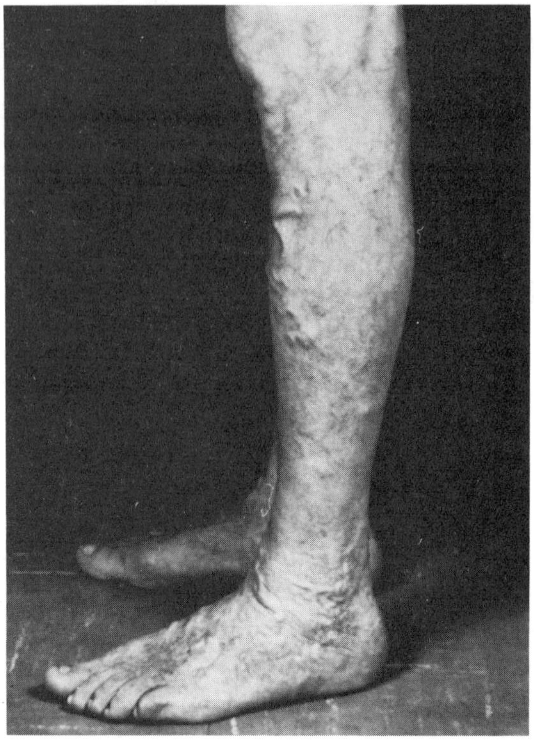

Figure 6-4 Varicose veins with venous star, a result of increased pressure in the vein.

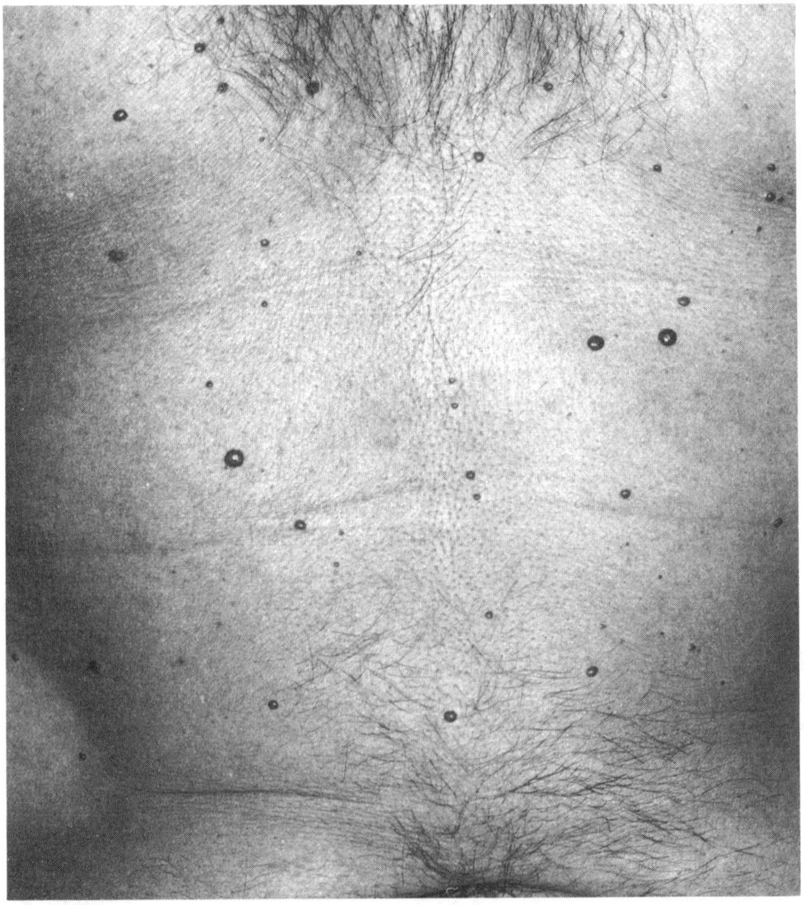

Figure 6-5 Cherry angioma. Multiple small red papules commonly occur on the trunk. (From T.P. Habif, *Clinical Dermatology,* 2nd ed., St. Louis: Mosby Year Book, Inc., 1990.)

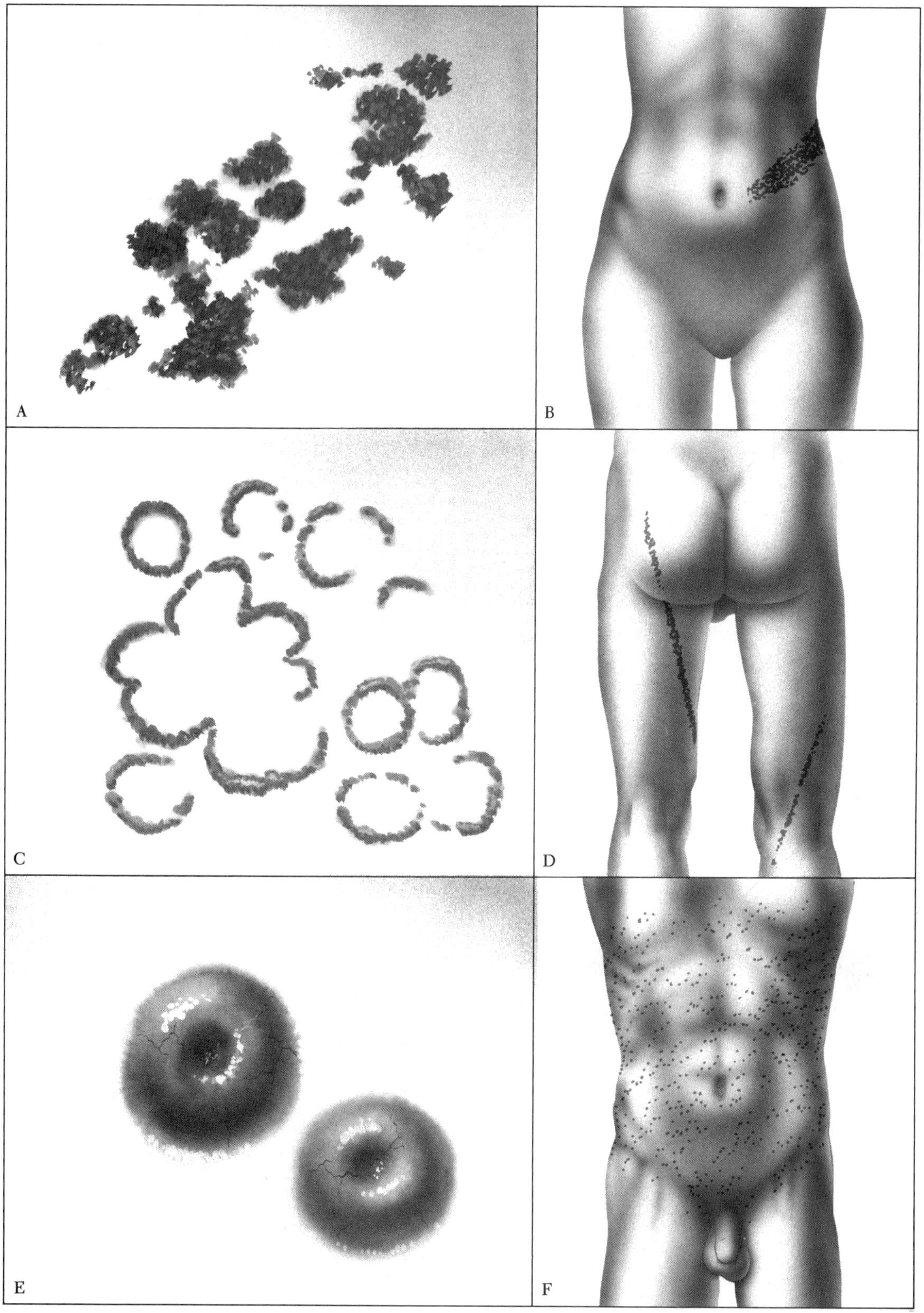

Figure 6-6 Configurations of skin lesions. **(A)** Grouped. **(B)** Zosteriform (follows a nerve route). **(C)** Annular and polycyclic (round). **(D)** Linear (in a line). **(E)** Iris cluster (central lesion with ring encircling it). **(F)** Generalized (diffuse over body or anatomic area).

herpes zoster, scabies, and seborrheic dermatitis are seen in Figs. 6-10, 6-11, and 6-12, respectively. Intertrigo, a red scaly maceration of the skin in areas of opposing surfaces, is commonly seen on the neck, axillae, and groin of infants because of moisture and constant irritation. Such maceration may be observed in these body areas in obese persons.

When documenting observed lesions, you must be able to use terminology to describe the type of lesion present as well as the pattern and the anatomic location. Fig. 6-13 and Table 6-3 illustrate types of skin lesions divided into two groups: primary lesions and secondary lesions; the latter result from changes that occur because of underlying primary lesions. Characteristics of skin lesions to be documented are

1. color—pink, red, yellow, brown, black, green
2. type—macule, papule, wheal, scale, ulcer, scar, and so on
3. pattern—annular, linear, clustered, bull's eye, and so on
4. bodily area—generalized, on exposed surfaces, faces, on the extensor surfaces of the joints, in skin fold areas, and so on

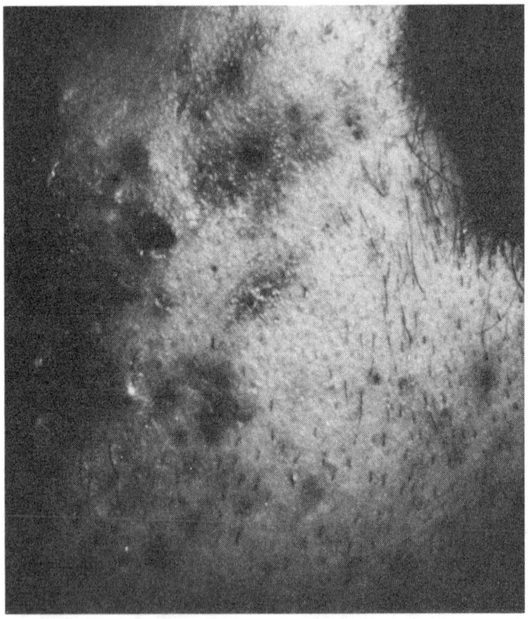

Figure 6-7 Severe acne vulgaris on the face. (Courtesy H. Gallego, M.D.)

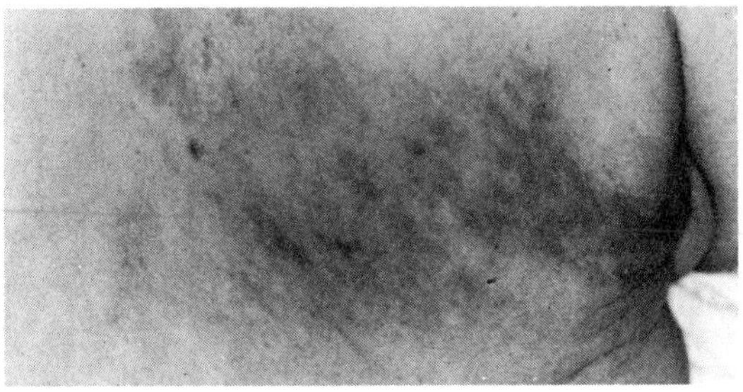

Figure 6-9 Herpes zoster.

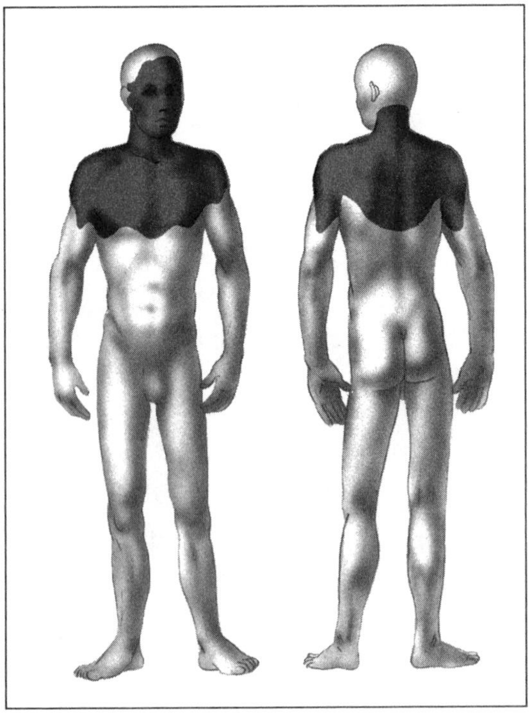

Figure 6-8 Common anatomic areas of acne.

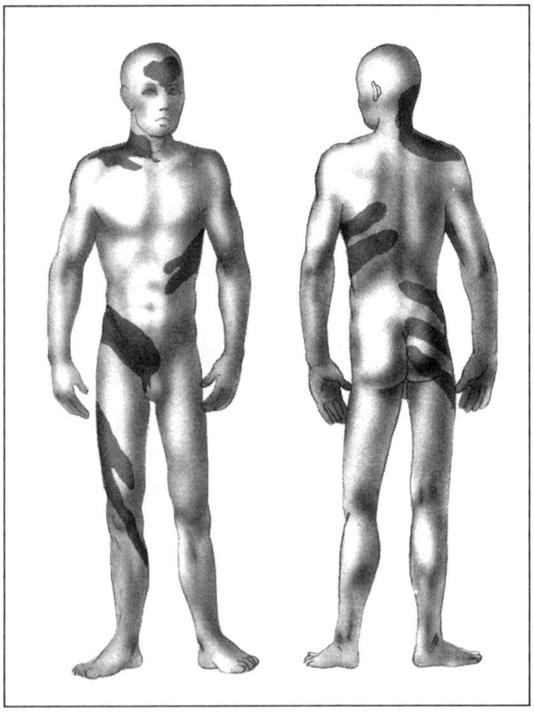

Figure 6-10 Body patterns of herpes zoster.

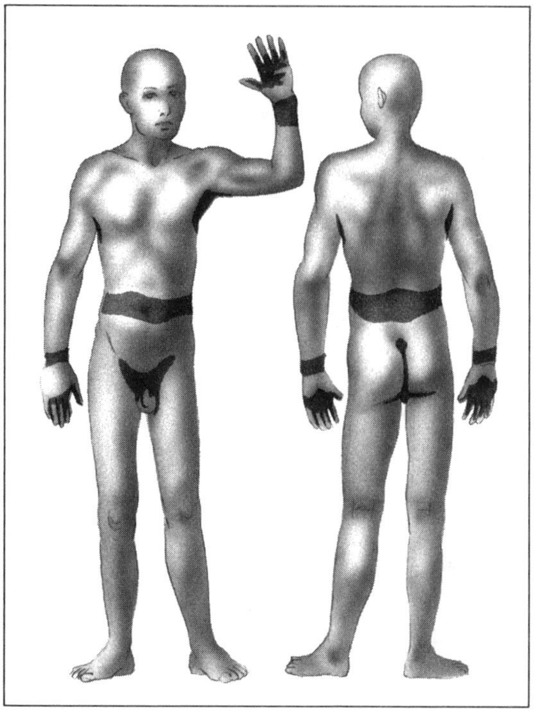

Figure 6-11 Common anatomic areas of scabies lesions.

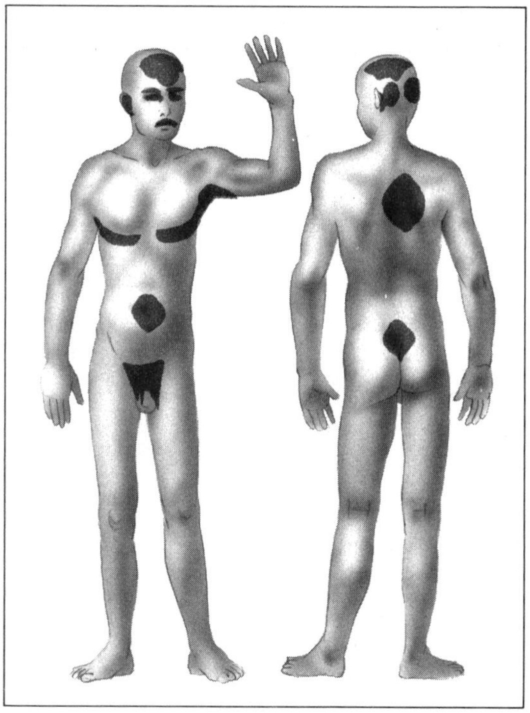

Figure 6-12 Common anatomic locations of seborrheic dermatitis.

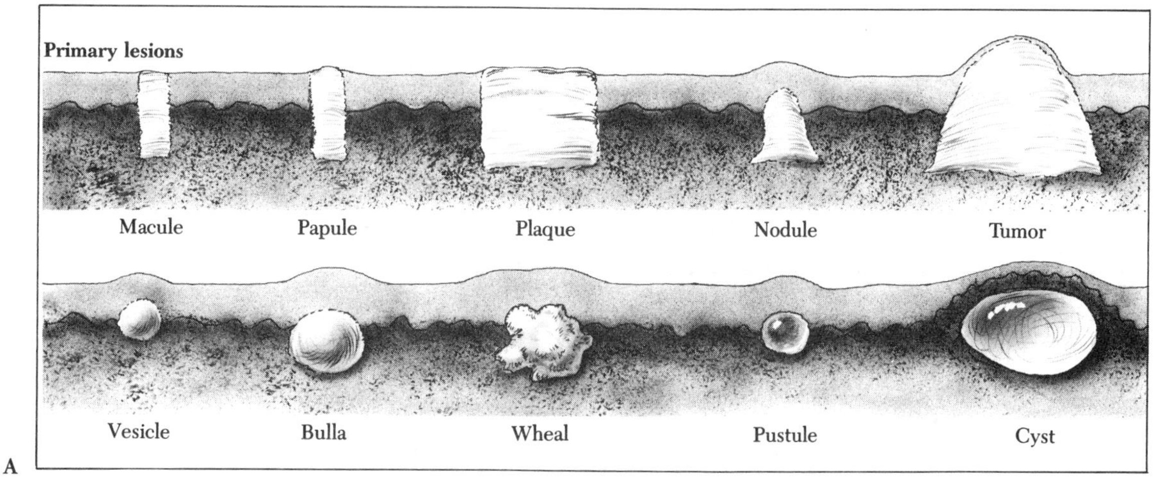

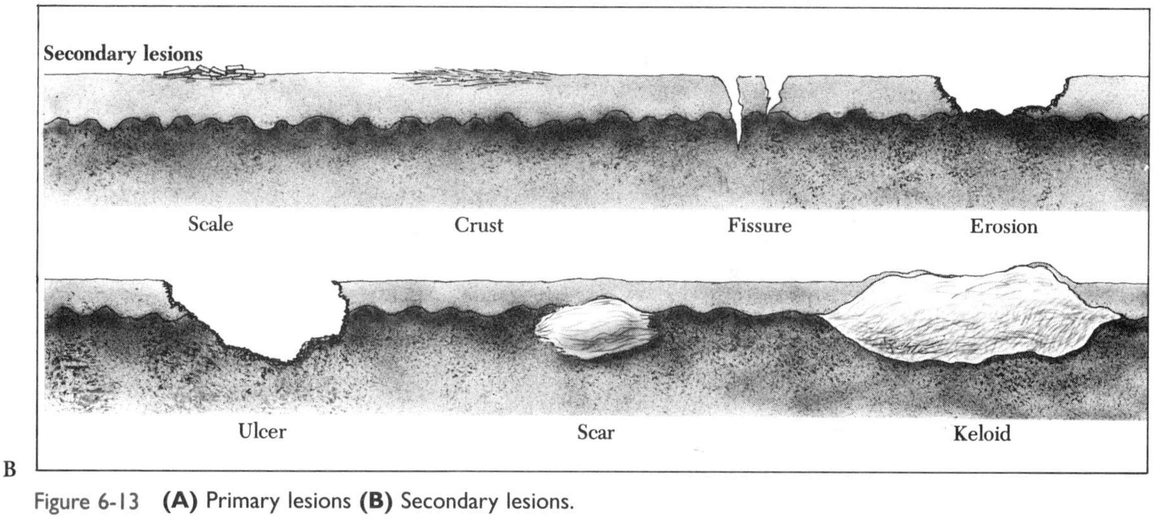

Figure 6-13 **(A)** Primary lesions **(B)** Secondary lesions.

Table 6-3 Primary and Secondary Skin Lesions

Primary lesions		
Type	Definition	Examples
Macule	A flat, nonpalpable area of change in skin color less than 1 cm in diameter	Measles, scarlet fever (Fig. 6-15), freckle, flat nevus, drug rash
Papule	A solid elevation of skin less than 1 cm in diameter, caused by thickening of the epidermis; definitely palpable	Wart, raised scaly area of psoriasis, pityriasis rosea
Vesicle	An elevation of the skin less than 1 cm in diameter, caused by clear fluid filling the upper layers of skin; palpable	Fever blister, chickenpox, smallpox, poison ivy, second degree burn, herpes simplex, herpes zoster, eczematous dermatitis, tinea corporis (Fig. 6-16)
Nodule	A solid mass less than 1 cm in diameter, extending deeper into dermis than a papule; moves with skin when palpated (some may extend into subcutaneous tissue; when palpated at this level skin will slide over nodule)	Area of poorly absorbed injection, dermatofibroma, subcutaneous nodule in rheumatic fever (especially with severe carditis and generally near occipital protuberances or over joints)
Plaque	Like a macule or papule but larger than 1 cm in diameter	Vitiligo, mongolian spot, plantar wart, xanthoma, psoriasis, pityriasis rosea, discoid lupus erythematosus
Bulla	Like a vesicle but larger than 1 cm in diameter, palpable	Pemphigus, some lesions in contact dermatitis, burn, sunburn, poison oak, poison ivy, bullous impetigo; on palms and soles with scarlet fever or congenital syphilis
Tumor	Like a nodule but larger than 1 cm in diameter; may be firm or soft	Lipoma, fibroma, carcinoma
Pustule	Like a vesicle or bulla but pus-filled	Acne, impetigo (Figs. 6-17 and 6-18), furuncles (arising from hair follicles), carbuncles (arising from sebaceous glands)
Wheal	A circumscribed elevation of the skin caused by escape of serum into the dermis (the larger the amount of the edema, the paler the wheal on a red to pale color continuum)	Urticaria, insect bite, poison sumac, poison ivy
Cyst	An encapsulated, fluid-filled area in the dermis or subcutaneous tissue (generally nontender and may transilluminate light)	Sebaceous cyst, epidermoid cyst

Secondary lesions		
Type	Definition	Examples
Scale	A flake of desquamated dead epithelium	Psoriasis, seborrheic dermatitis, pityriasis rosea, exfoliative dermatitis
Excoriation/ erosion	An absence of superficial epidermis	Superficial scratch, syphilitic chancre
Crust	A dried serum or blood exudate as found on the surface of an abrasion or excoriation or on the site of ruptured blisters	Fever blister, impetigo
Fissure	A crack in the epidermis	Chapping, cracking of lips as seen in severe dehydration or fever
Ulcer	A necrotic loss of epidermis	An open sore seen sometimes on the leg with sickle-cell anemia or on the leg and pressure areas with vascular insufficiency
Scar (cicatrix)	A connective tissue replacing skin damaged to depth of dermis during healing process	Healing site of trauma, wound, or surgery
Keloid	An overproduction of scar tissue that has a red, raised, smooth appearance, contains blood vessels, is sometimes irritable; has high incidence of occurrence in African-Americans	Keloid

5. size—if applicable, chart width, length, and depth measurements of masses.
6. mobility—if applicable, chart whether masses are fixed or movable.
7. consistency—if applicable, chart stony hard, firm, or soft quality of masses.

Palpation

Temperature—Skin is palpated for changes and whether a change, hyperthermia or hypothermia, is generalized or localized. Normal skin has a generalized warmth to the touch.

Texture—Normal skin is smooth to the touch. The characteristics of roughness and dryness generally seem to go together.

Moisture—Skin is normally dry without excessive perspiration.

Testing for skin turgor will reveal the moisture content and mobility of the tissues. Pinch the skin over the inner forearm or over the sternum and note how rapidly it returns to place. Normal skin returns almost immediately. Poor skin turgor observed in severe dehydration remains folded for 30 seconds or longer. Poor skin turgor is present with cachexia and also commonly found in elderly clients.

Decreased tissue mobility is noted with edema. Edema can sometimes be detected by inspection, but to determine whether it is pitting edema requires palpation. The tissue is pressed firmly for 10 seconds; if it does not return rapidly to the normal contour, pitting edema is present (Fig. 6-14). Pitting edema usually occurs first in dependent parts of the body. Thus, if there are no visible signs of edema, the sacrum and tibial aspects of the legs as well as the ankles should be carefully palpated to check for pitting. Generally one of two classifications—time and extent—are used to document the degree of pitting edema.

Time classification

0	No pitting
1+	Trace
2+	Moderate, disappears in 10 to 15 seconds
3+	Deep, disappears in 1 to 2 minutes
4+	Very deep, disappears in 5 minutes

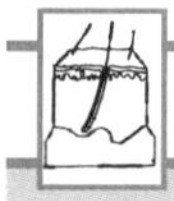

Technique of Palpation of the Skin

1. Use most sensitive area of hand for the particular characteristics.
2. Characteristics: temperature (dorsum of hand), texture (fingertips), skin turgor, abnormalities

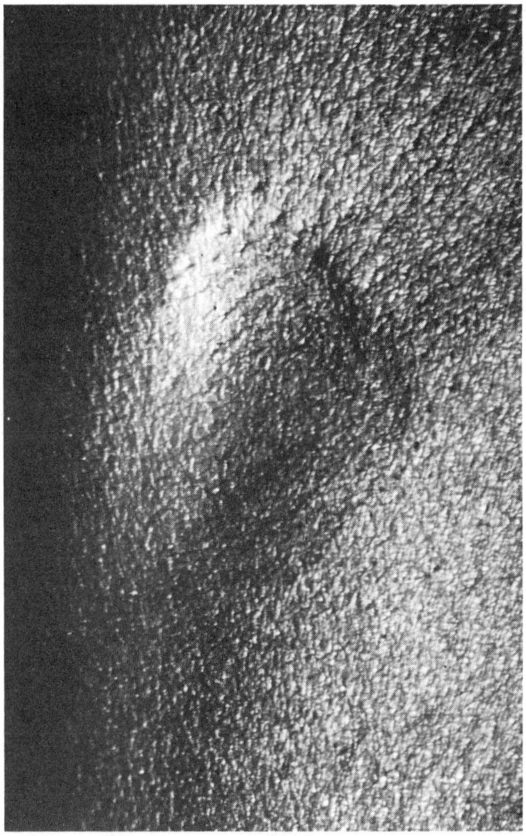

Figure 6-14 Indentation of pitting edema.

Extent classification

1+	Shallow pit formed by thumb pressure
2+	Deep pit formed by thumb pressure
3+	Signs of pitting in a dependent part of the body (e.g., limb is one and a half times the normal size)
4+	Generalized deep pitted edema accompanied by ascites (as in severe congestive heart failure)

- Any skin lesions should be carefully described using the terminology presented earlier in this chapter.
- Any recently appearing lesion should be regarded with suspicion. In particular, with the physical signs of nodule, telangiectasia, and ulceration of sun exposed areas, the client must be referred to a physician.
- Any recent change in the size or color of a wart or mole warrants consultation.
- Any nodular black-gray lesion with an irregular margin and rough, uneven surface needs medical evaluation.
- Any lesion that is constantly being irritated or that bleeds needs further evaluation by a physician.

These lesions could possibly be a basal or squamous cell carcinoma (Figs. 6-19 through 6-21) or a malignant

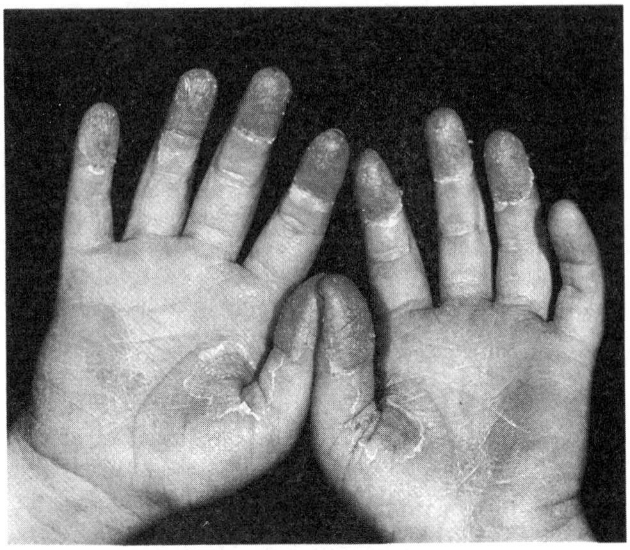

Figure 6-15 Scarlet fever. Desquamation of the hands. (From T.P. Habif, *Clinical Dermatology,* 2nd ed., St. Louis: Mosby Year Book, Inc., 1990.)

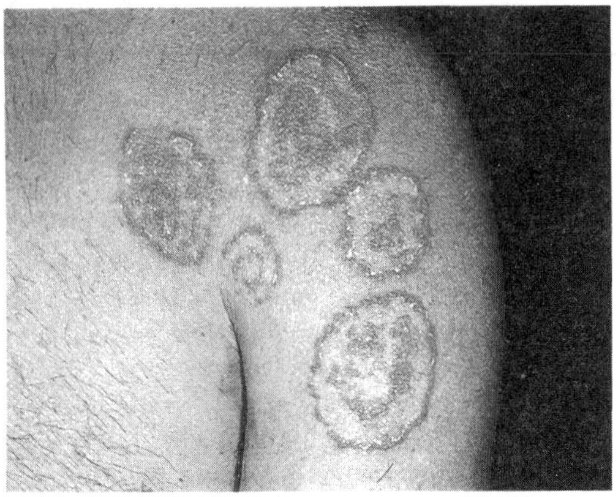

Figure 6-16 Tinea corporis. A classic presentation with an advancing red scaly border. The reason for the designation "ringworm" is obvious. (From T.P. Habif, *Clinical Dermatology,* 2nd ed., St. Louis: Mosby Year Book, Inc., 1990.)

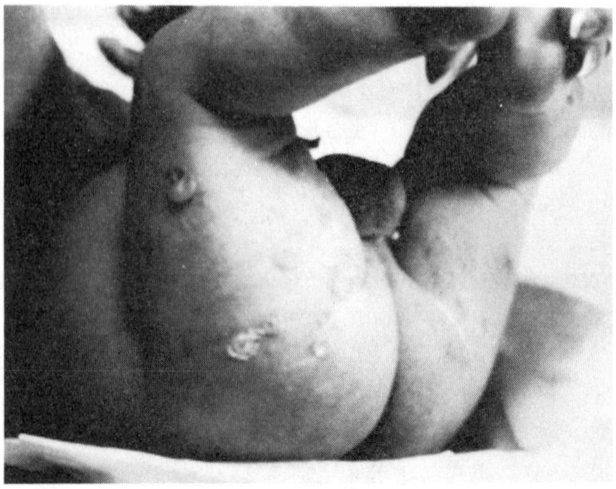

Figure 6-17 Impetigo contagiosa: bullous form. (Courtesy B. Hoggarth, M.D.)

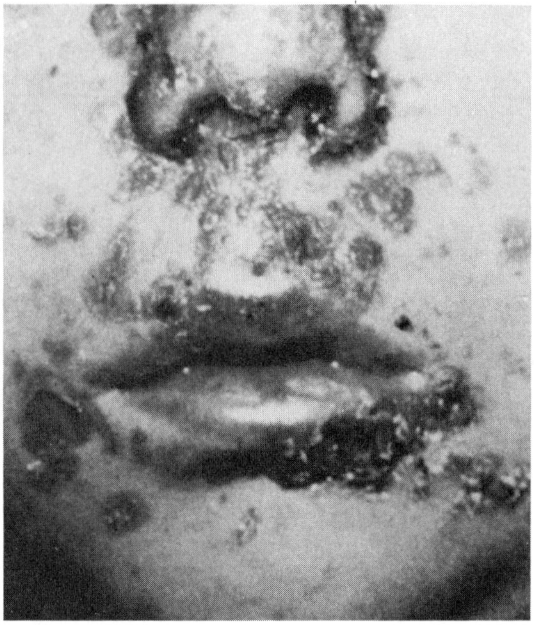

Figure 6-18 Impetigo contagiosa: vesiculopustular form. (Courtesy B. Hoggarth, M.D.)

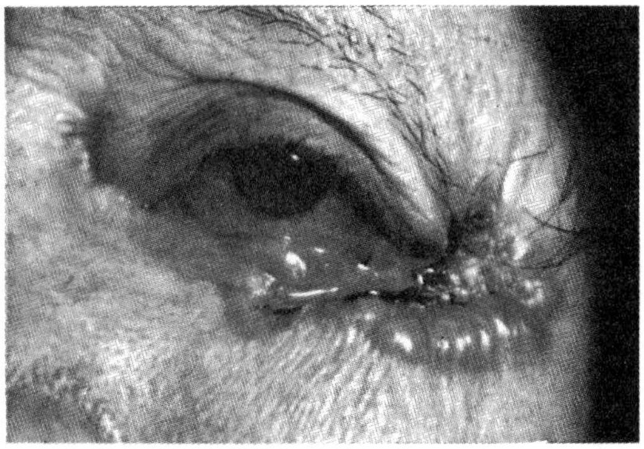

Figure 6-19 Basal cell carcinoma.

melanoma (Fig. 6-22). Other common abnormalities of the integument are seen in Table 6-4. The assessment and nursing management of insect infestations and viral, bacterial, and fungal skin alterations are provided in Appendix E.

Hair

Inspection and Palpation

Color and Texture

- Note the color of the hair.
- Ask if the client uses dyes or rinses, as allergies to them often cause rashes and itching on the scalp, face, ears, and neck.
- Note the texture of the hair.
- Note the distribution of the hair.

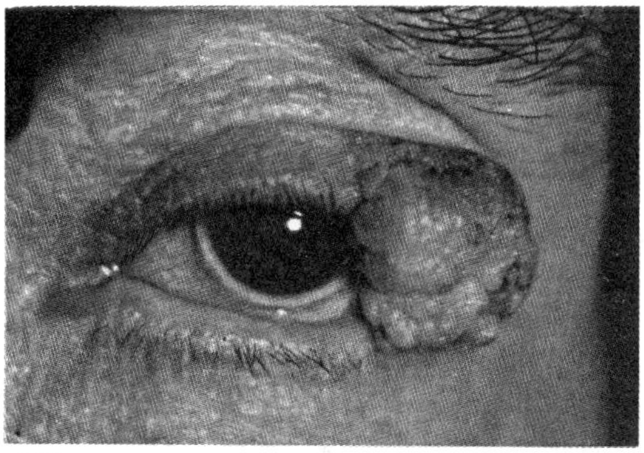

Figure 6-20

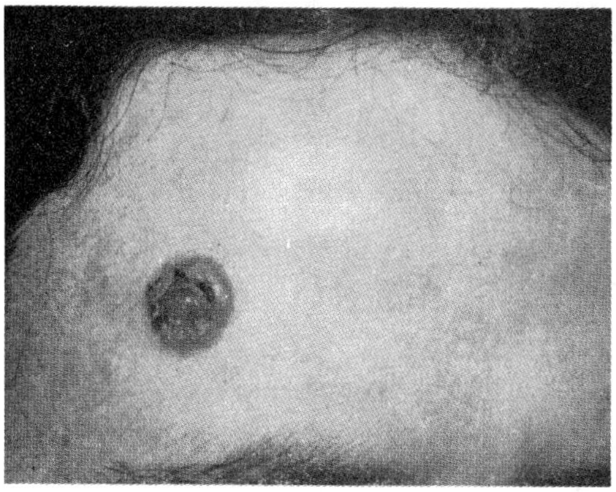

Figure 6-21 Basal cell carcinoma on forehead.

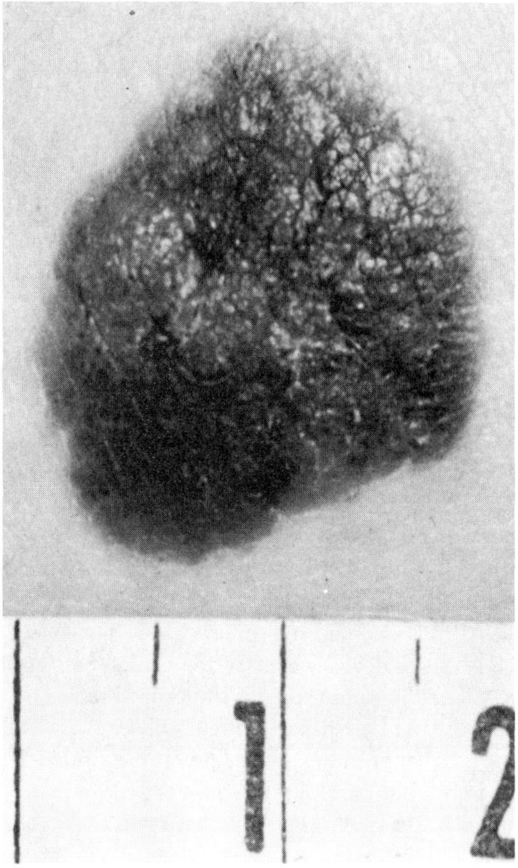

Figure 6-22 Melanoma.

Table 6-4 Other Common Abnormalities of the Integument

Terminology	Characteristics	Comments
Edema	Tissue fluid accumulation, localized or generalized	Check degree of edema and presence of pitting edema.
Diaphoresis	Increased perspiration	Assess for pain, anxiety, fever, high metabolic rate.
Rough, dry skin	Localized or generalized	Assess for exposure to soap, bubble bath, wool, cold, wind, loss of body fluids.
Hirsutism	Increased body hair	Assess for adrenocortical dysfunction, changes in mustache or beard growth and pubic hair pattern.
Alopecia	Decreased or absent body hair	Assess for anxiety, debilitating illness, high fever, starvation, and hypopituitarism.

Technique of Inspection and Palpation of the Hair

1. Adequate lighting and exposure
2. Alternate processes: (a) Inspect and palpate hair of each particular anatomical part of the body as the physical assessment proceeds; or (b) inspect and palpate hair of the entire body of the client.
3. Characteristics: color, texture, distribution, abnormalities

Hair color varies widely, from pale blond to dark black, and it may be changed readily with dyes and rinses. Graying of the hair is a common sign of aging, but it may occur prematurely as a hereditary condition or at birth in albinos. Scalp hair may be fine or coarse. Hyperfunction of the sebaceous glands causes hair to be oily, particularly close to the scalp. This oiliness is common in both boys and girls during adolescence. Body hair is usually very fine, although hair in the pubic and axillary areas is coarse.

The newborn baby is covered with lanugo, a downy hair over the entire body. Within a few weeks' time, the majority

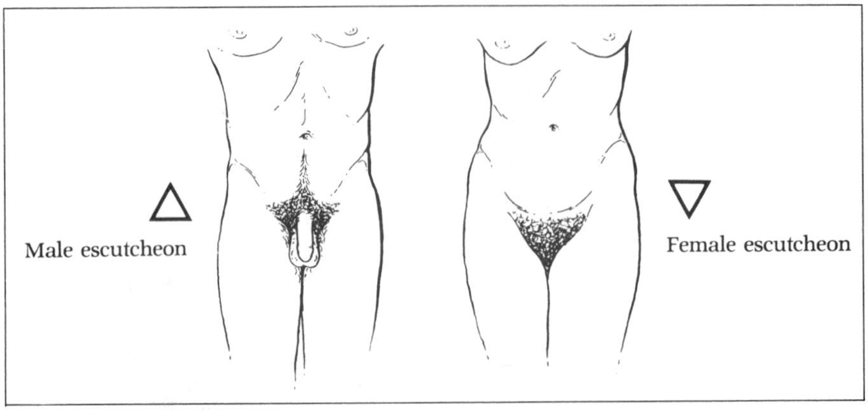

Figure 6-23 Normal hair distribution in adult men and women. Changes may signal hormonal abnormalities. (Reproduced with permission from Judge, R.D., Zuidema, G.D. and Fitzgerald, F. (eds.). *Methods of Clinical Examination* (4th ed.). Boston: Little, Brown, 1982.)

of this hair is lost. Body hair growth begins to develop at puberty in both sexes, but growth patterns differ in males and females. Males normally have more facial and body hair. Both sexes develop axillary and genital hair growth at puberty, but the pubic hair distribution differs.

The male pubic hair pattern resembles a diamond, with the top of the diamond extending to the umbilicus. The female pubic hair pattern is like an inverted triangle, having a straight horizontal plane approximating the level of the pubes (Fig. 6-23).

Nails

Inspection and Palpation

The normal color of the nails is a pinkish white. Occasionally, normal dark vertical bands of hyperpigmentation may be observed in persons of the African race (Fig. 6-24). Generally, nail texture is smooth. Parallel longitudinal ridges may develop in the older adult as part of the aging process and are not significant of any deficiency (Fig. 6-25). The normal angle between the nail and nailbed is 160 degrees (Fig. 6-26). With trauma or decreased circulation, the nails will become thicker than normal.

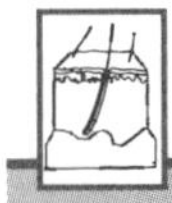

Technique of Inspection and Palpation of the Nails

1. Adequate lighting
2. Characteristics: color, texture, nail/nailbed angle, capillary refill, thickness, abnormalities
3. Test capillary refill time of fingernails and toenails.

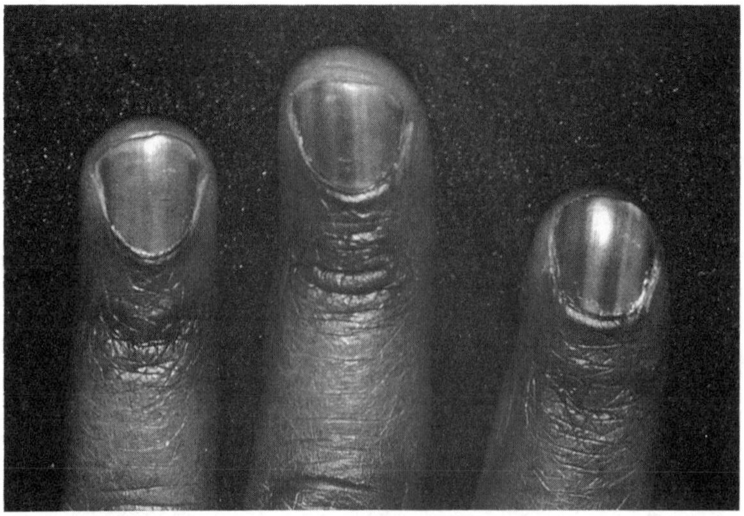

Figure 6-24 Pigmented bands occur as a normal finding in more than 90% of persons with African ancestry. (From T.P. Habif, *Clinical Dermatology,* 2nd ed., St. Louis: Mosby Year Book, Inc., 1990.)

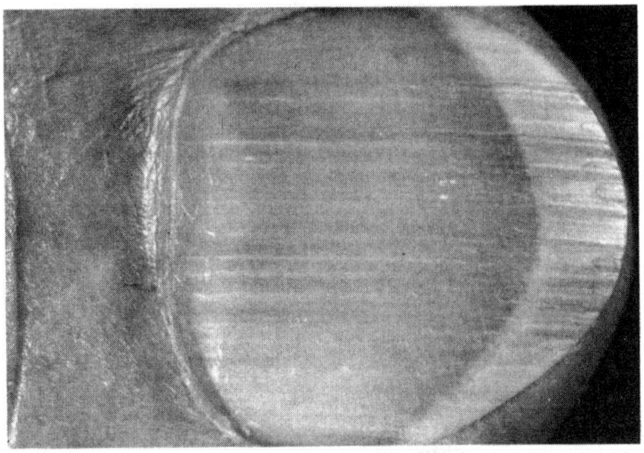

Figure 6-25 Longitudinal ridging. Parallel elevated nail ridges are a common aging change. This change does not indicate any deficiency. (From T.P. Habif, *Clinical Dermatology*, 2nd ed., St. Louis: Mosby Year Book, Inc., 1990.)

Because the nail plate is translucent, it affords a window to the underlying capillary bed, and the status of circulation to the extremities can be determined. With pressure, blanching of the capillary bed beneath the client's fingernail or toenail should occur (Fig. 6-27). On release of the pressure, the color should return immediately.

With chronic decreased oxygen levels, clubbing of the nails may be observed. The nails are one of the first places of the body where cyanosis is detected. In early clubbing, the angle is 180 degrees, and the nail appears flattened and even with the nailbed; the nail plate is spongy upon palpation. A simulation of the sponginess of the nail plate in early clubbing can be created by squeezing both the left and right sides of a nail with your thumb and middle finger of the opposite hand and then palpating at the cuticle area with your index finger. The angle in late clubbing is greater than 180 degrees, and the nail plate is visibly swollen (Figs. 6-26 and 6-28).

CLINICAL CORRELATIONS

Color Changes of the Integumentary System

Pallor is associated with such conditions as chronic disease, anemia, and shock where appreciable decreases in hemoglobin exist. It is also present in anxiety, fear, and syncope as a result of the peripheral vasoconstriction that occurs with stress. Paleness also may exist with edema that tends to mask the red hemoglobin tint of the skin.

Intermittent pallor or cyanosis of the extremities may suggest peripheral vascular problems. If only the fingers and toes are involved, it may be Raynaud's disease. Raynaud's disease is due to arteriolar spasm, which is aggravated by emotion or exposure to cold; it is more common in young girls, rarely occurring in boys or men.

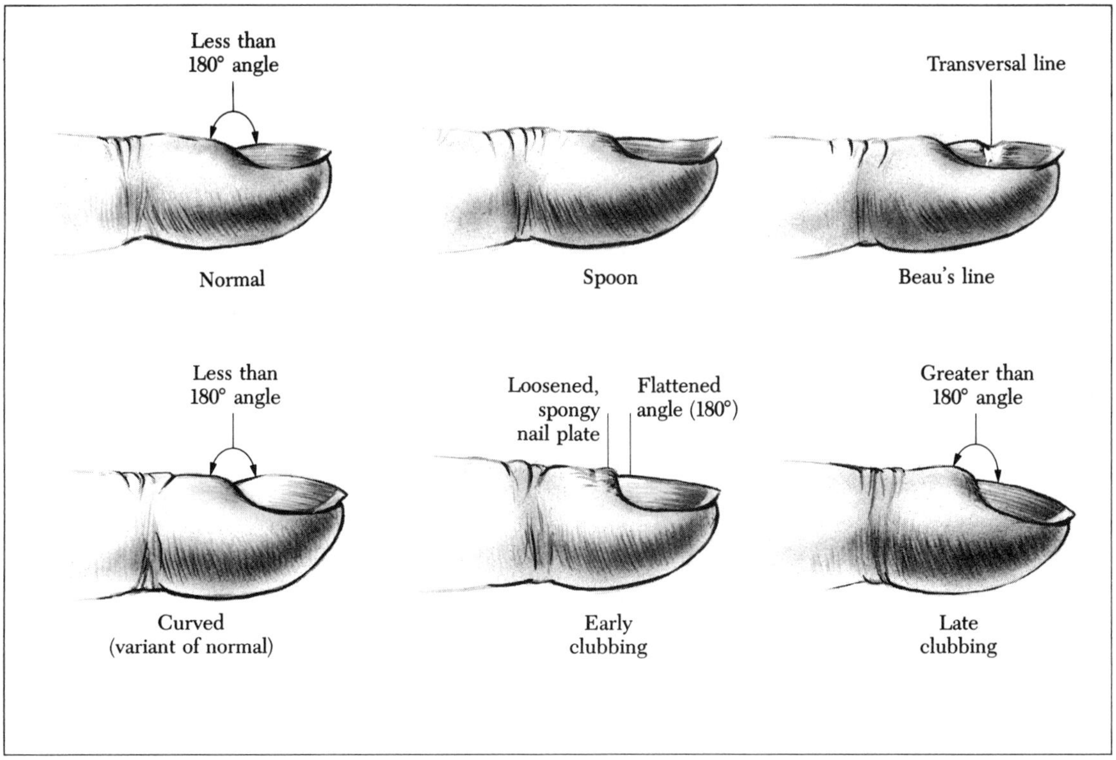

Figure 6-26 Normal and abnormal nails.

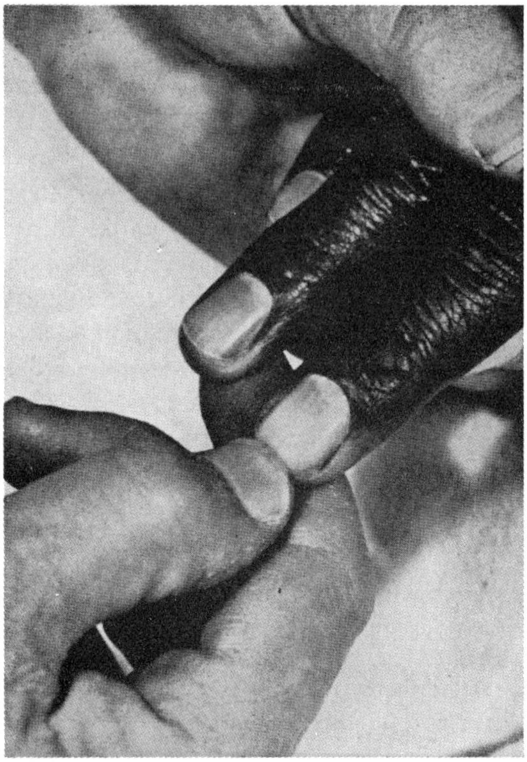

Figure 6-27 Technique for assessing capillary refill.

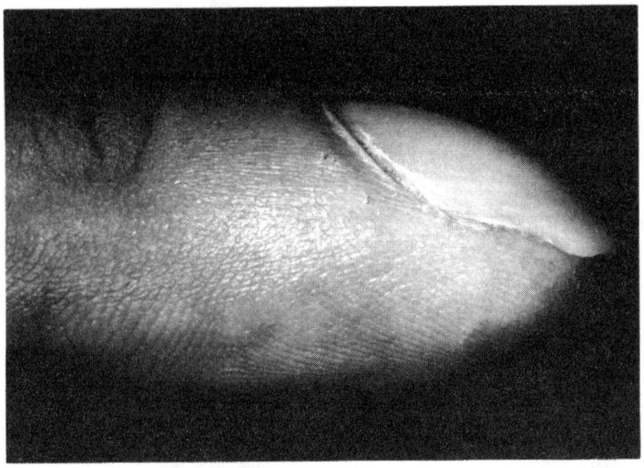

Figure 6-28 Finger clubbing. The distal phalanges are enlarged to a rounded bulbous shape. The nail enlarges and becomes curved, hard, and thickened. (From T.P. Habif, *Clinical Dermatology,* 2nd ed., St. Louis: Mosby Year Book, Inc., 1990.)

Lack of skin pigmentation occurs with albinism and vitiligo. The incidence of albinism tends to be high in equatorial areas. In the United States, the incidence of albinism is approximately one of every 20,000 people. Albinism is an abnormal but nonpathologic depigmentation of the skin, eyes, and hair. Frequently, albinos also show signs of photophobia and nystagmus because the choroid lining of the eye is not adequately protected from light. As children, albinos may have body image problems, as they may be the focus of ridicule and are unable to participate in some sports due to poor vision. Most albinos are considered legally blind and thus cannot get a driver's license. There are persons who believe that Noah of the Bible may have been an albino because of descriptions of his white hair and "fire in his eyes."

RECORDING OF FINDINGS

Normal findings are presented in the first column. The second column contains a recording of abnormal signs and symptoms manifested by a client prior to undergoing an incision and drainage of an abscess.

Skin *Inspection:* Color pink and heavily freckled; clear without excoriations, fissures, scars, or lesions; extremities pink without edema *Palpation:* Good skin turgor; warm and smooth to touch	**Skin** *Inspection:* A localized 2 × 3-cm erythematous area left midaxillary region *Palpation:* Above described left midaxillary region indurated; hot to touch; extremely tender; onset within a 24-hour period.
Hair *Inspection:* Normal distribution, full, and glossy, light brown hair *Palpation:* Normal texture—soft, flexible	**Hair** *Inspection:* Sparse, gray hair *Palpation:* Brittle
Nails *Inspection:* No deformities; no clubbing; no cyanosis *Palpation:* Good capillary refill	**Nails** *Inspection:* Bites nails; no clubbing; no cyanosis *Palpation:* Good capillary refill

Vitiligo is an acquired loss of pigmentation that presents itself as milky white patches of the skin, usually on exposed areas of the body (Fig. 6-29). It is an idiopathic affliction that is most common in tropical zones and among those of African ancestry. Vitiligo of the scalp is accompanied by depigmentation of the hairs of the affected area. The areas of depigmentation do not tan with exposure to the sun.

Cyanosis, a bluish discoloration of the skin, is commonly seen with heart and lung disease and with congenital defects such as atrioseptal heart defects (right-to-left shunts) and methemoglobinemia. A bright cherry red flush or patches on the face, neck, and chest, accompanied by deep, difficult respirations are suggestive of carbon monoxide poisoning.

Ecchymosis accompanies bleeding disorders such as hemophilia, anemia, leukemia, and hepatic dysfunction and is observed in clients who are taking high doses of anticoagulants. Ecchymosis is characteristic of meningococcic, streptococcic, and staphylococcic septicemias.

One cause of jaundice is the hemolysis of red blood cells. Hemolysis happens in hemolytic disease and in diseases caused by certain pathologic organisms (certain streptococci and staphylococci, tetanus bacilli, and diphtheria bacilli). Jaundice can follow severe burns and the intravenous administration of a hypotonic saline solution or of distilled water. All intravenous solutions must be isotonic to the blood; otherwise, the red blood cells expand from the osmotic influx of fluid and eventually rupture, releasing hemoglobin. The liberated hemoglobin is removed from circulation primarily by the liver and the spleen. The iron content is stored, and the non-iron-containing pigment is converted into bilirubin.

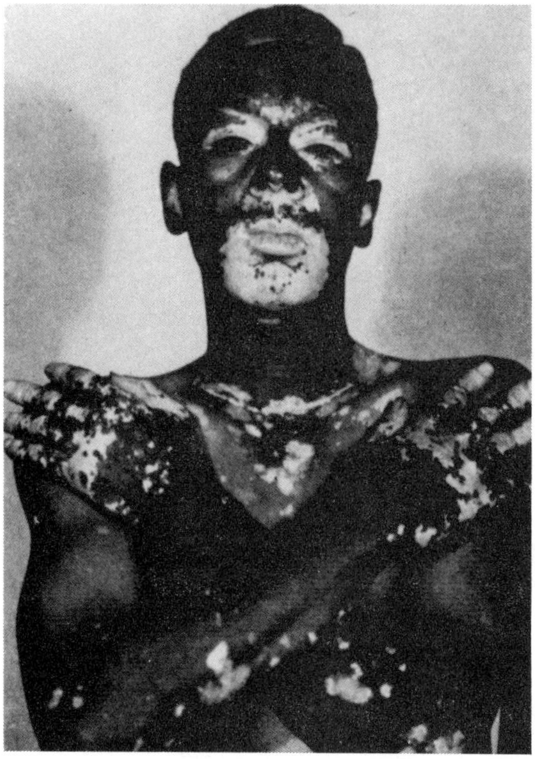

Figure 6-29 Vitiligo. Note symmetrical white patchy distribution.

Jaundice can also be caused by any condition that results in increased serum bilirubin, such as cirrhosis or biliary obstruction. It is also commonly observed in infectious mononucleosis; in this disease, abnormal liver function tests are found in about 90% of the cases.

A yellow tint to the skin is seen with chronic renal disease. It does not involve the sclera or mucous membranes. A bronze tan color of the skin may be present with Addison's disease (hypoadrenocorticism) and with some pituitary tumors. In these conditions, the darker coloring involves the areolae, genitals, and perineum, but it is also more prominent at the pressure and friction points of the body (elbows, buttocks, inner thighs, and axillae). The palmar creases are generally markedly darker and appear as dark brown streaks. It is also fairly common for the exposed areas of the body (face, neck, and arms) to have a darker hue and accompanying black freckles.

A generalized bronze hue is sometimes observed in hyperthyroidism and is characteristic of hemochromatosis, a rare disease that occurs 10 times as frequently in men as women and that develops chiefly after the fourth decade of life. Hemochromatosis is accompanied by hepatomegaly, diabetes mellitus, and often, cardiac failure.

Vascularity Changes

The normal vascularity observed will be masked or diminished with tissue edema; however, increased vascularity is commonly seen on the abdomen when the client has severe ascites. An increase in vascularity may accompany tumors and malignant skin lesions. When atrophy of muscles occurs, increased vascularity is observed. An example of this is the blood vessels seen through the thin, fragile skin of the older adult.

Skin Lesions

Annular and arciform lesions are characteristic of dermatologic reactions to some drugs. This format of lesions is also seen in urticaria and psoriasis. This pattern and/or an iris cluster is characteristic of erythema multiforme (Figs. 6-30 and 6-31). An iris grouping appears as a bull's-eye pattern. Often, zosteriform groupings are observed in diseases such as metastatic breast carcinoma, but these lesions, which are arranged in broad bands, are most typical of herpes zoster (see Figs. 6-9 and 6-10), and the band follows the line of nerve disease distribution. A linear or straight-line grouping is seen with lymphangitis and poison ivy lesions.

The moist areas behind the ears, in the axillae, under pendulous breasts, in the umbilici, in the groin, in the gluteal folds, and of the perianal region are common sites for cutaneous moniliasis (Fig. 6-32). The butterfly lesion characteristic of lupus erythematosus occurs chiefly on the forehead

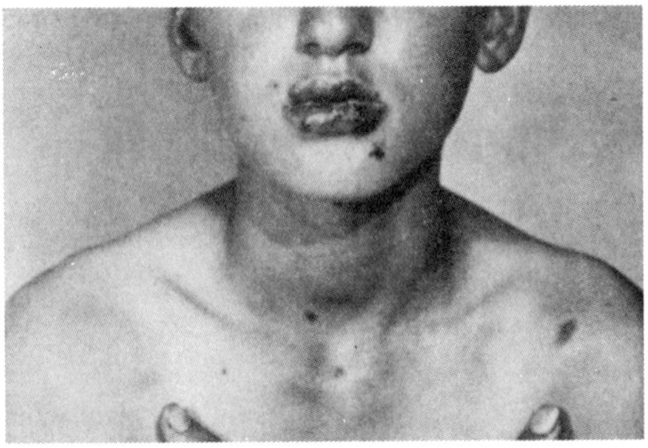

Figure 6-30 Papules of erythema multiforme on skin and lips.

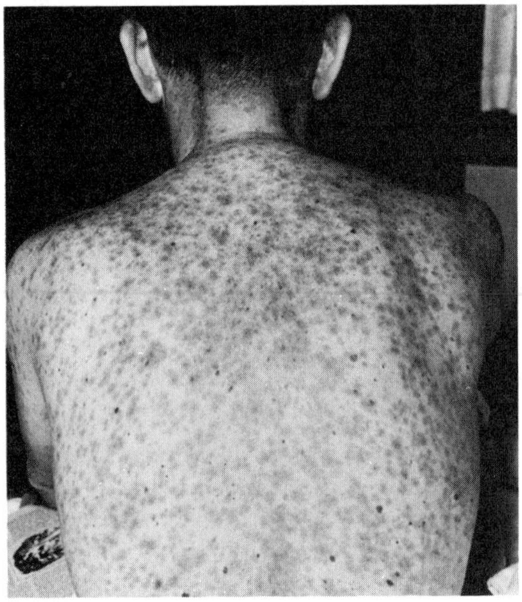

Figure 6-31 Erythema multiforme.

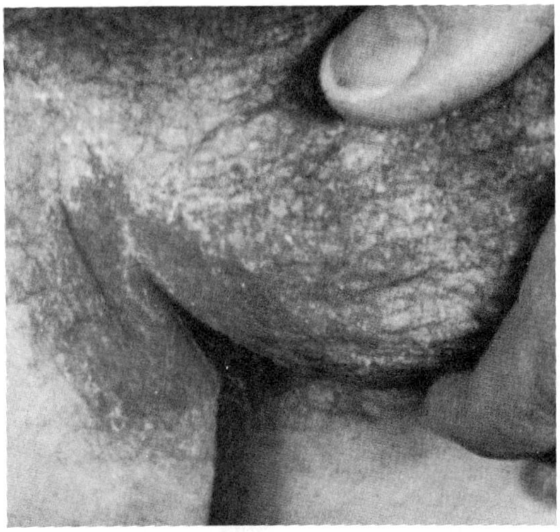

Figure 6-32 Monilial intertrigo, a type of lesion found in moist areas of the body.

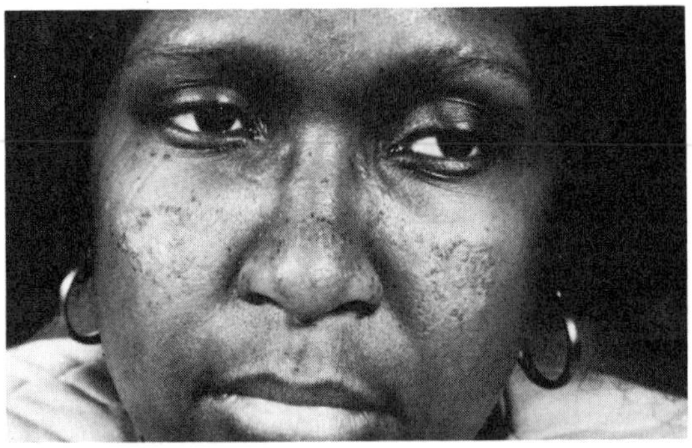

Figure 6-33 Butterfly lesion.

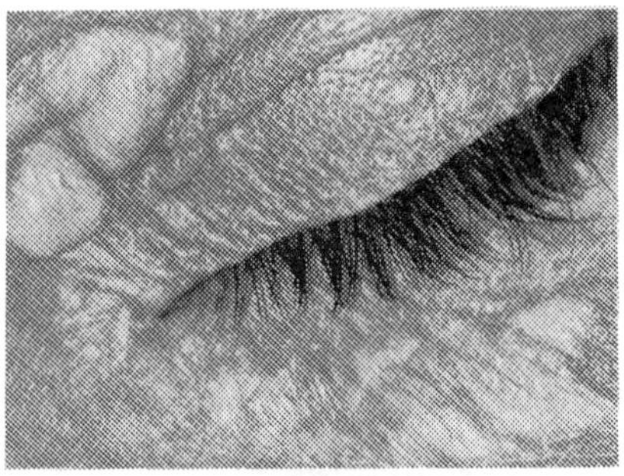

Figure 6-34 Xanthelasma consists of one or more bright yellow, sharply marginated plaques with no epidermal change, usually occurring on the eyelids. All patients with xanthelasma should be investigated for evidence of plasma lipid abnormalities.

and cheeks (Fig. 6-33). Xanthomas, yellow plaques of lipoid deposits, may be seen as secondary signs of uncontrolled diabetes mellitus and usually appear over the hands, about the nasal bridge, and on the eyelids (Fig. 6-34).

Petechiae are tiny reddish purple hemorrhagic spots that occur as a result of capillary bleeding (Fig. 6-35). They are seen in thrombocytopenic purpura (inadequate or defective platelets), hepatic dysfunction, and conditions in which increased capillary permeability is present, such as leukemia and subacute bacterial endocarditis. These small hemorrhagic spots may indicate an increased tendency for bleeding or an embolus to the skin.

Spider angiomas are caused by an excess of ketosteroids. Such an excess occurs with liver dysfunction because it is the liver that metabolizes the ketosteroids.

It is important to carefully assess and recognize signs of malignancy. Malignancies involving the skin are malignant skin melanoma, basal cell carcinoma, and squamous cell carcinoma. Suspected malignancies warrant medical referral (Table 6-5).

Palpation Changes of the Integument

Generalized hyperthermia of the skin occurs with sunburn or conditions in which there is an increased metabolic rate, such as fever, hyperthyroidism, and strenuous exercise. Localized areas of skin hyperthermia are found at sites of

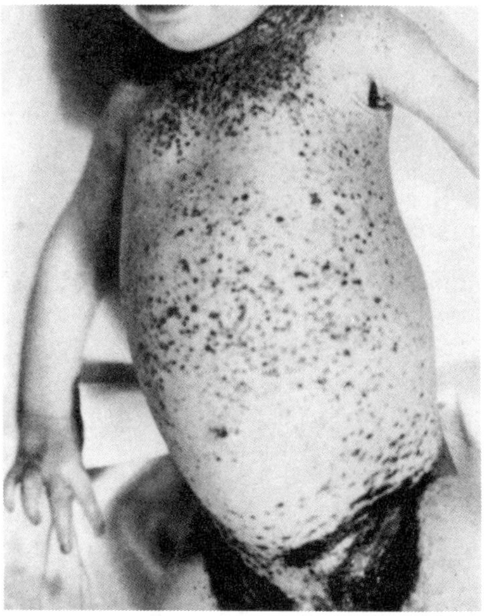

Figure 6-35 Petechiae. These small hemorrhagic spots are caused by capillary bleeding.

inflammation, such as phlebitis, furuncle, or a localized burn. A localized, hot, painful, indurated area is characteristic of cellulitis.

Generalized hypothermia is observed in shock, where there is a general decrease of peripheral blood flow. Localized areas of coolness suggest peripheral vascular disease.

Touching the skin surface of an individual with severe hyperthyroidism is like rubbing your hand over a piece of velvet. The texture of the skin in hypothyroidism, on the other hand, is quite rough to the touch. A roughness of the skin is also characteristic of hyperkeratosis; of skin reactions to such materials as soap, bubble bath, or wool; and of the irritating and drying effects of cold, wintry winds.

Diaphoresis can be seen in clients with pyrexia or thyrotoxicosis. Increased perspiration also results from stimulation of the nervous system, as from pain and anxiety.

Decreased tissue mobility is noted in conditions such as scleroderma and with edema. Edema formation can result from increased hydrostatic pressure within the vascular system (as in hypertension), increased venous pressure (as in

Table 6-5 Common Color-Change Abnormalities of the Skin

Terminology	Characteristics	Comments
Albinism	Depigmentation of skin, eyes, and hair	Nonpathologic; photophobia and nystagmus may accompany defective visual acuity. Assess body image concerns.
Vitiligo	Milky white patches usually on exposed areas	Idiopathic; more common in tropical zones and in African-Americans. Assess body image concerns. May be familial and may occur in hyperthyroidism, pernicious anemia, diabetes mellitus. May be caused by trauma or autoimmunity.
Mongolian spots	Blackish blue areas of lower back and buttocks	Nonpathologic; disappears in early childhood. Predominantly in African-American, Native American, and Asian newborns.
Jaundice	Yellow pigmentation of skin, mucous membranes, sclerae	Best observed in natural sunlight. Pathologic state.
Cyanosis	Bluish coloration: lips, earlobes, nailbeds, under tongue	Check for heart, lung abnormalities and type of medications client is taking. Pathologic state.
Carotenemia	Yellow pigmentation of skin—does *not* involve sclerae and mucous membranes; usually on palms, soles, and face	Check for increased carotinoids in diet, signs of diabetes mellitus, myxedema, hypopituitarism.
Erythema	Redness of skin	Assess for sources of irritation, inflammation, infection, heat, chilblain, increased vascularity, exposure to carbon monoxide gas.
Ecchymosis	Black-and-blue marks	Assess for trauma, other signs of bleeding disorder, hepatic dysfunction.
Malignant skin melanoma	Rough uneven surface, irregular notched edges, variegated coloring (red, white, blue, and black appearing lesions)	Referral needed.
Basal cell carcinoma	Generally on sun-exposed areas; central indentation of circumscribed lesion or central ulceration	Early detection enhances prognosis. Referral needed.
Squamous cell carcinoma	Firm lesion that eventually ulcerates	Leukoplakia may precede lesion. Early detection enhances prognosis. Referral needed.

congestive heart failure or in obstruction of venous or lymphatic return by tumors or in inflammation), increased capillary permeability (as with burns, allergies, insect bites, electrolyte retention, hyperaldosteronism, cortisone therapy, and renal shutdown, or just prior to or during the menses), and a decrease in osmotic pressure within the vascular system due to a decrease in serum protein (as in kidney disease or in the hypoproteinemia of starvation or liver disease).

Changes of the Hair

In regard to texture, dry brittle hair may be seen in hypothyroidism, but it is most frequently caused by overuse of hair dyes and of curling or straightening preparations. In hyperthyroidism, the hair has a very fine texture.

A client with hair distribution more like that of the opposite sex may have endocrine problems. Hirsutism in women and children caused by androgens will assume the distribution pattern of the normal adult man. This condition is observed in clients with masculinizing ovarian tumors, adrenocortical tumors, and Stein-Leventhal syndrome (Fig. 6-36). In hypopituitarism, there is a general decrease in or absence of body hair. A total absence of body hair, alopecia totalis, is rare, and the loss of hair may or may not be permanent (Fig. 6-37). Alopecia totalis may result from poor nutrition, serious illness, high fever, starvation, or nervous disease, or from chemotherapy and radiation therapy.

Changes of the Nails

Nails normally grow about 0.1 mm/day. The nails grow more slowly and become thick and yellow when lymphatic circulation is impeded.

Figure 6-26 shows Beau's line, a transverse white line or indentation that appears during an acute illness. Beau's line may reflect an earlier systemic disease or may be evidence of local trauma. As the nail grows, the line moves toward the distal end of the finger and is eventually trimmed off.

Paronychia is inflammation of the nail and surrounding tissue. In the acute stage, there is tissue erythema and pus along the area of the cuticles (Fig. 6-38A). With chronic paronychia, the cuticle is missing and there are raised horizontal ridges of the nails (Fig. 6-38B). A herpes simplex viral infection of the fingers seen in health care workers is known as herapetic whitlow (Fig. 6-39).

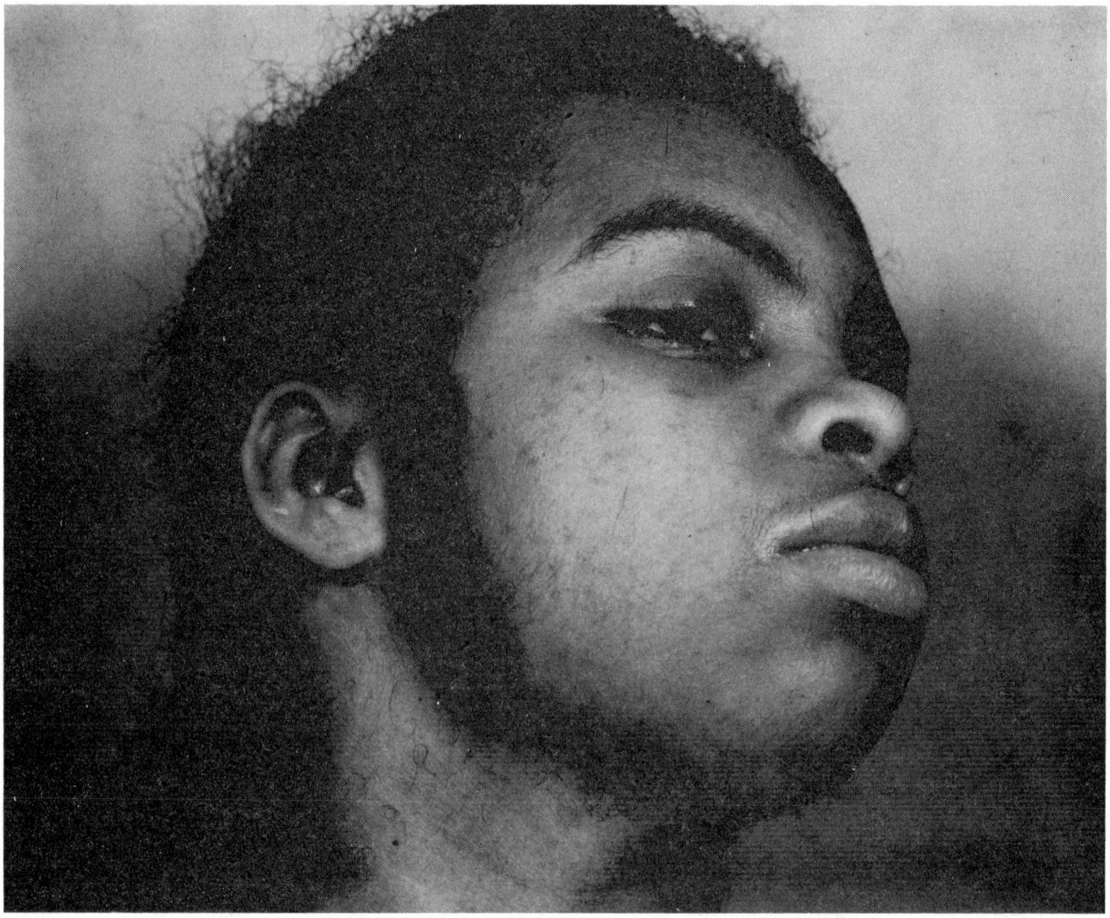

Figure 6-36 Hirsutism in young female. Note beginning mustache and beard growth.

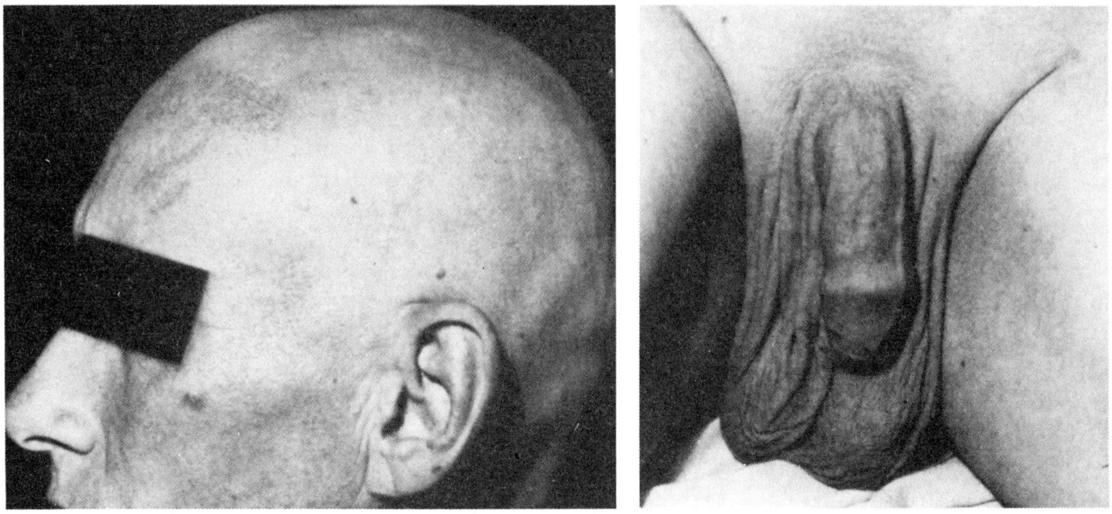

A B

Figure 6-37 Alopecia totalis of **(A)** the head and **(B)** the genitals. This rare condition may be permanent in some instances.

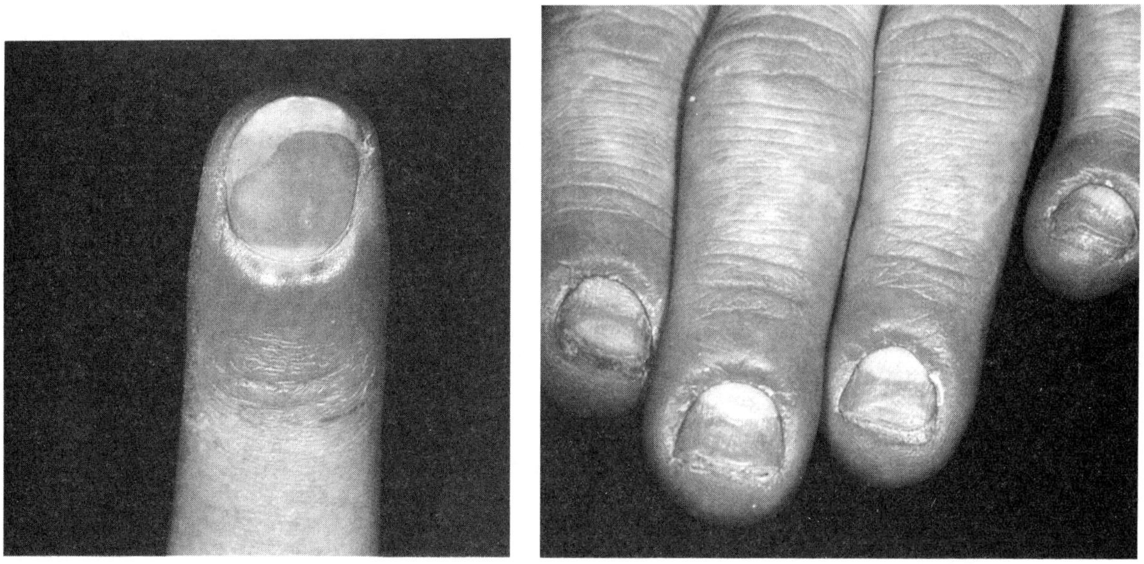

A B

Figure 6-38 **(A)** Acute paronychia. Erythema and purulent material occur at the proximal nail fold. **(B)** Paronychia, chronic inflammation with raised horizontal ridges and absence of cuticles. (From T.P. Habif, *Clinical Dermatology,* 2nd ed., St. Louis: Mosby Year Book, Inc., 1990.)

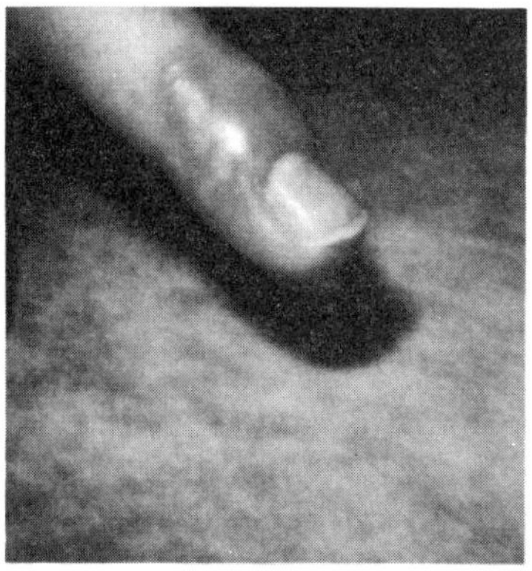

Figure 6-39 Herapetic whitlow, an HSV infection of the fingers, is a recognized hazard among ICU nurses, surgeons, anesthesiologists, and dentists. (From M. Auvenshine and M. Enriquez: *Comprehensive Maternity Nursing,* 2nd ed., © 1990 Boston: Jones and Bartlett Publishers. Reprinted with permission.)

Spoon nails, characterized by a concave profile, may be observed in prolonged iron deficiency anemia. Curved nails, a variant of the normal, can be differentiated from clubbed nails in that, even though they manifest a convex curve and look similar to clubbing, the angle between the nail and nail bed is still less than 180 degrees and within the normal range.

In early clubbing, the angle between nail and nail bed straightens out to 180 degrees. In late clubbing, the angle increases to greater than 180 degrees. Clubbing of the nails usually occurs first in the thumbs and index fingers and later involves the remaining fingers and the toes. Once the cause is eliminated, the clubbing is reversed.

There are several conditions in which clubbing occurs. The most common condition is pulmonary disease, such as emphysema, chronic obstructive lung disease, bronchiectasis, and pulmonary tumor. The second most common condition is cardiovascular disease, including subacute bacterial endocarditis and congenital heart disease with cyanosis. Clubbing may also be present with thyrotoxicosis, cirrhosis, and chronic obstructive jaundice. Clubbing may also be an inherited trait.

Pitting of the nails commonly accompanies psoriasis and fungal diseases of the nails. A ridging containing hypertrophy of the nails can result from dermatologic conditions, ischemia, direct trauma, and bacterial and fungal infections. Brittle, frayed, or terraced nails are occasionally observed in thyrotoxicosis, malnutrition, iron deficiency, and calcium deficiency, and with x-ray irradiation.

Splinter hemorrhages, reflected as red or brown streaks, may be nonspecific, although they are commonly observed in subacute bacterial endocarditis and trichinosis.

Although many of the previously described changes in nails accompany pathologic conditions, they are not necessarily diagnostic of these conditions. Such changes may occur in the normal individual.

SUMMARY

The integument is considered to be the body's most important organ. In this chapter, the structures and function were presented. The three basic layers were described, with emphasis on appearance and function. The entire assessment process begins with considering size, shape, and symmetry of the portion of the body being examined, followed by assessment of the outside surface, the skin. Because each area of the integumentary system has different characteristics, similar and dissimilar methods for examining the skin, hair, and nails were presented. Examples of causes and underlying mechanisms of abnormal changes and diseases of the integumentary system were discussed in the clinical correlations section.

DISCUSSION QUESTIONS/ ACTIVITIES

1. State the characteristics of the skin that are assessed.
2. Describe the technique used to test skin turgor and the normal finding.
3. What is the criterion for documentation of poor skin turgor?
4. Diagram the following patterns of skin lesion: annular grouping, iris cluster/bull's-eye pattern, zosteriform pattern, linear.
5. Define the following types of skin lesions:
   a. Primary lesions—macule, papule, vesicle, nodule, plaque, bulla, tumor, pustule, wheal, cyst.
   b. Secondary lesions—scale, excoriation/erosion, crust, fissure, ulcer, scar (cicatrix), keloid.
6. Give an example of a primary lesion changing into a secondary lesion.
7. Describe a skin lesion by using the criteria presented in this chapter.
8. Perform the techniques used for assessing skin turgor and capillary refill.
9. State the areas of the body where the following skin lesions commonly occur: acne, cutaneous moniliasis, butterfly lesion, xanthomas, intertrigo.
10. Define *leukoplakia* and describe what it looks like.
11. Describe the characteristics of a basal cell carcinoma, squamous cell carcinoma, and malignant skin melanoma lesion.
12. When assessing the integument, what are some questions you might ask a client?

REFERENCES

Allison, S. D., and Wong, K. L. 1968. Skin cancer: some ethnic differences. In *Environments of man,* ed. J. B. Bresler. Reading, Mass.: Addison-Wesley.

CHAPTER

7

Assessment of the Head and Neck

Learning Objectives

1. Identify the characteristics of the head, face, and neck that are assessed in inspection, palpation, and auscultation.
2. Differentiate between hereditary alopecia and alopecia areata.
3. Describe the procedure for palpating the lymph nodes of the neck.
4. Name the lymph nodes of the neck as you point out their locations.
5. Describe approaches for palpation of the thyroid gland.
6. Describe the dangers that are inherent in improper palpation of the carotid arteries.

Assessment of the head and neck begins with inspection of gross appearance—that is, size and contour. Palpation is performed simultaneously with a more detailed inspection of specific parts of the head and neck. During the examination of these anatomic areas, you will be evaluating portions of several body systems, including the skin, hair, lymph, endocrine, and cardiovascular systems.

STRUCTURE OF THE HEAD

The size and shape of the cranium may not be the same in all clients, but identical structures should exist. The regions of the head are identified by the underlying bone structures (Fig. 7-1).

CHARACTERISTICS AND TECHNIQUES OF EXAMINATION

The head is examined by inspection and palpation. Most often, inspection and palpation are used simultaneously when assessing the head. Percussion and auscultation are used only infrequently.

Inspection and Palpation of the Head

- Note the size, shape, and symmetry of the head.
- In infants under age 2, measure the head circumference at the level of the eyebrows anteriorly and the protuberance of the occipital base posteriorly. This measurement is then compared with set standards (see Chapter 18).
- The fontanelles are measured next. The anterior fontanelle is about 4 to 6 cm in each dimension at birth and closes

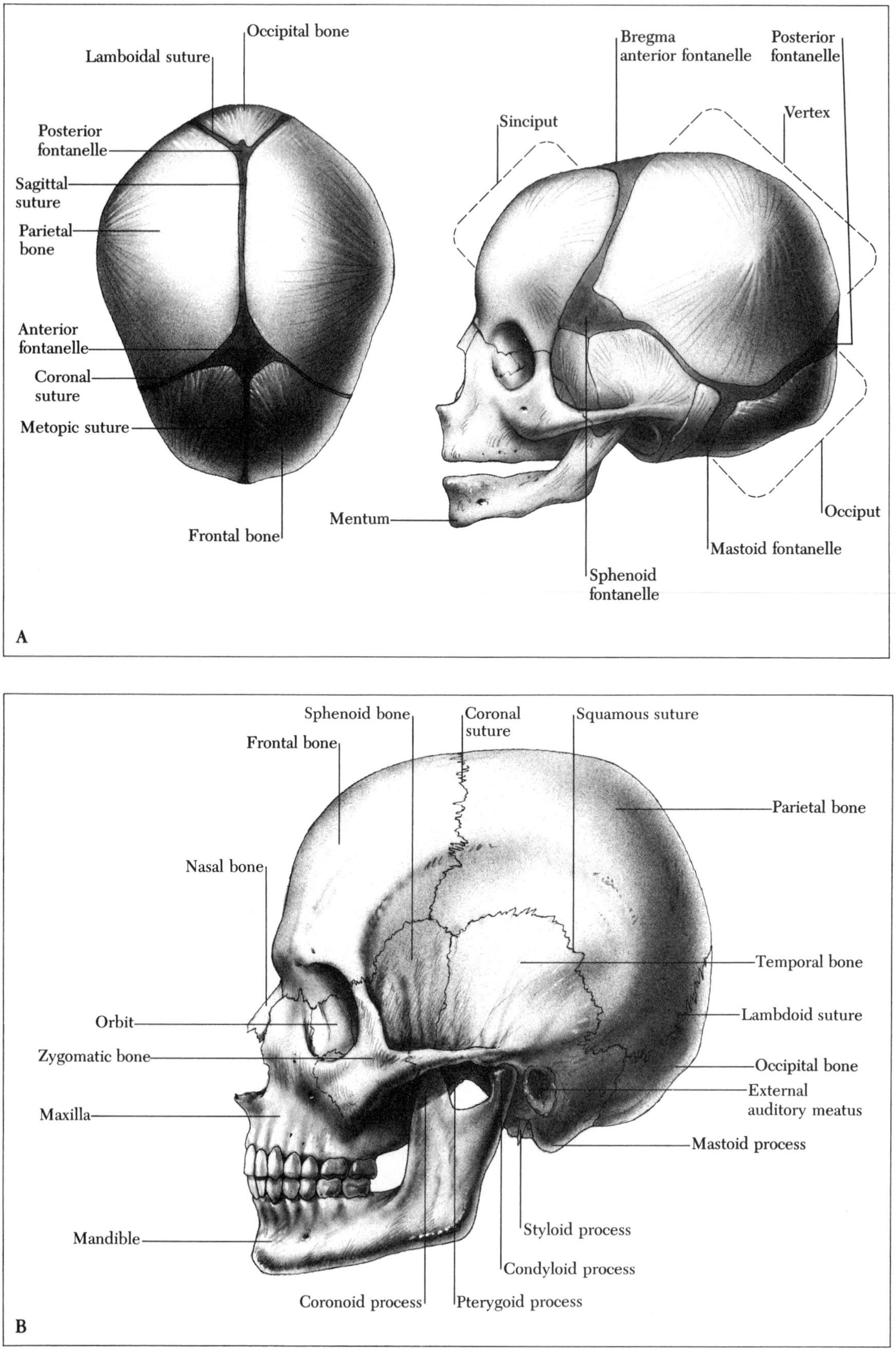

Figure 7-1 **(A)** Top and side view of an infant head. **(B)** Regions of an adult head.

Technique of Inspection and Palpation of the Head

1. Inspection of size and shape of head
2. Palpation of hair with gentle, rotating motion of fingertips
3. Inspection and palpation of scalp, noting texture
4. Abnormalities

by age 18 months. The posterior fontanelle is about 0.5 to 1 cm at birth and closes by age 2 months.

- Inspect the condition of the hair and scalp; the hair is normally full and glossy; the scalp is clean and free of lesions.
- Palpate the hair and scalp. There should be no skin lesions, masses, or tenderness.

The normal skull is usually round, with prominences at the frontal bone and the parietal bone. The sagittal suture, which runs from the anterior to the posterior portion of the cranium, is often palpable. There is a definite protuberance of the occipital bone, and the prominent mastoid bones can be noted behind each ear. Premature closure of the sutures in the child results in distinctive asymmetry of the head.

Palpation of the infant's head may reveal certain conditions that are normal until a certain age. For example, cephalhematoma—localized swelling of the scalp in newborns—may persist up to 3 months of age. Caput succedaneum—edema and bruising of the scalp over a portion of the occipitoparietal region—disappears in the newborn after about 1 week.

The condition of the hair and scalp gives important clues about an individual's health. Palpation is best accomplished by using the fingertips and a gentle rotating motion. The color, texture, and amount of hair should be noted. In the newborn, all of the original hair is shed within a few months, and sometimes the new hair is a different color. When examining an adult's hair, the hair color is difficult to determine because so many people use hair dyes. Permanents and dyes tend to make the hair dry and brittle. Dry, brittle hair is also a common sign of aging.

Alopecia—loss or thinning of hair—is a common condition. The most common type is hereditary alopecia, which is manifested in baldness that occurs late in life or prematurely. It is characterized by thinning of the hair and recession of the hairline and eventually occurs in about 80% of the male population. Hereditary alopecia is always bilaterally symmetric on the anterior portion of the skull (Fig. 7-2).

Inspection of the Face

- Observe facial expressions and movements.
- Note overall facial symmetry; inspect for any bulging, sunken areas, and drooping.
- Inspect for color, texture, edema, and lesions.

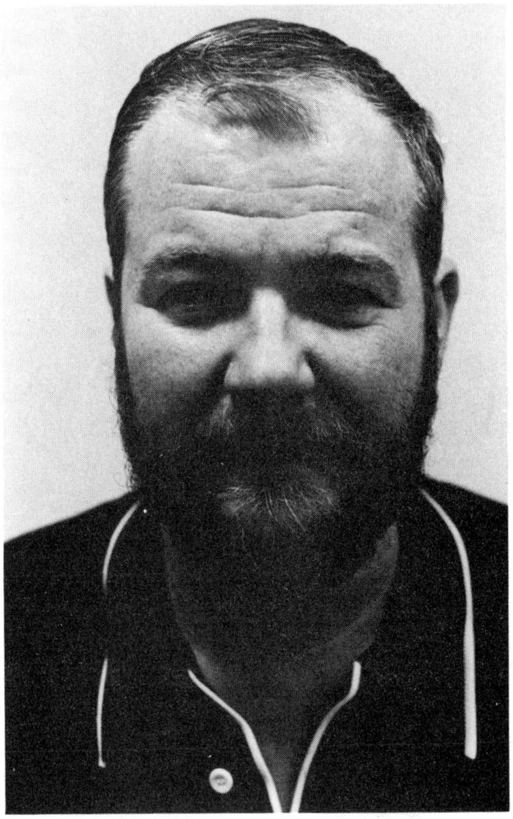

Figure 7-2 Example of hereditary alopecia. Note the symmetry of the receding hairline.

Technique of Inspection of the Face

1. Adequate lighting
2. Facial expression
3. Facial symmetry
4. Skin temperature, texture, and color
5. Abnormalities

You can learn a great deal from careful inspection of the face. Facial expressions may reveal depression, anxiety, hostility, disgust, or embarrassment. It is important to note such manifestations as grimacing, excessive blinking, or continual smiling. Such behaviors may indicate illness and may supply information on how the client feels as a person.

STRUCTURE OF THE NECK

For descriptive purposes, the neck is divided into three triangles (Fig. 7-3). The triangle beneath the mandible—the submandibular triangle—is bordered by the digastric muscles. The middle of the neck is defined by the thyroid cartilage and the suprasternal notch. The anterior cervical

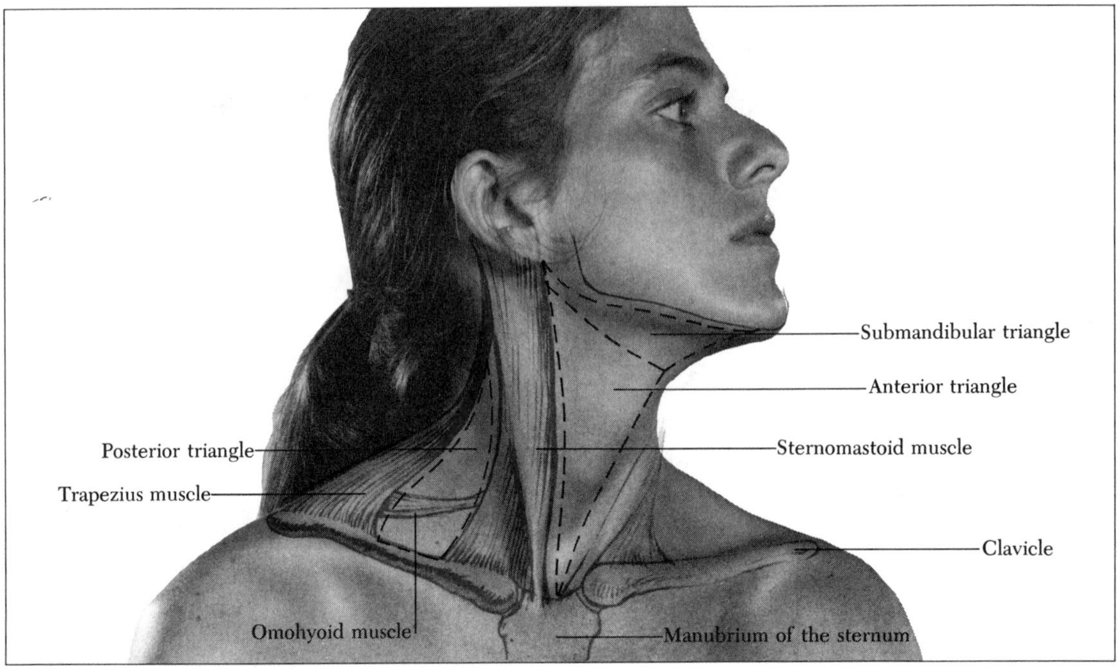

Figure 7-3 Diagram of anterior neck.

triangle is bounded by the submandibular triangle, laterally by the sternocleidomastoid muscle, and medially by the midline of the body. The posterior triangle is situated between the sternocleidomastoid and the trapezius muscle. The supraclavicular fossa is between the clavicle and the insertion of the sternocleidomastoid muscle, and the suprasternal notch is immediately above the manubrium of the sternum. The anterior midline structures of the neck are illustrated in Fig. 7-4. These structures include the hyoid bone, thyroid cartilage, cricoid cartilage, thyroid gland (lobe and isthmus), trachea, and the sternocleidomastoid muscle.

The groups of lymph nodes located in the neck are evident in Fig. 7-5. The lymph nodes function to filter the blood, engulf microorganisms, and produce lymphocytes and monocytes. Careful investigation of the areas of lymph drainage is a valuable diagnostic tool in the detection of acute inflammation, infection, metastatic carcinoma, and systemic diseases.

Figure 7-6 shows the location of the blood vessels of the neck. The carotids are the major arteries through which blood is circulated to the brain, the jugular veins are useful indicators of the efficiency of the heart and vascular systems.

Technique of Inspection of the Neck

1. Face the client directly.
2. Have client look straight ahead.
3. Characteristics:
   Size and symmetry of neck
   Position of trachea
   Visibility of thyroid gland
   Visibility of venous pulsation and distention

CHARACTERISTICS AND TECHNIQUES OF EXAMINATION

The three methods used in assessing the neck are inspection, palpation, and auscultation.

Inspection

- Inspect the position of the head. If the muscles of the neck are shortened on one side or are in spasm, the head will be tilted to one side.
- Note the size and symmetry of the neck. Asymmetry of the neck may result from edema, masses, or displacement of the trachea.
- Inspect for the thyroid gland.
- Look for pulsations in the neck region and jugular vein distention.

In normal individuals, the thyroid gland is not visible; thus, enlargement of the thyroid gland should be easy

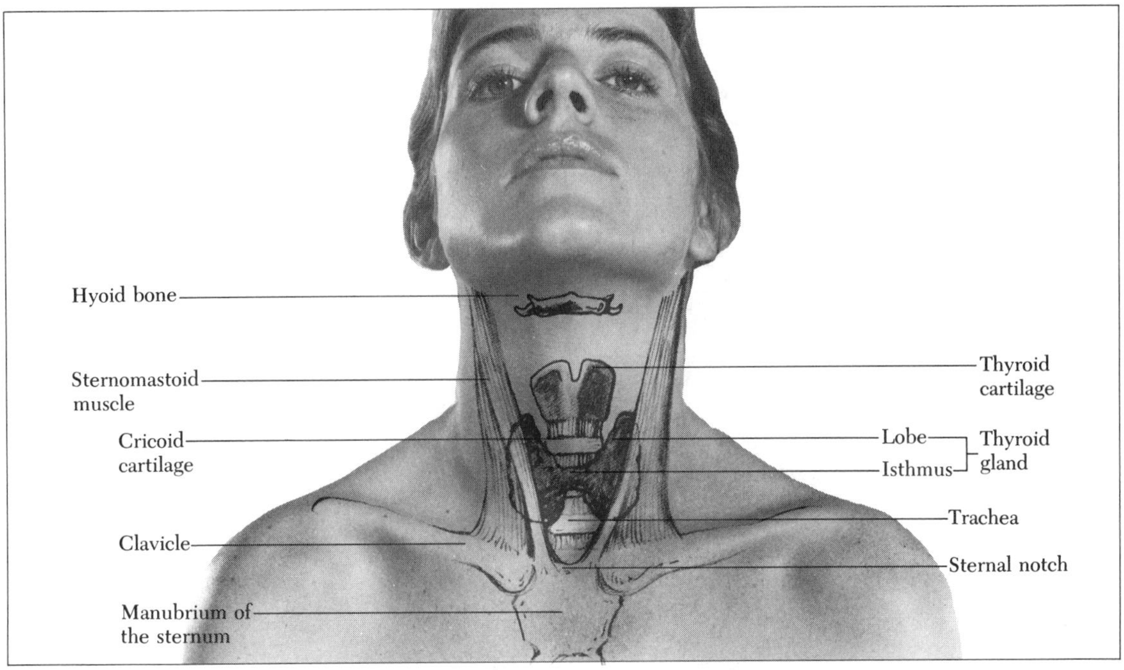

Figure 7-4 **Anterior midline structures of the neck.**

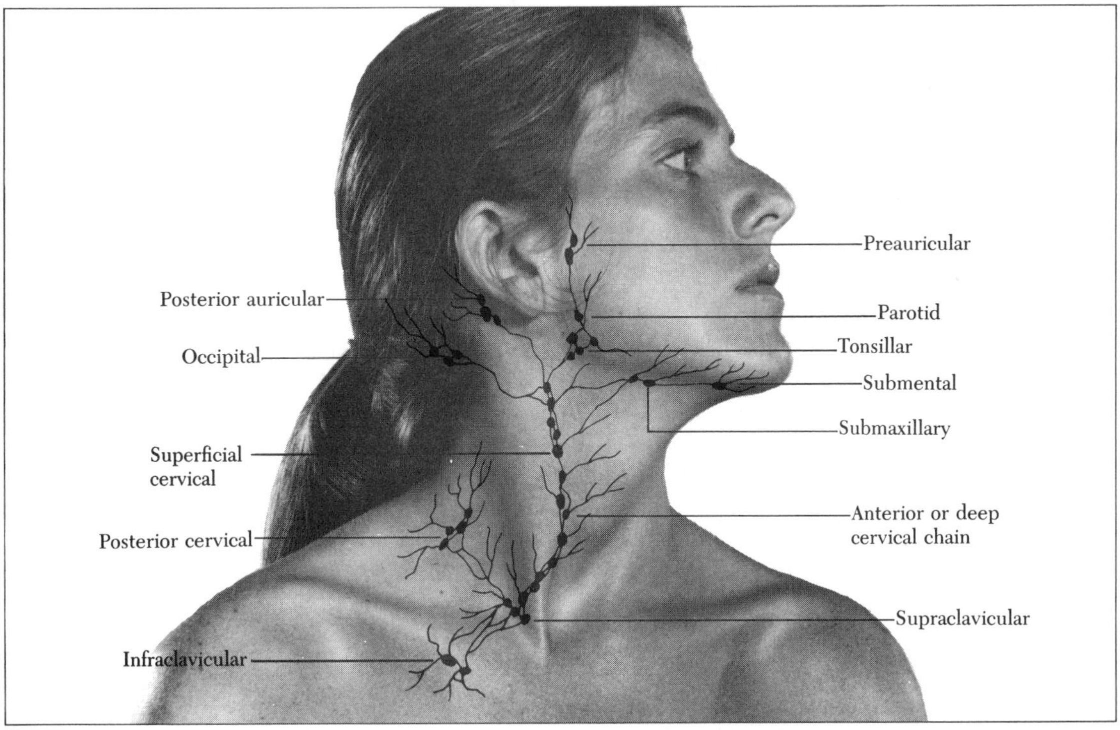

Figure 7-5 **Location of the lymph nodes of the neck.**

to note on inspection. The thyroid cartilage (Adam's apple) is normally visible and rises on swallowing. Venous pulsations and distention should not occur when the client is in an upright position. The trachea is normally midline.

Palpation and Auscultation

In this section, palpation and auscultation are discussed together because the findings from palpation often determine whether auscultation of the area is necessary.

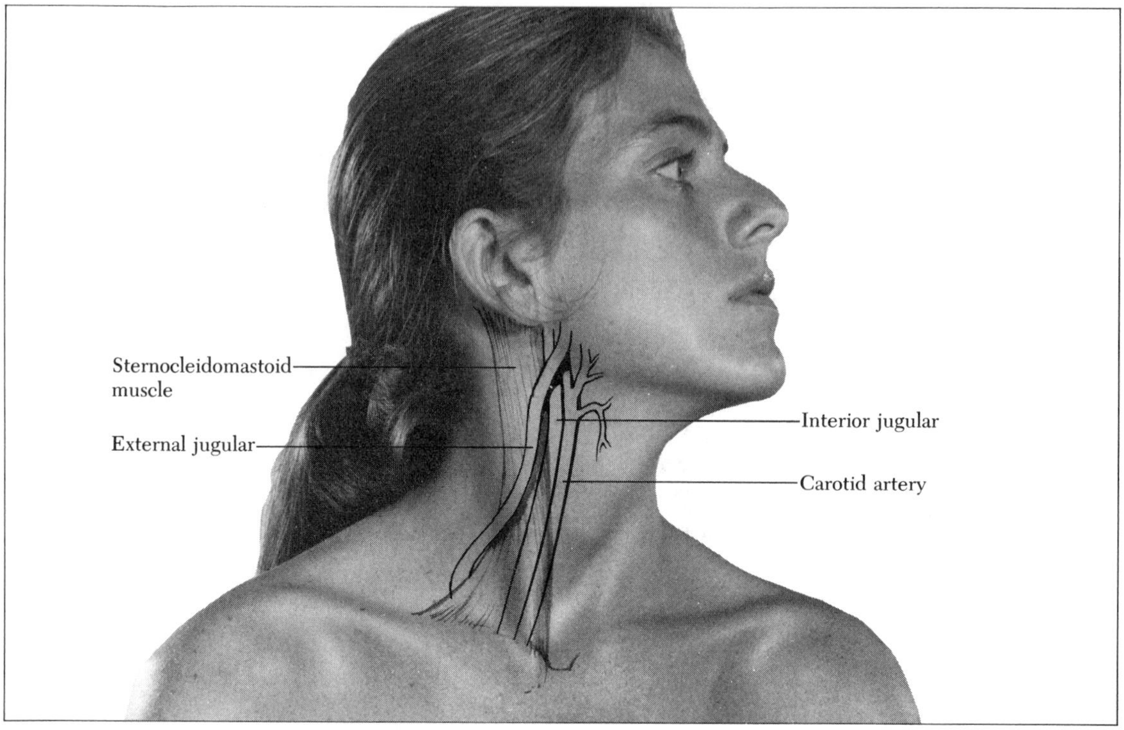

Figure 7-6 Location of blood vessels of the neck.

- Palpate the three triangular areas of the neck for tenderness or masses.
- Move the client's head and neck through the normal range of motion: rotation (side to side), flexion (chin to chest), hyperextension (tilted backward), and lateral flexion (ear to shoulder).
- Palpate the lymph nodes and the parotid gland.
- Place your index finger in the suprasternal notch and slide it to the right and then to the left of the trachea to gauge the space on either side. The trachea is normally midline; thus, the space between the trachea and the sternocleidomastoid muscle should be approximately the same on both sides.
- Palpate the thyroid gland.

There is normally no tenderness or masses in the neck region. On passive movement, the neck is normally supple, allowing this assessment to be performed easily. If the client has arthritis of the cervical spine, he will turn at the shoulders rather than turn his neck.

The lymph nodes and parotid gland should be palpated using a gentle to-and-fro or rotary motion with the fingertips. The nodes are generally palpated beginning with the occipital nodes and then the preauricular and posterior auricular nodes, the parotid gland, the posterior cervical, anterior cervical, submaxillary, submental, tonsillar, and supraclavicular nodes. To best palpate the supraclavicular nodes, it is helpful to have the client place his hands on his thighs and move his elbows and shoulders forward. This posture will relax the skin over the supraclavicular areas and provide more direct access to the lymph nodes.

Nodes are not normally palpable in the healthy individual, but enlarged nodes may be found as the result of an old infection. In such cases, a history of illnesses and injuries is helpful in differentiating active from previous pathologies. In children, cervical lymph nodes may be normally palpable until around 12 years of age.

If a mass is detected, it must be palpated to determine its size, location, consistency, mobility, and tenderness. Lymph nodes may be discrete or matted together; they may be extremely hard, moderately hard, soft, or cystic.

When palpating the thyroid gland from behind the client, the client's head is placed on a forward incline, tilted slightly toward the side to be examined. For example, do the following to palpate the right lobe:

- Use the middle and index fingers of both of your hands to locate the thyroid cartilage. The isthmus of the thyroid gland is about 1 cm below this cartilage (Fig. 7-7A).
- Use the index and middle fingers of your left hand to displace the thyroid cartilage to the client's right. Place the index finger of your right hand next to the trachea of the client's right to displace the sternocleidomastoid muscle as the client flexes his head forward and tilted slightly toward the right to relax the sternocleidomastoid muscle.

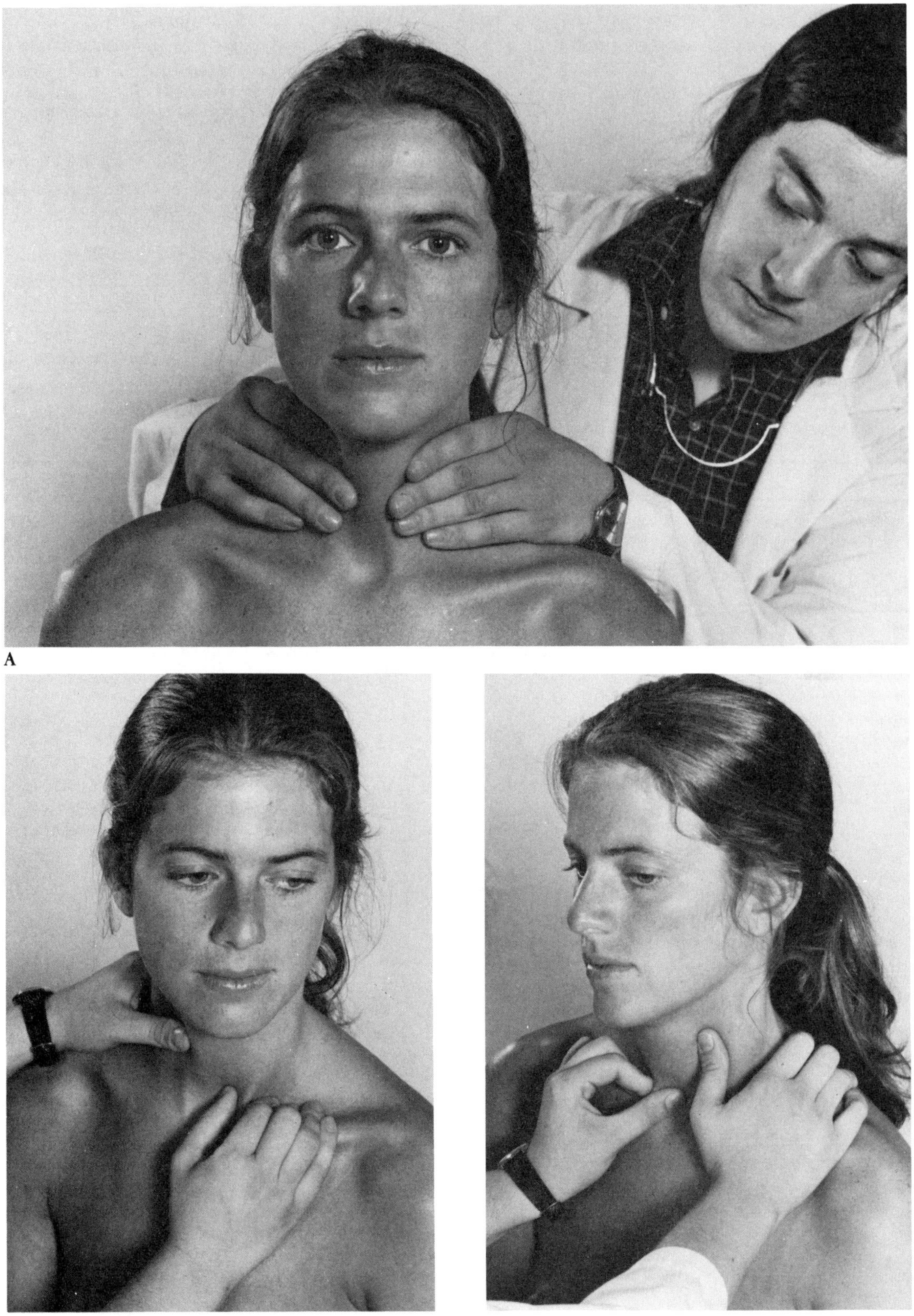

A

B C

Figure 7-7 **(A)** Palpation of the thyroid from behind. **(B)** Palpation of thyroid right lobe. **(C)** Palpation of thyroid left lobe.

- You may feel the upward movement of the right lateral portion of the thyroid gland and the thyroid cartilage as the client swallows.
- Repeat the examination on the client's left side.

Generally the normal thyroid gland is nonpalpable.

Do the following to palpate the thyroid gland from a frontal approach:

- Position your right thumb against the left side of the cartilage and place and second and third fingers of your right hand behind the sternocleidomastoid muscle (Fig. 7-7B,C).
- Feel for the lateral lobe with your left thumb as the client swallows.
- The procedure is reversed to palpate the left lobe.

The thyroid should be examined for size, consistency, and the presence of nodules. If the gland is enlarged, place the stethoscope over it and listen for a bruit.

- Palpation of the carotid arteries should normally reveal bilateral equality.
- Do not palpate both carotid arteries simultaneously.
- If there is weakness or absence of a carotid pulse, listen over the carotids with the bell of the stethoscope.

Palpating one carotid artery at a time allows full patency of the other artery to transport blood and oxygen to the brain. Carotid massage, which may occur inadvertently, may be hazardous in some cases because it lowers pulse rate. Common abnormalities of the head, face, and neck are shown in Table 7-1.

Table 7-1 Common Abnormalities of the Head, Face, and Neck

Terminology	Characteristics	Comments
Microcephalus	Small skull less than two standard deviations below mean for age and sex	Check for history of brain damage; mental retardation common.
Hydrocephalus	Enlarged head caused by blockage of cerebrospinal fluid in ventricular system	Early sign is dilated scalp veins.
Acromegaly	Overgrowth of cartilage and bones; elongation of jaw; enlarged ears, nose, hands, and feet	Increase in hat and glove size. Pressure of thickened cranial bones can cause increased intracranial pressure; excessive growth hormone in the adult.
"Bossing"	Bulging appearance of forehead; enlargement of frontal and parietal bones	Vitamin D deficiency (rickets), congenital syphilis common causes.
Seborrhea (dandruff)	Dry flakes or greasy crusts and scales; pruritus; remissions; exacerbations; accompanies oily skin	Excessive secretion of sebaceous glands. Check seborrheic areas other than scalp, i.e., chin, lateral nasal folds, center of chest and back, axillae, groins.
Wens	Movable, nontender, single, or multiple masses on scalp	Blockage of sebaceous gland of the scalp
Alopecia areata	Patchy loss of scalp and facial (beard) hair	May accompany fungal infections, secondary syphilis, and chromosomal disorders.
Edema	Generalized facial puffiness, periorbital, moon facies	Check for further signs of trauma, inflammation, nephrotic syndrome, myxedema, congestive heart failure.
Asymmetry	Unilateral ptosis of facial muscles with drooping of eyelid and corner of mouth	Check for signs of local trauma, Bell's palsy (facial nerve damage), and cerebrovascular accident.
Xanthomas	Yellow, raised plaques common on eyelids, nasal bridge, around tendons, i.e., knuckles, large joints	Lipoid deposits. Check for history of diabetes mellitus, hypercholesteremia; check cholesterol blood level.
Lymphadenopathy	Enlarged lymph nodes	Check for additional signs of infection and inflammation. Be aware of potential metastatic disease.
Goiter	Enlarged thyroid gland	Common with iodine deficiency diet and diets of cabbage, turnips, and broccoli; hyperthyroidism; sulfonamides; thiourea drugs
Carotid bruit	Buzzing sound auscultated over carotid artery	Check for signs of brain ischemia, e.g., syncope, vertigo, headache. Common in carotid stenosis, hyperthyroidism.

Technique of Palpation of the Neck

1. Observe active and passive range of motion: rotation, flexion, hyperextension, and lateral flexion
2. Palpate using fingertips.
3. Characteristics:
   Three triangular areas: submandibular, anterior, and posterior cervical
   Lymph nodes: preauricular, postauricular, occipital, submental, submaxillary, tonsillar, anterior cervical, posterior cervical, supraclavicular, infraclavicular
   Parotid gland
   Trachea
   Thyroid gland
   Carotid arteries

Technique of Auscultation of Neck

1. Warm stethoscope with hand.
2. Apply bell lightly with edges touching skin.
3. Decision making:
   Auscultate for hum when enlarged thyroid.
   Auscultate for bruit when carotid pulse is weak or absent.

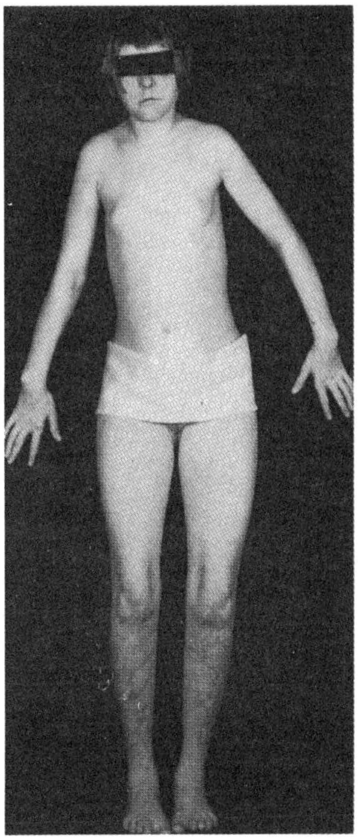

Figure 7-8 A 19-year-old woman with microcephalus and mental retardation.

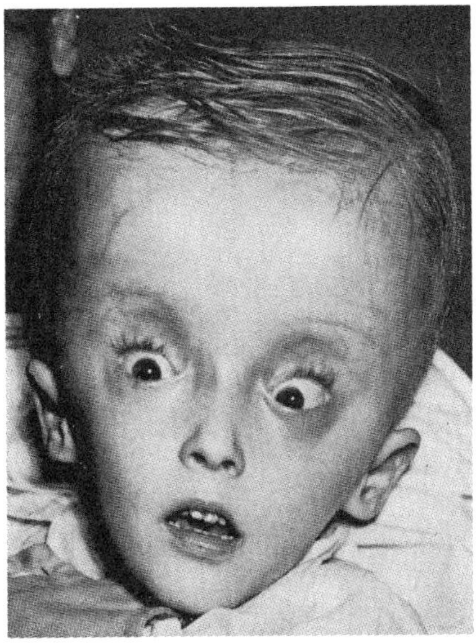

Figure 7-9 Hydrocephalus of severe grade preventing ossification of skull.

CLINICAL CORRELATIONS

Head

Abnormalities in the size and shape of the cranium can be seen in conditions such as microcephalus and hydrocephalus (Figs. 7-8 and 7-9.) An early sign of hydrocephalus is dilated scalp veins.

Deviations from normal findings of the head include bulging fontanelles, which occur with increased intracranial pressure. Depressed, sunken fontanelles occur with dehydration. Larger than normal fontanelles that are delayed in closure may be an indication of hydrocephalus, rickets, hypothyroidism, or osteogenesis imperfecta, as well as of chronic increased intracranial pressure. Increases in the size of this fontanelle may also indicate increased intracranial pressure.

In adults, conditions that affect size and shape of the head include acromegaly, a deformity caused by excessive secretion of the growth hormone (Fig. 7-10). In acromegaly, the skull enlarges and thickens. The cranial bones may become so thick that they cause increased intracranial pressure. Vitamin D deficiency (rickets) can cause enlargement of the frontal and parietal bones. Congenital syphilis may also produce enlargement of the frontal bones. Such bulging of the frontal bones is known as "bossing." Trauma or tumors of the skull often create obvious distortions and may be observed or palpated.

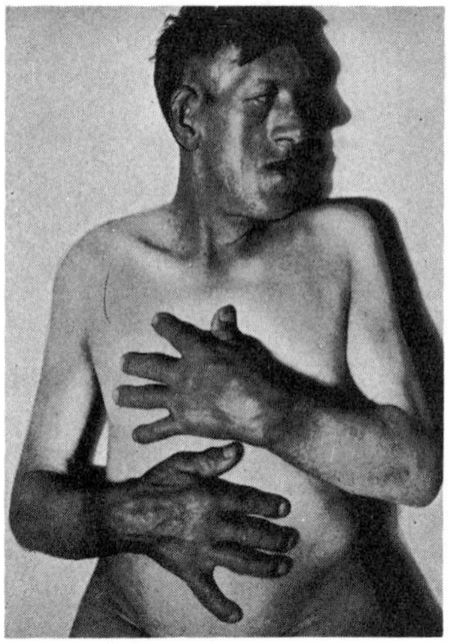

Figure 7-10 Acromegaly.

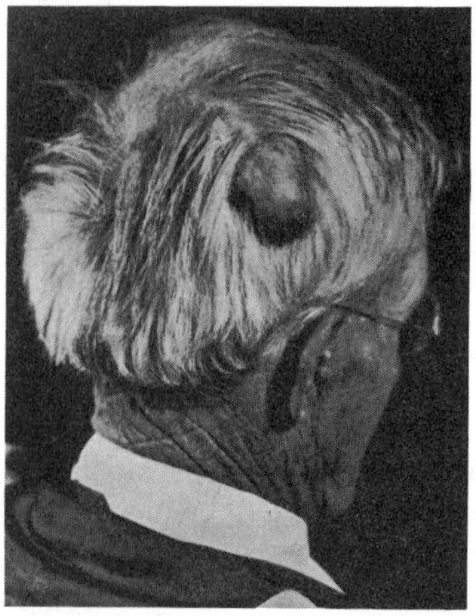

Figure 7-12 Sebaceous cyst of the scalp.

Hair

Dry, brittle hair is a sign of myxedema. Fine, soft hair is characteristic of hyperthyroidism. Toxic alopecia—the rapidly occurring loss or thinning of hair secondary to severe illness—does not occur symmetrically. Alopecia areata is depicted in Fig. 7-11; it is a patchy loss of hair from the scalp and often from the beard. Alopecia areata is frequently observed in fungus infections and secondary syphilis. In a child, uneven distribution of hair may indicate chromosomal disorders.

Scalp

Flaking or crusts on the scalp may indicate seborrhea, eczema, or an allergic response to hair care products. Sebaceous cysts or wens, which result from the occlusion of glands, can be found on any part of the body, but are often found in the scalp. They present as smooth, round nodules on the skin (Fig. 7-12).

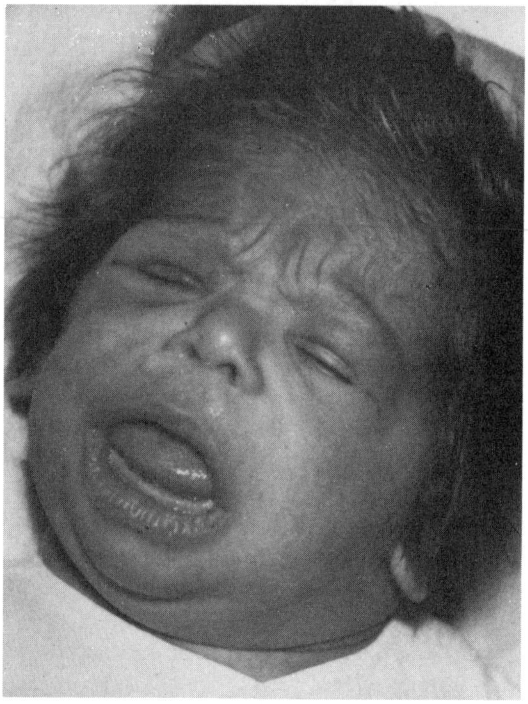

Figure 7-13 The facies of an infant with myxedema.

Face

Many physical conditions can affect the face. A cerebrovascular accident or damage to a facial nerve could result in drooping of one side of the face. Drooping eyelids with an accompanying heaviness to the face may indicate myasthenia gravis. Hormonal imbalances may cause puffiness of the entire face; edematous eyelids; thick tongue; the coarse, dry skin of myxedema (thyroid deficiency) (Fig. 7-13); and the startled, anxious appearance of the exophthalmic client with hyperthyroidism (Fig. 7-14). Cushing's syndrome—hyperfunction of the adrenal glands—is accompanied by a characteristic "moon face" and prominent jowls.

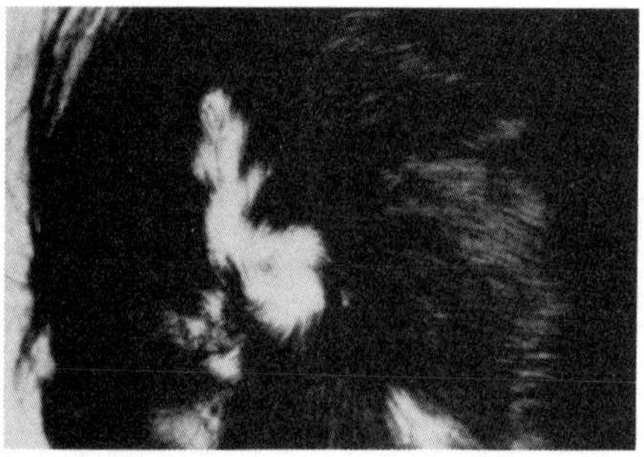

Figure 7-11 Alopecia areata due to secondary syphilis. Note the moth-eaten appearance.

Severe debilitating disease, such as dehydration, starvation, and fever, can produce the cachectic facies, characterized by sunken eyes, hollow cheeks, and dry, roughened

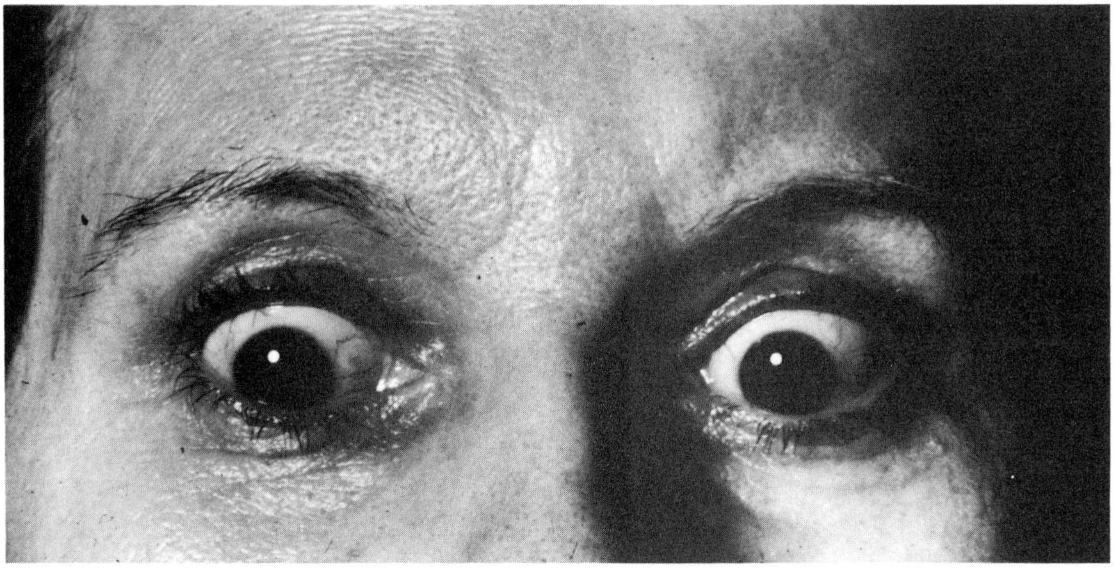

Figure 7-14 Exophthalmos of Grave's disease. Note the staring, startled appearance and wide palpebral fissures.

skin. Systemic disease can also produce changes in the face. Atrophy and tightening of the skin occurs in scleroderma (Fig. 7-15). Edema of the face may indicate kidney disease or congestive heart failure. The eyelids and surrounding tissues of the eyes are especially prone to edema; orbital edema is often the first sign of fluid retention.

Lesions

Xanthomas are circumscribed collections of lipids that may occur anywhere on the body but are commonly found on the eyelids, particularly near the inner canthus. They can be flat or elevated, and they vary in size. Occasionally, they are associated with a disease such as cholesteremia or diabetes mellitus, but frequently there is no associated disease process (see Fig. 6-34).

Nevi and the lesions of acne may be noted on the face as well as elsewhere on the body. Such changes in facial skin pigmentation as pallor, cyanosis, jaundice, and rubor indicate impaired health.

Lymph Nodes

The location of enlarged lymph nodes may give a clue to the origin of the problem. Occipital node enlargement may be due to scalp infections, whereas posterior auricular lymphadenopathy may indicate ear infection. Enlarged, tender cervical glands should direct your attention to the mouth and pharynx. Enlargement of the anterior cervical nodes may suggest respiratory infection. Submaxillary and submental node enlargement may reflect inflammation of the mouth. Enlarged, tender parotid glands often indicate

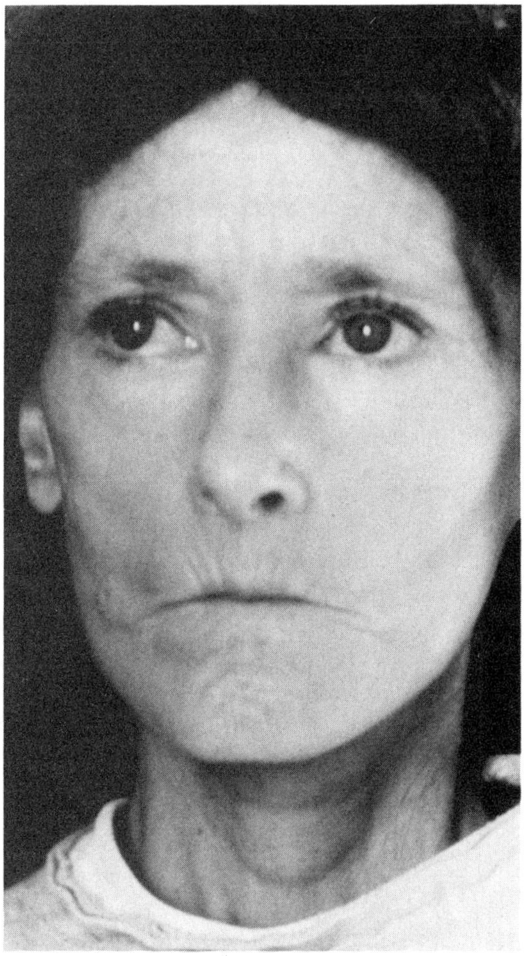

Figure 7-15 Facial changes in scleroderma. Note the drawn, pursed lips. (© Arthritis Foundation 1981.)

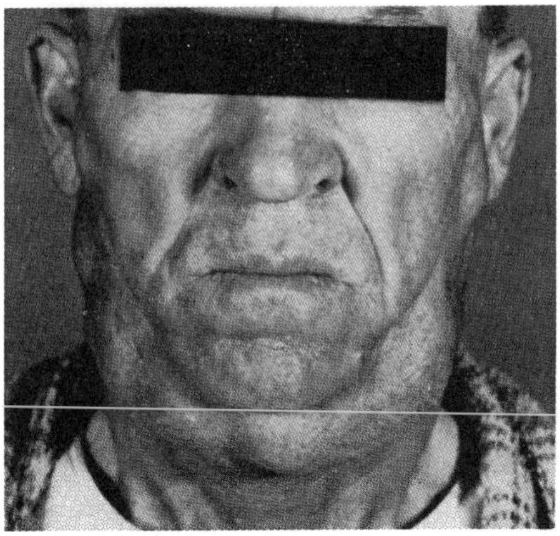

Figure 7-16 **Hodgkin's disease manifests as a collar of enlarged lymph nodes. Enlargement of preauricular nodes is also visible.**

mumps, a contagious infection. This disease is rarely seen because of the success of widespread vaccination programs.

Enlargement of the lymph nodes can be either local or widespread. Lymphadenopathy can accompany other signs of inflammation. Rapidly enlarging nodes may indicate antibody formation, and they may be quite tender. If the skin overlying the node is inflamed, the node is probably infected. Enlargement of nodes in more than one site may also be due to metastasis (e.g., Hodgkin's disease) (Fig. 7-16). Malignant infiltration of the nodes can occur without any accompanying signs of inflammation.

Lymph nodes that are nontender, hard, and matted together suggest metastatic disease. In acute inflammation, the nodes are usually rather soft and tender with enlargement. In chronic infection, as in tuberculosis, the nodes tend to be tender, firm, and matted together.

Thyroid

A systolic bruit may be heard in thyrotoxicosis because of increased blood flow through the tissues; this bruit will not have a cardiovascular origin. The thyroid may be enlarged in simple goiter, in inflammation, and in the presence of tumors (Fig. 7-17). Thyroid disorders are the most common endocrine disorders in children. Figure 7-18 illustrates a normal thyroid gland, thyroid enlargement, a thyroid nodule, and a multinodular thyroid gland as situated in the anterior, central region of the neck.

Carotid Arteries

With carotid stenosis, a cardiovascular bruit may be detected. You can create an artificial stenosis by placing gentle pressure over the healthy carotid, taking care not to apply so much pressure that the flow is cut off entirely. If you listen with the bell of the stethoscope above the point of pressure, you will be able to hear the artificially produced bruit.

Technique of Palpation of the Thyroid

1. Posterior approach: head slightly forward and tilted toward side being examined; index finger placed high to retract the sternocleidomastoid muscle; middle and ring fingers over the lateral portion of thyroid. Index and middle fingers displace the thyroid cartilage on the contralateral side. Have client swallow as each side is examined.
2. Frontal approach: head slightly tilted toward side being examined; thumb anterior to sternocleidomastoid muscle; two to three middle fingers behind sternocleidomastoid muscle. Thumb and fingers positioned same on opposite side of neck to displace thyroid cartilage.

Trachea

Deviation of the trachea from its midline position can be caused by local tumors in the neck, a thyroid enlargement, an aortic aneurysm, or by lung pathology. A tracheal tug is the downward movement of the trachea occurring with systole and is reflective of an aortic arch aneurysm.

SUMMARY

This chapter described the assessment of the head and neck. The head is examined by inspection and palpation, which are often used simultaneously. Careful inspection of the face can yield much important information about the client's state of health.

Examination of the neck requires three techniques: inspection, palpation, and auscultation. Because many structures must be assessed in this rather small area, the examiner must have a thorough understanding of the anatomy if a comprehensive examination is to be obtained. Examples of clinical diseases and the correlate findings of the head and neck examination were presented.

DISCUSSION QUESTIONS/ ACTIVITIES

1. Why is it important to palpate the client's head during the health examination?

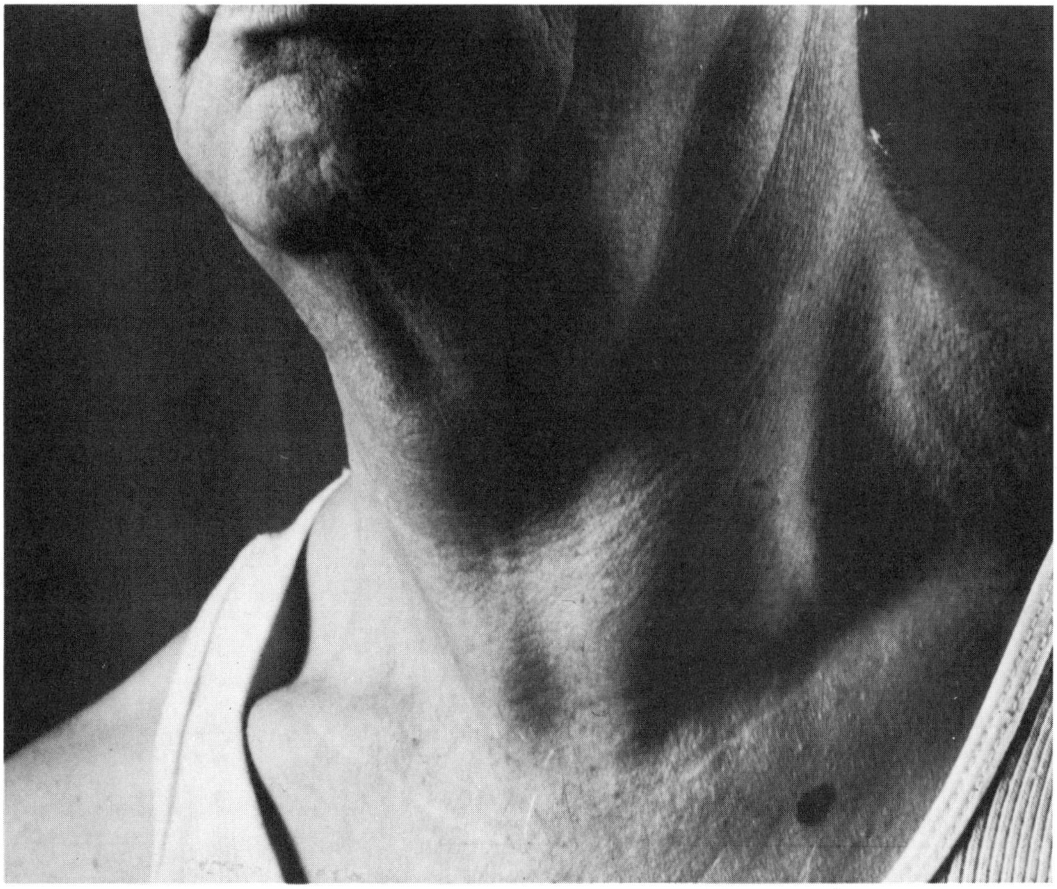

A

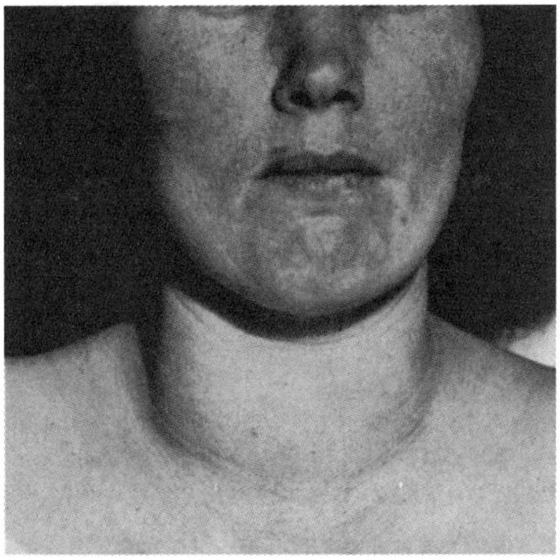

B

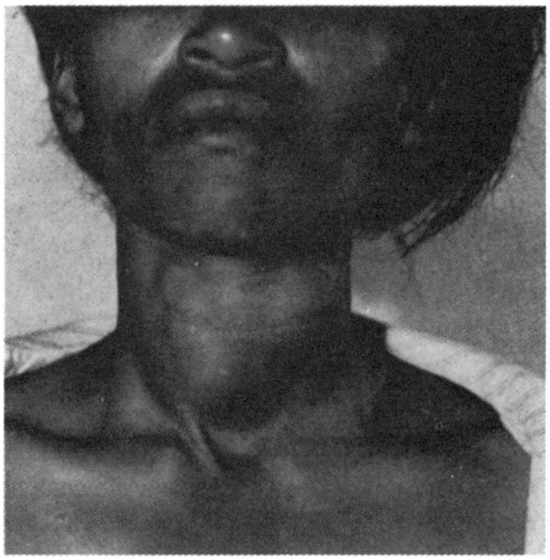

C

Figure 7-17 Thyroid disorders. **(A)** Enlarged thyroid. Note swelling at the site of the thyroid isthmus and on either side of the trachea. **(B)** Diffuse colloid goiter of moderate size. **(C)** Toxic modular goiter.

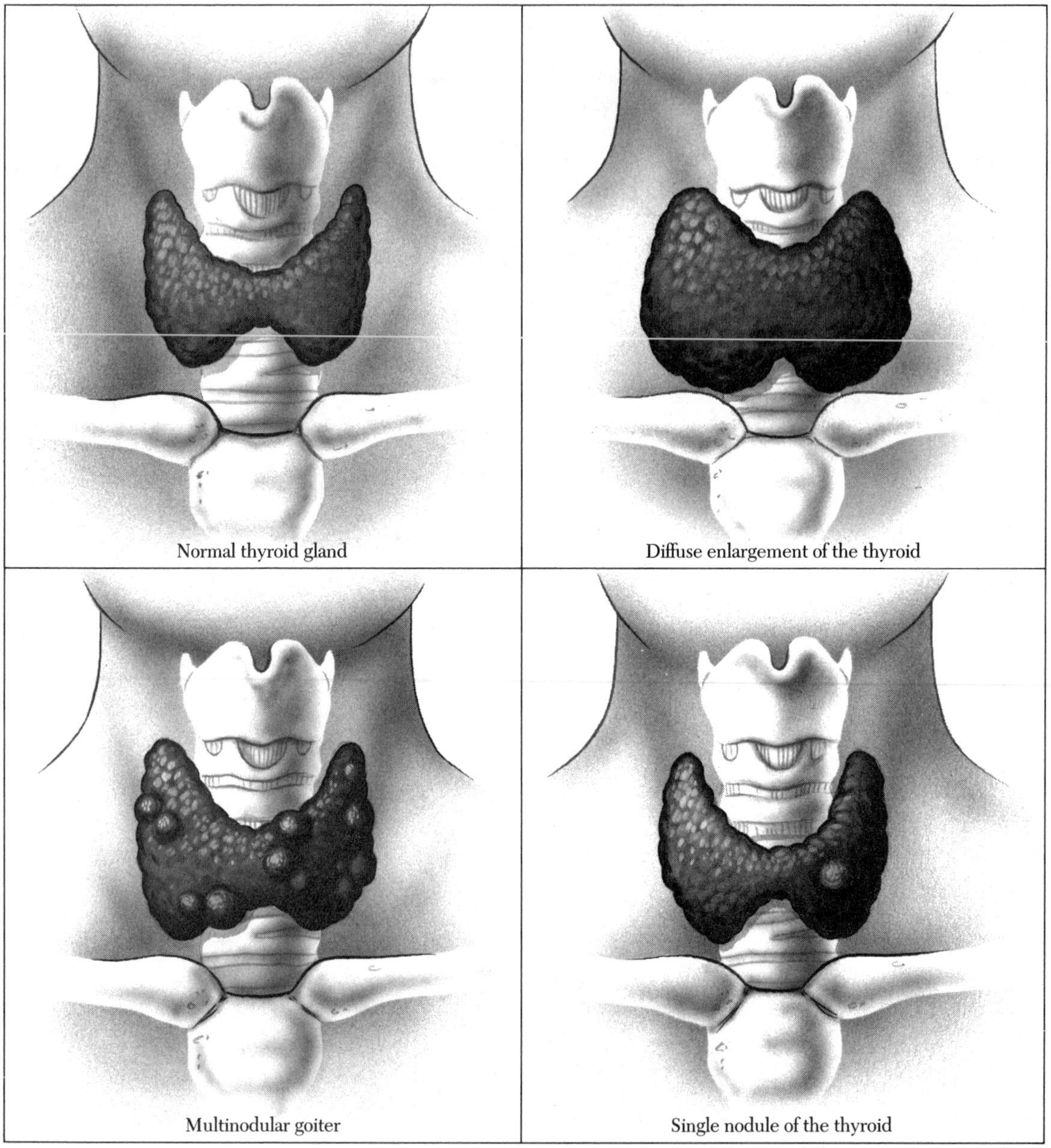

Figure 7-18 Anatomic position of the normal thyroid gland and pathologic thyroid findings.

2. Discuss various changes in the face that might indicate a change in the client's health status.
3. Role-play how you would approach the examination of a client who is wearing a wig.
4. How would you determine whether a client is using hair dye?
5. Demonstrate the normal range of motion of the neck.
6. List the areas of the neck that must be examined for lymph node enlargement.
7. List the aspects of enlarged lymph nodes that must be documented.
8. Demonstrate the technique you would use to palpate the thyroid gland.
9. Discuss the rationale for auscultation of the carotid arteries.
10. Palpate the lymph nodes of the neck in several children and adults. Discuss the differences.
11. Perform a physical assessment of the head, neck, and face of a client, peer, or relative; document your findings.

RECORDING OF FINDINGS

Normal findings are presented in the first column. The second column contains findings of a client in whom a change in the thyroid gland was noted during the health examination.

Head
Inspection: Normocephalic, atraumatic; frontal hereditary alopecia. Scalp clear.

Palpation: No lumps; no tenderness

Face
Inspection: Symmetrical; no muscular weakness; no involuntary movements; no facial edema; skin pink; no lesions noted.

Neck
Inspection: Symmetrical; no masses.

Palpation: Supple with normal range of movement; thyroid nonpalpable; no lymphadenopathy; no venous distention; carotids equal bilaterally and of good quality; trachea midline

Auscultation: No carotid bruits; no thyroid hum

Head
Inspection: Normocephalic, atraumatic; normal hair distribution. Scalp clear.

Palpation: No lumps; no tenderness

Face
Inspection: Symmetrical; no muscular weakness; no involuntary movements; no facial edema; skin pink; no lesions noted.

Neck
Inspection: Symmetrical; no masses.

Palpation: Supple with normal range of movement; thyroid enlarged, 1.5-cm mass with small, extremely hard, nontender, fixed nodules on right lobe; no lymphadenopathy; no venous distention; carotids equal bilaterally and of bounding quality; trachea midline.

Auscultation: No carotid bruits; no thyroid hum

CHAPTER

8 Assessment of the Eye

Learning Objectives

1. Describe the structure and function of the eye.
2. Identify the structures of the eye that are examined by inspection and palpation.
3. Demonstrate the techniques used for examining the pupils, extraocular muscles, visual fields, and visual acuity.
4. State when a Hirschberg's test and cover test must be performed.
5. Describe the technique used in conducting the ophthalmic examination.
6. Identify the normal parameters of the ophthalmoscopic examination of the eye grounds.
7. Discuss the relationship between the ophthalmic examination and the client's level of wellness.

The eye is complex and fascinating. Figure 8-1 illustrates several views of the eye and its main structures. Assessment of these structures are considered separately throughout this chapter.

STRUCTURE AND FUNCTION OF THE EYE

The eye is a sphere almost 1 inch in diameter. The greatest portion of this sphere is recessed in the bony orbit that protects it. Only a small portion of the anterior eye is visible. Figure 8-1 shows that the eyeball is covered by three coats of tissue: the *sclera,* the *choroid,* and the *retina.* The sclera is the outermost coat. The anterior portion of the sclera is referred to as the *cornea.* The cornea lies over the *iris* and is transparent. The rest of the sclera is opaque and appears white on inspection.

The choroid coat, the middle layer, contains a great deal of pigment and a large number of blood vessels. The choroid also provides special structures in its anterior portion. Foremost is the iris, which contains the pigments responsible for eye color. The iris consists of smooth circular and radial muscles arranged to form a round structure with an opening in the middle: the *pupil.* The involuntary muscles of the iris react to autonomic nervous system stimulation and regulate the size of the pupil. Posterior to the iris the choroid thickens into the *ciliary body,* which is composed of ciliary muscles. These involuntary muscles control the shape of the *lens,* the biconvex body that is part of the refracting mechanism of the eye. The ciliary muscles change the thickness of the lens to accommodate near and far vision. A circular ligament attached to the ciliary body holds the lens in place.

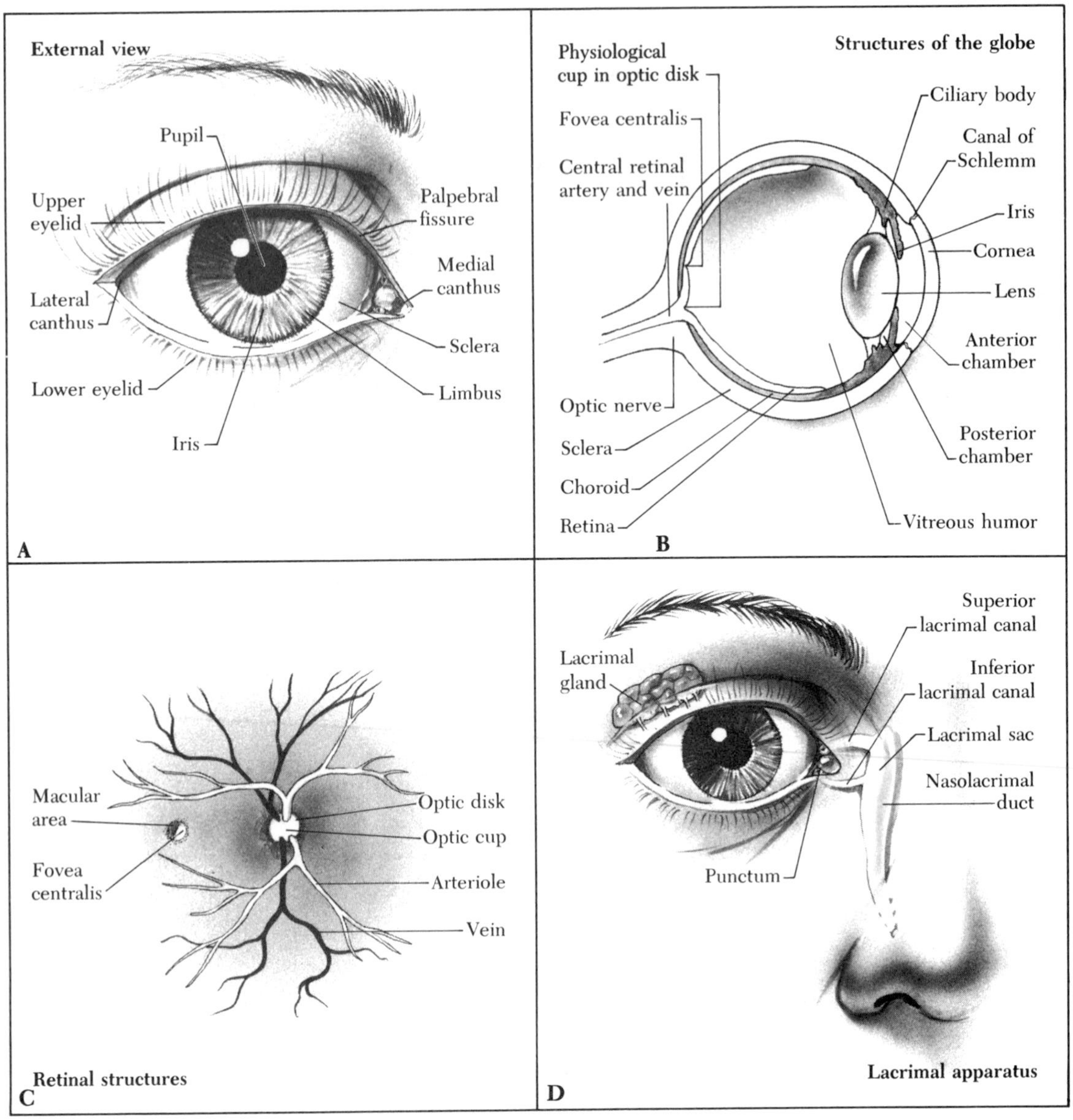

Figure 8-1 The eye. **(A)** External view. **(B)** Structures of the globe. **(C)** Retinal structures. **(D)** Lacrimal apparatus.

The retina, the innermost coat of the eye, is composed of nervous tissue that receives the visual images. The *fovea centralis,* a slight depression at the lateral posterior of the eye, marks the point of central vision. The area of the retina immediately surrounding the fovea centralis is called the *macula. Rods* and *cones* are the photoreceptor neurons that constitute the visual receptors of the retina. The rods respond to low-intensity light and shades of gray, while the cones respond to bright light and color. The rods are almost absent from the macula and increase in density toward the periphery of the retina. The cones are most densely concentrated in the fovea centralis. The fact that the rods are more responsive to shades of gray and are located away from the center of the retina can be illustrated by a simple experiment. The next time you are driving at night, tilt your head down so that your eyes will have to move upward to see the road in front of you. This will cause the image of what you are seeing to fall more toward the lower periphery of your retina and be received chiefly by the rods. You will find that you are much better able to see, even when there is another car approaching.

The small circular area in the medial posterior part of the retina is called the *optic disk.* It is here that the *optic nerve* emerges from the eyeball. The arteries and veins that provide the blood supply to the eye also enter and leave at this point.

The anterior compartment of the eye has two subdivisions: (1) the *anterior chamber* between the back of the

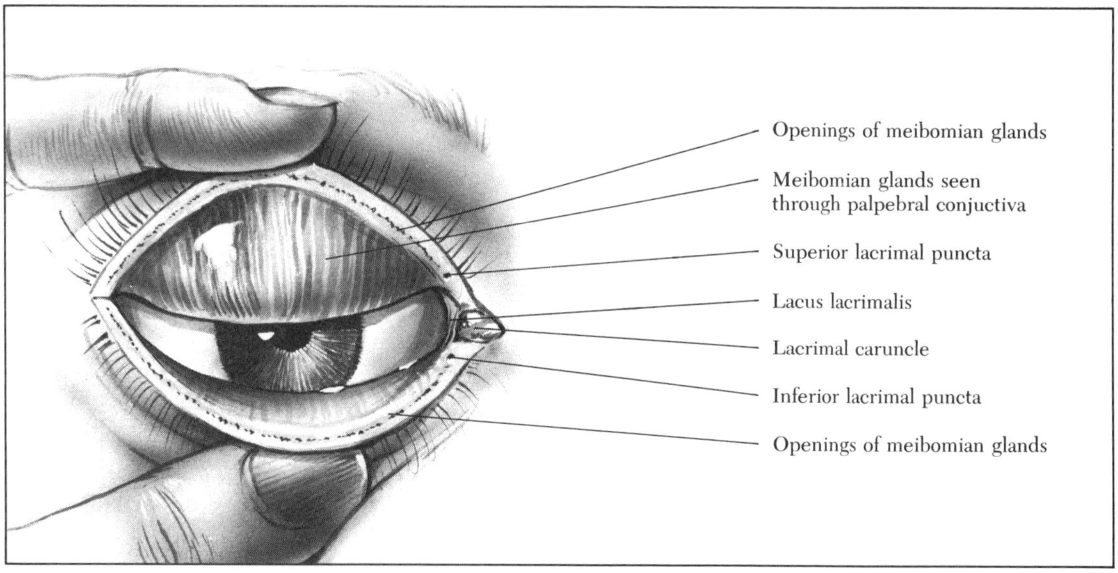

Figure 8-2 Structure of the eyelid.

cornea and the front of the lens and (2) the *posterior chamber* between the iris and the front of the lens. Aqueous humor, manufactured by the ciliary bodies, fills both of these compartments. It circulates from the posterior chamber to the anterior chamber and is then absorbed into the venous blood through the *canal of Schlemm,* which is located laterally between the junction of the sclera and the cornea. The posterior compartment of the eye contains vitreous humor, a gelatin-like substance that provides sufficient intraocular pressure to prevent the eyeball from collapsing.

The *lacrimal glands,* which produce tears, are situated in the upper lateral bony orbit. From this site the tears are carried through small ducts to the conjunctiva to keep the surface of the eye moist and to wash away particles. Excess tears are gathered by the *puncta,* which can be seen as two small dots at the medial *canthus* of the eye. From the puncta the tears pass through the lacrimal canals into the *nasolacrimal duct.* All of the tear ducts are lined with a mucous membrane that is an extension of the mucosa that lines the nose. When this membrane becomes swollen, the nasolacrimal ducts become plugged, causing tears to overflow onto the cheeks instead of draining into the nose as they normally should. Thus, an overflow of tears does not ordinarily occur except when the passageway into the nose is blocked or when tears are overabundant, as with crying or reaction to a foreign particle in the eye.

The eyelids gain their shape from the tarsal plate, a ridge of thick connective tissue. Figure 8-2 indicates that the *meibomian (sebaceous) glands* lie in vertical columns within the tarsal plates, forming light yellow streaks. These glands open onto the posterior portion of the lid margins. The space between the open eyelids is called the *palpebral fissure.* Under normal conditions, the open eyelids are equally separated. The lower lid should meet the iris, with the upper lid covering a small fraction of the iris (23 mm). The underside of the lids are lined by the *palpebral conjunctiva.* The *bulbar conjunctiva* covers the eye up to the limbus (corner of the cornea and sclera).

The extrinsic muscles of the eye are attached to the outside of the eyeball and to the bones of the orbit. They are voluntary muscles responsible for eye movement, and they are innervated by the somatic fibers of the 3rd, 4th, and 6th cranial nerves (Figs. 8-3, 8-4). Normally, these muscles are able to move the eyes in six basic directions.

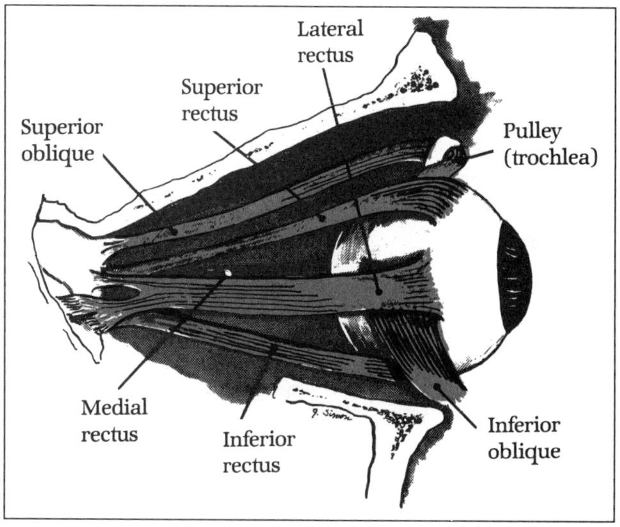

Figure 8-3 Extraocular muscles of right eye. (From *Physical Assessment in Nursing Practice,* 4th ed., Sana, J.M. and Judge, R.D. Copyright © Boston: Little, Brown 1982.

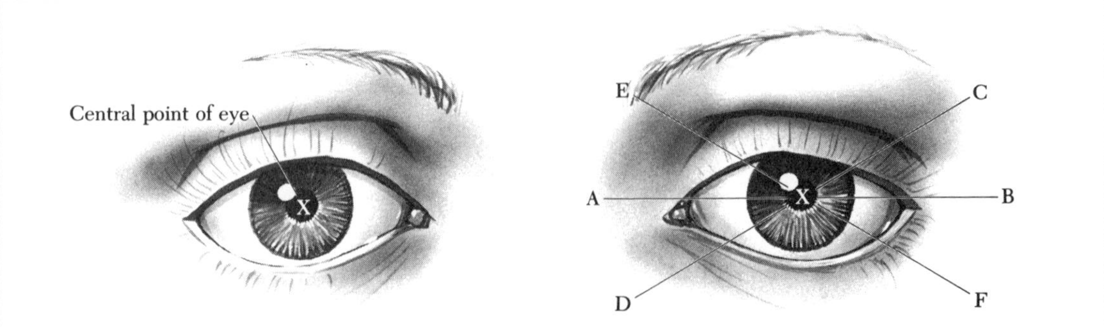

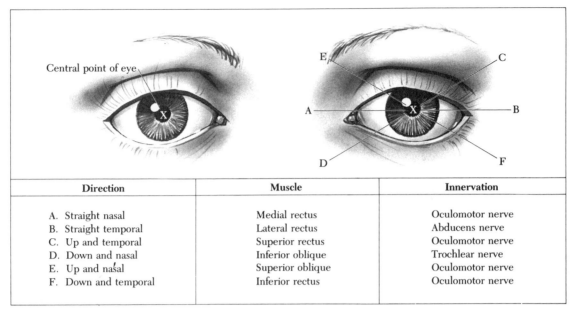

Direction	Muscle	Innervation
A. Straight nasal	Medial rectus	Oculomotor nerve
B. Straight temporal	Lateral rectus	Abducens nerve
C. Up and temporal	Superior rectus	Oculomotor nerve
D. Down and nasal	Inferior oblique	Trochlear nerve
E. Up and nasal	Superior oblique	Oculomotor nerve
F. Down and temporal	Inferior rectus	Oculomotor nerve

Figure 8-4 Cardinal positions of the eye.

Techniques for Inspection and Palpation of the Eye

1. Adequate lighting
2. Fullness of eyebrows
3. Lacrimal apparatus: raise eyelid; check between upper lid and eyeball; apply finger pressure to lacrimal sac.
4. Eyelids: evaluate and observe:
   a. Palpebral fissure
   b. Position
   c. Conjunctiva:
      (1) palpebral: gently evert upper lid.
      (2) bulbar: separate lids; have client look down and to both sides.
   d. Sclera
   e. Cornea: use oblique lighting.
   f. Pupils—equal, round.
   g. Pupillary reaction to light: bring penlight from lateral side to focus on pupil.
   h. Consensual reaction: note response of the pupil of one eye as light is focused on the opposite eye.
   i. Accommodation: tell client to look at distant spot, then at finger 15 cm away from and lateral to face.
   j. Convergence: have client follow your finger as it is moved inward to 2 to 3 inches from the tip of the client's nose.
5. Extraocular muscles: face client directly; have client follow finger or pencil through six cardinal positions.
6. Intraocular pressure: have client close eyes; place tip of thumb and index finger lightly on eyelid; palpate gently for consistency.
7. Visual fields: face client directly at 2 ft away; ask client to cover one eye. Cover your opposite eye; have client fix gaze on your uncovered eye; place outstretched arm equidistant between client and you. If client is unable to see your fingers at this point, move your wriggling fingers toward the nose. Repeat same procedure, moving hand from the 8 axes of the visual field of the eye being assessed. Repeat the procedure for the opposite eye.

CHARACTERISTICS AND TECHNIQUES OF EXAMINATION

Inspection and Palpation

As you examine each part of the eye, you will find it less tiring for the client and more systematic to perform inspection and palpation simultaneously. This approach also allows you to complete the examination of one part of the eye before moving to another part.

Lacrimal Apparatus

- Raise the eyelid and look between the upper lid and the eyeball to check whether the lacrimal gland is enlarged.
- Apply finger pressure to the lacrimal sac at the inside of the lower inner orbital rim. This action will express any existent mucopurulent drainage of infection from the punctum.

Eyelids

- Inspect the eyelids for lesions, turning of the lid either inward or outward, spasms, ptosis, and edema.
- Never press on an injured eyeball. If you determine that the eyeball has been penetrated or has a foreign object embedded in it, stop the examination at once and notify an ophthalmologist.
- Examine the palpebral fissures. Normally, they are equally separated.
- Observe for lid lag. There should be none.

Have the client look downward as you observe his eyes. If a rim of the sclera is seen above the iris as the eye moves downward, lid lag is present (Fig. 8-5).

Conjunctiva

- Evert the upper lids and inspect the palpebral conjunctiva. The surface of the palpebral conjunctiva is normally pink.
- Examine the bulbar conjunctiva.

There are normally many small blood vessels visible on the bulbar conjunctiva. Redness can result from serious eye diseases; however, individuals who are very tired or who have eyestrain will develop redness of the bulbar conjunctiva.

Figure 8-6 illustrates the technique used to evert the upper lid.

- With the client looking *downward,* hold the eyelashes gently forward and upward while placing pressure on the upper tarsal border with an applicator.
- When the lid is everted, hold the lashes to the brow and inspect the conjunctival surface.
- To return the lid to its normal position, merely ask the client to look upward. If this does not invert the lid, take hold of the lashes and gently pull forward.

The bulbar conjunctiva can be observed by separating the lids and having the client look down and to both sides.

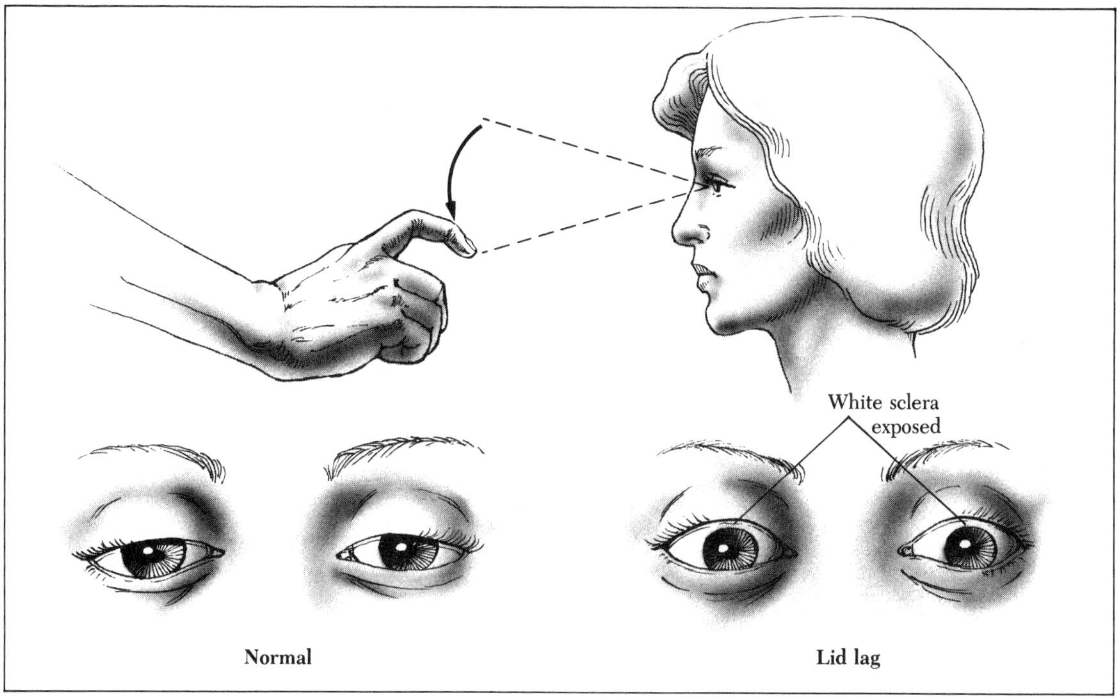

Figure 8-5 Lid lag.

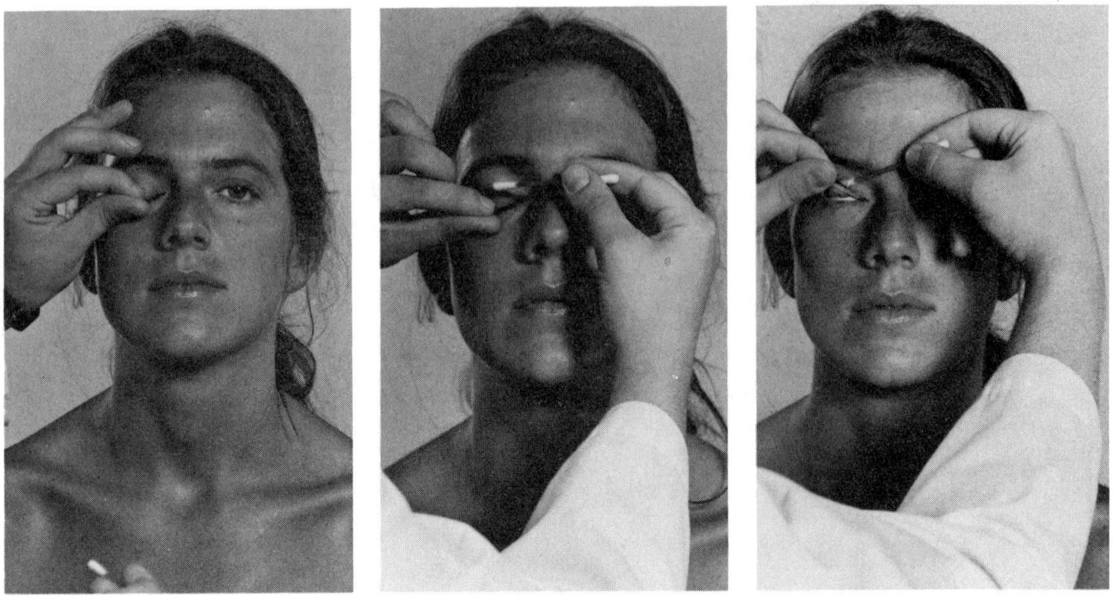

A B C

Figure 8-6 Technique for everting the upper eyelid. **(A)** Lid pulled down as client looks downward. **(B)** Pressure applied over tarsal border. **(C)** Lid gently pulled downward and flipped upward.

Sclera

- Observe the sclera. Normally, the sclera is white.
- In occasional African-Americans, the sclera has a gray-blue hue that is generally recorded as "muddy."

Cornea

- Note the surface and clearness of the cornea. The cornea is normally smooth and transparent. The normal eye has a moist glossiness.
- Test the corneal reflex.

Inspect the cornea from an oblique view by shining a penlight on it. Superficial irregularities can be detected in this manner. In older whites and African-Americans, an arch or circle of cloudy white-gray-blue material may be found encircling the periphery of the cornea; this phenomenon is called *corneal arcus* or *arcus senilis* (Fig. 8-7). This condition is insignificant unless observed in younger people.

The corneal reflex should be tested late in the examination of the eye by touching a wisp of cotton to the center of the cornea and observing for rapid lid closure. Figure 8-8 illustrates this technique. You should approach the client from the side, because the client's seeing the cotton wisp near her eye might in itself cause blinking. Test both eyes; they should have equal reaction.

Pupils

- Note whether the pupils are PERRLA (pupils equal, round, react to light and accommodation).

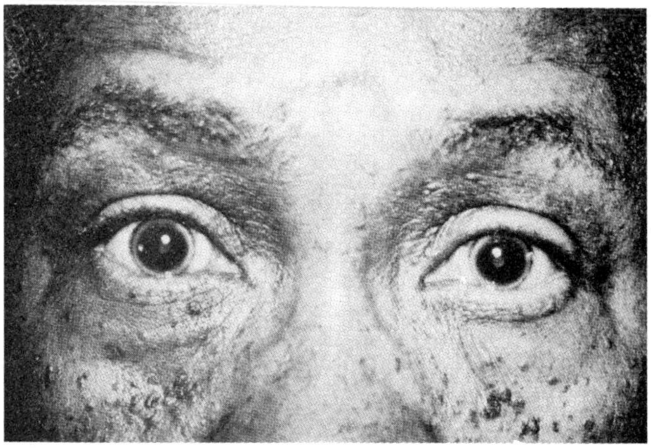

Figure 8-7 Arcus senilis.

Inequality in pupil size is called *anisocoria.* Unequal pupils are always considered abnormal and in need of further investigation. There is a nonpathologic condition, however, called *Adie's syndrome* in which one pupil is dilated. It is observed in young women (Fig. 8-9).

- To test for direct pupillary reaction, stand on one side of the client and focus a penlight on the pupil. The normal pupillary reaction is constriction.
- To test for consensual reaction to light, perform the same procedure but observe the opposite pupil; it should also constrict, even though no direct light is focused on it.
- Perform these tests on both eyes.

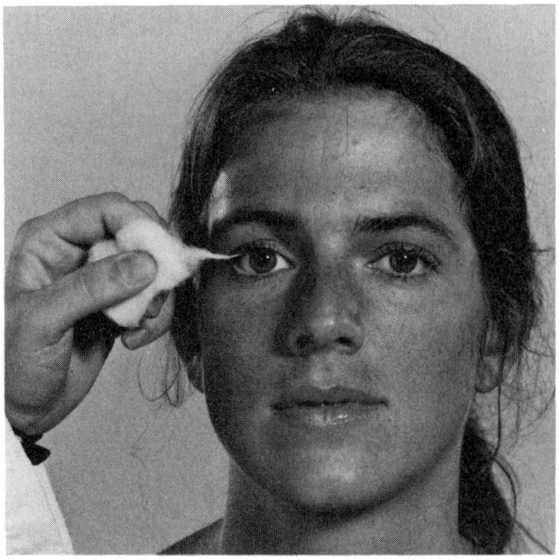

Figure 8-8 Technique for testing corneal reflex.

When the optic nerve is diseased, the affected eye will have no direct reaction to light, although it will react consensually if the unaffected eye is stimulated. When the affected eye is stimulated, however, the unaffected eye will not react consensually.

Accommodation is the phenomenon whereby the pupils dilate to bring in more light when looking at a distant object. As the eyes focus on a near object, the pupils should narrow.

- Test for accommodation.
- Have the client look at a distant point and then at your fingers or a pencil held about 15 cm (6 in.) away from and lateral to his face.
- A bright toy held afar and then quickly brought toward a child's eyes also provokes pupillary contraction.
- Observe for convergence.

As the eyes focus on a near object, both eyes move medially and the pupils constrict; this phenomenon is normal and is called *convergence reaction.*

The important points in checking for accommodation response are to verify its presence and determine whether it is equal in both eyes. It is important to recognize that older persons often do not accommodate well and will show a slower, sluggish response. In the infant, the accommodation reflex is present by the age of 6 months.

Extraocular Muscles

To test whether the extraocular muscles are functioning normally, follow this procedure:

- Face the client and ask her to follow a finger or moving object (e.g., pen, pencil) that is held at least 30 cm (12 in.) or more from her face.
- Move the finger or object through the six cardinal positions illustrated in Fig. 8-4.
- With a child, it is best that you to place a free hand on the top of its head so that only the eyes move and not the head.
- Observe for nystagmus.

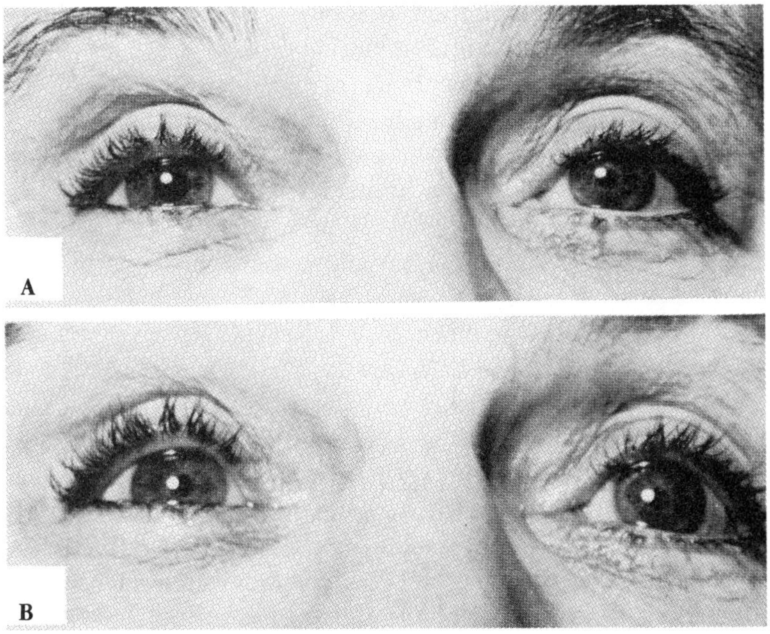

Figure 8-9 Adie's pupil. **(A)** Unilateral tonic pupil. **(B)** Constriction following instillation of Mecholyl.

The eyes should follow the movement smoothly and symmetrically. Inability to move the eye in one of these directions indicates weakness or paralysis of the muscle or damage to the cranial nerve that innervates a particular muscle that corresponds to the particular cardinal position (Fig. 8-10). While performing this test, also observe for nystagmus, an involuntary rhythmic back and forth movement of the eye in a lateral or vertical direction. Although it often occurs temporarily on extreme lateral gaze in persons with normal muscles, it can be the result of a neurologic condition.

If the eye movement is not conjugate (eyes move as a pair symmetrically) or the client reports diplopia or appears to have eyestrain, a Hirschberg test or parallel eye test (see Figs. 18-13 and 18-14) and a cover test (discussed in Chapter 18) are warranted.

Intraocular Pressure

- Palpation of intraocular pressure (Fig. 8-11) provides only a crude measurement but may alert you to any abnormality in consistency.
- Increased tension feels similar to the consistency of palpating the tip of your nose.
- Routine tonometry, using a pen-like instrument that measures the resistance to a puff of air on the cornea, is performed every 2 to 3 years on all clients over 40 years of age to detect the beginning stage of glaucoma.

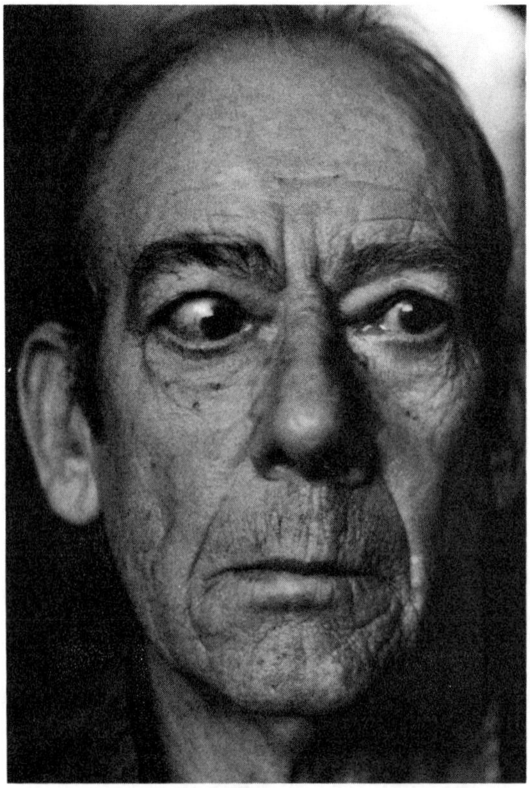

Figure 8-10 **Left lateral gaze dysfunction of rectus eye muscle due to abducen (CN VI) involvement.**

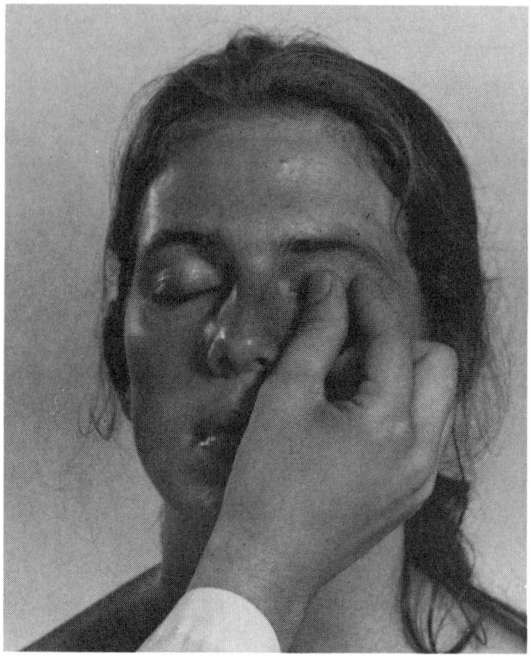

Figure 8-11 **Palpation of intraocular pressure.**

Visual Fields

A crude estimate of the peripheral fields of vision can be obtained by a technique called *gross confrontation.* Using this procedure, you are comparing your own field of vision with the client's. Not always performed routinely, it needs to be performed with a client suspected of having a visual problem, on the older adult who is at higher risk for glaucoma, and on the client with neurologic symptoms. Figure 8-12 illustrates this procedure.

- Stand face to face with the client, about 2 feet apart, with your eyes level with the client's.
- Have the client focus on your eyes.
- Have the client cover one eye, and you cover your opposite eye.
- Move your wiggling fingers or an object midway between you and the client in eight axes from the periphery, as shown in Fig. 8-13.

The horizontal field of vision is smaller because of interference by the eyebrow, nose, and cheekbone. Therefore, as your fingers move forward from the top of the client's head he should be able to see them at about a 50-degree angle. The field of vision is about 60 degrees medially and about 70 degrees downward. The lateral field of vision is 90 degrees; thus, with normal visual field range, both you and the client will immediately see your fingers.

Visual Acuity

It is crucial that children between the ages of 1 and 6 have annual visual screening, as these years constitute the critical

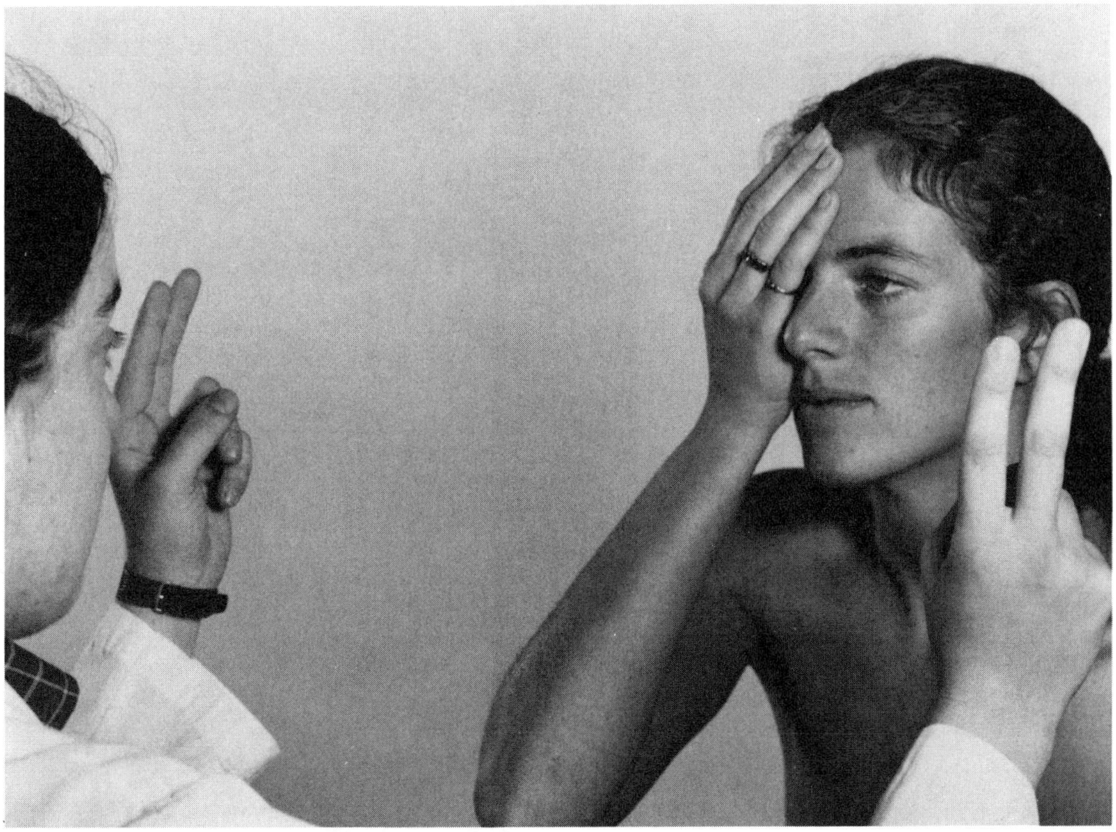

Figure 8-12 Gross confrontation technique.

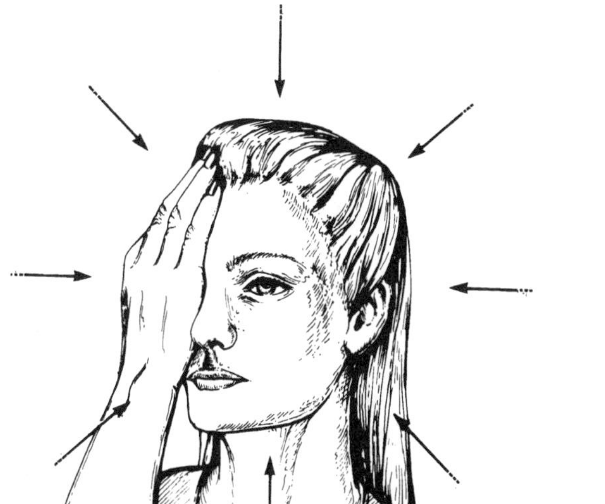

Figure 8-13 Visual field axes.

period of development of acute vision. Early detection is imperative to counteract permanent visual defects. Because preschool visual screening in the United States is presently inadequate, parents may wish to perform vision screening tests with home eye test kits obtained from the National Association for the Prevention of Blindness (16 E. 40th Street, New York, NY). Slight defects must be assessed further by an ophthalmologist.

Testing of visual acuity with the older child and the adult is accomplished by using a Snellen eye chart (Fig. 8-14).

- Have the client stand 20 feet from the chart and cover one eye.
- Have the client read the numbers from the top of the chart downward.
- Then have the client cover the opposite eye and read the chart again.
- Have the client read the chart again with both eyes uncovered.
- If the client wears lens for far-distance vision, repeat the preceding steps with the client wearing her glasses. (Reading glasses often blur distant vision.)
- Record the last line of which the client can read at least 50% of the numbers. Always record whether corrective lenses are worn during the examination.
- Any recording greater than 20/40 is referred for ophthalmologic assessment.

The recording is a fraction. The numerator expresses the distance to the chart (20 feet), and the denominator, listed

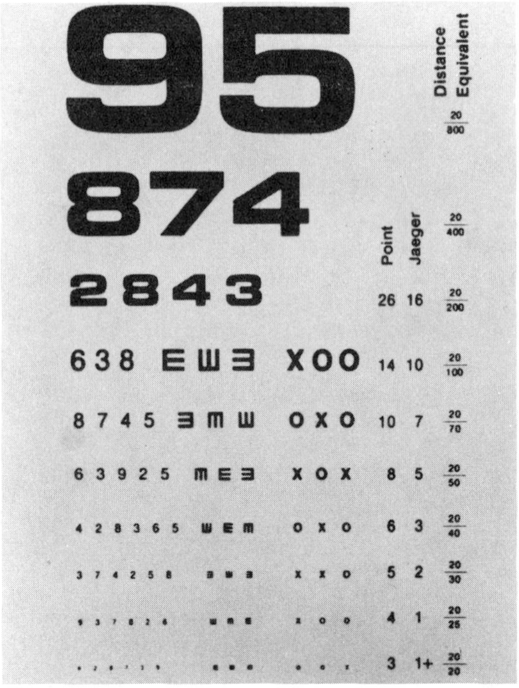

Figure 8-14 Example of an eye chart.

by each line on the chart, represents the distance at which the average eye can read that particular line of the chart. Therefore, a recording of 20/40 means that the client is 20 feet away from the chart and can read the line that the average eye can read at 40 feet. A recording of 20/200 indicates that at 20 feet the client can read only the largest number of the chart. This number can be seen at 200 feet by a person with normal vision.

For preschoolers and people who cannot read, a chart on which the letter E is arranged in different positions and in various sizes can be used. In this situation, the client merely points to the direction in which the legs of the E are facing.

The results of visual acuity testing are recorded for each eye and for both eyes: for example, OD (right eye) 20/30; OS (left eye) 20/20; and OU (both eyes) 20/20.

Near vision can be tested with a hand-held card that is 14 inches away from the client's eyes. If one is not available, use a newspaper or magazine. If the client wears reading glasses, test his near vision while he is wearing the glasses; he should be able to read newspaper-size print with no difficulty.

Table 8-1 describes the range of visual acuity, lists symptoms of visual conditions, and provides corrective methods. Legal blindness is defined by either limited visual fields of less than 21% in the better eye or by visual acuity of 20/200 in the better eye as corrected by glasses.

Color Vision

There are generally two rows of letters underlined on the Snellen chart—one underlined in red and the other by a green stripe. A gross test of color vision is to ask the client to read the line that has a green stripe under it. A more accurate method is to use color plates. A number or figure of a primary color—red, green, or blue—is placed in a variegated maze of color. The client with normal color vision readily sees the number or figure. Color vision should be tested throughout life because disease can affect color vision as can inherited color blindness. The latter is a condition affecting mostly white males because the defective gene is carried on the X chromosome. By receiving only one X chromosome, males have the likelihood of having the defective gene expressed, whereas in the female receiving two X chromosomes, one is more likely to be normal and will dominate the defective gene.

A Word on Diagnosis

Age-related macular degeneration most often strikes after age 60. The only early symptom tends to be blurred vision, but as more and more cells of the macula are destroyed, people may begin to see a small blind spot in the middle of their field of vision. As the disease becomes increasingly severe, straight lines often appear crooked.

You can use the grid to keep an eye on your own vision at home. While covering one eye, look at the dot in the center. Then do the same with the other eye. If in either case the lines surrounding the dot appear wavy, blurry, or distorted, you should have your eyes examined by an ophthalmologist.

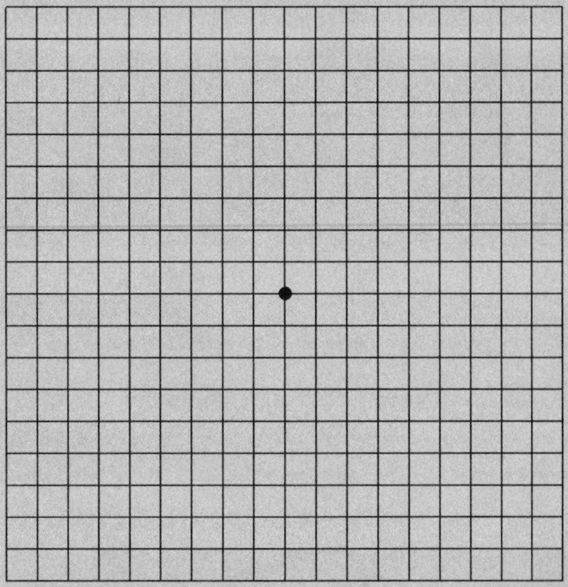

Source: Tufts University *Diet & Nutrition Letter* 12(11) 1995. Reprinted with permission, *Tufts University Diet & Nutrition Letter*, 53 Park Place, New York, NY 10007.

Table 8-1 Types of Visual Acuity

Condition	Interpretation	Signs and symptoms	Treatment
Emmetropia 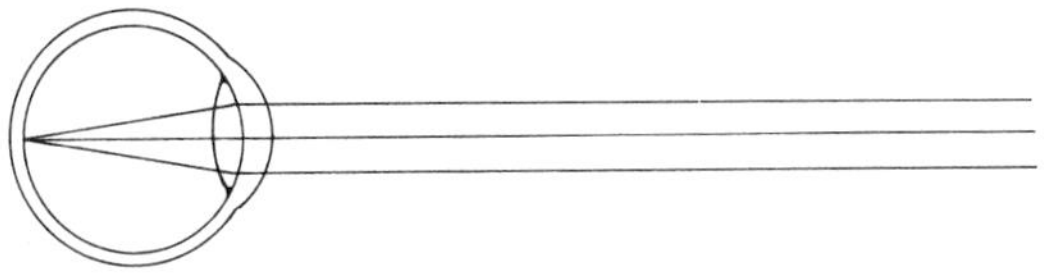	Ideal eye	None: light is focused on retina easily by accommodation	None
Hypermetropia (Hyperopia) 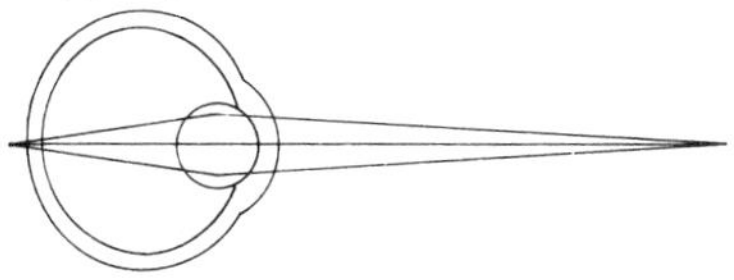 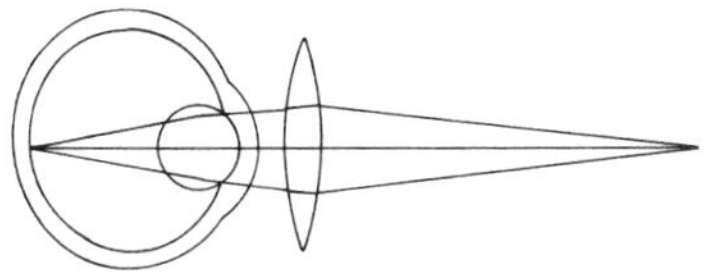	Far-sighted eye; light is brought to focus behind the retina	Eyestrain; may be blurring of vision, headache, nausea	Convex lens
Myopia 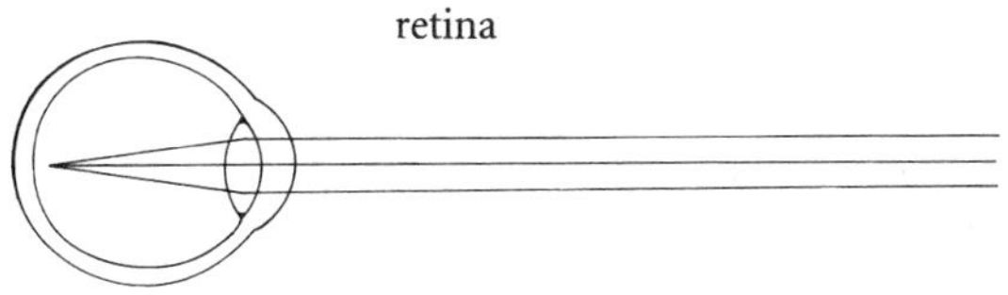 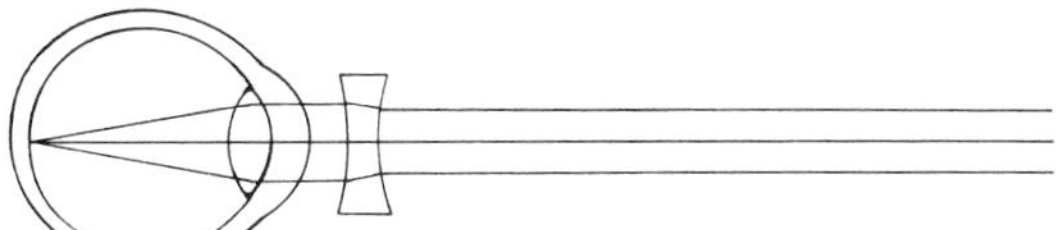	Near-sighted eye; light is brought to focus in front of the retina	Defective vision; eyestrain not as frequent as noticed in hyperopia	Concave lens
Astigmatism 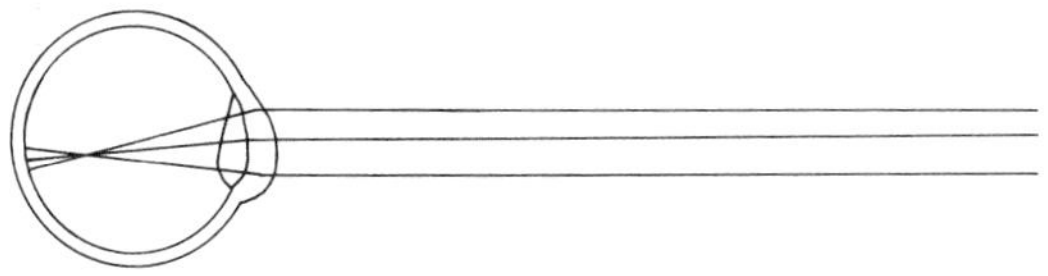 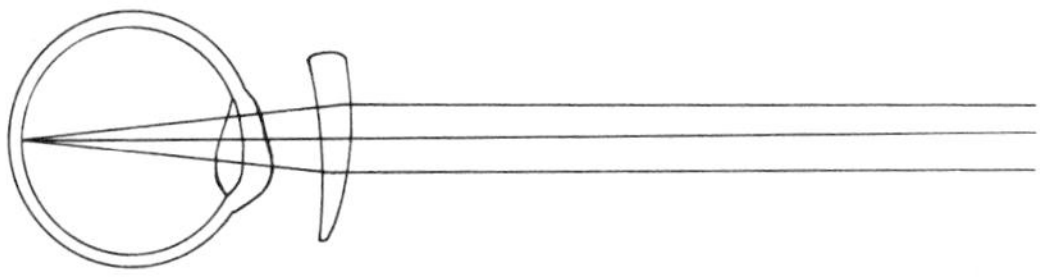	Abnormal curvature of cornea or lens	Defective vision; images do not focus properly on retina (irregular astigmatism may follow corneal injury or ulcer)	Corrective lenses (cylindrical, thick); glasses worn continuously in high degrees; in lower degrees only for work causing eyestrain
Presbyopia	"Old sighted" eye; physiologic process in which lens begin to lose elasticity and ciliary muscles begin to weaken, resulting in gradual loss of accommodation; usually affects persons past the age of 45	Inability to read without holding reading material over 30 cm away from the eye	Glasses for near work; bifocals (distant correction plus magnifying lenses at the bottom for near vision)

OPHTHALMOSCOPIC EXAMINATION

The ophthalmoscopic examination of the eye requires a great deal of practice, so the beginner should not become discouraged. You can practice and get the feel of the instrument by using it to read the newspaper.

Careful examination of the interior eye will assist in detecting not only eye diseases but also systemic disease. Several structures are examined through the ophthalmoscope: the lens, retina, optic disk, arteries, veins, and macula.

Conducting the Examination

The posterior eye (fundus) is best examined when the pupil is dilated, but dilation is not performed routinely during health assessment unless the client's history or other physical findings indicate that a more thorough examination is needed. If so, refer the client for examination by a physician or an ophthalmologist, whichever is more appropriate with regard to your findings.

For optimum viewing of the eye grounds (fundus), the room should be darkened (pupil will be dilated). Blinking of the client's eye can interfere with the examination. Movement will cause the beam of examining light to move out of alignment with the client's pupil.

- Slightly elevate the client's upper lid with the thumb of your free hand. The remainder of your free hand can be rested on the client's head and will serve to steady it.
- Instruct the client to gaze straight ahead over the shoulder of whichever hand you are using to hold the instrument.
- Face the client in either a sitting or standing position.

Technique for the Ophthalmoscopic Examination

1. Darken room.
2. Face client, sitting or standing.
3. Holding ophthalmoscope in right hand, use your right eye to examine client's right eye. Repeat for left eye, using left hand and left eye to client's left eye.
4. Place index finger on focus wheel.
5. Hold ophthalmoscope firmly against your brow.
6. Position viewing aperture in front of your eye.
7. Hold client's upper eyelid open with thumb of your "free" hand.
8. Direct beam of light into client's pupil from distance of 30 cm and find red reflex.
9. Move closer with red reflex toward the client's pupil until client's and your foreheads are almost touching.
10. Note characteristics of retina, disk, and vessels.

- Your hand holding the ophthalmoscope, your examining eye, and the client's eye to be examined should all be on the same side of the body. In other words, your right hand holds the ophthalmoscope while your right eye examines the client's right eye (Fig. 8-15). Failure to use this procedure will result in an uncomfortable collision with the client's nose.
- If, for some reason, you can use only one examining eye, you can avoid collision by examining the client's opposite eye while she is in the supine position. This approach is illustrated in Fig. 8-16. In this position, the client's opposite eye can be approached from the head of the examining table; this upside-down approach places your nose lateral to the client's head.
- Most practitioners who wear glasses or contact lenses do not remove them while performing the examination. However, myopic and hyperopic conditions of the examiner and/or client can be corrected by lens settings. Start with the red lens if it is known that the client is myopic. Clients with *severe astigmatism* wear their contact lenses or glasses for the ophthalmoscopic examination; in this case, the diopter settings of the scope cannot correct the severe distortion.
- Set the lens wheel at zero, and then adjust to the setting that provides the best viewing.
- Place your index finger on the lens wheel to allow for focusing.
- Brace the head of the ophthalmoscope solidly against your brow, with the viewing aperture positioned in front of your eye.
- Direct the beam of light into the client's pupil from a distance of about 30 cm; a red reflex from the healthy fundus will be seen to fill the eye; the red reflex should be clear and free from opacities.
- Many clients experience benign, annoying vitreous floaters; floaters are translucent specks of protein or cells that drift within the vitreous humor and are seen as dark specks between the lens and retina. Have the client move his eyes to stir the eye fluid and move the floater out of the way.
- Move closer following the red reflex until your forehead is almost touching the client's forehead.
- Have the client look in various directions or move the ophthalmoscope so you can inspect the entire fundus.

Minus numbers (red) focus further away; plus numbers (black) focus nearer. The red reflex must be kept in focus until your forehead is almost touching that of the client. If you lose the focus, move back and begin again. Absence of the red reflex indicates poor positioning of the ophthalmoscope or an abnormality of light transmission through the lens. To recognize abnormalities of the eye grounds, you must have a clear understanding of the appearance of the normal fundus.

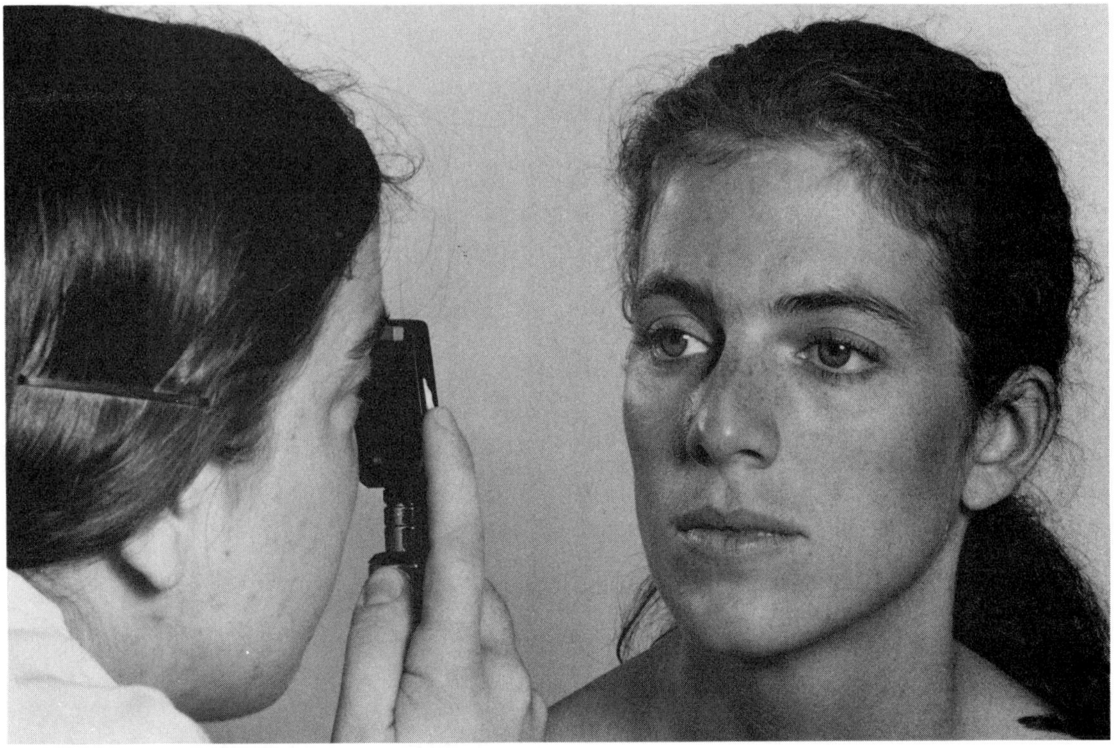

Figure 8-15 Same-eyes examination technique.

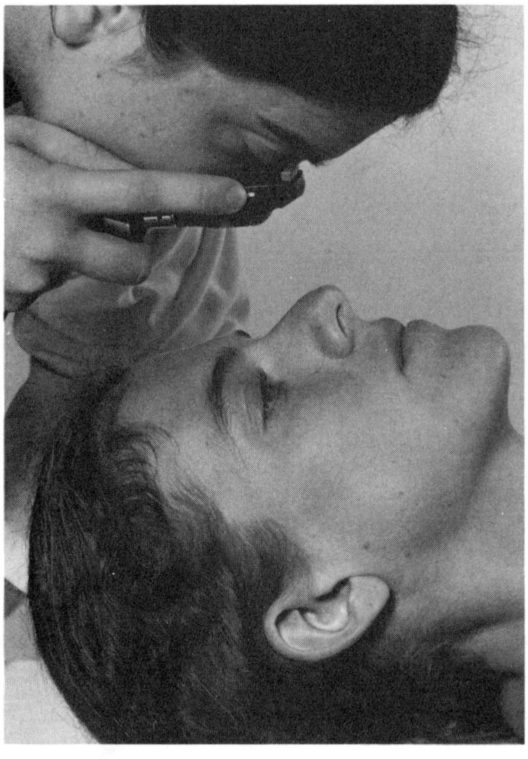

Figure 8-16 Inverse head-of-bed approach.

Examination of the Fundus

Examination of the fundus begins with the location and assessment of the *optic disk.* The disk is situated more nasally on the retina and normally appears round or vertically oval with flat discrete edges. It is a creamy yellow or pinkish yellow color and is about 1.5 mm in diameter.

The diameter of the disk, referred to as DD (disk diameter), is a unit of measure used to document the location and diameter of lesions (distance in DDs from the optic disk margin). Abnormal findings are also located according to the hour sign on the face of a clock (e.g., dark red spot ¼ DD in size, 1 ½ DD away @ 3:00).

- To visualize the disk, direct the light of the ophthalmoscope from about 15 degrees temporal to the straight-ahead gaze of the client.

Most disks have a funnel-shaped depression in the temporal side that presents as a white or pale yellow area; it does not extend completely to the disk margin. This is referred to as the *physiologic depression,* or *physiologic cup. Vessels* can be seen emerging from the cup and extending to the periphery of the retina.

Arteries are bright red and reflect a streak of narrow white light. They are approximately a quarter smaller in diameter than the veins. Veins lack a central white reflex stripe and are larger and darker red than arteries (Fig. 8-17). Usually, at the proximal end of veins, light pulsation can be visualized; this pulsation is normal and helps to differentiate veins from arteries. Retinal arteries do not pulsate.

The arteriovenous decussations (where the arteries and veins cross) should be carefully observed for any indentation (nicking) or displacement (humping). These do not normally exist in the healthy individual.

If you have difficulty finding the optic disk, follow a vessel. The vessel will become larger as it approaches the optic disk, and will eventually meet and enter the disk.

The entire fundus should be examined by having the client rotate the eye so that different areas can be explored. The macula should be examined last, as it is the point most sensitive to light.

The macula is a small area about 1-DD wide and approximately 2 to 3-DD temporal to the disk and in the same horizontal plane. It is a slightly deeper red color than the surrounding fundus. It is avascular, and the bright spot in the middle represents reflected light from the fovea centralis. This area is examined last as it is light-sensitive, causing the client's eyes to tear. To easily locate the macula, have the client look directly at the scope.

The pigmentation of the fundus can vary and still remain within normal limits. Generally, the darker the skin, the darker the fundus, and vice versa. Figure 8-18 shows a normal fundus in a white person, while Fig. 8-19 shows a normal African-American fundus, which has a darker blue tint. Occasionally, a thickened, pigmented retinal epithelium may appear as a black ring or crescent at the edges of the scopic view.

The optic nerve fibers are myelinated up to the point that they emerge into the retina. In some individuals, the myelination of these fibers continues beyond the lamina cribrosa, producing a striking appearance. This is a normal variation in which semi-opaque white brushes project from about the disk, partially or completely obscuring the retinal vessels and disk margin (Fig. 8-20).

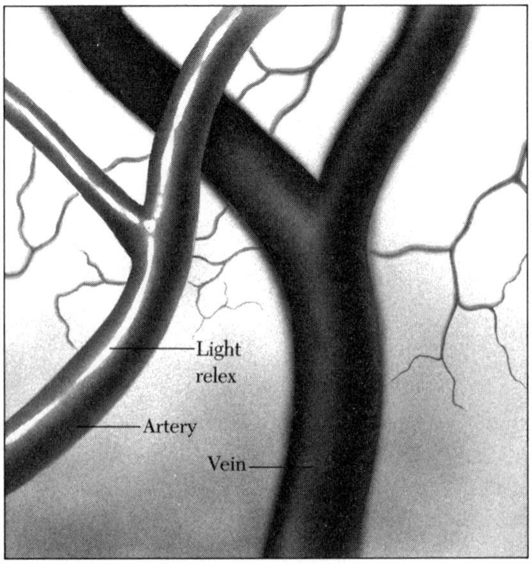

Figure 8-17 Normal retinal artery and vein.

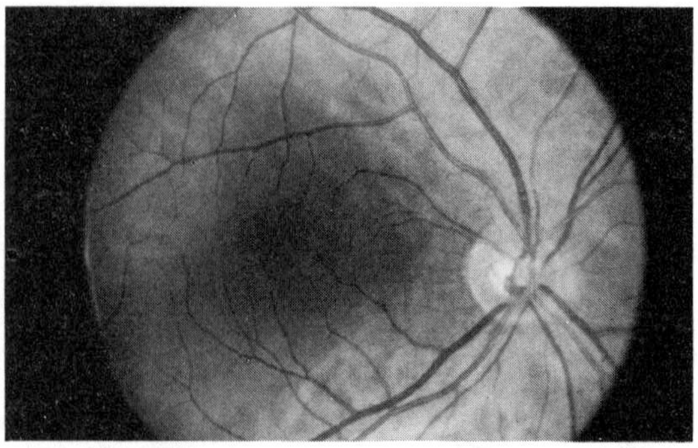
Figure 8-18 Caucasian fundus. (See also endsheet plate 1.)

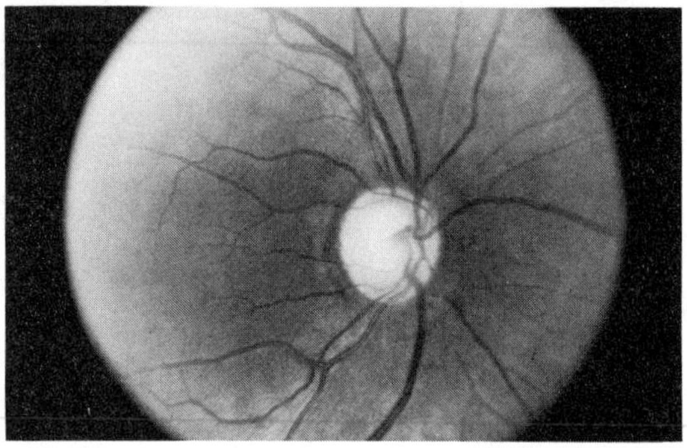
Figure 8-19 African-American fundus. (See also endsheet plate 2.)

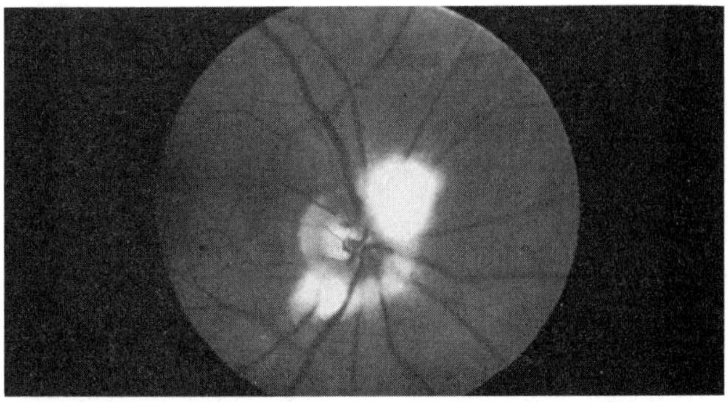
Figure 8-20 Nonpathologic myelinated fibrination always seen extending from the optic disk.

CLINICAL CORRELATIONS

External Eye Conditions

A *hordeolum* (style) is an infection of one of the meibomian glands of the eyelid (Fig. 8-21). It may suppurate with appli-

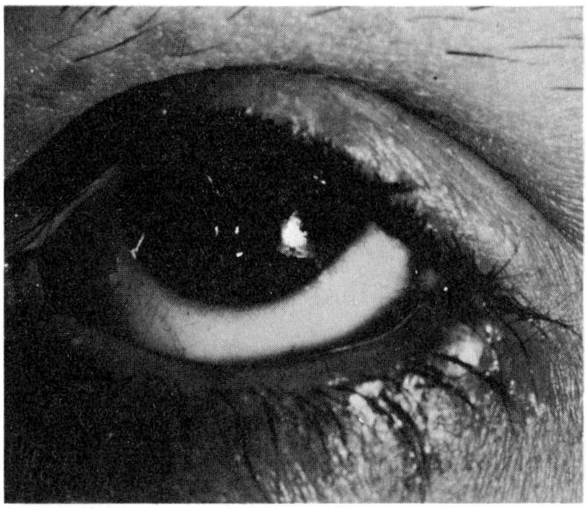

Figure 8-21 Hordeolum (stye).

cation of warm compresses or may need treatment with an antiseptic and antibiotic. Generally, a hordeolum resolves in 7 to 10 days.

A *chalazion* is a cyst of a meibomian gland that will be seen to bulge through to the surface of the eyelid (Figs. 8-22 and 8-23). Occasionally, it may become infected, but initially it appears as a hard, painless lump. Unlike a hordeolum, it will not subside or rupture on its own. It needs to be removed surgically.

Positional defects of the lids include *entropion* (inward rolling of the lid) and *extropion* (outward rolling of the lid) (Fig. 8-24). These defects often can be detected in elderly persons; the eye may become easily infected or irritated. The defects can be repaired surgically. *Blepharospasm,* an involuntary twitching of both eyelids, may occur in elderly clients. It maybe an isolated phenomenon due to eyestrain or nervous irritability, or it may be related to involvement of the facial nerve.

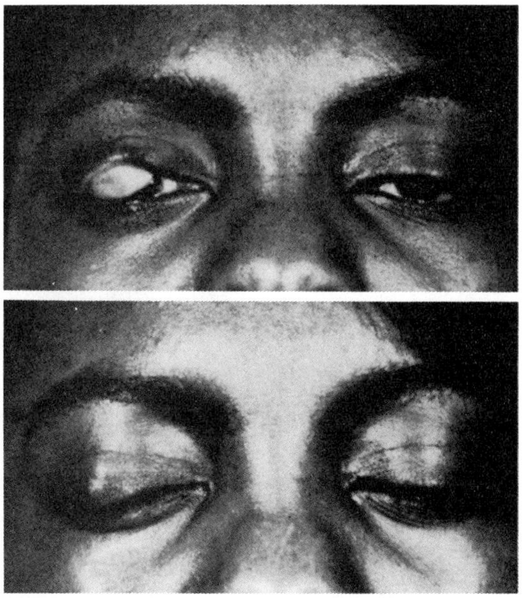

Figure 8-22 Chalazion of right upper eyelid. Note the small, firm bulge slightly lateral to the midline of the eyelid.

Blepharitis, inflammation of the lid margins involving the lashes, appears as erythema, scales and crusting exudate often caused by bacterial infection and allergies. A chronic type may occur with scalp and eyebrow seborrhea (dandruff) (Fig. 8-25).

Edema of the eyelid often indicates systemic problems such as renal diseases, heart failure, allergy, and thyroid deficiency, as well as direct trauma to the eye.

When the eyelids are closed, they should meet completely. In clients with *exophthalmos,* a protrusion of the eyeball(s), the palpebral fissure is wider than normal (see Fig. 7-14 on page 165). The client often cannot close the lids completely.

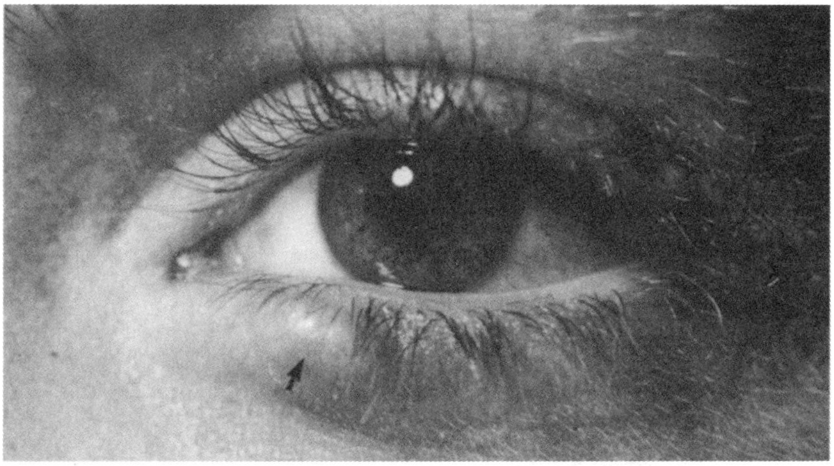

Figure 8-23 Chalazion of left lower lid seen externally. (From Sana, J.M. and Judge, R.D. *Physical Assessment for Nursing Skills* (2nd ed.). Boston: Little, Brown, 1982, p. 151.)

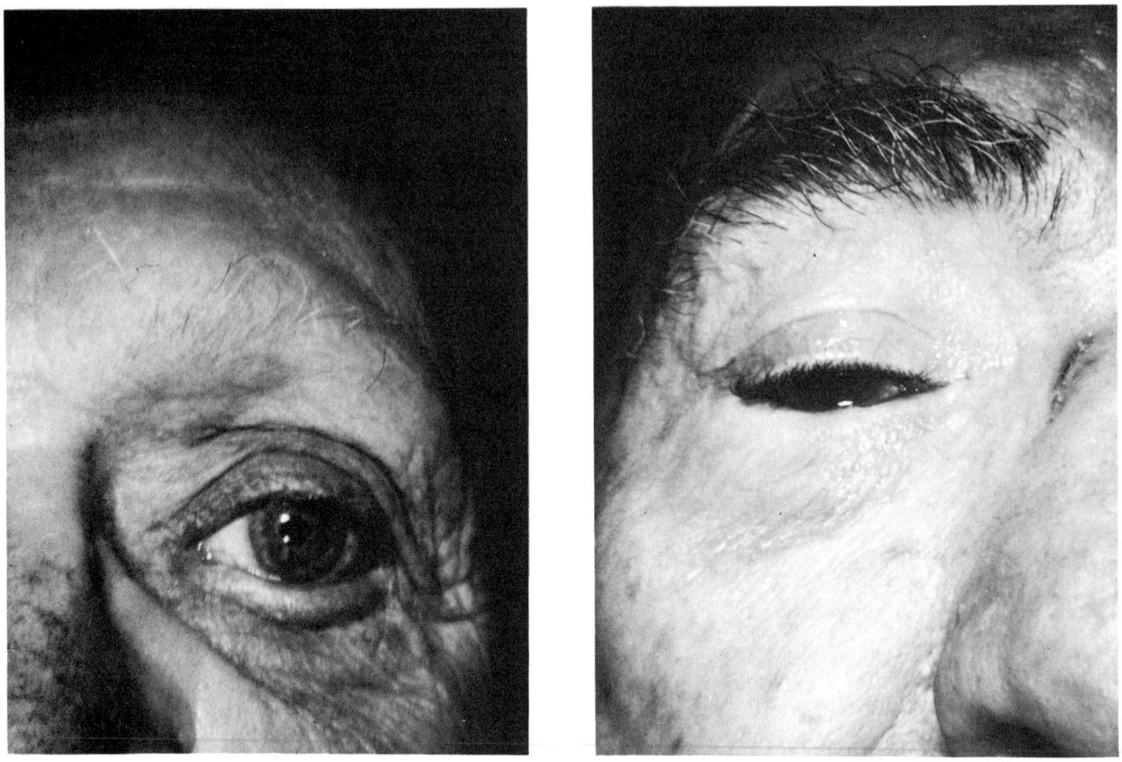

A B

Figure 8-24 **(A)** Extropion of left lower eyelid. **(B)** Entropion of right lower eyelid.

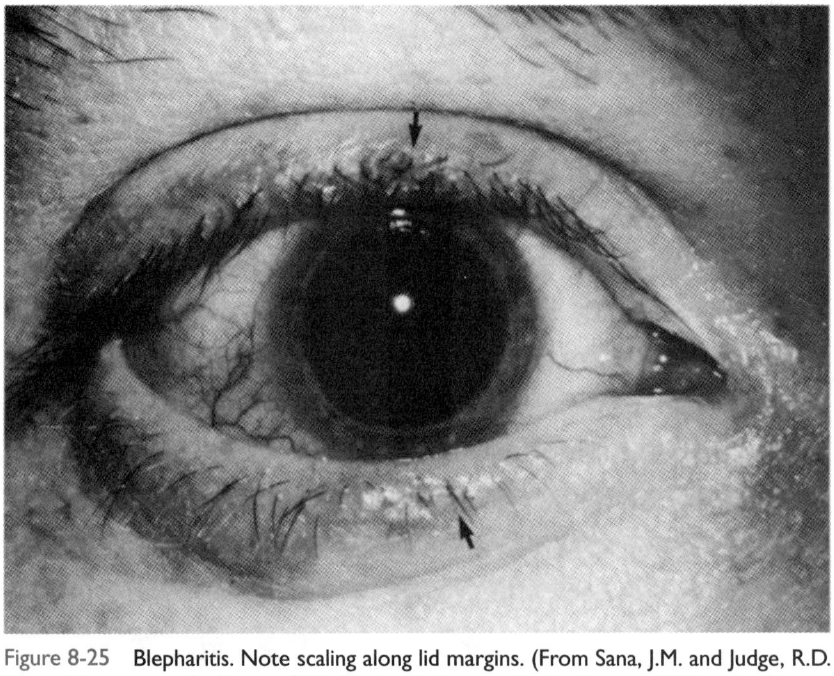

Figure 8-25 Blepharitis. Note scaling along lid margins. (From Sana, J.M. and Judge, R.D. *Physical Assessment for Nursing Skills* (2nd ed.). Boston: Little, Brown, 1982, p. 147.)

Unilateral exophthalmos usually results from inflammation or infection within the orbit or an orbital tumor; however, Graves' disease may manifest unilaterally, but is not the rule. Additionally, clients with hyperthyroidism may display lid lag.

Ptosis, drooping of the eyelid, can result from muscular weakness, interference with the oculomotor nerve, or interference with the sympathetic nerves that maintain the smooth muscle tone of the eyelid (Fig. 8-26). In Bell's palsy, a disease affecting the 7th cranial nerve, the palpebral fissure is widened and the eyelid will not close. The lower lid sags, and when an attempt is made to close the eyes, the eye on the paralyzed side is seen to roll upward. Partial ptosis may reflect Horner's syndrome, which involves the cervical sympathetic nerves. Marked ptosis of an upper eyelid associated with decreased pupillary light reaction may be an early indication of oculomotor paralysis.

The palpebral conjunctiva of anemic clients generally appears very pale. An erythematous and swollen palpebral conjunctiva indicates irritation or inflammation. With inflammation of the bulbar conjunctiva (conjunctivitis), the vessels become engorged, and there is redness, swelling, and pain (Fig. 8-27). The inflammation pattern can be peripheral injection, as seen in Fig. 8-27, or central injection, wherein the inflammation appears to radiate from the iris. Serious diseases, such as iritis, keratitis, and glaucoma, can also cause redness and require prompt evaluation and treatment by an ophthalmologist. Conjunctivitis or pinkeye caused by bacteria and viruses is highly contagious. Ophthalmic antibiotics resolve bacterial infections.

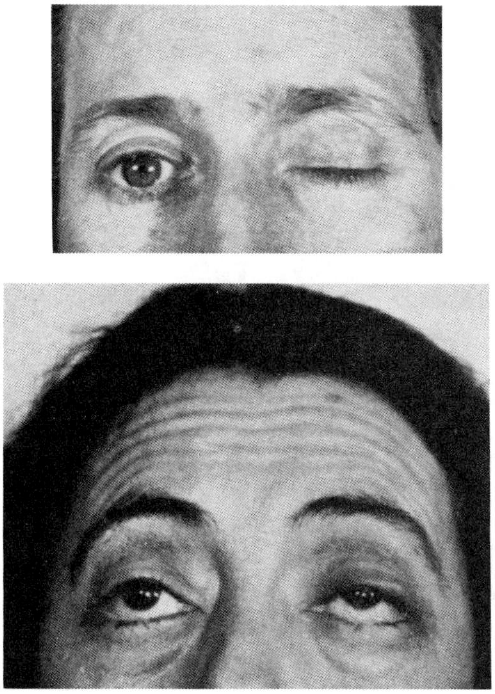

Figure 8-26 Ptosis of left eyelid as a result of oculomotor nerve paralysis.

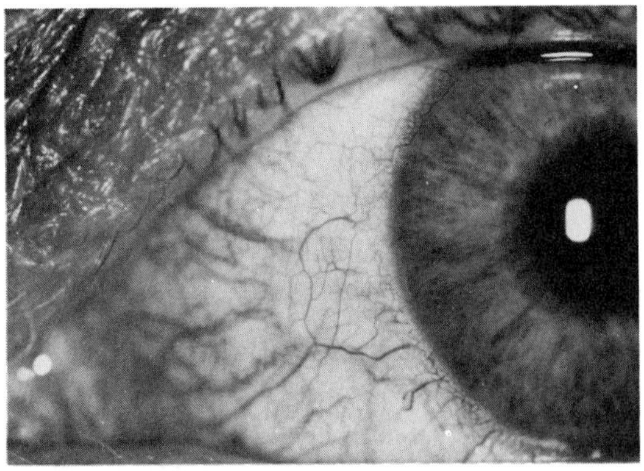

Figure 8-27 Conjunctivitis. (See also endsheet plate 3.)

Subconjunctival hemorrhage resulting from trauma, increased venous pressure, or hemorrhagic disorders produces a red patch, which is usually in an exposed section of the bulbar conjunctiva (Fig. 8-28). This bright red patch of varying size will most often be reabsorbed within a few days.

A triangular thickening of the bulbar conjunctiva extending from the inner canthus toward the center of the cornea is called a *pterygium* (Fig. 8-29). If vision is impaired, it may require surgical treatment.

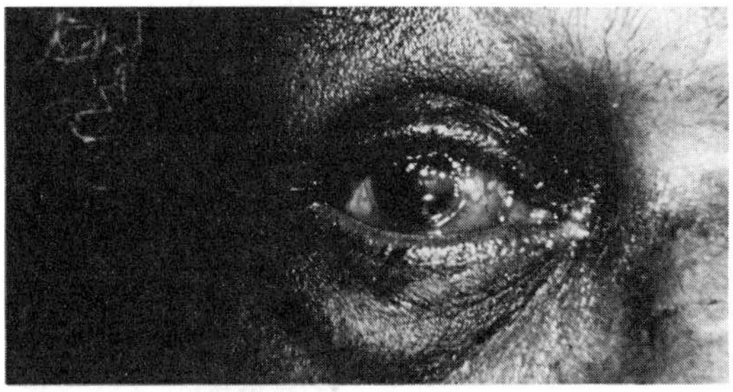

Figure 8-28 Hemorrhage. (See also endsheet plate 4.)

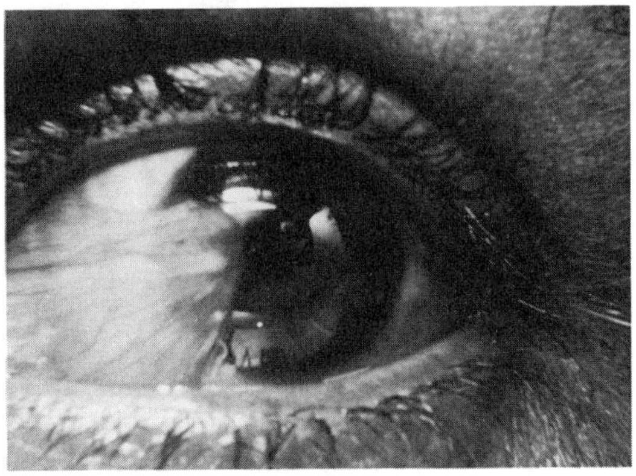

Figure 8-29 Pterygium. (See also endsheet plate 5.)

Scleral Changes

In hepatitis, the sclerae may become a bright yellow; in obstructive jaundice, greenish yellow; and in pernicious anemia, lemon yellow. Cyanosis and pallor also may be detected by careful observation of the sclerae.

Corneal Changes

A dullness may be noted in nutritional deficiencies (especially avitaminosis A), glaucoma, and hypercholesteremia. Any ulceration or opacity is abnormal. Pain, photophobia, and redness of the bulbar conjunctiva accompany active ulcerations. Yellow opacities usually indicate active ulcerations, whereas bluish white opacities indicate healed ulcerations. Abrasions are almost impossible to detect with superficial light and need to be stained with fluorescein, which will produce a brilliant yellow-green indication of the abrasion. This staining technique is not part of a routine physical assessment process; when this procedure is warranted, it should be performed only if you have been specially trained in the technique.

Diseases of the cornea are often severe. *Trachoma,* relatively rare in the United States, causes more blindness in the world than any other condition. Trachoma is a chronic infection of the conjunctiva caused by microorganisms. In the United States, it has a higher incidence among Native Americans and Mexican-Americans. Corneal ulceration, which can result in corneal perforation, is a major cause of blindness in the United States. It can be precipitated by a number of causes, including allergy, diabetes mellitus, and trauma.

Kayser-Fleischer rings—brown-green rings of pigment around the corneal limbus—are of pathologic significance. They occur in Wilson's disease, which manifests serious neurologic and liver degeneration.

Absence of the corneal reflex due to lack of corneal sensitivity indicates injury of the sensory component of the 5th cranial (trigeminal) nerve; however, failure of lid closure may be due to injury of the motor component of the 7th cranial (facial) nerve.

Pupillary Changes

In clients with head injury, the pupils may be small and unreactive to light, dilated and fixed, or unequal. Drugs also cause pronounced effects on the pupil. Morphine constricts the pupils, whereas cocaine dilates them by stimulating the sympathetic nerve endings. Dilated unreactive pupils are observed in conditions of anoxia or in deep barbiturate poisoning. Cranial tumors can produce dilation or constriction of the pupils, depending on where they are located in the cranium.

In chronic syphilis, the pupils are usually small and irregular and do not dilate in response to mydriatic drugs. The pupils fail to react to light but do accommodate. This phenomenon is termed the *Argyll Robertson pupil.*

Changes in the Lens

The lens are viewed through the pupil and are normally of a clear transparency that decreases with aging. Cataracts are

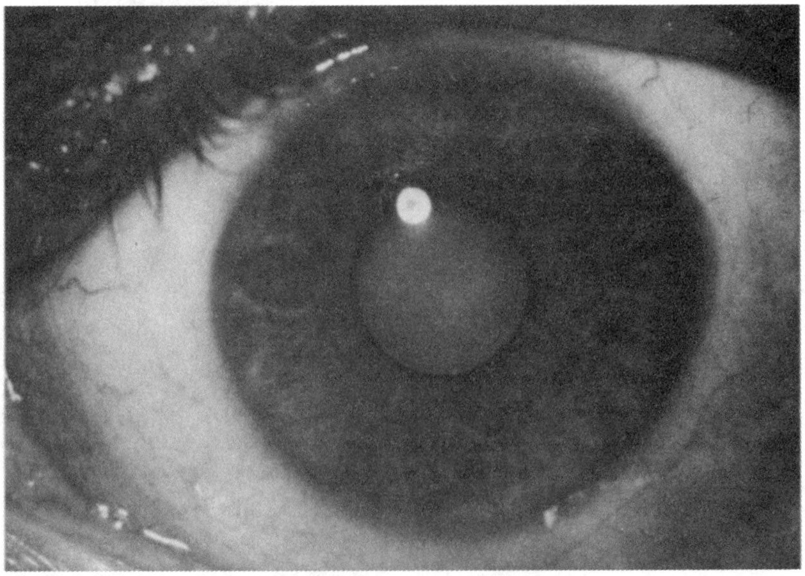

Figure 8-30 Cataract. Note light reflex on upper edge of pupil. (From: Sana, J.M. and Judge, R.D. *Physical Assessment for Nursing Skills* (2nd ed.). Boston: Little, Brown, 1982, p. 153.)

opacities of the lens that appear as cloudy, spoke-shaped, nuclear or central opacities (Fig. 8-30). Approximately 1.25 million people are blinded annually by cataracts. They can be congenital, but they are usually caused by the aging process; other etiologies are infection, radiation, ultraviolet radiation, prolonged steroid hormone therapy, and a secondary complication of diabetes mellitus.

Intraocular Pressure

Softness is indicative of dehydration. Increased intraocular tension may indicate glaucoma, a serious condition in which unchecked pressure can lead to blindness. If glaucoma is discovered early, it is possible to prevent further damage to the retina by the use of medications or special surgical procedures. Because glaucoma has a higher incidence in the middle-aged and elderly population, it is important that routine tonometry be performed every 2 to 3 years on all clients over 40 years of age. Any significant reduction of the client's field of vision should be confirmed by an ophthalmologist. Glaucoma is a common, serious condition that restricts visual fields.

Changes in color vision can occur anytime in life from such conditions as macular degeneration, retrobulbar neuritis, optic nerve disease, toxic amblyopia, and lesions at the optic chiasmal site.

Age-related macular degeneration is the leading cause of irreversible blindness among older Americans; it mostly occurs after 60 years of age. Eating green leafy vegetables and foods containing betacarotene may prevent the degenerative process.

CLINICAL CORRELATIONS OF OPHTHALMOSCOPIC EXAMINATION FINDINGS

If there are diffuse, dense opacities in the client's eye, a dull red or black reflex is observed. Black spots appearing against the red reflex are produced by opacities in the lens or vitreous humor.

The dark spots, when visualized, can be clearly focused by moving the ophthalmoscope back and forth. Once they are focused, ask the client to look slightly upward. Spots on the cornea or anterior lens move upward, whereas vitreous opacities remain stationary.

The red reflex provides information about the condition of the transparent portions of the eye. Small cataracts, corneal scars, and opacities produce a shadow in the red reflex. Hemorrhage and extensive cataracts may completely block the reflex.

The major abnormalities affecting the optic disk are papilledema, optic atrophy, and glaucomatous cup. *Papilledema* (choked disk) is a serious condition in which either unilateral or bilateral swelling and elevation of the nerve head is seen, with the retinal vessels bending sharply over its edge. Signs of papilledema are blurred or fuzzy margins of the optic disk, filling in of the physiologic depression, full and tortuous retinal veins, and absence of venous pulsations. Many disease states produce papilledema, but the most common are increased intracranial pressure (from brain tumor, hydrocephalus, meningitis, or subarachnoid hemorrhage) and severe hypertension. The presence of papilledema (Fig. 8-31) is often the first sign of a serious condition.

RECORDING OF FINDINGS

Normal findings are presented in the left column. The second column contains recordings for a client who was later medically diagnosed as being hypertensive.

Eye
Inspection: Eyes moist and glossy. Eyebrows full; lashes present; no orbital edema; equal separation of palpebral fissures; no lid lag; no ptosis; conjunctiva pink without bulbar injection; sclerae white; cornea clear; PERRLA/consensual reaction; convergence WNL; EOMs intact; no nystagmus; no strabismus; visual fields normal by gross confrontation; OD 20/20, OS 20/20, OU 20/20 without corrective lenses. Fundoscopy: red reflex clear; disk well demarcated, pinkish yellow color; A/V 2:3; no AV nicking; no hemorrhages; no exudates.

Palpation: Ocular tension—soft on palpation.

Eye
Inspection: Dull appearance. Eyebrows full; lashes present; no orbital edema; equal separation of palpebral fissures; no lid lag; no ptosis; conjunctiva pink without bulbar injection; sclerae white; cornea clear; PERRLA/consensual reaction; convergence WNL; EOMs intact; no nystagmus; no strabismus; visual fields normal by gross confrontation; OD 20/20, OS 20/20, OU 20/20 with corrective lenses. Fundoscopy: red reflex clear; blurred disk edges; narrowed copper-wire arteries; AV nicking; flame-shaped hemorrhages ½ DD away at 4:00; diffuse cotton-wool patches.

Palpation: Ocular tension—soft on palpation.

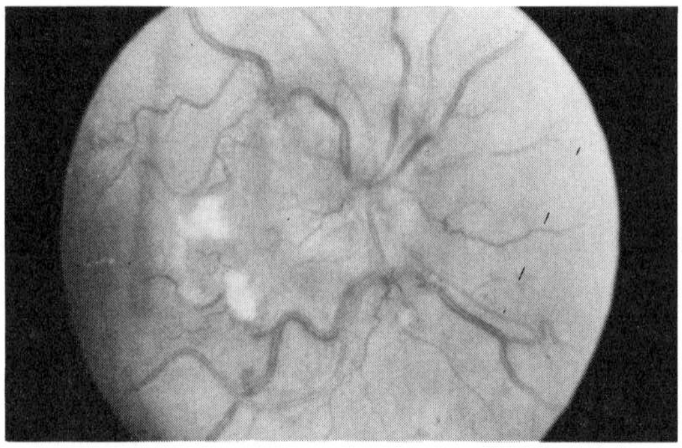

Figure 8-31 Papilledema. Note blurring of disk and tortuous veins. (See also endsheet plate 6.)

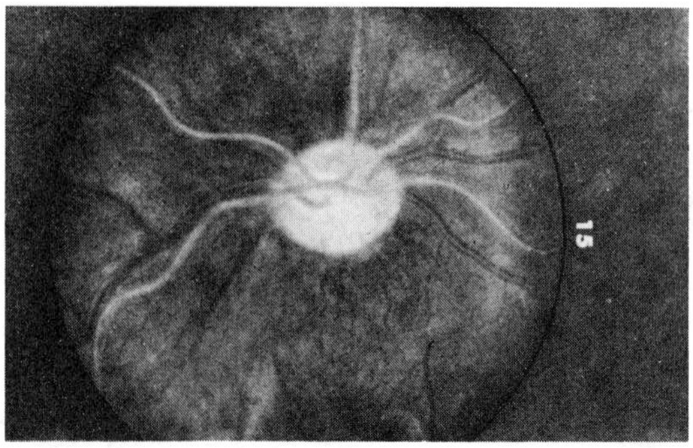

Figure 8-33 Copper-wire arteries. (See also endsheet plate 8.)

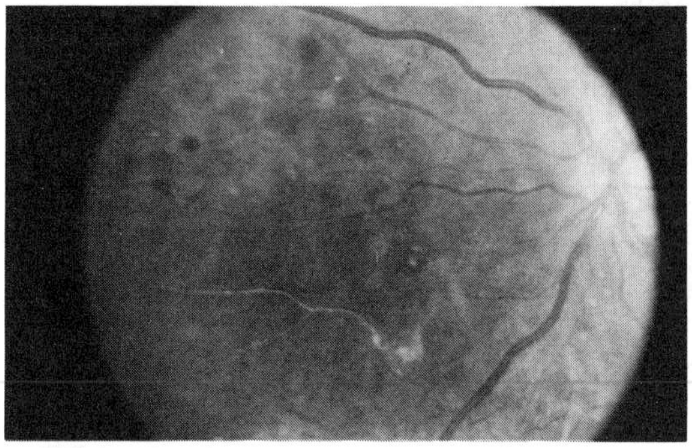

Figure 8-34 Silver-wire arteries. (See also endsheet plate 9.)

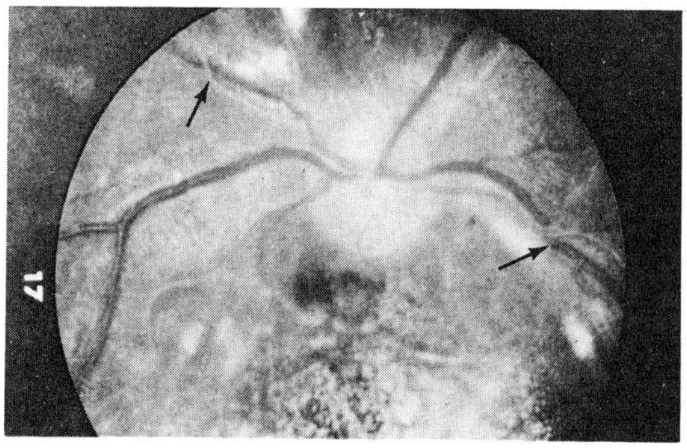

Figure 8-35 AV nicking. (See also endsheet plate 10.)

Optic atrophy results from partial or complete compression (death) of the optic nerve and can cause blindness. It is presented as pallor or a chalky whiteness of the disk. This condition can be caused by severe papilledema, glaucoma, or tumors of the brain. Nerve degeneration occurs in conditions such as multiple sclerosis and in rare cases may be hereditary. Optic atrophy is frequently observed in tabes dorsalis.

Glaucomatous cup (Fig. 8-32) is a diagnostic sign of glaucoma. The cup may be deep and is bluish white, with the vessels disappearing behind the edge of the cup.

The small retinal vessels are most sensitive to disease processes. The walls of the arterioles are transparent when viewed by the ophthalmoscope; you will see a column of blood. In arteriosclerosis, usually occurring with hypertension, the lumens of the vessels are narrowed due to fibrous tissue replacement. The light reflection becomes brighter. In moderate disease, the arteries may be a burnished copper (copper-wire arteries) (Fig. 8-33). Later, in far-advanced arteriosclerosis, they appear as widened white strips (silver-wire arteries) (Fig. 8-34). In addition, the arteries will disappear sooner than the veins, as both project out toward the periphery of the fundus.

When the arteries become thick and stiff, they cause deflection of a vein as they cross it. This condition is referred to as *arteriovenous (AV) notching* or *nicking* (Fig. 8-35). With AV nicking, a portion of the vein on either side of the overlying artery is not visible.

Tortuous and engorged veins are often observed in atherosclerosis, diabetes mellitus, multiple myeloma, polycythemia, and leukemia. Venous distention can occur in congenital heart disease, diabetes mellitus, and leukemia (Fig. 8-36).

Hemorrhages and exudates are always pathognomonic. The shape of the hemorrhage indicates the depth at which it occurs in the retina. Superficial hemorrhages are flame-shaped, and deeper ones are more round and blotchy (Figs. 8-37 and 8-38). Small, rounded hemorrhages are seen in

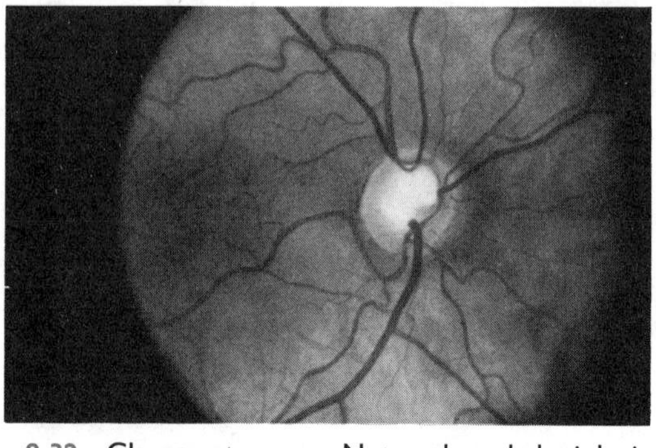

Figure 8-32 Glaucomatous cup. Note enlarged physiologic cup and arching of vessels over disk's edge. (See also endsheet plate 7.)

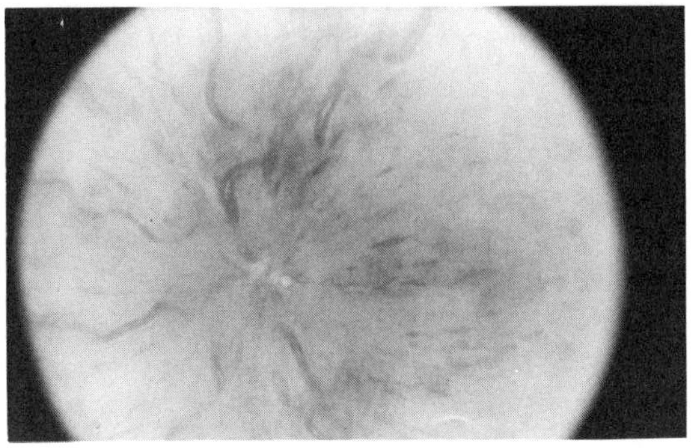

Figure 8-36 Tortuous vein distention. (See also endsheet plate 11.)

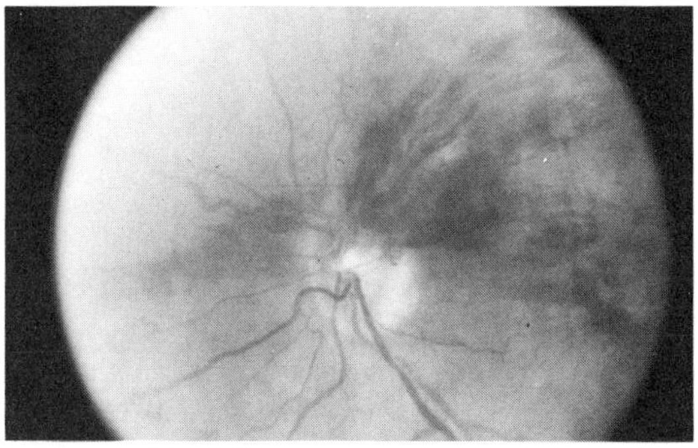

Figure 8-37 Blotchy hemorrhage. (See also endsheet plate 12.)

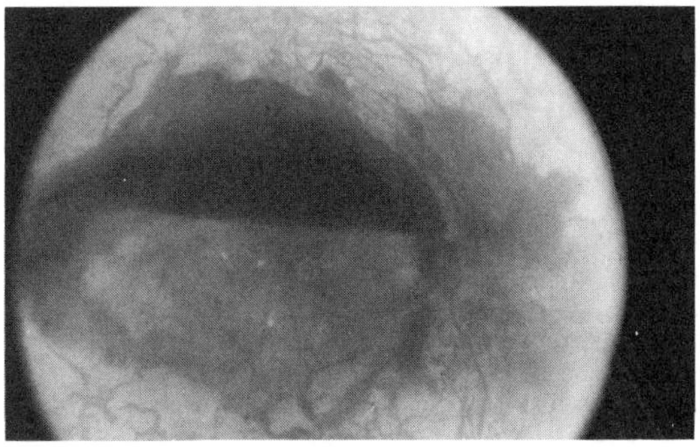

Figure 8-38 Blotchy hemorrhage. (See also endsheet plate 13.)

diabetes mellitus, whereas flame-shaped hemorrhages are seen in hypertension. The presence of microaneurysms, tiny discrete red dots with smooth edges, is often suggestive of venous occlusion or diabetes mellitus, in which they occur chiefly around the macula. They may be difficult to distinguish from small hemorrhages, but it is helpful to know that hemorrhages usually have irregular and slightly blurred edges.

Exudates, which occur in many systemic diseases (e.g., diabetes mellitus and hypertension), are dense, grayish, lo-

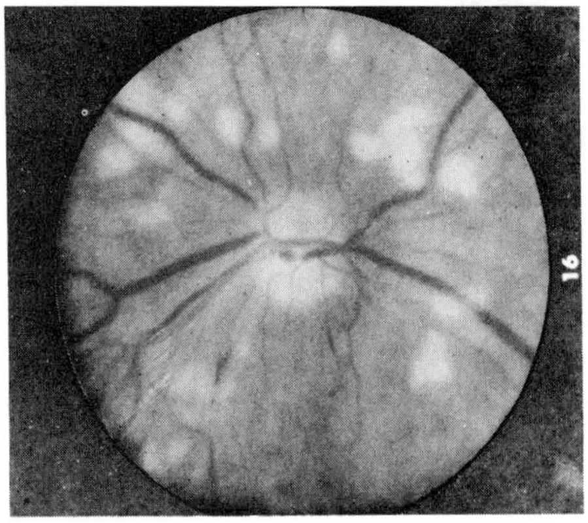

Figure 8-39 Cotton-wool patches (soft exudates). (See also endsheet plate 14.)

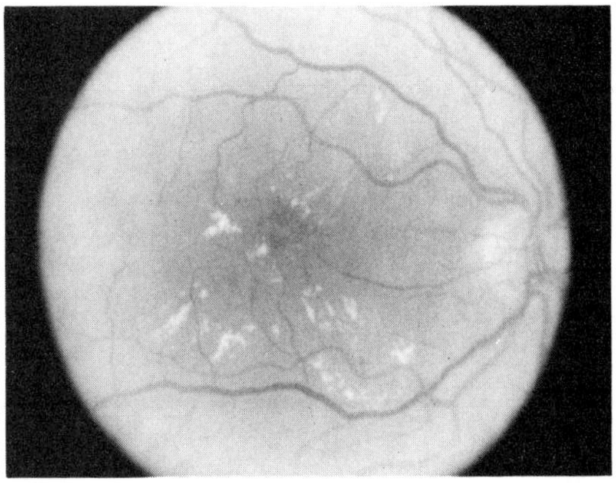

Figure 8-40 Hard exudates. (See also endsheet plate 15.)

calized retinal infiltrates. There are two types: soft and hard.

The soft exudates, often termed *cotton wool patches* (Fig. 8-39), are gray-to-white fluffy, indistinct areas. Soft exudates are arteriolar microinfarctions. They are often accompanied by microaneurysms. Cotton wool patches occur in hypertension, subacute bacterial endocarditis, and lupus erythematosus, and with papilledema, regardless of its cause.

Hard exudates (Fig. 8-40) are numerous, small, whitish yellow spots with distinct edges and smooth solid-appearing surfaces. Hard exudates are thought to be intraretinal lipoid or colloid deposits in old deep hemorrhages.

Drusen, often seen in older clients, are benign degenerative hyaline deposits in the fundus. They are either gray or yellowish spots and are almost always symmetrically located in both eyes. Drusen are distributed in a haphazard formation, whereas hard exudates usually form circular or linear patterns, but, even so, it is difficult to differentiate between them. Drusen are not pathognomonic, nor do they affect vision.

Moderate retinal detachment may appear as an area out

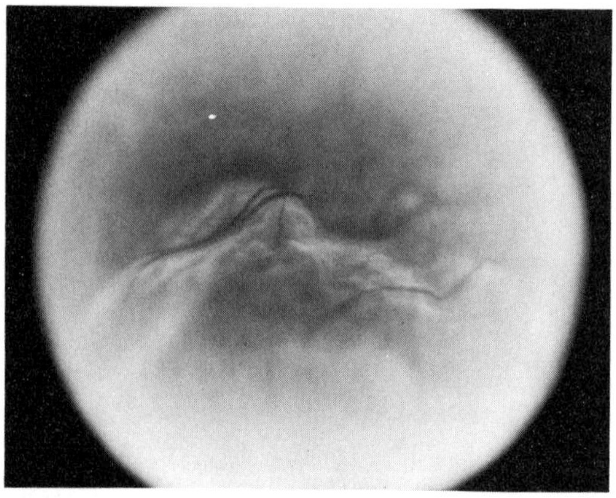

Figure 8-41 Detached retina. (See also endsheet plate 16.)

of focus in comparison with the remainder of the fundus. There may be a dramatic onset of flashers and floaters. As the retina becomes more widely separated, it presents as a wrinkled gray sheet (Fig. 8-41). Retinal detachment is usually idiopathic, although underlying tumors, injuries, or postretinal hemorrhage may be causes.

SUMMARY

This chapter described assessment of the eye. Because the eye is a complex organ, each part of the eye was examined separately in a systematic manner. Inspection and palpation are the initial techniques used and are performed simultaneously. The lacrimal apparatus, eyelids, conjunctiva, and cornea are inspected and palpated. The pupils are assessed for light reaction, size, and accommodation. Special techniques are used to check the extraocular muscles and intraocular pressure. Visual field examination and testing of visual acuity and color vision are part of the assessment. The ophthalmoscopic examination is used to assess landmarks within the eye and reveals many types of health conditions. Examples of abnormal examination findings are correlated with selected disease and injuries.

DISCUSSION QUESTIONS/ ACTIVITIES

1. In the following diagram, identify the components of the eye.

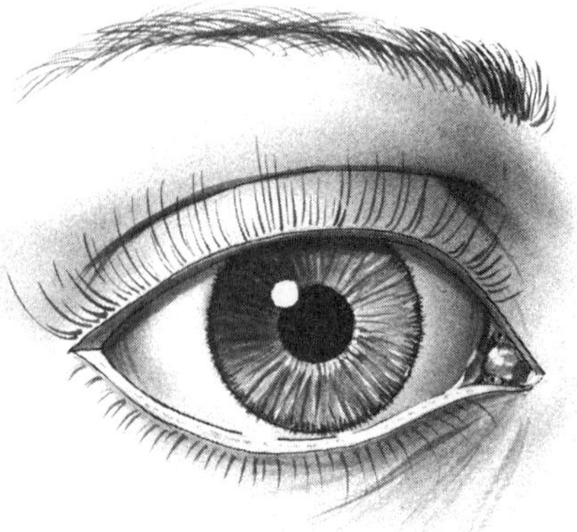

2. Describe the procedure for examining the external eye.
3. Discuss common abnormalities found in the following areas: eyelids, conjunctiva, sclera, cornea, lens.
4. Demonstrate how you would evert the palpebral conjunctiva of the upper eyelids and the lower eyelids.
5. Demonstrate how you would test for direct pupillary reaction and for consensual reaction to light.
6. Demonstrate the technique you would use to test for accommodation and for extraocular muscle movement.
7. Demonstrate the use of the Snellen chart for testing visual acuity.
8. State why color vision is routinely tested, and the significance of color blindness.
9. How would you assess near visual acuity if you did not have a hand-held vision card?
10. Demonstrate the technique used to assess peripheral vision.
11. Demonstrate the technique for using the ophthalmoscope.
12. Describe how you would locate the following: red reflex, optic disk, macula.
13. Discuss what is meant by the following terms: AV nicking, cotton wool patches, exudates, flame-shaped hemorrhage, glaucomatous cup.
14. What means would you use to test the vision of a preschool child?

CHAPTER

9 Assessment of the Ear, Nose, Mouth, and Pharynx

Learning Objectives

1. Review the structure and function of the ear, nose, mouth, and pharynx.
2. List the characteristics of the ear, nose, mouth, and pharynx that are noted during inspection.
3. Describe the technique of using the otoscope in the examination of the auditory canal and tympanic membrane.
4. Explain the Weber and Rinne tests and the normal finding of each.
5. Discuss the techniques of palpation and transillumination in assessing the maxillary and frontal sinuses.
6. Recognize the normal findings regarding the ear, nose, lips, gums, buccal mucosa, teeth, tongue, palate, and oropharynx.

This chapter describes assessment of the ears, nose and mouth, and pharynx. The structure and function of each anatomic area is discussed, followed by an explanation of the special techniques needed in assessing the area. The otoscope is used to facilitate examination of these structures.

STRUCTURE AND FUNCTION OF THE EAR

The ear consists of three parts: the external ear, the middle ear, and the inner ear (Fig. 9-1). The external ear has two parts: the flap on the side of the head called the *auricle*, or *pinna*, and the *external auditory canal*, a tube leading from the auditory meatus (opening) to the temporal bone. The auditory canal in children is horizontal, but in adults it is angulated inward, forward, and then downward (Fig. 9-2). Its length is about 3 cm. The external ear is separated from the middle ear by the *tympanic membrane* (eardrum).

The middle ear contains three auditory ossicles (bones): the *malleus* (hammer), the *incus* (anvil), and the *stapes* (stirrup). There are four openings into the middle ear: one from the external canal—the opening covered by the *tympanic membrane* (eardrum), in which the handle of the malleus is embedded; two from the internal ear—the *oval window*, into which the stapes fits, and the *round window*, which has a membrane covering; and one from there—the opening that extends from the middle ear to the nasopharynx. The *eustachian tube* is important in the equalization of pressure between the inner and outer surfaces of the tympanic membrane.

The normal eardrum is pearly gray. There are three landmarks on the drum (Fig. 9-3): (1) the annulus, which forms

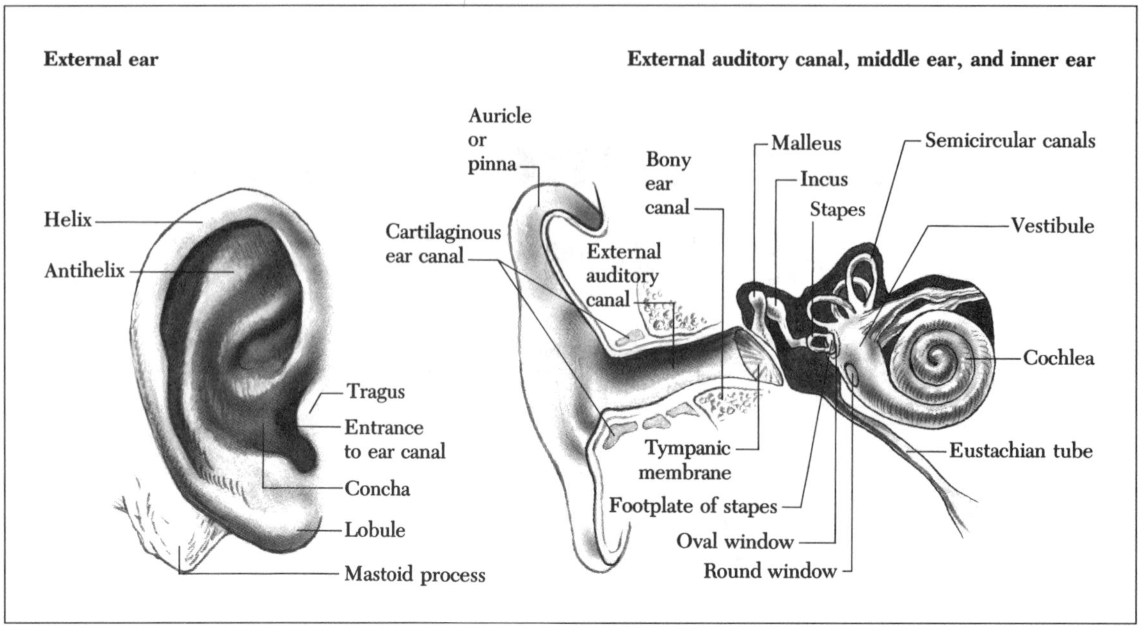

Figure 9-1 Diagram of the ear.

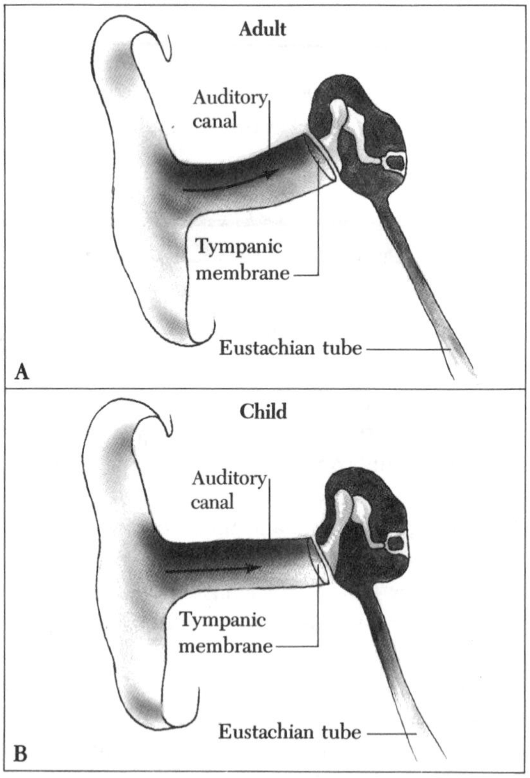

Figure 9-2 Differences in the auditory canals of **(A)** an adult and **(B)** a child.

the outer border of the drum and is a paler color than the remainder of the membrane; (2) the malleus, which angles downward posteriorly from the annulus to a point at the center of the tympanic membrane, and (3) the light reflex, which is a bright cone-shaped reflection of light in the lower

The Physiology of Hearing

For hearing to occur, the auditory area of the cerebral cortex must be stimulated. The process of hearing begins when sound waves are picked up by the pinna and are channeled into the auditory canal, where they strike the tympanic membrane, setting up vibrations. When the membrane vibrates, the malleus vibrates, establishing a chain reaction in the incus and stapes, with the latter vibrating against the oval window. It is at this point that the sound waves begin to move through conduction of fluid. The transmission of the impulses continues through the cochlear duct, the organ of Corti, and the cochlear nerve (a division of the 8th cranial nerve) to the brain stem; through the medulla, pons, midbrain, and thalamus; and finally to the auditory area of the temporal lobe.

anterior aspect of the tympanic membrane. It is located at the 5 o'clock position in the right ear and at the 7 o'clock position in the left ear.

The inner ear consists of a bony labyrinth with a membranous labyrinth inside. The bony labyrinth contains the *vestibule*, the *cochlea*, and the *semicircular canals*. The membranous labyrinth consists of the *utricle* and *saccule*, two sacs that are inside the vestibule and that line the cochlear duct (of the cochlea) and the endolymphatic duct (of the semicircular canals). Within the walls of the utricle and saccule are *macula utriculi* and *macula sacculi*, respectively; these are sensory epithelia whose functions are to conduct impulses to the brain that allow for a sense of position of

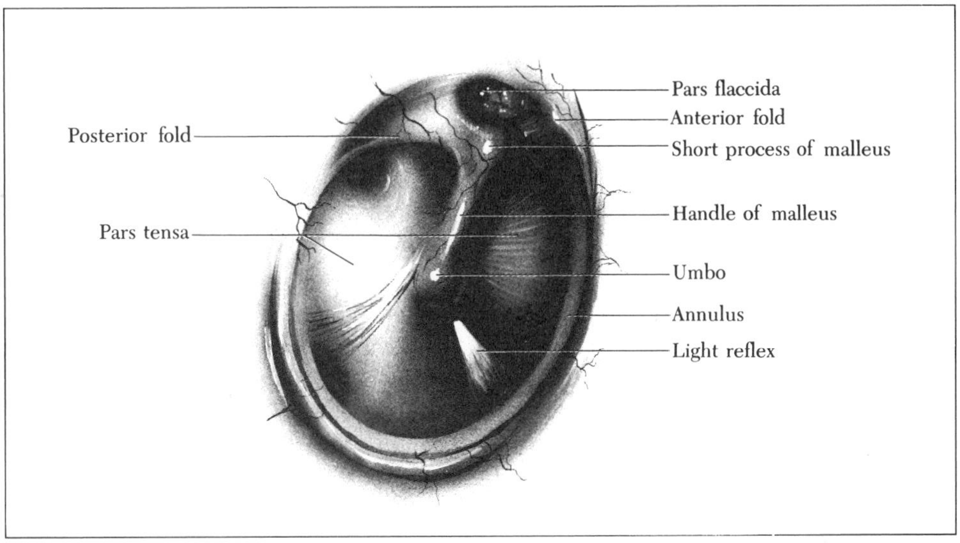

Figure 9-3 Diagram of the right eardrum.

the head. Within the cochlea is the hearing sense organ, the *organ of Corti.* It is from here that impulses are conducted to the brain, producing the sensation of hearing. These semicircular canals contain receptors that function as organs for the sense of equilibrium.

By examining the ear, you are able to view only the external portion, the auditory canal, and the tympanic membrane. Conditions involving the middle ear cannot be visualized but may be reflected by the tympanic membrane.

CHARACTERISTICS AND TECHNIQUES OF EXAMINATION

Inspection and Palpation

- Note the size, shape, and position of the ears on the head.
- Check that the helix is in line with the eyebrows.
- Inspect the pinna, and palpate it for lesions or nodules.
- Check that the cartilage of the ear is stiff but not rigid.
- Press on the tragus to check for tenderness.
- Palpate the antrum of the mastoid bone for tenderness.
- Examine the canal and the tympanic membrane with the otoscope.
- Choose the largest speculum that will fit the canal comfortably.
- Position the client's head so it is tipped sideways toward the opposite shoulder to facilitate examination (Fig. 9-4).
- Hold the otoscope with the handle pointing up; this way your hand can be held closely against the client's head, and the otoscope will move with the client's head movement, and trauma to the canal or eardrum is avoided.
- To steady the head of the child during otoscopic examination, position the child's head sideways on the examining table (Fig. 9-5).

Technique for Inspection and Palpation of the Ear

1. Note position and size.
2. Palpate for lesions or nodules.
3. Palpate tragus and antrum of mastoid bone for tenderness.
4. If necessary, gently remove cerumen.
5. Choose speculum of appropriate size.
6. Tip client's head sideways (toward opposite side being examined).
7. Child's head lying sideways on table.
8. Ask client to hold very still.
9. Grasp auricle of ear being examined between thumb and forefinger.
10. Adult—pull auricle upward, back, and slightly outward.
11. Child—pull auricle back and outward.
12. Gently insert speculum (follow progress with eye).
13. Examine external canal.
14. Examine tympanic membrane.
15. Test for hearing loss:
    Rinne test—strike tuning fork and place handle to mastoid process; when vibration stops, hold tuning fork before pinna (repeat for other ear).
    Weber test—strike tuning fork and place in center of forehead or middle top anterior skull.
    Gross tests: whispered voice, watch tick

- Instruct the client to hold his head very still.
- Grasp the auricle between your left thumb and forefinger.
- Because the adult ear canal angulates, pull upward ("up" for "grownups") and backward and slightly outward on

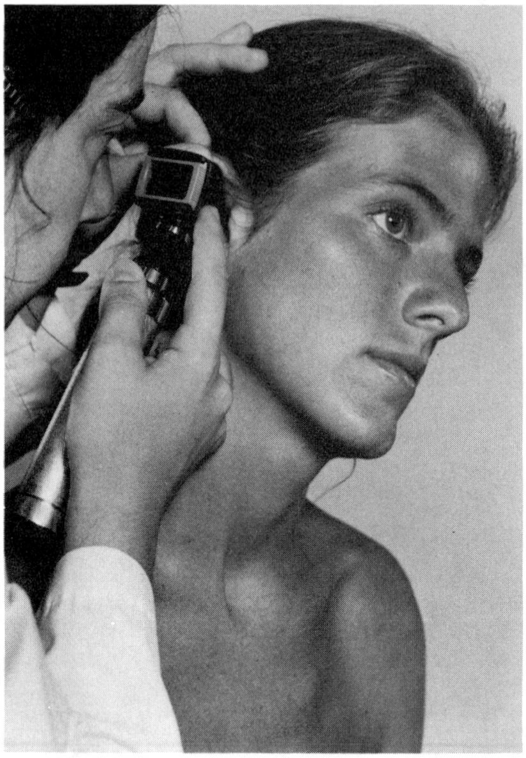

Figure 9-4 Examination of the auditory canal and tympanic membrane.

the auricle to view the tympanic membrane. For children, pull backward and outward.

- Gently insert the speculum into the canal with your right hand.
- Never insert the speculum into the auditory canal without following its progress with your eye.
- Gentleness is important, because halfway to the tympanic membrane, pressure from the speculum can be quite painful.
- Examine the external canal for erythema, swelling, patency, amount of cerumen, discharge of any type, and foreign bodies.
- Inspect the tympanic membrane for color, bulging, retraction, lesions, and perforations.
- To test the mobility of the drum, instruct the client to pinch his nose closed and blow against closed lips. A normal drum will bulge outward. Do *not* perform this test with clients who have an obvious ear disease.

To visualize the canal, you may have to remove excessive cerumen (earwax) that may be blocking your view (Fig. 9-6). This can be accomplished with gentle and careful use of a cotton-tipped applicator or with irrigation using warm water, mineral oil, or a commercial preparation (e.g., Ceruminex) designed specifically for this purpose. Cerumen may be dry and flaky or range from moist honey-colored to very dark brown. The majority of people have moist cerumen with color that varies in the range relative to the individual's skin pigmentation.

Hearing Acuity

Hearing loss can be determined by testing with a tuning fork (Fig. 9-7). The Rinne test detects conduction deafness. The Weber test detects conduction deafness or sensorineural deafness.

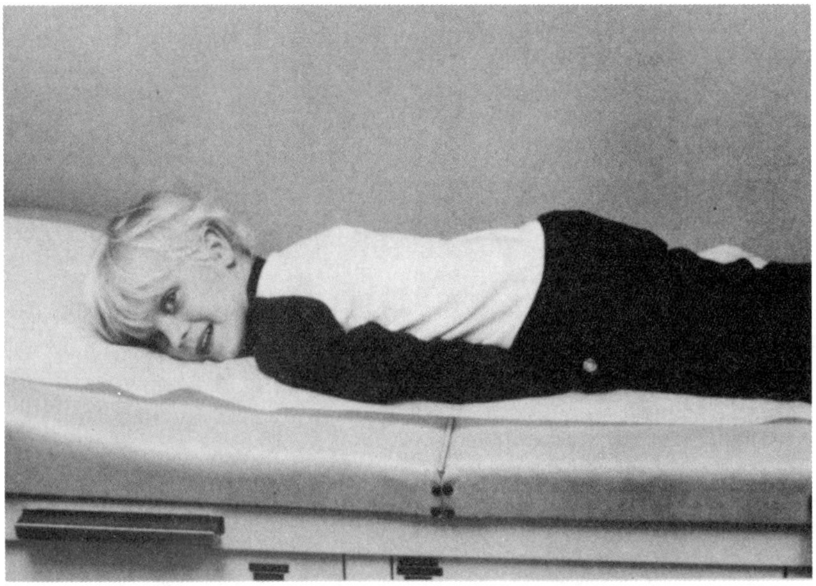

Figure 9-5 Positioning of a child for otoscopic examination. (From Sana, J.M. and Judge, R.D. *Physical Assessment for Nursing Skills* (2nd ed.). Boston: Little, Brown, 1982, p. 449.)

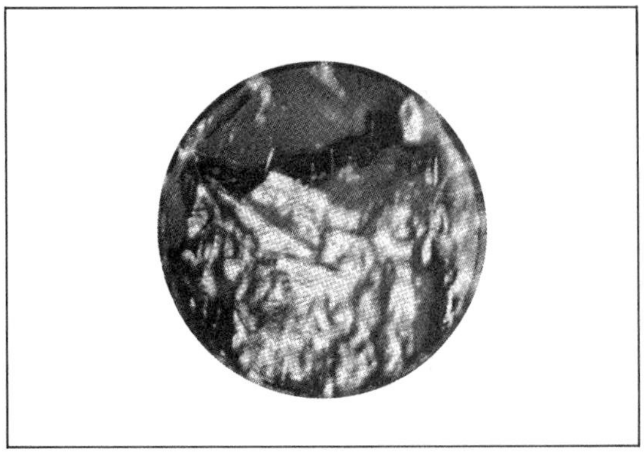

Figure 9-6 Otoscopic view revealing excessive cerumen.

To perform the Rinne test, use a no. 512 (preferably) up to a no. 1024 fork.

- Strike the tuning fork, and place the handle to the mastoid process (Fig. 9-8A).
- Ask the client to indicate when she can no longer hear the sound.
- When this point is reached, immediately place the vibrating head of the tuning fork near to the external ear (Fig. 9-8B).
- Ask the client if she can hear it at this location.

Normally, sound transmitted through air is heard better than sound transmitted through bone, so the client should continue to hear the sound. If so, the test is referred to as being positive.

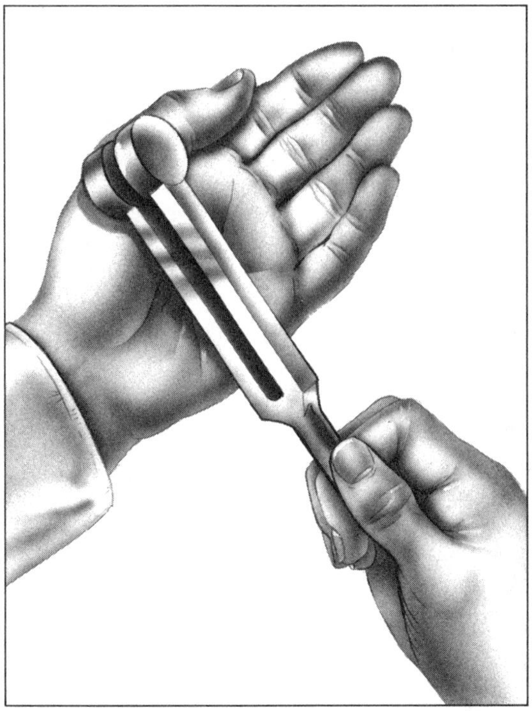

Figure 9-7 Technique for using a tuning fork in the Rinne test. The ends of the tuning fork are pinched and the fork is tapped against the heel of the hand.

Recording of a positive Rinne test usually takes the following form: *AC* > *BC* (air conduction is greater than bone conduction). If the Rinne test is negative (the sound cannot be heard when the fork is brought before the ear), bone

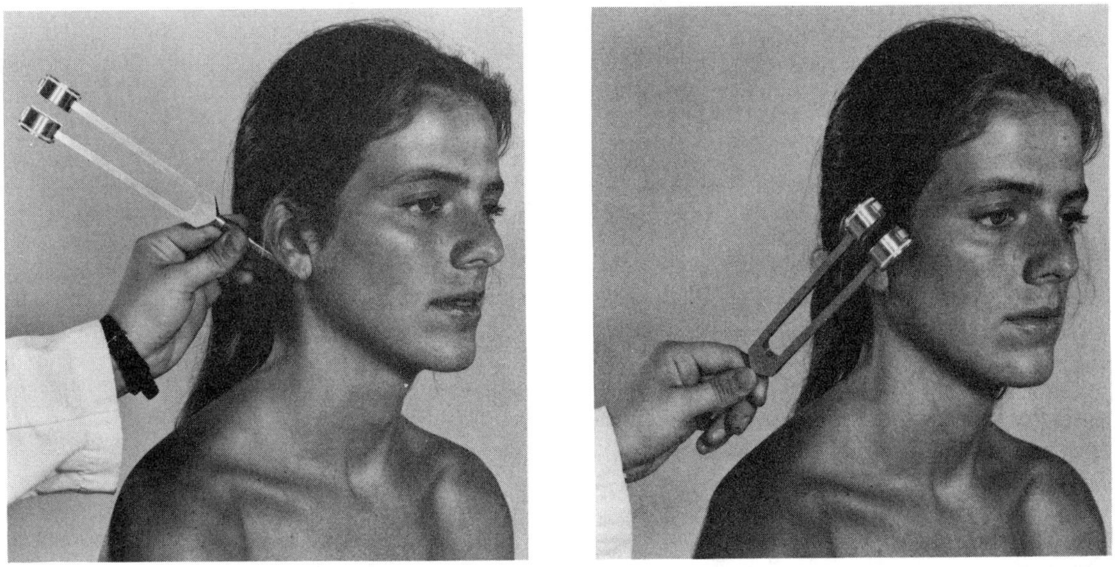

A B

Figure 9-8 The Rinne test. **(A)** The tuning fork is placed on the mastoid process and the client is asked to indicate when she can no longer hear the sound. **(B)** The tuning fork is placed next to the external ear as soon as the client says she cannot hear the bone-conducted sound.

conduction is greater than air conduction; this means that a conduction defect exists.

To perform the Weber test, use a no. 512 (preferably) up to a no. 1024 fork.

- Strike the tuning fork, and place it in the center of the client's forehead or in the middle top anterior portion of the skull (Fig. 9-9).
- Ask the client where she hears the sound, that is, whether she hears the sound better in one ear or the other. The normal client will hear the sound equally in both ears or may state that she hears the sound "all over" her head.

With pathology, the client will readily answer that she hears the sound better in one ear than in the other. Thus, any need for concentrated thought or hemming and hawing by the client denotes the absence of pathology. Recording of a normal testing is, "Weber test—no lateralization."

Two gross tests of hearing are the whispered or spoken-voice test, the finger-rubbing test, and the watch-tick test.

- With the whisper test, approach the client from the side or from behind so that she cannot read your lips.
- Direct your whispered voice toward the ear being tested.
- To prevent the client's other ear from picking up the sound, muffle the sound for the other ear by lightly rubbing the palm of your hand over it or placing a finger in the external auditory canal and gently wiggling it during the testing.
- As with the testing of the eyes, the testing of the ears should be done one ear at a time.
- The client with normal hearing acuity should be able to hear your whispered voice in a quiet room at a distance of 2 feet from the ear.

If the client cannot hear the whispered voice, then repeat by using the spoken voice, then a loud voice. Document accordingly which voice volume the client was able to hear.

The finger-rubbing—rubbing your thumb and middle finger together much like the motion of snapping your fingers—normally can be heard 12 inches away from the ear. Additionally, the watch-tick test is simply an evaluation of the client's ability to hear a watch ticking as it is moved away from her ear. Because this method tests only high-frequency sounds, it is a poor test to use exclusively.

In young children, you can carefully observe responses to loud noises, whispers, and watch ticking and note their ability to make verbal sounds. Cooperation with the Rinne and Weber testing can be elicited from children as young as 2 years old. Younger infants can be tested with an automated sensor called the cribogram, which can test several newborns at once. It records the physical movements before, during, and after a sound is presented through a nearby microphone. Hearing loss is detected through analysis of the recordings.

If you discover evidence of hearing loss as a result of the gross tests or tuning fork tests, you should refer the client to an audiologist for further quantitative measurements. Because audiologists do not have a medical background, the

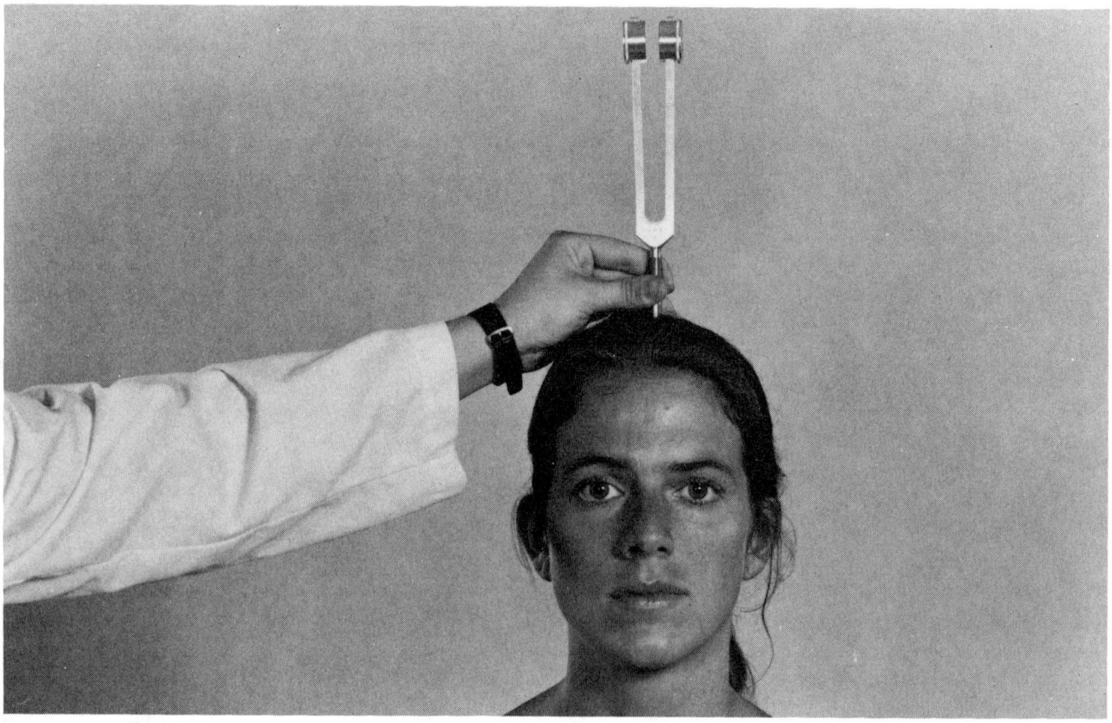

Figure 9-9 The Weber test.

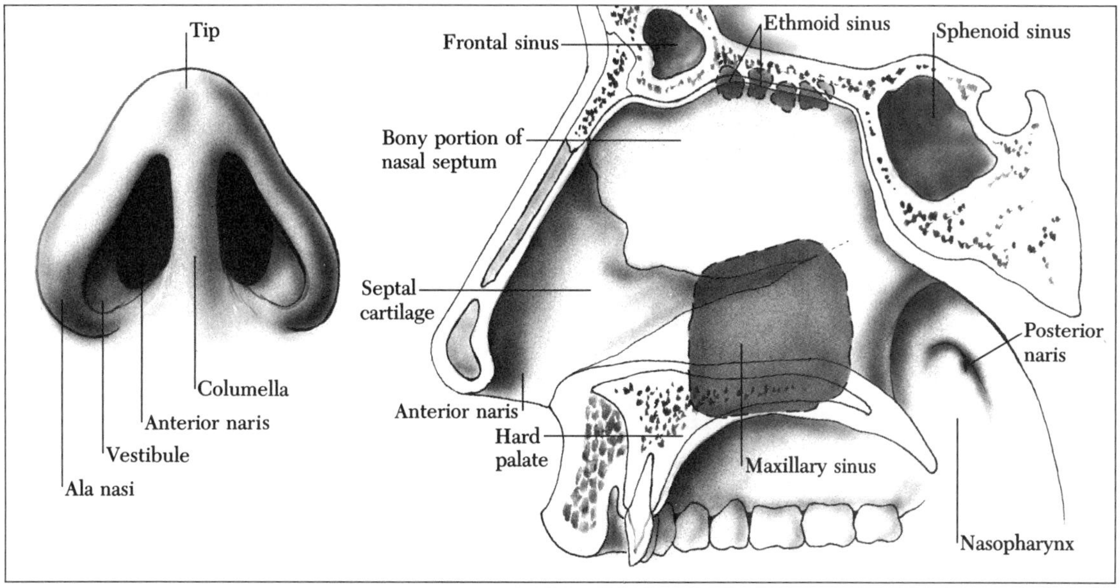

Figure 9-10 Cross-section of the nose.

client should be referred to a physician if diagnosis and treatment of ear disease are required. If a specialist seems warranted, refer the client to an otologist (a physician with advanced education in this field).

STRUCTURE AND FUNCTION OF THE NOSE

Figure 9-10 illustrates two nasal chambers, called *nares.* They open externally through the nostril (*anterior nares*) and posteriorly through the *nasopharynx* (via the *posterior nares*). The nasal chambers are lined with respiratory mucosa except anteriorly, where there is epithelium (skin) containing sebaceous glands and multiple coarse nasal hairs. These hairs are very important in the filtering of the entering air. The two nasal chambers are separated by the *nasal septum,* which is composed of cartilage and bone. The olfactory hair cells, the receptors for the sense of smell, are located in the superior portion, which is lined with neuroepithelium. This highly vascular membrane is continuous with the external skin and the internal mucous membrane lining the sinuses.

Figure 9-11 shows the superior posterior portion of the nose, which contains the *inferior, middle,* and *superior turbinates.* These bones increase the mucous membrane surface of the nasal passages and slightly obstruct the current of air flowing through them. The mucous membranes also serve to moisten and warm the inhaled air. The cleft between these bones is referred to as a *meatus.* Each meatus is named after the adjacent turbinate.

The paranasal sinuses (see Fig. 9-10) are air-filled cavities within the bones of the skull; they are lined with mucous membrane. Only the frontal and maxillary sinuses can be easily examined. The *maxillary sinuses* are located on either side of the nose in the maxillary bones. The *frontal sinuses* are located in the lower forehead between and above the eyes. The *ethmoid sinus* is between the eyes over the roof of the nose. The *sphenoid sinus* is posterior to the ethmoid and maxillary sinuses. One of the functions of the sinuses is to give timbre and resonance to the voice.

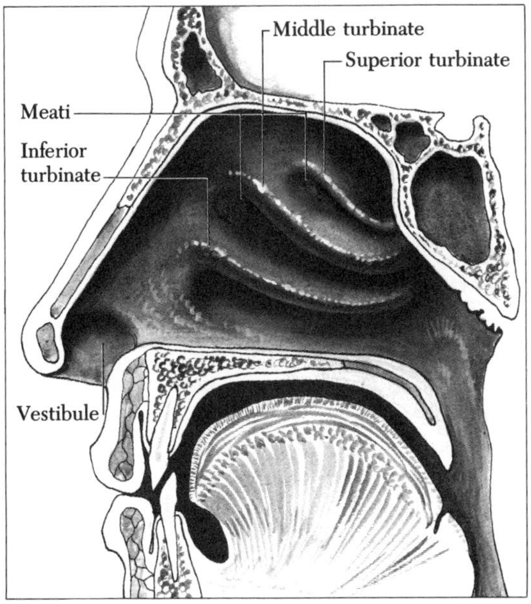

Figure 9-11 Cross-section of the nose showing turbinates and meati.

Technique of Inspection and Palpation of the Nose

1. Carry out a visual inspection.
2. Lightly palpate if indicated.
3. Put large, short speculum on otoscope.
4. Lift tip of nose and insert speculum in nares (repeat with other nares).
5. Inspect mucous membrane for:
   Color
   Discharge
6. Inspect septum.
7. Look for large inferior turbinate and middle turbinate.
8. Palpate and percuss sinuses:
   Frontal
   Maxillary
9. Transilluminate
   Maxillary sinuses—place bright lighted attachment on handle of otoscope into mouth and have client close mouth or place very bright penlight externally over maxillary sinuses while viewing buccal mucosa for transillumination.
   Frontal sinuses—press very bright light under superior orbital ridge.

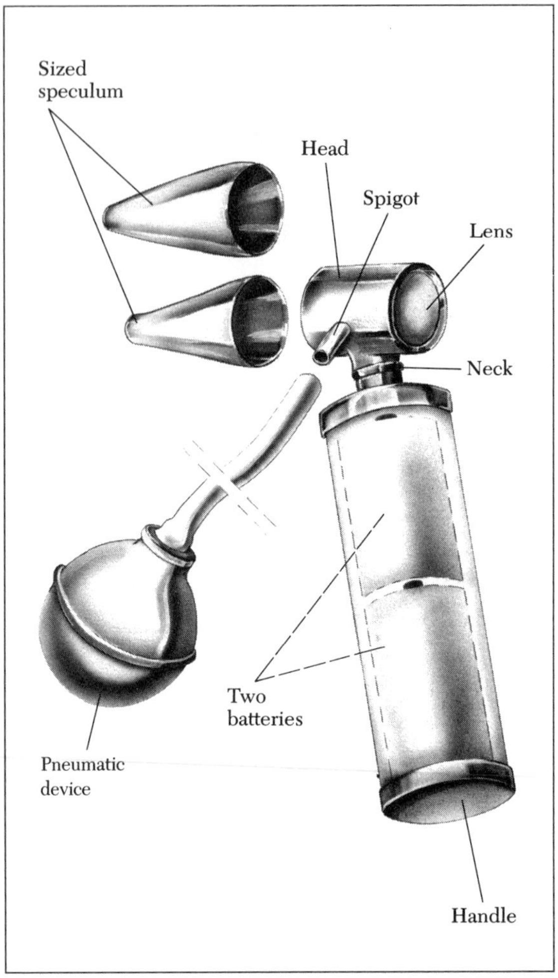

Figure 9-12 The large speculum of an otoscope can be used as a nasal speculum.

CHARACTERISTICS AND TECHNIQUES OF EXAMINATION

Inspection

Simple inspection of the external nose is usually adequate unless injury has occurred. In that case, light palpation will elicit the location of pain and tenderness. The nose is examined by using a penlight or an illuminated nasal speculum (Fig. 9-12). The large, short speculum on the otoscope can be used.

- Visualization is facilitated by lifting up the tip of the client's nose with your thumb before inspecting with your penlight or introducing the speculum and holding it in this position during the examination (Fig. 9-13).
- If a speculum is used, avoid touching or injuring the septum.
- Inspect the mucous membrane for changes from its normal red color.
- Note the presence and character of any discharge.
- In most adults, the septum is not completely straight; it usually deviates toward one of the passages.
- Inspect the septum for perforations.
- In the superior posterior area, look for the large inferior turbinate, which is ordinarily easy to see.
- The middle turbinate can be viewed most of the time unless there is swelling of the mucosa, a condition common in certain climates.
- Never attempt to push the speculum past a swollen turbinate.
- The posterior turbinate is rarely seen because of its position.
- If obstruction is suspected, hold a naris closed by pressing the tip of your index finger on the side of the nose and having the client inhale deeply (once) through his nose. Repeat this procedure on the opposite side.

Palpation

- Palpate or lightly percuss the maxillary and frontal sinuses (Fig. 9-14A) with the fingertips, as demonstrated in Fig. 9-14B.
- The sinuses are normally nontender; pain usually indicates sinusitis.
- The ethmoid sinus can be examined only by intranasal inspection.

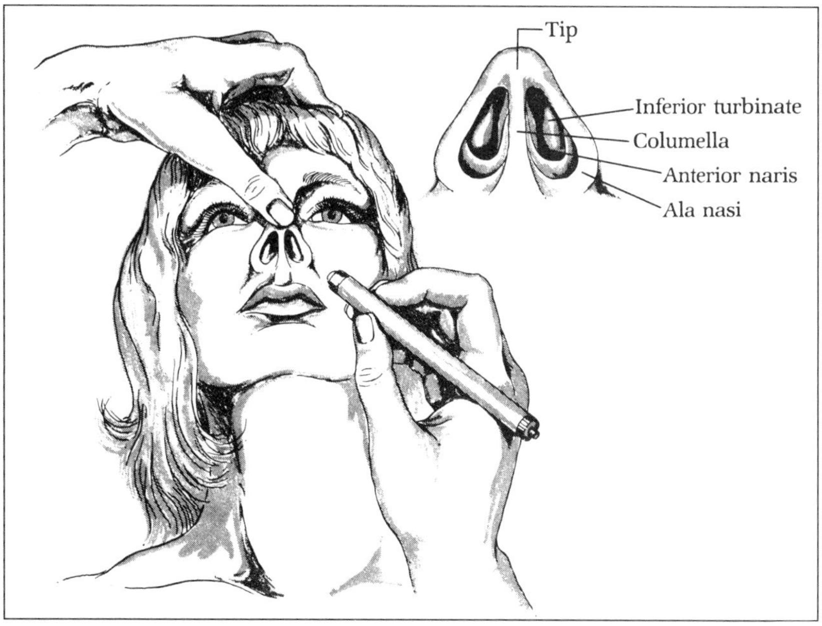

Figure 9-13 Technique for penlight examination of nasal septum and mucosa. (From Sana, J.M. and Judge, R.D. *Physical Assessment for Nursing Skills* (2nd ed.). Boston: Little, Brown, 1982, p. 188.)

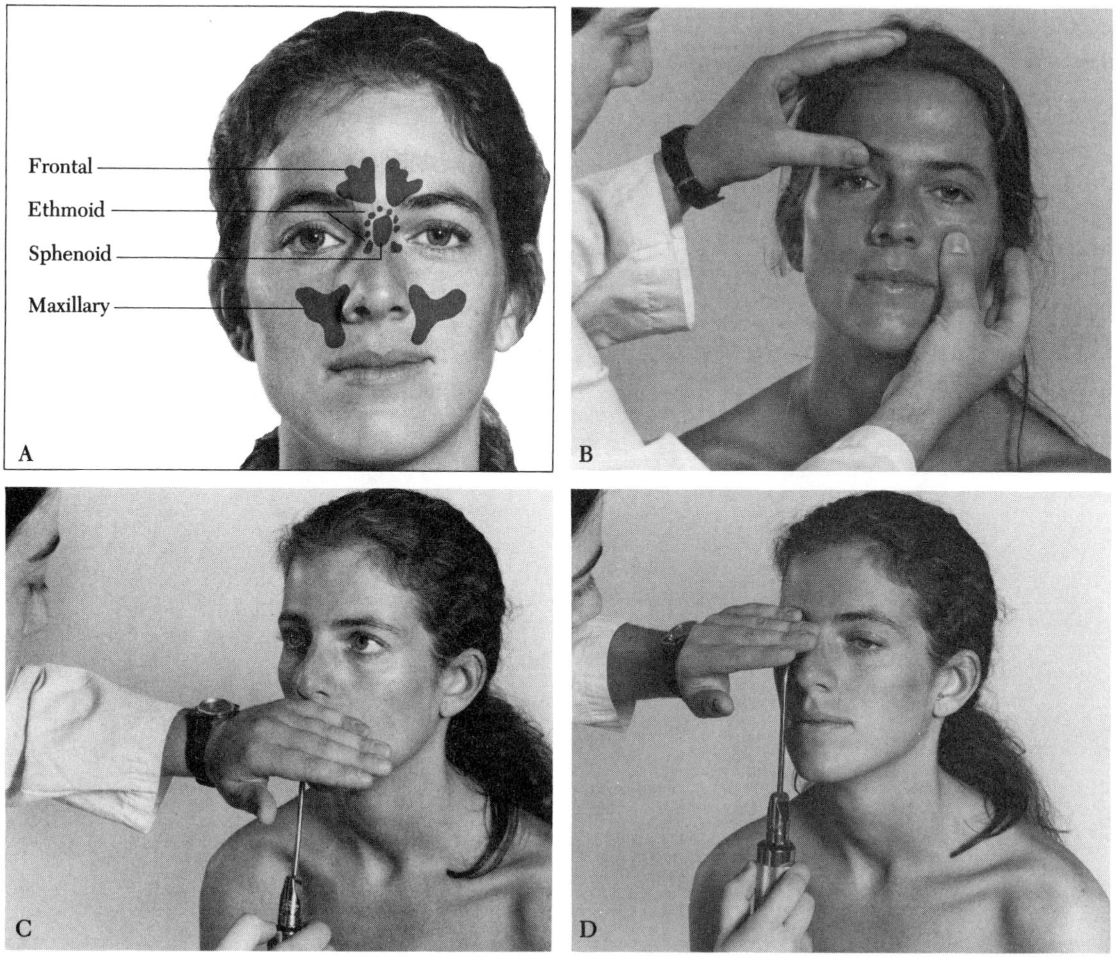

Figure 9-14 Palpation and transillumination of the sinuses. **(A)** Sites of sinuses. **(B)** Palpation is done with the left thumb on the right frontal sinus and the right thumb on the left maxillary sinus. **(C)** Transillumination of the maxillary sinuses. **(D)** Transillumination of the frontal sinus.

Transillumination

Transillumination of the sinuses generally is performed if the client has tenderness or other signs of sinusitis. Figure 9-14C illustrates transillumination of the maxillary sinuses.

- Place a very bright light into the client's mouth and have her close her lips.
- Normally, the air-containing sinuses light up symmetrically.
- If one or the other contains fluid, it will be darker than the other. Figure 9-14D shows how to transilluminate the frontal sinuses by pressing the lighted attachment on the otoscope handle under the superior orbital ridge.

Technique for Examination of Mouth and Pharynx

1. Inspect lips.
2. Use bright light, gloves, and tongue blade to examine
   Gums
   Mucous membrane
   Teeth
   Tongue:
   color size
   texture symmetry
   deviation lesions
   Palate and uvular reflex
   Oropharynx
   Tonsils—insert tongue blade deeply to each side. (Try not to elicit gag reflex, unless a problem is suspected.)
3. Palpate the oral structures wearing a glove.

STRUCTURE AND FUNCTION OF THE MOUTH AND PHARYNX

Figure 9-15 depicts the buccal cavity, which is made up of the cheeks, the tongue and its muscles, the hard and soft palates, and the teeth. Its entire surface is lined with mucous membrane. The floor of the mouth consists of the tongue and underlying muscles. The rough elevations on the tongue are called *papillae.* Beneath the tongue is a tissue fold, the *frenulum,* that connects the tongue to the floor of the mouth. On either side of the frenulum, presenting as small elevated dark dots, are the *submandibular duct.* The ducts of the *parotid glands* open into the *buccal mucosa* at a point opposite the upper second molar. The *hard palate,* anteriorly, is composed of bone; the *soft palate,* posteriorly, is composed of muscle in the shape

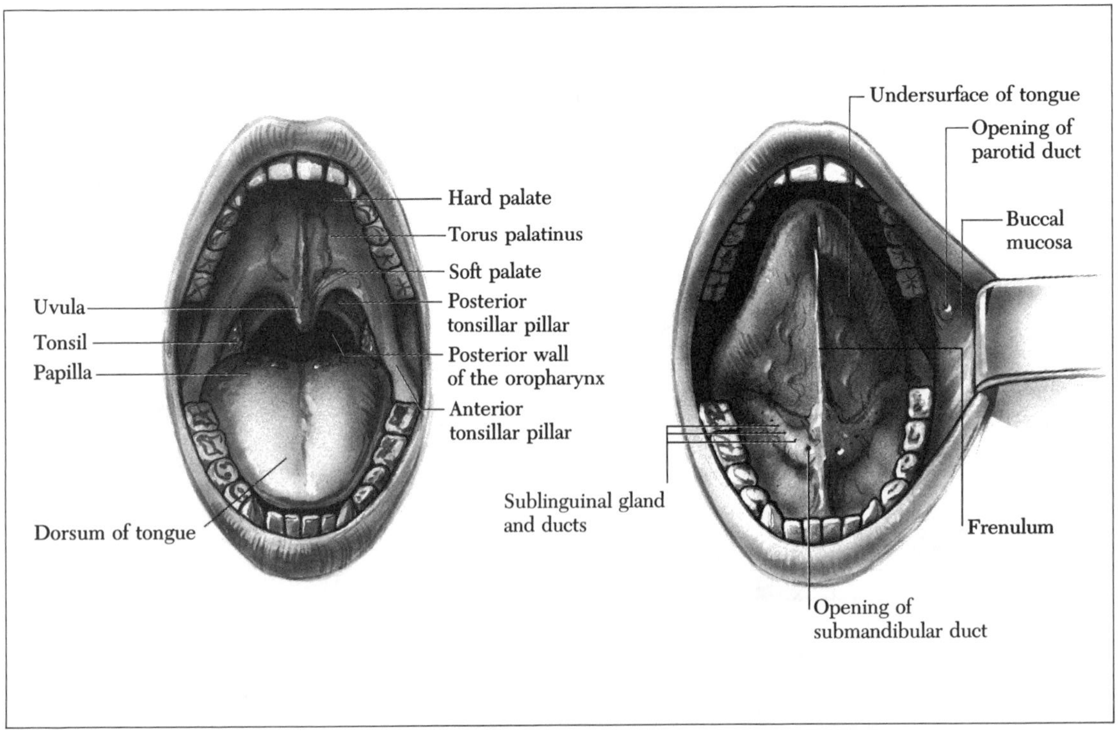

Figure 9-15 The buccal cavity.

Table 9-1 Approximate Age of Tooth Eruption

Deciduous teeth		Permanent teeth	
Name	Erupt (age in months)	Name	Erupt (age in years)
Lower central incisors	5–9	First molars	6–7
Upper central incisors	8–12	Central incisors	7–8
Upper lateral incisors	10–12	Lateral incisors	7–8
Lower lateral incisors	12–15	First premolars	9–10
Anterior (first) molars	12–15	Second premolars	9–10
Canines	18–24	Canines	12–14
Posterior (second) molars	24–30	Second molars	12–15
		Third molars	17–25

Source: From Thomas, C.L. (ed.): *Taber's Cyclopedic Medical Dictionary*, ed. 17, F.A. Davis, Philadelphia, 1993.

of an arch on either side. These arches are known as the *palatine arches.* The inferior portion of the arch is called the *anterior tonsillar pillar.* The arches lead to the oropharynx, at which point they become the *fauces,* which is where the tonsils are located. Posterior to the arch is the *posterior tonsillar pillar.* The *uvula* projects downward from the middle of the soft palate.

Children may be born with teeth or may not have any tooth eruption until about 16 months of age. The average child at 1 year of age generally has six teeth; at 18 months, 12 teeth; at 2 years, 16 teeth; and at 2½ years, 20 teeth. The first set of teeth (deciduous teeth) are temporary; they are shed and replaced by a second set of permanent teeth. The approximate ages for specific tooth eruption are presented in Table 9-1. The 32 permanent teeth, 16 in each jaw, are identified in Fig. 9-16.

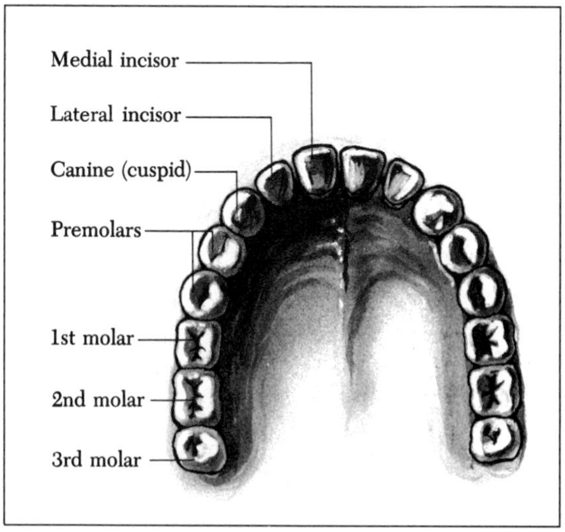

Figure 9-16 The permanent teeth.

The throat, or pharynx, is lined with mucous membrane and extends from the base of the skull to the esophagus. It has three divisions: (1) the *nasopharynx,* located behind the nose; (2) the *oropharynx,* posterior to the mouth; and (3) the *laryngopharynx,* which is posterior to the larynx. The adenoids are located on the roof of the nasopharynx, and the tonsils are on either side of the oropharynx. These organs are responsible for guarding the body against organisms entering the mouth and throat.

CHARACTERISTICS AND TECHNIQUES OF EXAMINATION

Lips

Examination of the mouth and pharynx begins with inspection of the lips.

- Note the color of the lips.
- Inspect for any signs of inflammation or the presence of any lesions, such as pustules, ulcers, fissures, or desquamation.
- Herpes simplex, commonly known as "cold sores" or "fever blisters," is seen in a majority of the population. The lesions can occur on both the lips and the face; they appear as clear vesicles.
- Observe for symmetry of the lips. Small degrees of asymmetry are difficult to see.
- Asymmetry may be accentuated by asking the client to smile or by having him clench his teeth with his lips open.

After examining the lips, proceed to the remainder of the mouth and pharynx, keeping in mind that the mouth is full of bacteria. Use a tongue blade and bright light, as well as gloves if inflammation is present. The tongue blade is used to retract the lips, cheeks, and tongue for proper visualization of all structures.

Gums

- Inspect the gums. In the healthy individual, they are pink and firm.
- Note the amount of salivation. There is very little in infants under 3 months of age but is observed during the teething process in children.
- Take note of the effect of drugs on salivation (e.g., the "dry" mouth of atropine).

Mucous Membrane

- Examine the mucous membrane lining the mouth. The membrane lining the cheeks is normally pink and clear of lesions.
- Fordyce's spots are small yellow spots that may be seen on the buccal mucosa opposite the molars. They are asymptomatic enlarged ectopic sebaceous glands in the mucosa and are present in most people.

Teeth

The condition of the teeth is a good indicator of the general health of the client.

- Inspect the teeth for caries and type of occlusion, and compare the number with the number that is average for the client's age.
- Yellow-brown teeth may be seen in infants and in women in the last trimester of pregnancy who have been given tetracycline. (This discoloration may persist for several years following cessation of the drug.)

Tongue

Thorough examination of the tongue requires palpation as well as inspection, because some diseases of the tongue have no surface manifestations and need to be felt to be detected.

- Inspect the tongue for color, texture, deviation, size, symmetry, fasciculations, and lesions.
- The tongue normally has a whitish coating through which the papillae show.
- The client should be able to move her tongue from side to side.
- When the client is instructed to stick out her tongue as far as possible, it should protrude in the midline.
- Ask the client to raise the tip of her tongue toward the roof of her mouth. Inspect the floor and the frenulum. The frenulum is normally loose and pliable.
- Palpate the sublingual glands. These glands are normally firm and uniform.

In adults, inability to extend the tongue may be the result of a neoplasm; in children, it may be due to a shortened frenulum. In the latter condition, speech defects may be noted, particularly in the pronunciation of the letters *d, t, th, n,* and *l.* Correction of this condition, commonly known as being "tongue-tied," consists of a small incisional loosening of the frenulum; this minor surgery is usually performed in the emergency room.

Palate

Congenital cleft palate is readily observable in the neonate. It is not unusual to see a bony protuberance in the midline of the palate in many of the adults you will examine; this projection is termed a *torus palatinus.*

- Tilt the client's head slightly back in order to see the palate.
- The soft palate is normally pink and has fine vessels under the mucosa.
- The hard palate is whiter, more irregular, and has rugae running transversely.
- The hard palate is also a good area in which to detect jaundice.
- Note whether there is any deviation of the uvula.
- When the client is asked to say, "aah," his uvula should rise in the midline.

Oropharynx

Testing of the gag reflex is not usually performed during a routine examination unless there are suspicious signs of abnormality, such as hoarseness, dysphagia, or uvular deviation.

- To inspect the oropharynx, the tongue blade must be inserted deeply.
- Press the tongue blade to the side of the tongue to avoid the gag reflex.
- Note symmetry, color, and any exudate, lesions, and edema.
- Inspect the tonsils; they are located on either side of the oropharynx. All lymphoid tissues, including the tonsils, are enlarged in the young child.

Following examination of the oropharynx and tonsillar areas, the gag reflex can be elicited if necessary by pressing on the posterior tongue with the tongue blade. Finally, wearing a glove, palpate the oral structures.

CLINICAL CORRELATIONS

Ears

Low set ears *may* reflect mental retardation, usually that resulting from congenital defects. This condition can be seen in children with Down's syndrome. *Tophi* are hard, pale, nontender collections of urate crystals that are commonly found on the helix of the pinna; they are usually associated with gout (see Fig. 9-17). The auricle of the ear should be stiff but not rigid. "Cauliflower ears," thickened and gnarled, are evidence of repeated trauma and are commonly seen in prizefighters. Very large ears are said to be observed in pernicious anemia.

Mastoiditis is no longer commonly seen because of the use of antibiotics, but tenderness in the mastoid process area is often associated with *acute otitis media* (middle ear infection) (Fig. 9-18).

In disease, changes in the color of the tympanic membrane and in the landmarks become significant (Table 9-2 and Fig. 9-18).

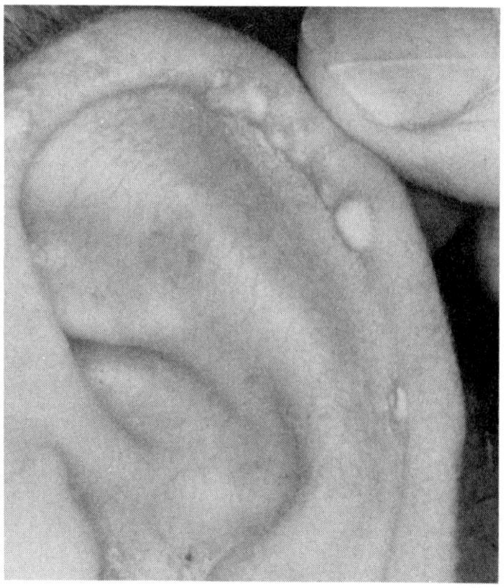

Figure 9-17 Gouty tophi of the ear. (© Arthritis Foundation 1981.)

Hearing loss may be classified according to the following four categories:

1. *Conduction deafness* refers to the hearing loss that occurs when there is interference with the functioning of the structures in the middle ear. The most common causes of middle ear deafness are otitis media, otosclerosis, and rupture of the tympanic membrane. Hereditary otosclerosis is the most frequent cause of progressive conduction deafness; it is the factor responsible for 50% of deafness in adults.
2. *Sensorineural deafness* results from disease occurring anywhere from the organ of Corti to the brain. Nerve deafness has many causes: heredity; rubella in the pregnant mother; chronic middle ear infection in childhood spreading to the inner ear; and exposure to loud noises, such as gunfire, dynamite blasting, and working with heavy equipment. Teenagers and others who listen to loud amplified music may develop a form of nerve deafness referred to as "rock and roll deafness."

Table 9-2 Pathologic Manifestations of the Tympanic Membrane

Manifestation	Cause	Condition
Yellow or amber	Serum or pus	Acute or chronic otitis media
Blue	Blood behind drum	Skull injury
Bright red	Inflammation	Acute otitis media
Bubbles behind drum	Serous fluid	Serous otitis media
Absent light reflex	Bulging of drum	Suppurative otitis media
White thick drum	Scarring of drum	Untreated infection
Chalky granulated nodule	Inflammation	Chronic inflammatory process
Malleus very prominent	Retraction of drum	Obstruction of eustachian tube
Dark areas	Perforation	Rupture of drum

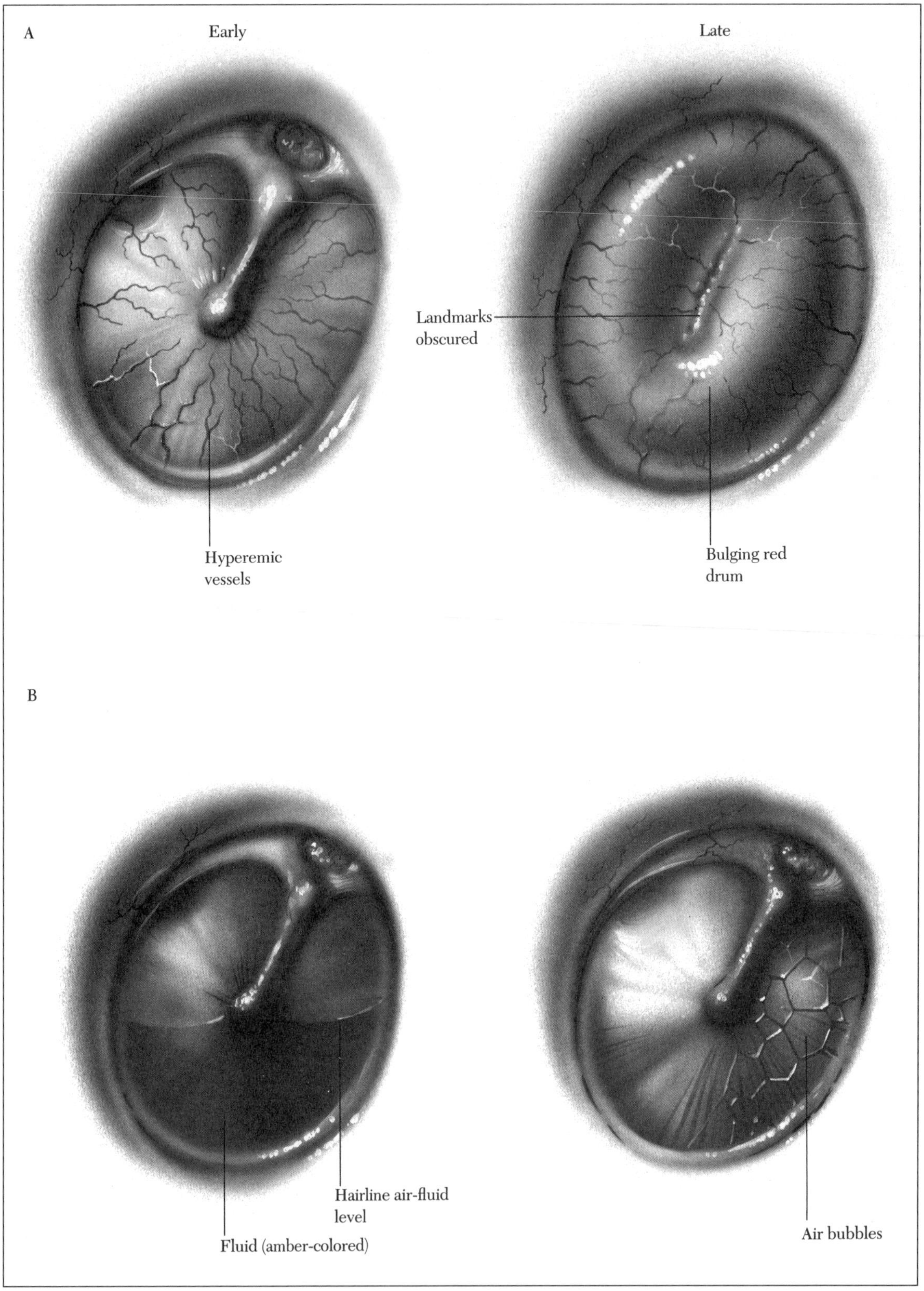

Figure 9-18 **(A)** Acute purulent otitis media. **(B)** Serous otitis media.

3. *Central deafness* occurs from damage to the auditory pathways or auditory center; this may happen with a cerebrovascular accident.

4. *Functional deafness* refers to cases in which there is no organic basis for the loss of hearing.

Using the Weber test if the client has conduction hearing loss in one ear, he will hear the sound better in that ear. This is because normal noise in the room tends to obscure hearing in the normal ear. The client with conduction loss will not hear the room noise and thus has a better chance to hear the bone-conducted sound. If the client has sensorineural loss, he will hear the sound better with the normal ear. A sensorineural loss manifests a positive Rinne *(AC > BC)* and an abnormal Weber (lateralizes to the good ear) (Table 9-3). Common pathologic conditions that require medical attention and treatment are otitis externa and otitis media.

Otitis externa, infection of the external ear, is most frequently seen in children and young adults in the summer season. It often occurs secondary to getting the ears wet, as with frequent swimming or hair washing. It may also be due to staphylococcal or Pseudomonas infection. With these infections, the ear canal is swollen and discharges purulent material. If pulling gently on the tragus elicits pain, the diagnosis is almost always external otitis.

The most common ear infection in childhood is probably simple *otitis media.* It tends to occur in the winter months. With this condition, the tympanic membrane is very erythematous, and there is pain in and about the ear; this pain can be severe. Fever and malaise, and sometimes GI problems, may accompany the infection. If the condition becomes subacute, persistent purulent drainage may result. Antibiotic therapy is required. The tympanic membrane can rupture and purulent discharge is released from the middle ear into the external canal. Rupture and recurrent middle ear infections result in chronic otitis media. The chronically infected ear is characterized by a persistent or recurring purulent, foul-smelling drainage, with or without pain, and by differing degrees of hearing loss, usually of the conduction type.

Trauma and rupture of the eardrum occur most often as a result of accident. People who clean their ears with cotton swabs or with sharp objects (e.g., hairpins) covered with tissue may inadvertently puncture the eardrum. This is as common in adults as in young children.

Health problems involving the endolymphatic system of the inner ear and the vestibular branch of the auditory nerve may be reflected in the sign of nystagmus and complaints of vertigo. Generally, with the ear, the nystagmus is horizontal; vertical nystagmus tends to occur with brainstem lesions. Retinal lesions may give rise to ocular nystagmus which is reflected by a slow rotary pattern.

Nose

Rhinitis, an inflammation of the mucous membrane of the nose, produces a definite erythematous and edematous mucosa. In allergy, however, the mucosa is bluish gray. Discharge is common in rhinitis and sinusitis. Severe chronic rhinitis is characterized by thick greenish discharge with an offensive odor.

Table 9-3 **Common Causes and Clinical Findings of Hearing Losses**

	Conduction loss	Sensorineural loss
Site of damage	External or middle ear	Inner ear or nerve (from the organ of Corti to the brain)
Etiology of dysfunction	Excessive cerumen, ruptured tympanic membrane, otosclerosis, otitis media	Exposure to loud noise—e.g., loud music, dynamite, jackhammer, gunshots, heredity, rubella in pregnant mother, chronic middle ear infection spreading to inner ear
Weber test Normal finding: does *not* lateralize	Lateralizes to affected ear because bone vibrations are detected better than normal without the distraction of environmental noise; you can simulate an external or middle ear conduction loss by occluding one ear with your finger, and you will experience the vibrations lateralizing to your occluded ear; in an absolutely quiet room, a normal finding of no lateralization will result.	Lateralizes to unaffected ear because bone vibrations are not conducted to brain due to inner ear or nerve damage
Rinne test Normal finding: *AC > BC*	Air conduction of the vibrations is blocked; therefore, bone conduction will bypass the external and middle ear and last longer *(BC > AC)*	Air conduction of the vibrations are longer than bone *(AC > BC);* therefore, the normal finding prevails, but hearing is diminished by both routes.

Perforation of the septum may result from continuous use of cocaine, continuous nose picking, syphilis, tuberculosis, systemic lupus, or nasal septal surgery. The anterior septum is a common site of epistaxis, which can be controlled easily. Bleeding from the posterior nares is frequently profuse and is more difficult to control. Epistaxis may occur from trauma, hypertension, coagulation disturbance, tumor, and acute rheumatic fever.

Purulent drainage from the middle meatus, the cleft-like area between the anterior and middle turbinates, indicates sinusitis. Nasal polyps appear as smooth, mobile, grayish white pale tumors. The polyps resemble peeled grapes, round and glistening, and are commonly found with allergic rhinitis and cystic fibrosis. Nasal obstruction will occur as they become larger. Carcinomas of the mucosa are unusual; such growths are gray-white and relatively insensitive.

Sense of smell may decrease with aging and the accompanying increase of hair growth in the nares, especially of elderly men, as well as with smoking and during bouts of colds.

Lips

Circumoral pallor or pale mucosa is seen in anemic states. Cyanotic lips accompany hypoxic states. Cherry red lips are characteristic of acidotic states and of aspirin or carbon monoxide poisoning.

Cheilitis, inflammation of the lip, can be caused by poor oral hygiene, by overexposure to sunlight or wind, or by the chemicals in lipsticks and other creams and cosmetics. It is also manifested in seborrheic dermatitis of the lips and in hypertrophy of the mucous glands and their ducts. *Cheilosis* is frequently seen in vitamin B–complex deficiency (especially that of riboflavin) and with monilial and other infections. This condition is characterized by reddened lips and cracks or fissures in the corner of the mouth that are generally very painful. Most tumors of oral cancer occur on the lips, primarily on the lower lip. A drooping of the lips on one side may indicate paralysis of the facial or trigeminal nerve.

Gums

Gingivitis, inflammation of the gums, may result from poor dental hygiene or may indicate the presence of a systemic disease. This condition is manifested by red, swollen, and bleeding gums. Vitamin C deficiency also causes reddened and hemorrhagic gums (Fig. 9-19).

Periodontitis, a serious inflammation of the periodontium caused by residual food, bacteria, and calcium deposits (tartar), can, if unchecked, spread inflammation to the bone in which the teeth are rooted, causing loosening and loss of teeth.

Gingival bleeding is present in leukemia, as is ulceration of other structures of the mouth, such as the buccal mucosa, the soft palate, the pharynx, or the tonsils. A dark line along the gingival margin is characteristic of both lead and bismuth poisoning (Fig. 9-20). However, a melanotic line may be found normally in the client of African ancestry.

Salivation

Excessive salivation (i.e., drooling) is observed during the teething process in children and in clients with *stomatitis* (inflammation of the mouth). Saliva may collect in the mouth as a result of pseudobulbar palsy, the dysphagia that occurs with 9th or 10th cranial nerve injury (the glossopharyngeal and vagus nerves).

Buccal Mucosa

With anemia, the oral mucosa may be pale. In Addison's disease, the oral mucosa undergoes pigment changes manifested by irregular spots or brown blotches. Koplik's spots, small bluish white spots within the lower lip and scattered about the mucosa at the level of the lower teeth, are visible early in measles and are pathognomonic of that disease. Red spots over the buccal mucosa and the palate are frequently an early sign of German measles. Petechiae may be evident in leukemia and in subacute bacterial endocarditis.

Leukoplakia (Fig. 9-21), a patchy white lesion on the mucous membrane of the cheeks, gums, or tongue, is usually raised and has well-defined borders. It can be caused by chronic irritation (as from smoking, chewing tobacco), poor nutrition (alcoholism), and syphilis, and may be associated with AIDS. These lesions can be precancerous. Leukoplakia is distinguishable from monilial infection in that the lesions cannot be peeled away. The milky curd-like lesions of *Candidiasis* (moniliasis; thrush) leave a raw, red area that may bleed when peeled off.

Teeth

Green, brown, or blue discoloration may be seen in erythroblastosis fetalis. Pitting, white spotting, or brown staining can be the result of excessive fluoride ingestion (Fig. 9-22). Defects of the enamel range from deep grooves or grooves around the surface of the crown to absent incisal edges or occlusal surfaces. These defects are associated with gastrointestinal disturbances or with deficiencies of calcium, phosphorus, or vitamins A and B. Pegged lateral incisors and notched central incisors (Hutchinson's teeth) are a sign of congenital syphilis (Fig. 9-23).

In young children, malocclusion can cause severe earaches. Improper occlusion may indicate neoplasms, although malocclusion of the permanent teeth in older children may be caused by persistent thumb sucking. Delay in the appearance of deciduous teeth may indicate such conditions as rickets, cretinism, congenital syphilis, or Down's syndrome.

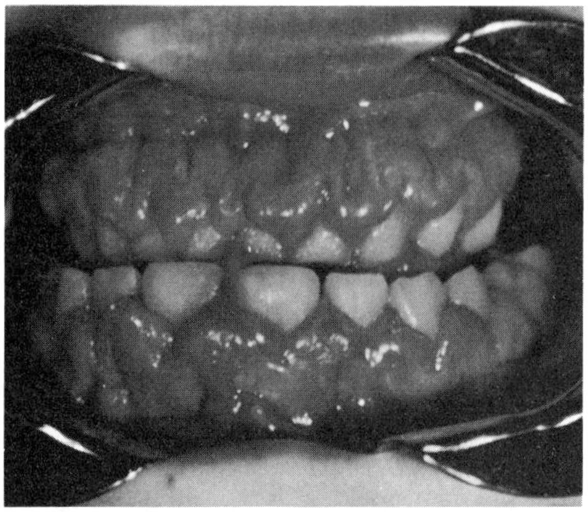

Figure 9-19 Hyperplasia of the gums in acute monocytic leukemia.

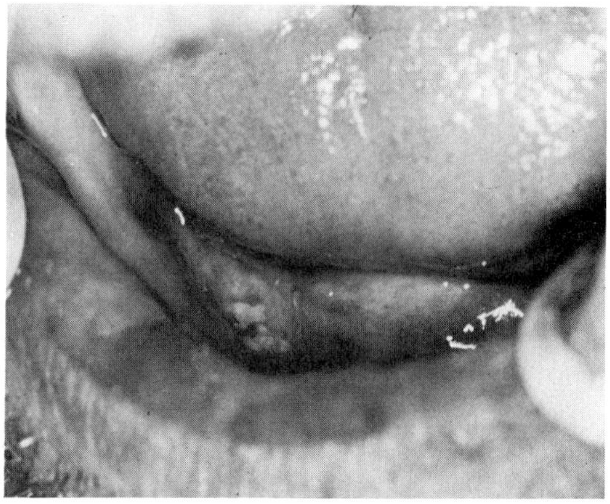

Figure 9-21 Leukoplakia under tongue.

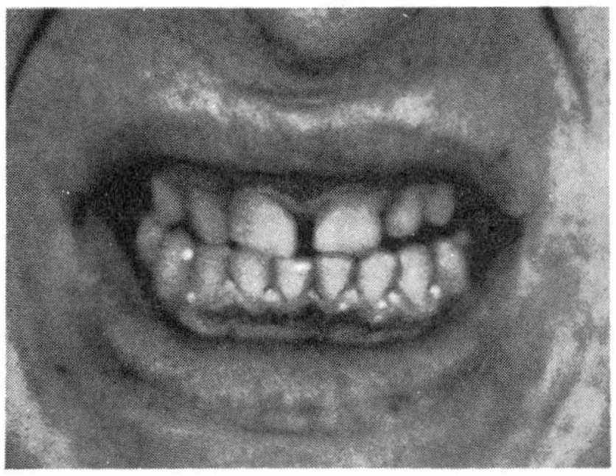

Figure 9-20 Lead line.

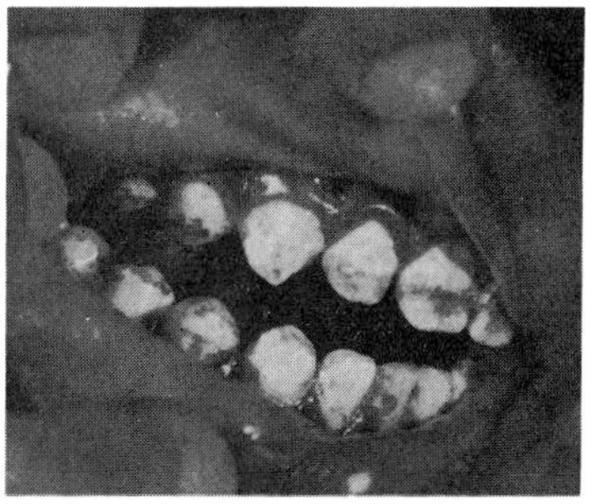

Figure 9-22 Mottled enamel due to fluoride in water.

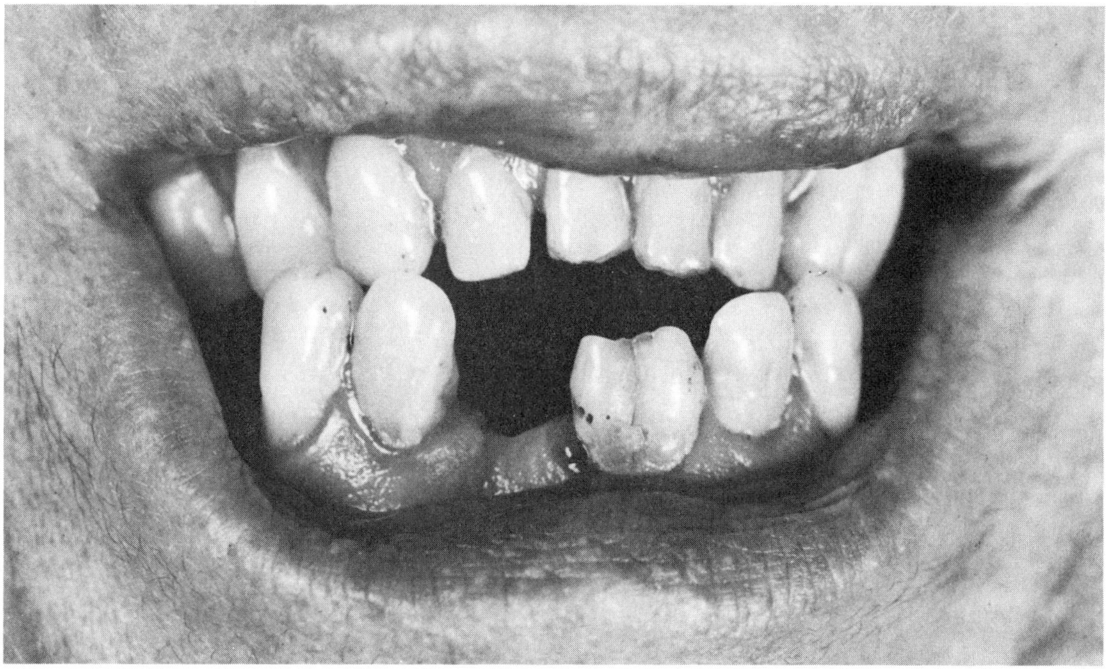

Figure 9-23 Hutchinson's teeth. Note notching of the central incisors and pegged lateral incisors.

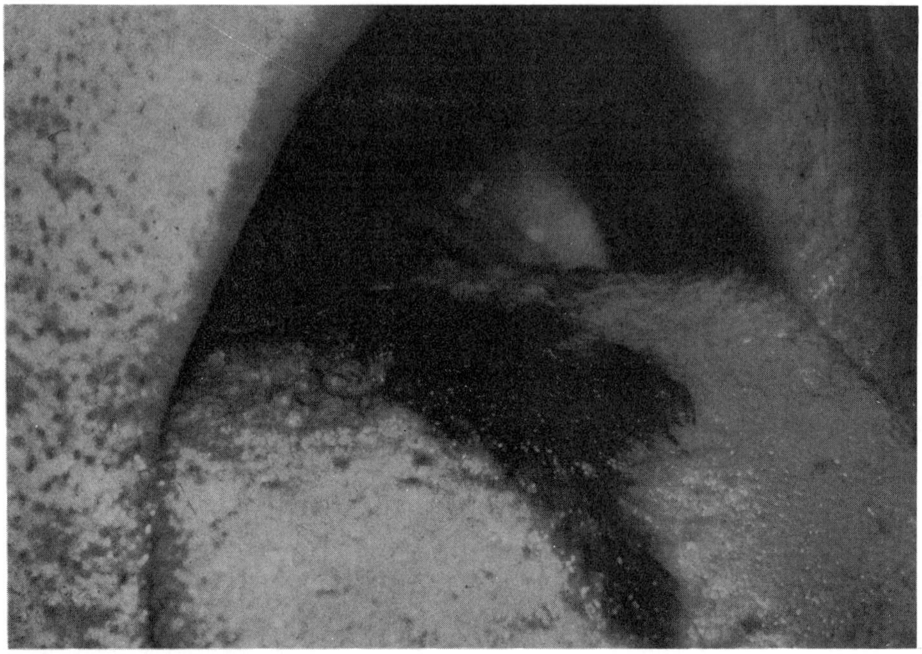

Figure 9-24 Hairy tongue. (From Prior, John and Silberstein, Jack S. *Physical Diagnosis,* 4th ed. St. Louis: CV Mosby Co., 1973, p. 146.)

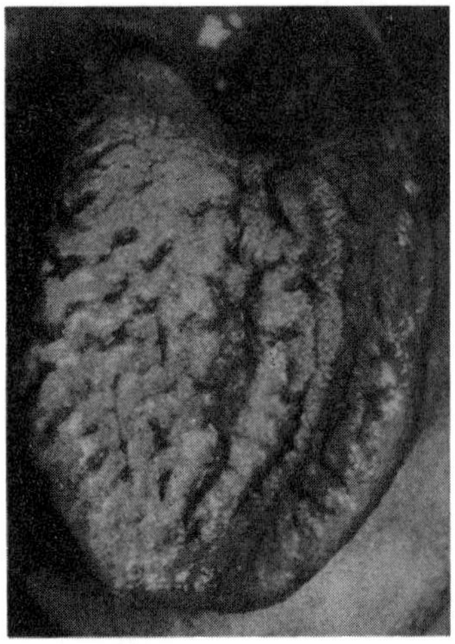

Figure 9-25 Scrotal tongue.

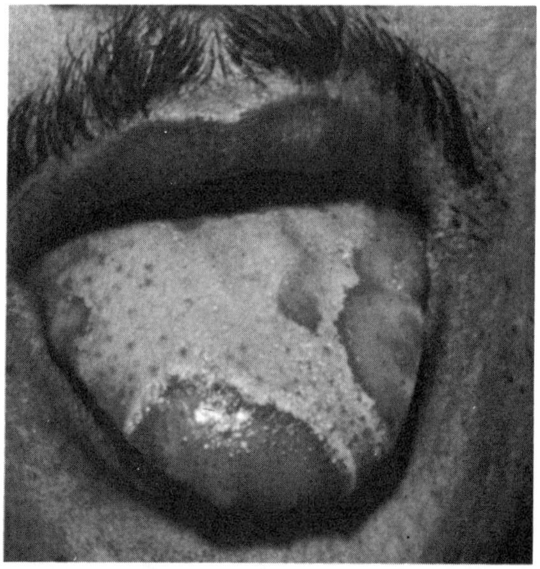

Figure 9-26 Geographic tongue.

Tongue

A sore, red tongue and diminished or absent papillae occur with pernicious anemia and with riboflavin and niacin deficiencies. A red, beefy tongue is characteristic of pernicious anemia. A black, hairy tongue can occur following the excessive use of antibiotics, mouthwash, smoking, or alcohol (Fig. 9-24). Deep fissures can indicate dehydration or malnutrition. Congenital fissures run horizontally across the tongue, whereas the fissures observed in dehydration run vertically (Fig. 9-25).

Normally, there are no fasciculations or tremors of the tongue. Fine tremor may be present in hyperthyroidism, and gross tremor is observed in cerebral palsy and alcoholism.

A small tongue may be seen with malnutrition and with paralysis of the hypoglossal nerve. A geographic tongue shows white, raised, geographically shaped areas that surround areas of tongue atrophy (Fig. 9-26). Deviation to one

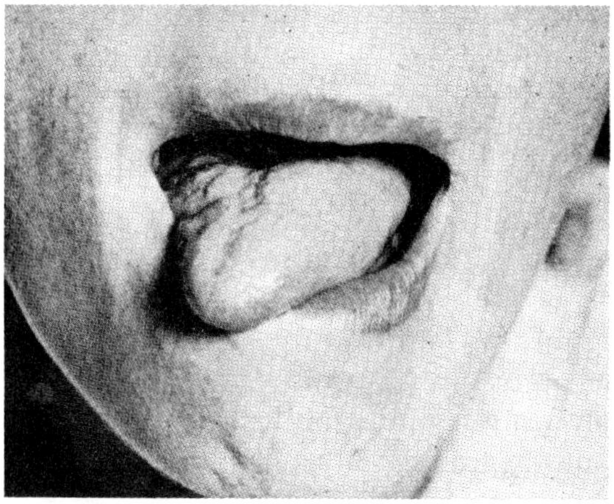

Figure 9-27 Deviation and atrophy of tongue due to paralysis of the hypoglossal nerve.

side may indicate hypoglossal nerve damage (Fig. 9-27). A large tongue may be an early sign of hypothyroidism or acromegaly. The tongue may also appear large in clients with mental retardation.

Asymmetry of the tongue may be due to nodules or growths or to neoplasms or bacterial or fungal diseases. Wear a glove to palpate such lesions.

Oropharynx

Uvular deviation suggests possible impairment of the 9th or 10th cranial nerve. Absence of the uvular reflex may also be an early sign of poliomyelitis or diphtheria.

The presence of pus or large amounts of mucus on the posterior wall of the pharynx is generally evidence of inflammation of the nasopharynx or of the sinuses.

RECORDING OF FINDINGS

Normal findings are presented in the left column. Abnormal findings are presented in the right column.

Ear

Inspection: Normal size and positioning, no deformities.

Palpation: No masses, lesions, or tenderness of tragus and mastoid process.

Percussion: Watch ticking heard bilaterally; Weber test—no lateralization; Rinne: *AC* > *BC.*

Fundoscopy: No cerumen or discharge; no redness or swelling of ear canals; TMs pearly gray color, no perforation; light reflex present.

Nose

Inspection and palpation: No tenderness or deformity; patent bilaterally, no perforations or deviation of septum; can identify alcohol; no redness, swelling, or discharge.

Percussion: Sinuses not tender. Frontal and maxillary sinuses transilluminate.

Mouth

Inspection: Lips pink, no cracks or fissures; buccal mucosa pink; soft and hard palate clear—no ulcers, sores, or lacerations; tongue normal—no cracks, fissures, or edema, protrudes in midline, no tremor; teeth in good condition, no caries or missing teeth.

Palpation: No nodules, no tenderness.

Pharynx

Inspection: Mucosa pink; uvula rises in midline on phonation; tonsils present without inflammation; gag reflex present.

Ear

Inspection: Normal size and positioning, no deformities.

Palpation: No masses or lesions; left ear: tragus painful to touch.

Percussion: Watch ticking heard bilaterally; Weber lateralizes to left ear; Rinne: *BC* > *AC.*

Fundoscopy: Canal reddened, eardrum yellow; light reflex absent; right ear pearly gray color, no perforation, light reflex present at 5 o'clock.

Nose

Inspection and palpation: No deformity; mucosal pallor and swollen with moderate amount of clear drainage; patent bilaterally; no perforations of septum; unable to identify alcohol and soap.

Percussion: Frontal and maxillary sinuses tender on light percussion and do not transilluminate.

Mouth

Inspection: Lips dry and cracked; buccal mucosa pale; soft and hard palate clear—no ulcers, sores, or lacerations; tongue midline without cracks, fissures, tremors, or edema; multiple dental caries; lower lateral incisors absent.

Palpation: No nodules; no tenderness.

Pharynx

Inspection: Mucosa red; uvular reflex present; tonsils enlarged and reddened; gag reflex present.

Acute tonsillitis presents as red, swollen tonsils. A white tonsillar membrane is found in diphtheria, infectious mononucleosis, leukemia, and beta streptococcal infection. Acute pharyngitis, a viral or bacterial infection, causes a bright fiery red pharyngeal membrane. The tonsils also become swollen, and flecks of exudate are visible.

In streptococcal sore throat, the pharynx is diffusely reddened, and the tonsils and tonsillar nodes beneath the angles of the mandible are enlarged. The uvula is edematous, and an exudate covers the tonsils and the pharynx. Streptococcal infection may also be asymptomatic; therefore, routine pharyngeal culturing is performed during seasons of highest incidence and in geographic areas of risk.

Absence of the gag reflexes may indicate a problem with the glossopharyngeal or vagus nerve. Table 9-4 provides further data about common abnormalities of the nose, mouth, and pharynx.

Table 9-4 Common Abnormalities of the Nose, Mouth, and Pharynx

Terminology	Characteristics	Comments
Nose		
Rhinitis	Erythema and edema of mucosa	Note thick, greenish, odorous discharge for chronic condition. Note bluish gray mucosa in allergic rhinitis.
Perforation of septum	Difficulty breathing, dryness of mucosa, epistaxis	Note hole in septum; look for habits including nose picking and/or cocaine use. History of venereal disease. History of nasal-septal surgery.
Sinusitis	Inflammation, drainage, pain over sinuses, fever, chills, headache	Check for causative agent: virus, bacterium, allergy. Presence of polyps, deviated septum, dental abscess in maxillary bone, or general debility.
Polyps	Smooth, mobile, pale tumors; bleed easily	Should be removed if possibility they will become malignant. Nasal obstruction as they grow larger.
Lips		
Herpes simplex	Cluster of clear vesicles on lips that rupture, ulcerate, and become crusted	Caused by invasion of virus, herpes simplex type 1 or 2.
Cheilitis or cheilosis	Red, cracked, dry, bleeding lips; painful cracks, fissures in corner of mouth	Check for poor oral hygiene, overexposure to sunlight, wind, or chemicals. Vitamin B complex deficiency, monilial infection, seborrheic dermatitis.
Gums		
Gingivitis	Red, swollen, bleeding	Note poor dental hygiene; check for systemic disease, Vitamin C deficiency.
	Dark line along gingival margin	Check for lead or bismuth poisoning.
Peridontitis	Red, swollen peridontium (tissues surrounding the tooth)	Note dental hygiene, calcium deposits. Be aware that teeth will be lost.
Excessive salivation	Drooling	Check for inflammation of mouth, 9th or 10th cranial nerve injury.
Mucous membranes		
Anemia	Pale mucosa	Assess for development of mouth lesions or ulcers.
Koplik's spots	Small bluish white spots on lower lip and mucosa of lower teeth	Check for measles, since these spots are diagnostic before rash appears.
Petechiae	Small, purplish hemorrhagic spots	Check for leukemia, subacute bacterial endocarditis.
Leukoplakia	Patchy, raised, white lesion on cheeks, gums, or tongue; has well-defined borders	Check for chronic irritation, poor nutrition, or syphilis. These lesions can be precancerous. Lesion cannot be peeled away as a monilial infection can.
Teeth		
Dental caries	Brown, gray, to gray-orange areas on tooth surfaces; size of area varies	Note dental hygiene. Some have a familial predisposition to caries. Check nutritional status.

Table 9-4 Continued

Terminology	Characteristics	Comments
Discoloration	Yellow-brown Green-brown	Check for use of tetracycline. Often seen in clients who had hemolytic disease as newborns.
	Pitting, white spotting, or brown	Excessive fluoride ingestion; dental plaque.
Defects in enamel	Deep grooves, absent edges of incisors or occlusal surfaces	Note history of gastrointestinal problems, deficiency of calcium, phosphorus, or vitamins A and B.
Hutchinson's teeth	Pegged lateral incisors Notched central incisors	Congenital syphilis.
Tongue		
Alteration in color	Red, sore, beefy papillae, decreased or absent	Check for pernicious anemia. Riboflavin and/or niacin deficiencies.
	Black, hairy	Note use of antibiotics.
	Bright red, dorsal surface resembles map	Geographic tongue (nonpathologic)
Alterations in contour	Deep vertical fissures Deep horizontal fissures	Check for dehydration, malnutrition Congenital defect (scrotal tongue)
Positional deviation	Tremors, fasciculations	Fine tremors may be present in hyperthyroidism. Gross tremors in cerebral palsy.
	Tongue doesn't protrude to midline or can't move from side to side	Possible hypoglossal nerve involvement
Asymmetry	Small tongue	Note malnutrition, paralysis of hypoglossal nerve.
	Large tongue	Hypothyroidism, acromegaly, mental retardation. Note nodules, growths—neoplasm, fungus, bacteria.
Palate		
Torus palatinus	Bony protuberence in midline of palate	Nonpathologic
Cleft palate	Fissure, which is bilateral or unilateral, forming a passageway between mouth and nose	Congenital anomaly
Deviation of uvula	Uvula does not rise in midline	Check for 9th, 10th cranial nerve involvement. Can be early sign of polio or diphtheria.
Oropharynx		
Acute tonsillitis	Red, swollen tonsils with yellowish exudate. Chills, including temperature, headache, pains and aches in back and extremities, pain when swallowing	Check for beta-hemolytic streptococcus, carditis, nephritis.
Infectious mononucleosis	White tonsillar membrane	Check for cervical, axillary, and inguinal lymphadenopathy or splenomegaly.
Acute pharyngitis	Bright, fiery red pharyngeal membrane, tonsils swollen with exudate; edematous uvula, white exudate covering tongue and tonsils; malaise, fever, dysphagia	Streptococcal infection

SUMMARY

In this chapter, assessment of the ear, nose, mouth, and pharynx was described. Examination of the ear involves assessing the external portion, the auditory canal, and the tympanic membrane. The otoscope is used to inspect internal structures. There are several tests that can be used in determining hearing loss. The techniques used for examining the nose are inspection, palpation, and transillumination of the sinuses. Examination of the mouth, including the lips, gums, teeth, and tongue, and of the palate and oropharynx consists mainly of inspection and palpation. Examples of clinical signs reflective of pathology in the ears, nose, mouth, and throat were given in the clinical correlations section.

DISCUSSION QUESTIONS/ ACTIVITIES

1. Discuss the anatomy of the ear and the physiology of the conduction of sound.
2. Describe the difference between the external auditory canals of the adult and of the child. How would this difference affect the examination of the ear of the child compared with that of the adult?
3. What is the light reflex, and where is it located?
4. Describe various manifestations of pathology that are reflected by the tympanic membrane.
5. Demonstrate the Rinne and Weber tests.
6. Demonstrate the technique for examining the ear.
7. Demonstrate the procedure for examining the nares.
8. Why is it often difficult to view the middle and superior turbinates?
9. Which paranasal sinuses can be examined easily? What is the procedure for this examination?
10. Discuss the rationale for having a client with dentures remove them during examination of the mouth.
11. What structures are examined in the oropharynx?
12. Describe leukoplakia and how it can be differentiated from monilial infection.
13. Describe the appearance of the normal tongue.
14. Describe some common abnormalities that may be found when examining the lips, buccal mucosa, tongue, and pharynx.

CHAPTER

10 Assessment of the Thorax and Lungs

Learning Objectives

1. Review the structure and function of the thorax and lungs.
2. Compare the shape of the thorax of the adult with that of the child.
3. State the characteristics of respirations that are noted on inspection.
4. Recognize the landmarks of the thorax used in documentation of physical findings.
5. Describe the norm and technique of assessing fremitus.
6. Describe the techniques of percussion and auscultation of the lung fields.
7. Identify the various percussion notes and breath sounds and the locations where they are normally heard on the thorax.
8. Explain the technique of determining the diaphragmatic excursion.
9. Identify the skeletal deformities of the thorax that are risk factors for healthy, adequate respiratory functioning.

Assessment of the thorax and lungs begins with noting the gross appearance of the thorax—its size and shape. Next, progressing from the outside, the skin is examined; then the muscles and bones are assessed, followed by examination of the lungs.

STRUCTURE AND FUNCTION OF THE THORAX

The thorax is a bony cage defined by the sternum, the costal cartilages, the ribs, and the bodies of the thoracic vertebrae. In the normal client, the thorax is cone-shaped, that is, narrow at the top and wide at the bottom. The thorax supports the bones of the shoulder and upper extremities and contains the lungs, heart, and upper portions of the major blood vessels.

The *sternum,* located at the anterior medial chest, is a flat narrow bone about 15 cm in length. It is divided into three parts: the upper part, or *manubrium;* the middle part, or *body;* and the lower part, or *xiphoid process* (Fig. 10-1). The upper seven costal cartilages are attached to the manubrium and body. The xiphoid process has no attached ribs but does provide for the attachment of some of the abdominal muscles. The thorax contains 24 ribs, with 12 on each side of the thoracic cavity. All of the ribs are attached to the vertebral column. The first seven pairs, which are connected to the sternum by means of the costal cartilages, are called *true ribs.* Of the remaining five pairs, called the *false ribs,* the upper three are attached to the costal cartilage of the next rib above. The two lowest ribs are termed *floating,* or *vertebral, ribs.* The spaces between the ribs are the *intercostal spaces.* The spaces are numbered by the space below the rib.

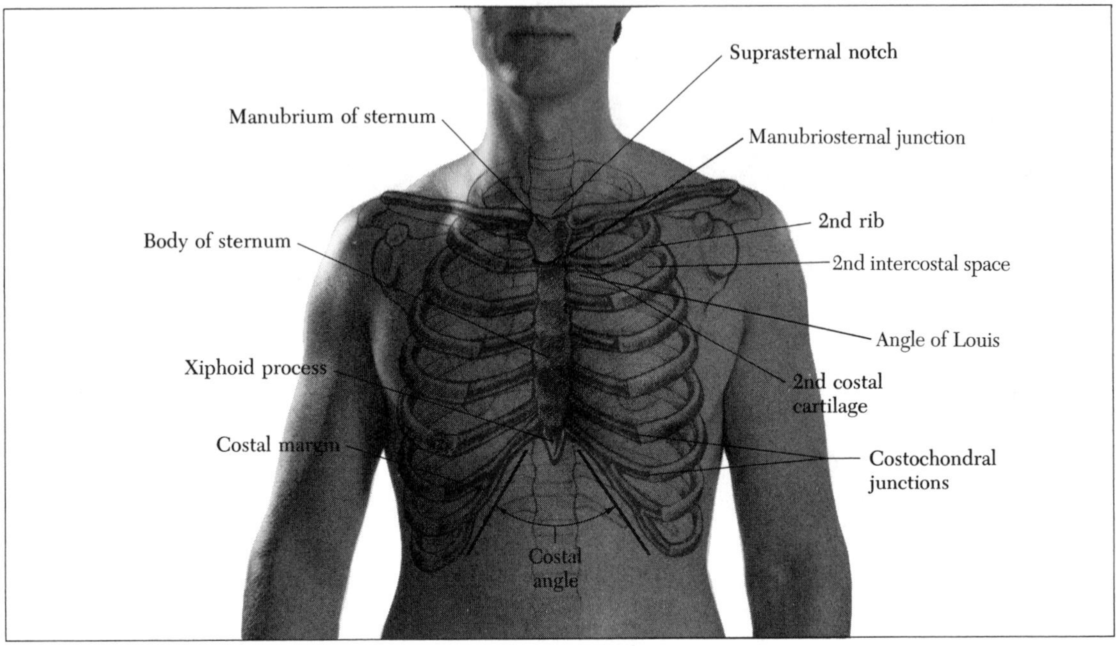

Figure 10-1 Anatomy of the chest.

For example, the space below the third rib is the third intercostal space.

STRUCTURE OF THE LUNGS

The lungs are elastic cone-like sacs that fill up the pleural section of the thoracic cavity. The base of the lungs extends to the diaphragm. The apices rise slightly above the clavicles. Both lungs lie against the rib cage anteriorly and posteriorly. Figure 10-2 illustrates the *trachea,* which brings air to the lungs and divides at the *hilum* into the right and left main *bronchi.* These further divide into *bronchioles* and finally terminate in the *alveoli* where the major act of respiration occurs—the diffusion of oxygen and carbon dioxide.

The *mediastinum* is the mass of tissues in the center of the thoracic cavity, dividing the lungs and containing the esophagus, trachea, and large vessels of the heart.

Figure 10-3 illustrates that the left lung is divided into two lobes—upper and lower—while the right lung is divided into three—upper, middle, and lower. The lungs are covered by the *pleura,* a smooth membrane. The lining of the thorax is the *parietal pleura,* the lung coverings the *visceral pleura.* The potential space between the two is termed the *pleural space.*

To locate findings in the thorax, you must understand the placement of the ribs. On the anterior chest, an important landmark is the *manubriosternal junction.* This ridge lies next to the second rib and forms the upper line of a right angle that is referred to as the *angle of Louis* (see Fig. 10-1). The second intercostal space lies within the angle of Louis. From this point of the identified second intercostal space, you can count the other spaces as necessary to identify the location of other structures within the thoracic cavity. This is also the area wherein the trachea bifurcates (see Fig. 10-3) and where the fifth thoracic vertebra is located in addition to the upper portions of the right and left atria. On the posterior portion of the chest wall, the 7th cervical vertebra is at the base of the neck and is the most prominent spinous process. Just below this is the 1st thoracic vertebra, which is often as evident as the 7th cervical.

The scapulae lie approximately between the second and eighth ribs and are about 4 cm from the midspinal line.

Certain anatomic landmarks (Fig. 10-4) are helpful in describing physical findings. On the lateral chest they are the *anterior axillary line* (AAL), the *midaxillary line* (MAL), and the *posterior axillary line* (PAL). On the anterior chest, these are the *midsternal line* (MSL), the *midclavicular line* (MCL), the *intercostal spaces* (ICSs), the *ribs,* the *suprasternal notch,* the *precordium,* and the *epigastric area.* On the posterior thorax, the *midvertebral line,* the *midscapular line,* and the *spinal vertebrae* serve as helpful landmarks.

CHARACTERISTICS AND TECHNIQUES OF EXAMINATION

Inspection

The assessment of the thorax is performed by using the technique of inspection. Palpation of the thorax occurs during the assessment of the lungs.

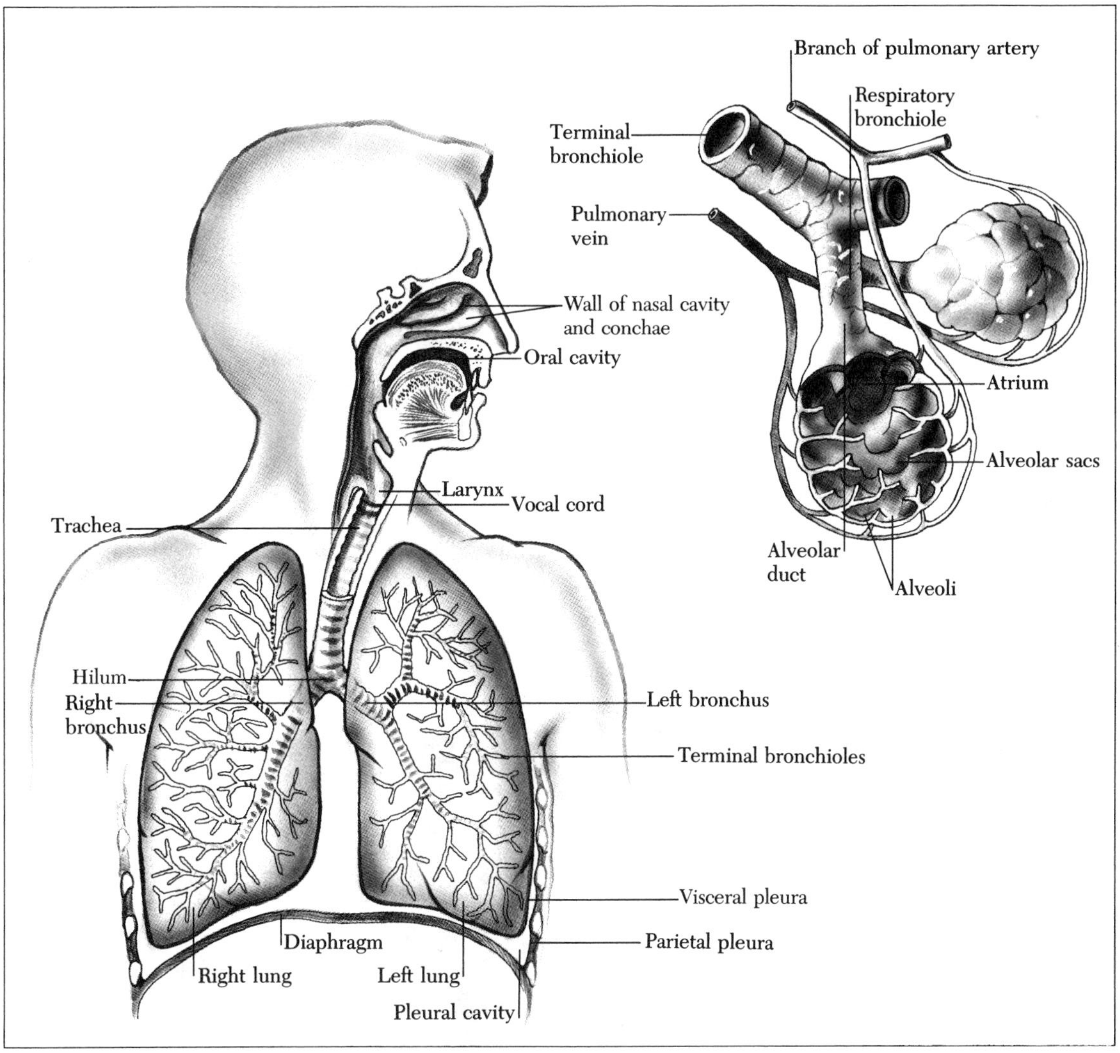

Figure 10-2 Structure of the lung, with detail of alveoli.

For the chest to be inspected adequately, the client must be stripped to the waist and lighting must be good. The chest may be examined with the client in the supine or the sitting position. If the client cannot sit up, be sure that his body is straight and is as flat as can be tolerated. Whether in the sitting or supine position, the client's back must be straight.

- Observe the anteroposterior (AP) diameter of the client's chest from a lateral position. This is the sideview distance from the sternum in the front to the vertebral column at the client's back.
- The AP diameter of the adult thorax should be less than the transverse diameter. The shape of the normal adult thorax is elliptic; the infant's is cylindric/round. Figure 10-5 shows cross sections of the shape of the thorax in the child and in the adult. An increased AP diameter is seen in the client in Fig. 10-16.

Technique for Inspection of the Thorax and Lungs

1. Provide adequate lighting and a warm room.
2. Bare the client to the waist.
3. Have client sit with back straight.
4. Characteristics: Symmetry, skin, AP diameter, scapulae, spine, respirations, abnormalities.

- With the child, at least until 2 years of age, the chest circumference should be measured at the level of the nipple line. The measurement should be approximately the same (± 2 cm) as the child's head size.
- Check for symmetry of the thorax. Minor degrees of asymmetry are not serious. The shoulders should be at one level, but in many clients, one shoulder may be slightly

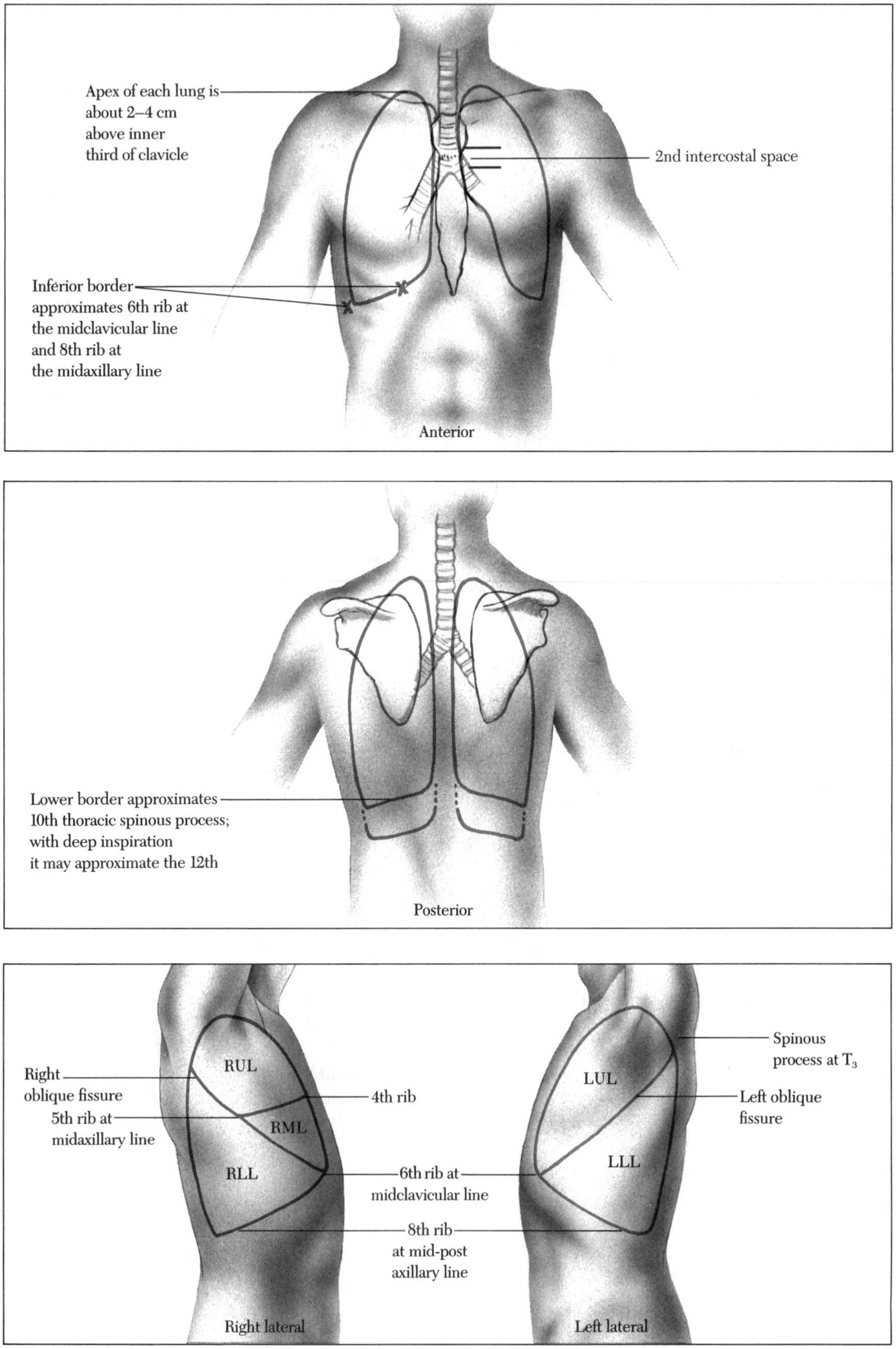
Apex of each lung is about 2–4 cm above inner third of clavicle
2nd intercostal space
Inferior border approximates 6th rib at the midclavicular line and 8th rib at the midaxillary line
Anterior
Lower border approximates 10th thoracic spinous process; with deep inspiration it may approximate the 12th
Posterior
Right oblique fissure
5th rib at midaxillary line
RUL
RML
RLL
4th rib
6th rib at midclavicular line
8th rib at mid-post axillary line
Spinous process at T_3
LUL
LLL
Left oblique fissure
Right lateral
Left lateral

Figure 10-3 Positions of the lungs and ribs.

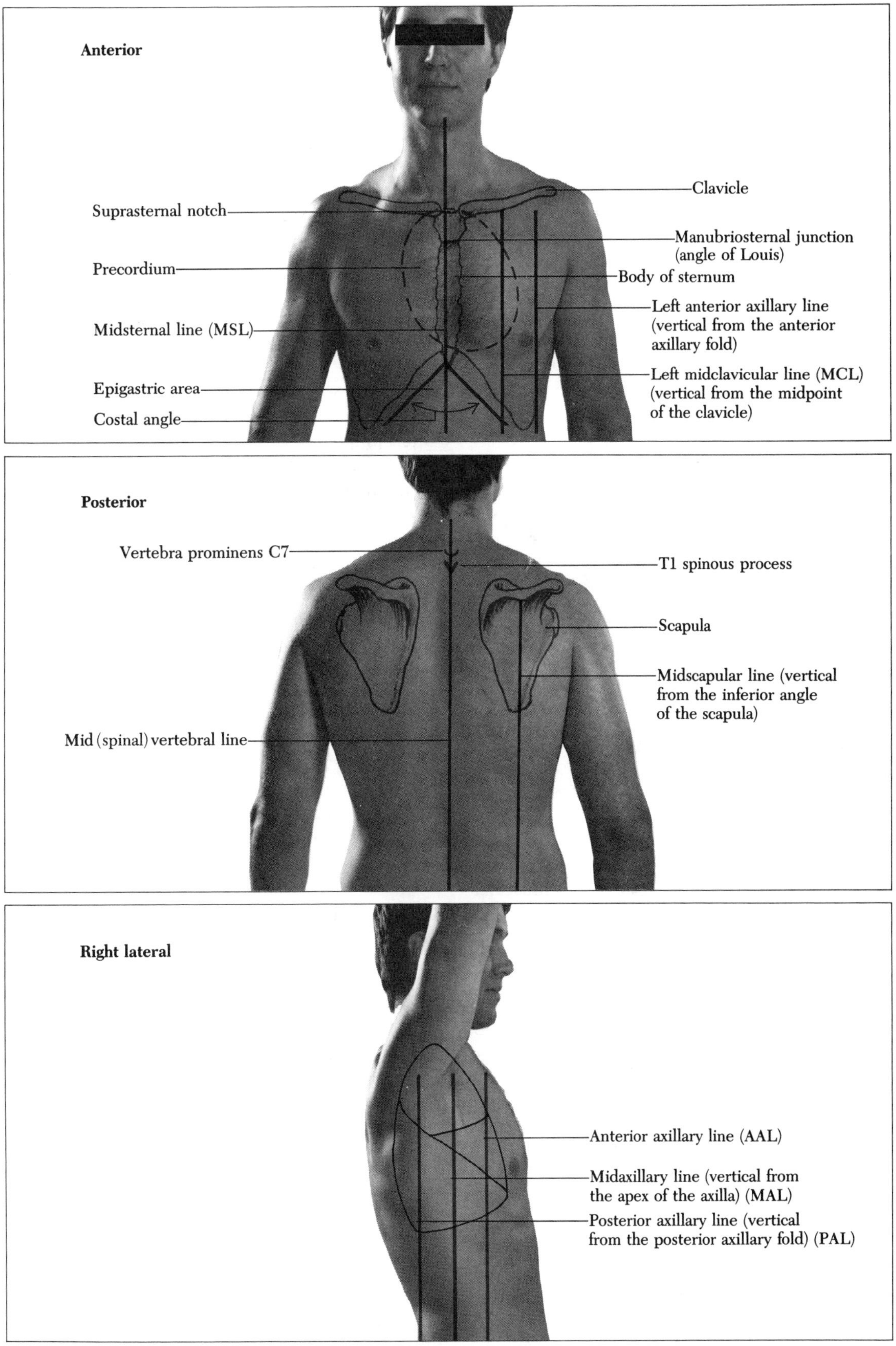

Figure 10-4 Topographic landmarks for physical assessment of the chest and respiratory system.

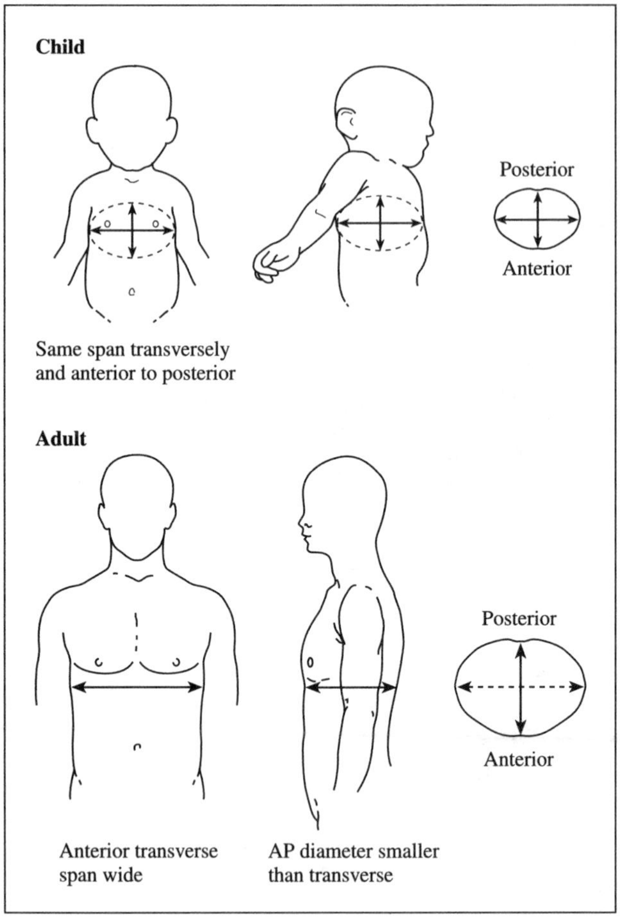

Figure 10-5 Normal shape and AP diameter of the thorax of a child and an adult.

lower than the other, which can be normal. Very often, the handedness of the client results in greater muscular development on one side.

- Check whether the scapulae are on the same level and if the spine is straight with a slight concavity at the thoracic area (Fig. 10-6).
- Examine the skin of the chest for hair, lesions, and vascularity. Males generally have more body hair than females. In the male, the hair growth is less abundant on the posterior aspect of the thorax in comparison with the anterior chest. In females, the amount of hair growth on the anterior and posterior thorax is essentially the same.
- Examine the respiratory accessory muscles of the neck and the rate, depth, and type of respiration (see box on page 222). The respiratory rate varies with age and activity. Respiration is usually diaphragmatic in males and costal in females.

The anxious client may complain of apprehension, shortness of breath, and a sense of suffocation. Sighing respirations often pinpoint the neurotic client; this kind of breathing may be described as overbreathing accompanied by a deep inspiration and a long sighing expiration. Decreased respiratory movement wherein inspiration is barely noticeable accompanies chest trauma, pain, pleurisy, consolidation, fibrosis, atelectasis, pneumothorax and chronic obstructive pulmonary disease (COPD). Table 10-1 lists common abnormalities of the thorax.

Palpation

Palpation is conducted by using the fingertips and ulnar or palmar aspects of the hands accordingly.

- Check to see if the trachea is midline. Palpation of the trachea should be performed to determine movement and possible presence of deviation. On inspiration, the trachea stretches downward. Insert your thumb and index finger about the trachea (between the trachea and the sternocleidomastoid muscles), just above the sternoclavicular

Table 10-1 Common Abnormalities of the Thorax

Terminology	Characteristics	Comments
Barrel chest	Increased AP diameter; chest has no apparent movement during respiration.	Seen with chronic pulmonary disease
Funnel chest	Lower sternum depressed; ribs flare outward.	Rickets, congenital abnormality
Retraction of ribs and intercostal spaces	Abdominal, intercostal, or supraclavicular muscles draw back during inspiration.	May be due to tumor, foreign body, secretions, chronic lung disease, collapsed lung, or fractured ribs.
Bulging of chest wall	Intercostal spaces protrude further forward than ribs on expiration.	Possibly due to enlarged heart, aortic aneurysm, pleural effusion, tension pneumothorax, chronic pulmonary disease
Rachitic rosary	Prominent costochondral junctions; knobs form at angles.	Long-standing vitamin deficiency such as rickets

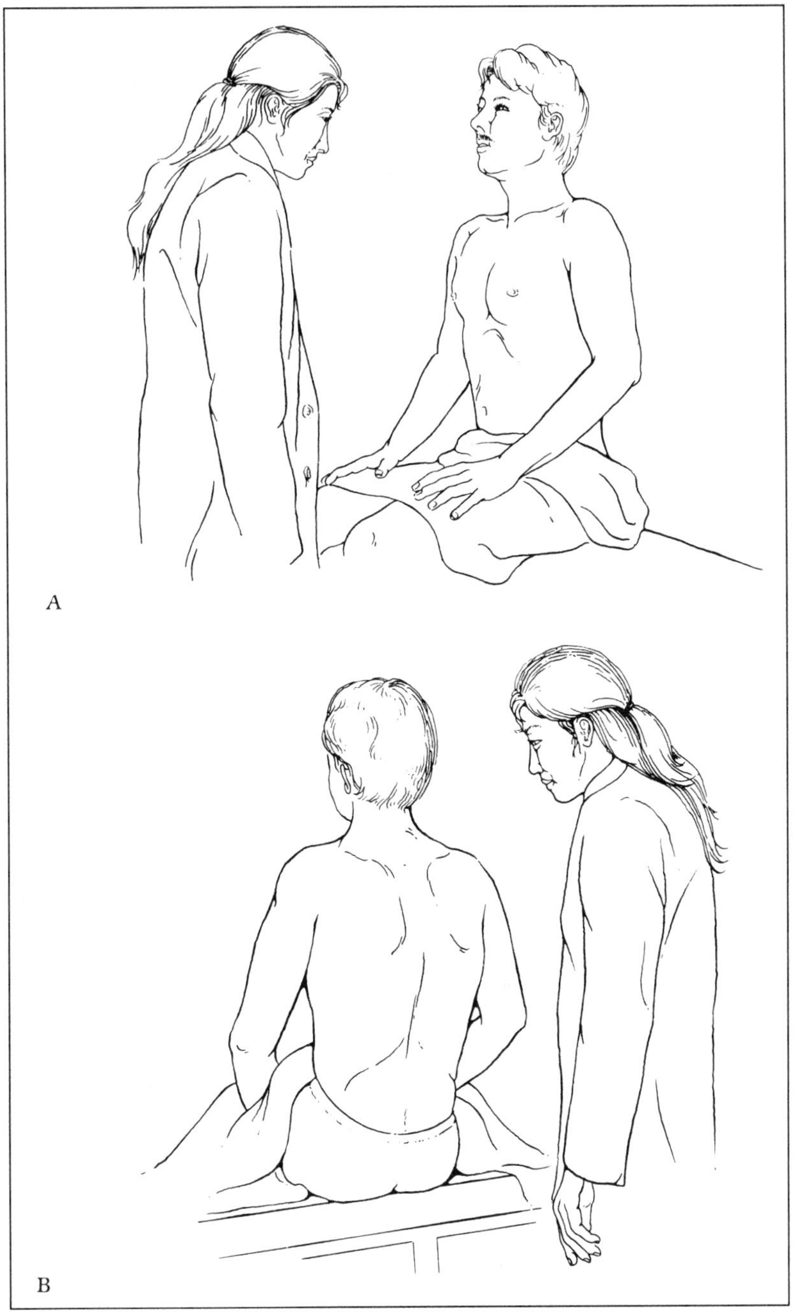

Figure 10-6 Examination of the thorax begins with careful inspection of both the **(A)** anterior and **(B)** posterior thorax. (From Judge, R.D., Zuidema, G.D., Fitzgerald F. (eds.). *Methods of Clinical Examination* (4th ed.). Boston: Little, Brown, 1982).

notch. If the trachea is deviated, you will be able to do this easily on one side but not on the other.

- The client with tracheal deviation warrants immediate referral to a physician.
- Determine whether both sides of the respiratory system expand equally. Check posteriorly and both superior anterior and costal margin movement on the anterior chest. Abnormalities are more likely to be detected anteriorly as there is more movement in the anterolateral thorax. Thoracic expansion is tested with both a normal and a deep inspiration. Normally there is about a 3-inch (7.6-cm) expansion.
- To check posterior expansion of the thorax, stand behind the client and place your hands over the lower posterolateral aspect of the thorax with your thumbs adjacent and near the spine, as illustrated in Fig. 10-7

Abnormal Breathing Patterns

The following terms are used when recording types of breathing patterns.

Dyspnea refers to a difficulty in breathing characterized by air-hunger or a desire for air. It is normal when due to vigorous work or athletic activity but can result from insufficient oxygenation of the lungs that occurs in circulatory disturbances, low hemoglobin, acidosis, and lesions in the medullar respiratory center. It can be either inspiratory or expiratory dyspnea. Inspiratory dyspnea may be accompanied by ICS retraction and stridor and be associated with obstruction of the airway (e.g., foreign body, tumor, posttracheal abscess, and severe inflammation). With expiratory dyspnea, the small bronchioles are obstructed as in asthma, bronchitis, and obstructive emphysema. It may be accompanied by ICS bulging. Dyspnea may also be a subjective feeling.

Stridor is the term used to characterize the high-pitched crowing sounds that occur with difficult inspiration; it is observed in children with croup and in aspiration of a foreign object.

Tachypnea describes increase in the respiratory rate 40 or more breaths/min. Clients with reduced compliance of the lungs, as in heart disease, tuberculosis, pleurisy, and atelectasis (collapsed lung tissue), tend to have rapid, shallow breathing. Tachypnea may also be seen with hysteria, neurasthenia, fever, pneumonia, hyperthyroidism, pleurisy, or in states of alkalosis. If tachypnea is prolonged, excessive loss of carbon dioxide may result.

Bradypnea is a decrease in respirations, as seen with drugs or brain tumors that depress the medulla in the brainstem.

Apnea is temporary cessation of breathing.

Hyperpnea is increase in the depth of respiration and is normal following exercise. It can be caused by pain, drugs, hysteria, and high altitude.

Technique for Palpation of the Thorax and Lungs

1. Gently palpate the bones of the thorax.
2. Palpate the equal expansion of the lungs.
3. Use palmar and/or ulnar aspects of your hands.
4. Have client say "99" or "blue moon."
5. Compare side to side.

and Fig. 10-8A. Have a small fold of skin between your thumbs. Have the client exhale and then take a deep inspiration; your thumbs should move apart at the same time and should be equal in the distance of their movement.

- The superior anterior thoracic expansion is assessed by placing your thumbs along both sides of the sternum at the level of the 4th-5th ICS, as seen in Fig. 10-8B.
- The costal margin movement is evaluated by placing your hands, with outspread fingers, on the lower anterolateral areas of the thorax, with your thumbs pointing toward the xiphoid process, as seen in Fig. 10-8C.

- Palpate the entire thorax for texture of the skin, any pulsations, pain or tenderness, swelling, masses, or crepitation.

The normal spoken voice produces palpable vibrations called *vocal fremitus,* or *tactile fremitus.* Fremitus is easy to palpate on the chest of the crying baby. Transmission of the tactile vibrations should be compared on both sides of the chest; that is, vibrations felt over the left lung field should be compared with those felt over the right lung field. Figures 10-9 and 10-10 illustrate how fremitus is detected with the ulnar aspect of the hands and with the palmar aspects of the fingers.

- The hands are placed on the corresponding sides of the posterior chest wall, and the client is asked to repeat words that normally set up increased vibrations, such as "99," "blue moon," or "1-2-3." The lateral aspects of the thorax, particularly the anterior thoracic area overlying the middle lobe of the right lung, should also be palpated.
- Fremitus is present in the normal lung. Low-pitched voices, generally found in men, will be more palpable. Fremitus also is more intense at the back of the neck, between the scapulae, and in the 1st and 2nd ICSs.

Percussion

Percussion is performed in the ICSs, avoiding the ribs, as percussion on the ribs will elicit dullness. Table 10-2 and Fig. 10-11 illustrate the percussion notes of a normal chest.

The percussion notes heard over the normal lung should be resonant. The sound is loudest where the chest wall is thinnest. Because the chest wall is thinner in children, the percussion notes over their lung fields are more resonant than those of adults.

Hyperresonance is the percussion sound heard over a hyperinflated lung, as in emphysema. Because there is little difference between resonance and hyperresonance, other

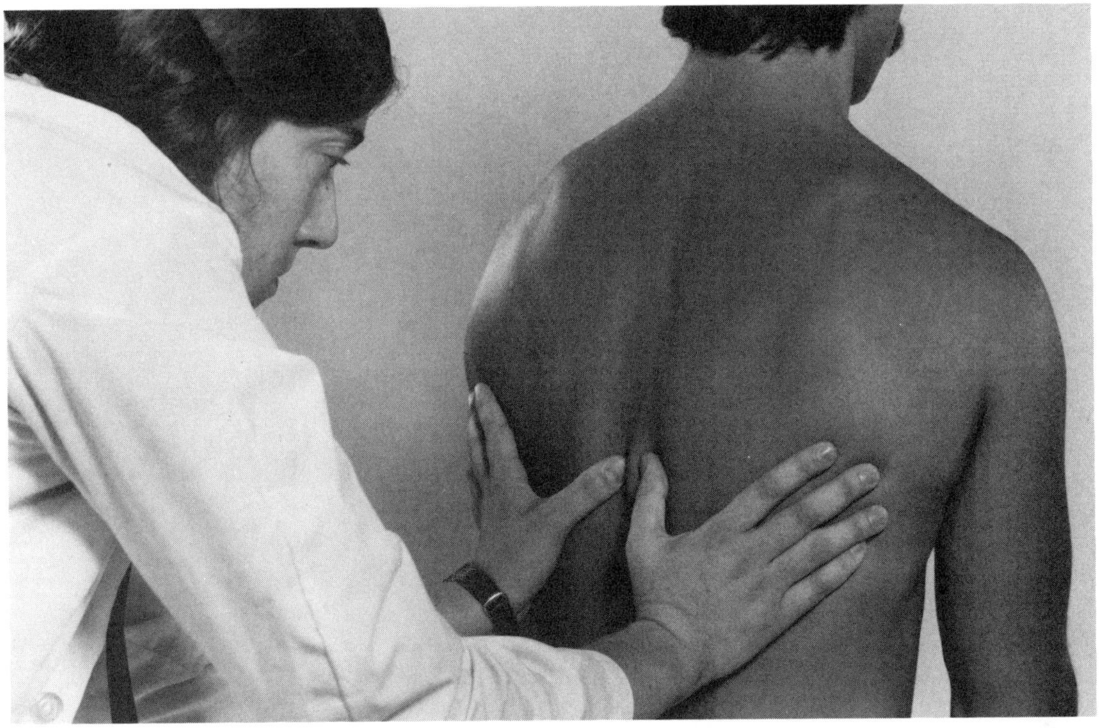

Figure 10-7 Technique for determining respiratory expansion.

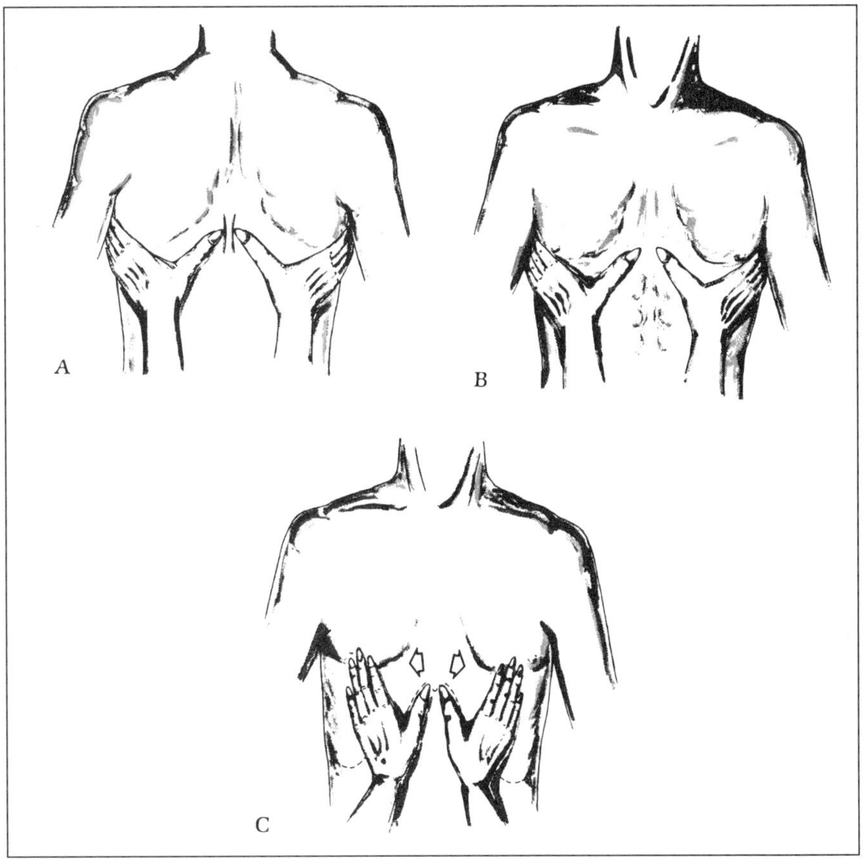

Figure 10-8 Testing inspiratory expansion. (From Sana, J.M. and Judge, R.D. *Physical Assessment for Nursing Skills* (2nd ed.). Boston: Little, Brown, 1982, p. 206.)

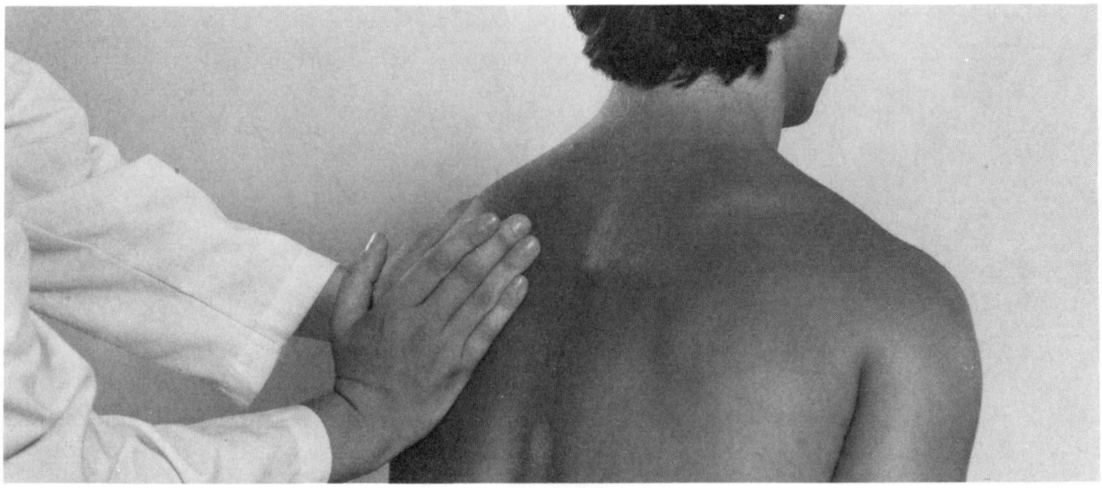

A

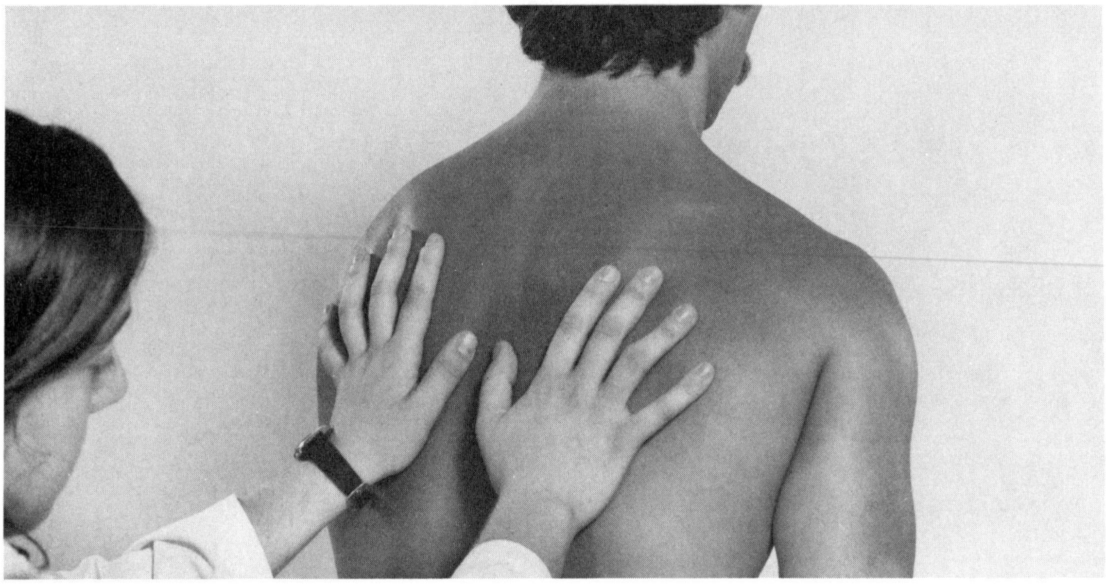

B

Figure 10-9 Palpation technique for fremitus. **(A)** Ulnar. **(B)** Palmar.

Table 10-2 Description of Percussion Notes

Note	Intensity	Pitch	Duration	Quality	Normal location
Flatness	Soft	High	Short	Extreme dullness	Thigh
Dullness	Soft	High	Moderate	Thudlike	Liver
Resonance	Moderate to loud	Low	Long	Hollow	Peripheral lung
Hyperresonance	Very loud	Very low	Very long	Booming	Child's lung
Tympany	Loud	High	Moderate	Musical, drumlike	Air-filled stomach

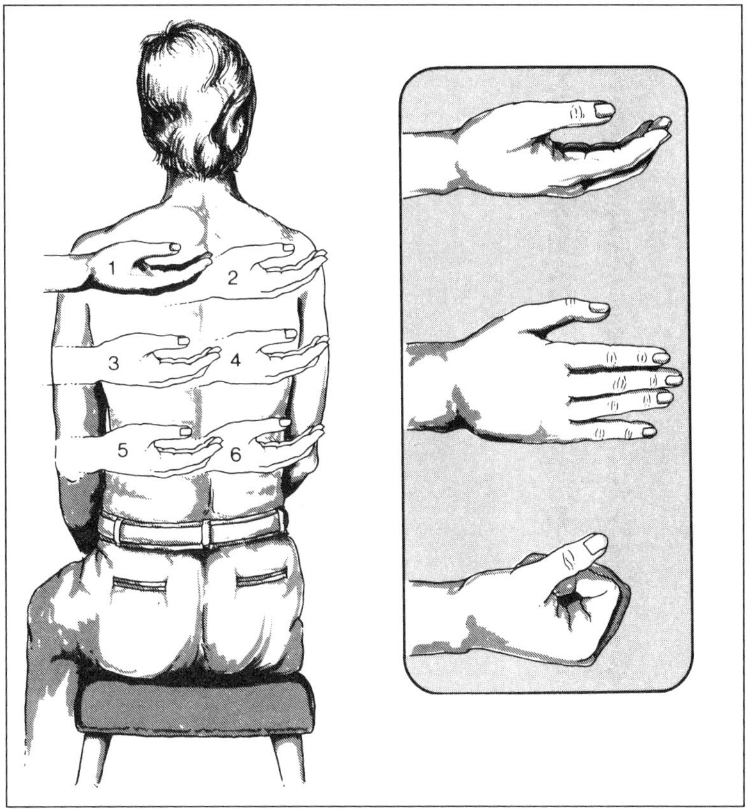

Figure 10-10 Hand positions that can be used to assess fremitus. (From Sana, J.M. and Judge, R.D. *Physical Assessment for Nursing Skills* (2nd ed.). Boston: Little, Brown, 1982, p. 208.)

Technique for Percussion of Lung Fields

1. Percussion done in the intercostal spaces.
2. For percussion of posterior wall, have client flex neck and lean slightly forward with arms folded at waist.
3. Percuss anterior, posterior, and lateral walls of the chest.
4. Proceed side to side on the anterior and posterior aspects at 2- to 3-inch intervals.
5. Proceed from axilla downward at 2- to 3-inch intervals to about the 10th rib for assessment of lateral aspects.
6. Decision making: Employ techniques of bronchophony, egophony, and whispered pectoriloquy over area(s) of abnormal percussion notes (see section "Other Techniques" later in this chapter).

clues may be needed to confirm hyperresonance. For example, a suspected hyperresonant percussion note may be more credible if there are accompanying signs of emphysema, such as a lowered diaphragm level below the tenth rib and a barrel chest. Dullness is percussed over solid organs such as the heart, liver, and spleen. On the posterior chest wall, dullness is encountered over the scapulae and the heavy shoulder muscles, as well as areas of consolidation.

When the client is lying on her side, there are areas of relative percussion dullness due to the effect of the mattress and body weight (Fig. 10-12). On the lower left anterior chest wall, tympany may be elicited because of the presence of a gastric air bubble.

Percussion of the lungs should be performed in a systematic manner on the anterior, lateral, and posterior walls of the chest. Figure 10-13 illustrates this procedure.

- Begin percussion on the anterior wall above the clavicles in the supraclavicular space and continue down to the diaphragm, as with palpating for fremitus.
- Compare one side of the chest with the other.
- Percuss the lateral chest wall beginning in the axilla and work down a few inches at a time to about the level of the tenth rib.

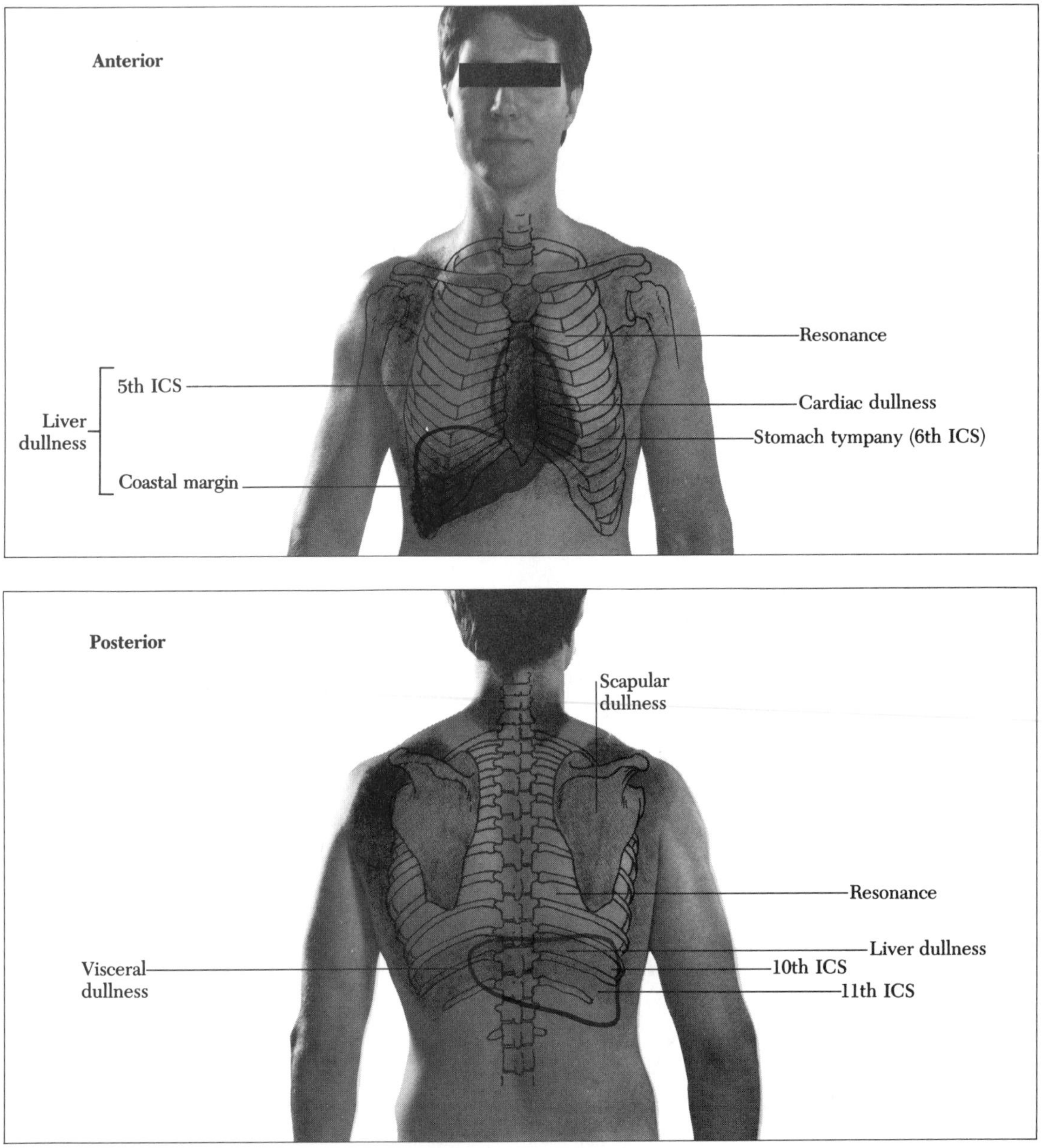

Figure 10-11 Normal percussion notes on the anterior and posterior chest.

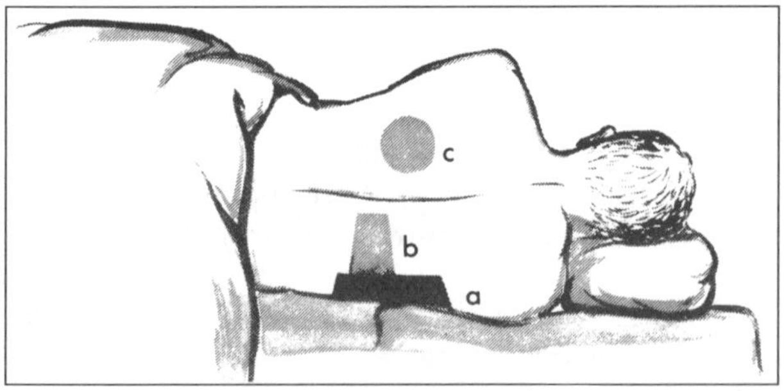

Figure 10-12 Quality of percussion note from the effect of side-lying position. **(A)** Zone of relative dullness due to deadening effect of mattress. **(B)** Zone of dullness due to compression of chest by weight of body. **(C)** Zone of dullness due to crowding of ribs. (From Sana, J.M. and Judge, R.D. *Physical Assessment for Nursing Skills* (2nd ed.). Boston: Little, Brown, 1982, p. 211.)

- When percussing the posterior chest wall, instruct the client to lean forward with arms folded at the waist and head flexed.
- Percuss the posterior chest on both sides beginning at the apices of the lungs, percussing the left side and then the right, each time moving downward toward the diaphragm.

The lowest point in the normal lung where resonance can be detected is at the diaphragm, which is at about the level of the eighth to the tenth rib (see Fig. 10-3). This border changes during inspiration (diaphragm moves downward, expanding the area for resonant percussion) and during expiration (diaphragm moves upward). As the lungs expand

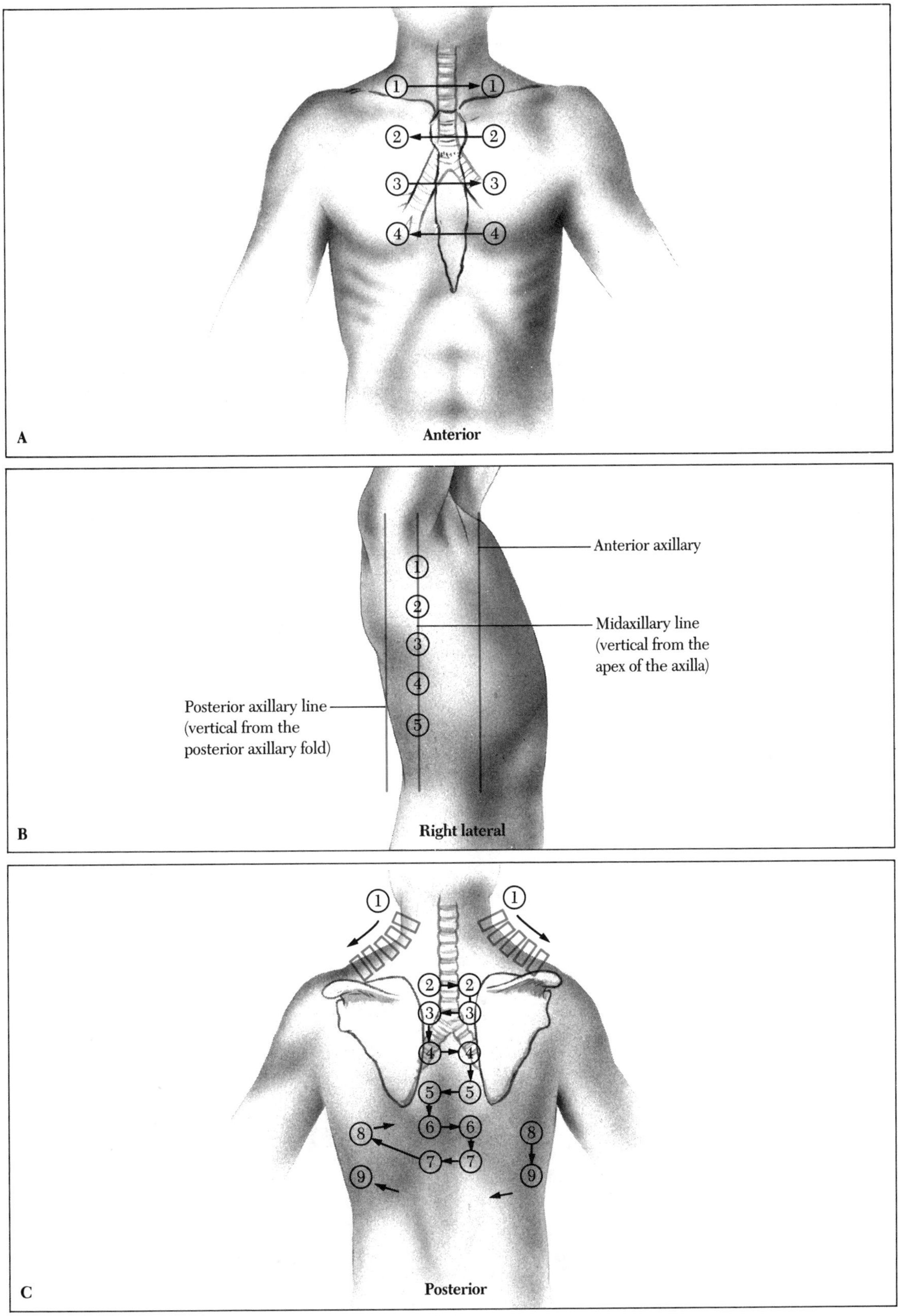

Figure 10-13 Method of thoracic percussion. **(A)** Percussion of anterior thorax. **(B)** Right lateral percussion. **(C)** Percussion of posterior thorax.

and deflate, the area of underlying lung tissue with the accompanying percussion resonance does the same. You may wish to locate the lower border of the lung by checking where the level of fremitus disappears; this will give you an approximation of at what point you will detect percussion dullness.

Figure 10-14 illustrates excursion of the diaphragm.

- Carefully observe the client so that she does not become hypoxic.
- Instruct the client to let you know immediately if she becomes dizzy.
- Ask the client to take a deep breath, let it out, and hold it at the end of expiration. Demonstrate this for the client. Then percuss down one side of the posterior thorax until dullness is found. Note this level of dullness; it identifies the lower lung base and the level of the diaphragm.
- Ask the client to take a deep breath and hold it. Repeat the percussion of the side to the border of dullness, which will normally be lower, since the lungs will have become expanded, and the diaphragm will have moved down in the normal respiratory system.
- Measure the distance from the first level of dullness to the second level of dullness; this is the diaphragmatic excursion.
- Repeat the same procedure on the other side of the posterior thorax.
- The diaphragmatic excursion of both left and right sides should be essentially equal. The normal diaphragmatic excursion is about 1 to 2 rib spaces in children and 3 to 6 cm in adults.

An athlete will ordinarily have a diaphragmatic excursion in the upper end of the normal range. Decreased diaphragmatic excursion is often seen in the elderly because of age-related enlargement of the alveoli and bronchial ducts.

Auscultation

The sounds heard by auscultation of the lungs are the result of the movement of air through the trachea, bronchi, and alveoli. Normal breath sounds are of three variations: vesicular breath sounds, bronchovesicular sounds, and bronchial sounds. You should listen over normal lung fields to begin to understand and identify these sounds.

Vesicular breath sounds, heard over most of the normal lung, result from air swirling through the bronchioles and alveoli. They are soft, low-pitched sounds often described as gentle sighing or as like a "breeze in the trees." They are basically an inspiratory sound because they reflect the passage of air into the alveoli. The best example of this sound can be heard at the base of the lungs. With vesicular breathing, the inspiratory phase is longer than the expiratory phase. Inspiration is usually higher pitched and louder than expiration. At times, expiration may be inaudible.

Bronchovesicular sounds are a mixture of vesicular and bronchial breath sounds. Normally, these sounds can be heard over the bronchi on each side of the sternum at the level of the first and second intercostal spaces; they are also heard posteriorly between the scapulae. The inspiratory and expiratory phases in bronchovesicular breathing are approximately equal and do not have a pause between inspiration and expiration.

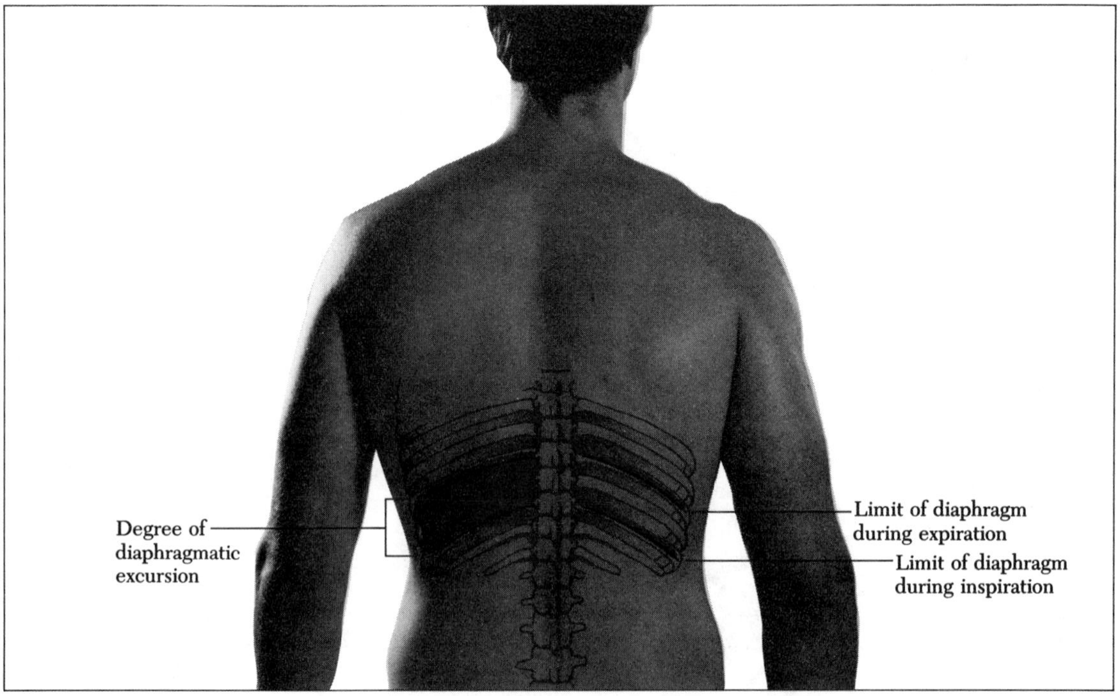

Figure 10-14 Method of determining diaphragmatic excursion.

Technique for Determining Diaphragmatic Excursion

1. Have the client take a deep breath and let it out.
2. Percuss downward from area of resonance.
3. Mark the level of dullness.
4. Ask client to take a deep breath and hold it.
5. Percuss from about 3 to 4 inches above the marked level of dullness.
6. Mark the new level of dullness and measure the distance downward from the first level of dullness.
7. Observe client for pallor and vertigo during procedure.

Technique for Auscultation of the Lungs

1. Warm stethoscope with hands.
2. Check that client's head is in midline position.
3. Ask client to breathe through open mouth and take slightly deeper than normal breaths.
4. Diaphragm of stethoscope is placed firmly on chest.
5. Proceed at 2- to 3-inch intervals side to side on anterior and posterior aspects of chest.
6. Proceed at 2- to 3-inch intervals from axillae to lung bases.
7. Decision making: Employ bronchophony, egophony, and whispered pectoriloquy techniques if abnormal ausculatory sounds are detected.

Bronchial sounds are moderately high-pitched sounds that result from turbulence of air as it passes through the bronchi. To understand how bronchial respirations sound, listen near the manubrium. These sounds are much louder than vesicular sounds and are characterized by a short inspiratory phase and a long expiratory phase.

Table 10-3 provides a tabular synopsis of the characteristics of normal breath sounds.

Tracheal sounds are loud and raspy. Listen directly over your trachea just below the larynx. Tracheal sounds have a loud, long inspiratory phase, a pause, and then a loud, long expiratory phase. *Tracheal sounds* ***never*** *are heard over* ***normal*** *lung fields.*Figure 10-15 shows locations of normal breath sounds of the neck and thorax.

In the adult bronchovesicular sounds are not heard in any areas of the normal lung other than those mentioned above. In the child the lung sounds are normally louder because of the thinness of the chest wall; therefore, the sound quality affords little diagnostic value.

Auscultate on the posterior chest wall from above the scapulae (this will include the apices of the lungs). Compare both sides of the chest as you auscultate first the left side and then the right side before moving down a couple of inches each time toward the base of the lungs.

Always place the stethoscope firmly against the chest wall. Without firm placement, chest hair may rub against the diaphragm, mimicking fine rales. If chest hair interferes with auscultation, moisten the hair with a wet washcloth; this will cause the hair to adhere to the chest, and there will be less movement of the hair directly on the diaphragm of your stethoscope. Avoid blowing or breathing on the stethoscope while auscultating, as this, too, will produce abnormal sounds.

To auscultate the client's breath sounds:

- Make certain that the client's head is in the midline position during auscultation. This is especially important with children because a slight turn of the head may narrow their flexible bronchi and decrease the breath sounds, suggesting possible pathology when none actually exists.
- Instruct the client to breathe normally through an opened mouth.

Table 10-3 **Characteristics of Breath Sounds**

Type	Description	Schematic representation	Normal location
Vesicular	Soft, low-pitched Inspiration *longer, louder,* and higher pitched than expiration		Heard over most of the chest and peripheral lung fields
Bronchovesicular	Higher pitched Inspiration and expiration have very *similar* pitch, *duration, intensity.*		Anterior—on either side of sternum around first and second interspaces; posterior—between scapula.
Bronchial	Blowing, hollow, and high-pitched *Expiration longer, louder,* high-pitched, tubular	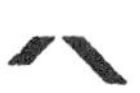	Anterior—near the manubrium midline on the chest. Abnormal when heard over lung field tissue.

Key: length = duration: long or short; thickness = loudness intensity.

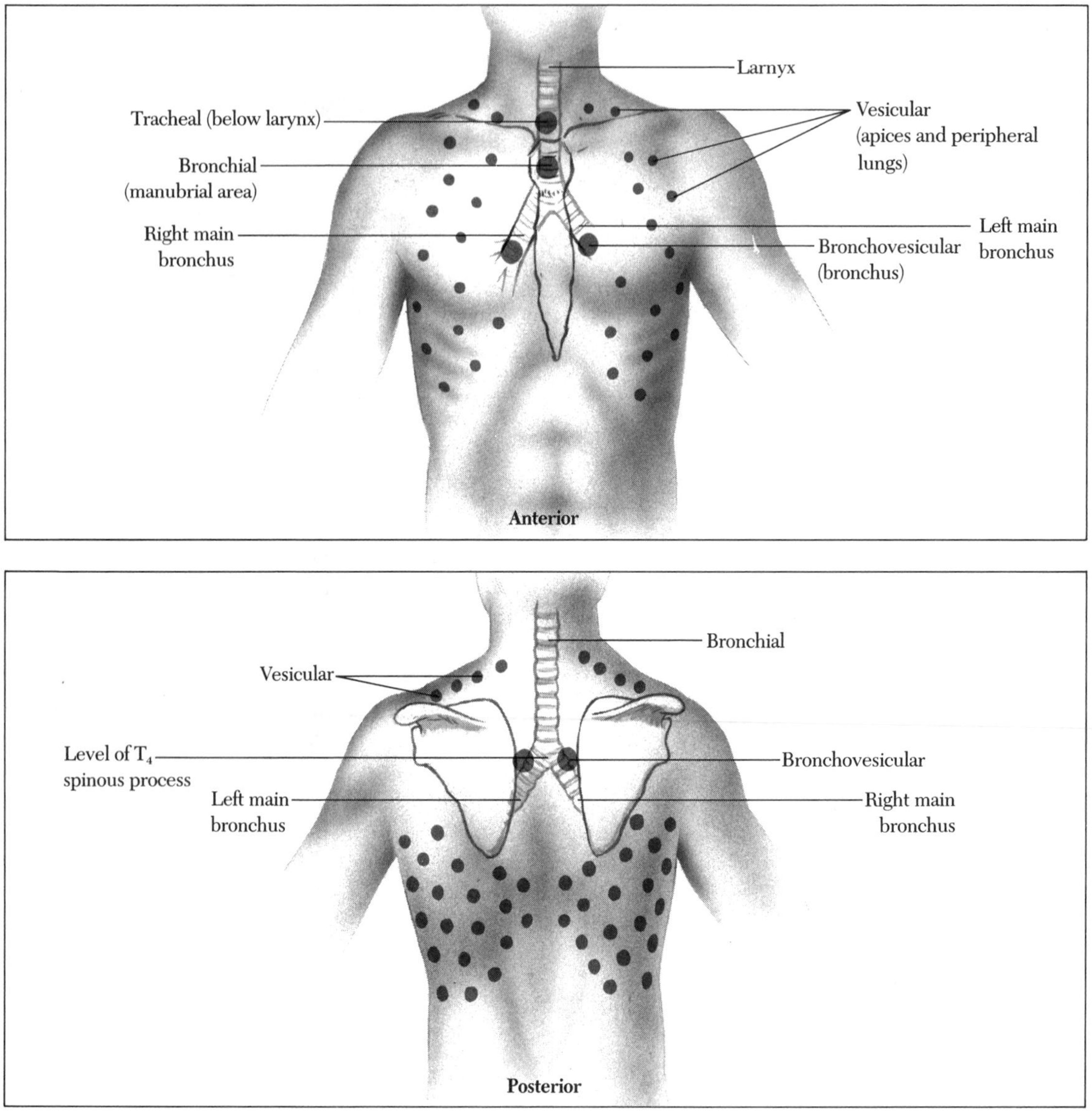

Figure 10-15 Locations of normal breath sounds of the neck and thorax (all small circles are vesicular).

- Place the diaphragm of the stethoscope *firmly* on the chest wall and begin listening to the anterior chest from slightly above the clavicles to include assessment of the apices to; Continue listening from the left lung to the right on down to the base of the lungs. Auscultation of the left lung is difficult on the anterior wall because the sounds from the heart interfere.
- Listen from under the axilla to the base of the lungs on both sides of the chest. This is important because sounds emanating from the right middle lobe can best be heard on the right lateral side of the chest.
- Auscultate the posterior chest wall from above the scapulae to include the apices of the lungs (see Fig. 10-3 for location of the apices of the lungs). Compare both sides of the chest as you auscultate first the left side and then the right side before moving down a couple of inches each time toward the base of the lungs.

The most common cause of changes in breath sounds is the presence of fluid in the lungs. Thus, bronchovesicular sounds heard at the base and the periphery of the lungs are present in such conditions as pneumonia and pleurisy.

Sounds not usually heard over the normal lung fields are referred to as *adventitious* (extraneous) *sounds,* such as *crackles* (rales, pronounced "rahls"), *wheezes* (sibilant and sonorous rhonchi), and *rubs.*

Crackles, or rales, are produced by movement of air into fluid-containing tissue. They are always considered abnormal, although transient fine crackles may be detected in clients who have been underventilating, such as bedridden elderly clients. A cough or a few deep breaths will expand the lung bases and eliminate these adventitious noises.

Crackles (rales) are classified in many ways, but the simplest and best is according to the sound pitch, which is termed *fine, medium,* or *coarse.*

1. *Fine crackles (crepitant rales)* are best heard at the end of inspiration and reflect the passing of air through fluid in the intricate alveoli of the lungs. The sound of a fine crackle can be simulated by holding several pieces of your hair close to your ear and rolling them back and forth between your thumb and index finger.
2. *Medium crackles (subcrepitant rales)* occur with the presence of increased fluid in the bronchi, as would exist in congestive heart failure, with pulmonary edema, and in bronchial inflammation (bronchiolitis, bronchitis). They sound like the fizz of a carbonated beverage, a bit louder than fine crackles.
3. *Coarse crackles (bubbling rales)* are produced by air passing through fluid-filled bronchi and the trachea. They are fairly continuous throughout inspiration and expiration and have a gurgling bubbly quality; the coarsest are characterized by the "death rattle."

Wheezes (musical or sibilant rales and sonorous rales), or rhonchi, occur when air passes through narrowed trachea, bronchi, and bronchioles. They occur in both phases of respiration but are more prominent during expiration, when there is more resistance. To accentuate these adventitious sounds, instruct the client to take a deep breath and then to force it out hard.

A wheeze or sibilant rhonchus is a high-pitched sound generally heard on inspiration and expiration as the air passes through partially collapsed or obstructed airways, whereas a sonorous (snoring) rhonchus is a low-pitched sound heard on expiration. Wheezes are characteristic of chronic bronchitis, cystic fibrosis, asthma, and foreign-body aspiration.

A pleural friction rub is caused by the rubbing together of the visceral and parietal pleurae. Normally, these two structures glide easily over one another. In cases in which there is inflammation of the pleura, as in pleurisy, the roughened, inflamed edges rub together, producing a characteristic grating sound. You can imitate this sound by laying the palm of your hand flat over your ear and then scratching the dorsum with a fingernail of your other hand.

A pleural friction rub is best heard in the lower anterior and lateral portions of the chest, as these are the areas of greatest thoracic movement. The rub is heard during both phases of respiration and increases in intensity during inspiration and with deep breaths. The sound also usually increases if the stethoscope is placed more firmly against the chest wall. This rub can be differentiated from a pericardial friction rub by asking the client to hold his breath. If the sound is still heard, it is a pericardial friction rub rather than a pleural friction rub.

Persistent smokers often have crackles that disappear after coughing. Crackles that disappear after coughing usually have no significance. In some instances, having the client cough at the end of expiration will loosen pulmonary exudates and produce inspiratory crackles. This maneuver will elicit the crackles that are an early sign of fluid accumulation.

Other Techniques

If abnormal percussion notes or abnormal lung sounds are discovered, you can perform three additional techniques: *bronchophony, whispered pectoriloquy,* and *egophony.* Although these techniques are not performed routinely in a screening examination, they can be used for further investigation of an abnormality discovered in the lung examination. The underlying scientific principle of these techniques is that fluid or consolidation will transmit the vibrations of the spoken or whispered voice through the lungs to the chest wall.

Both bronchophony and whispered pectoriloquy will aid in the detection of consolidation. In testing for bronchophony, the client is asked to softly repeat the numbers "1-2-3" several times. Normally you can hear the client's spoken word over a bronchus, but if you hear it clearly during these procedures through your stethoscope in the periphery of the lung, an abnormal condition is indicated.

In testing for whispered pectoriloquy, the client is asked to whisper so that the vocal cords are not used. The

Special Assessment Techniques of the Lungs

1. *Bronchophony:* Place diaphragm of stethoscope over abnormal area of lung field. Ask client to softly repeat "1-2-3." **Normal finding: "1-2-3" sounds muffled.** Presence of bronchophony is pathologic. Finding in bronchophony is clearly transmitted "1-2-3."
2. *Egophony:* Place diaphragm of stethoscope over abnormal area of lung field. Ask client to say "eeeeeee." **Normal finding: "eeeeeee" sound maintained.** Presence of egophony is pathologic and is reflected by the change of "eeeeee" to an "aaaaayyh" sound.
3. *Whispered pectoriloquy:* With the diaphragm of the stethoscope over an abnormal area of the lung, ask the client to whisper "1-2-3." **The normal finding is a muffled, whispered "1-2-3."** The pathologic presence of whispered pectoriloquy is reflected by sharp/distinct, clear transmission of the whispered "1-2-3."

client's whispered voice should be heard faintly and indistinctly through the chest wall. If the whispered words become distinguishable throughout the chest wall, abnormality exists.

Egophony is a form of bronchophony that uses the principle that fluid favors higher pitches and that it will alter the pattern of the spoken word. Ask the client to repeat the sound "eeee." If egophony is present, it will sound like "aaaa" through your stethoscope. This change of sound denotes abnormality. These abnormal sounds will be heard in varying degrees, depending on the amount of consolidation and fluid present.

Table 10-4 addresses assessment regarding oxygen supply and demand in relation to conditions for healthy lungs and conditions that alter function.

CLINICAL CORRELATIONS

Inspection

Acne lesions, seborrheic keratosis, and cafe au lait spots more often occur on the posterior aspect of the thorax. Dilation of superficial veins on the anterior chest wall is characteristic of superior vena cava obstruction.

Table 10-4 Assessing Problems of Oxygen Supply and Demand

Component of respiration	Conditions for healthy lungs	Conditions that alter function	Nursing assessment
Ventilation	Normal chest anatomy	Scoliosis Kyphosis	Inspection Structural deformity Tracheal deviation Use of accessory muscles Retractions Effect of position on breathing Depth of ventilation Length of expiration Abdominal distention Wounds, incisions Restrictive dressing Rate and pattern of ventilation Level of consciousness Neurologic examination Palpation Symmetry of chest excursion Crepitus Tactile fremitus Ausculation Breath sounds Adventitious sounds Voice sounds
	Intact and compliant chest wall	Flail chest Barrel chest	
	Functioning respiratory muscles receiving appropriate neurotransmissions	Spinal cord injury Guillain-Barré syndrome Muscle relaxants Status epilepticus Tetanus	
	Intact pleural membranes with negative intrapleural pressure	Pneumothorax Pleural effusion	
	Open and intact upper airways	Aspiration Laryngeal edema Bronchospasm	
	Compliant lung tissue	Atelectasis Fibrosis	
	Appropriate conscious control	Anxiety Plain on inspiration	
	Functioning chemical and neurologic systems	Cerebral anoxia High fever Barbiturates, opiates Anesthesia Acid-base imbalance Increased intracranial pressure	
Diffusion	Adequate O_2 and tension	High altitudes	Inspection Dyspnea Cough Sputum Vital signs Digit clubbing Cyanosis (a late sign) Palpation Tactile fremitus Ausculation Breath sounds Adventitious sounds Voice sounds
	Thin, healthy alveolar-capillary membrane	Thick alveolar-capillary membrane: fibrosis exudate	
	Adequate alveolar-capillary surface area	Lobectomy Chronic obstructive pulmonary disease	
	Adequate perfusion	Increased dead space	
	Adequate ventilation	Increased shunting	

Table 10-4 Continued

Component of respiration	Conditions for healthy lungs	Conditions that alter function	Nursing assessment
Oxygen transport to the tissues	Adequate RBC count and hemoglobin levels	CO poisoning Anemia Abnormal RBCs Left shift in oxyhemoglobin	Inspection Color of membranes, nailbeds, skin Capillary refill Restlessness Edema Bruising Palpation Peripheral pulses Skin turgor, temperature Ausculation Apical pulse Blood pressure Breath sounds
	Appropriate blood volume	Hemorrhage Dehydration	
	Adequate cardiac output	Cor pulmonale Shock	
	Appropriate hemostasis	Abnormal bleeding and/or clotting	
	Unimpeded blood flow	Thrombosis	

An increase in AP diameter will be seen in conditions such as emphysema, where the client exhibits the classic barrel chest (Fig. 10-16). In the child, a persistent round chest after the age of 6 suggests a chronic pulmonary disease such as asthma.

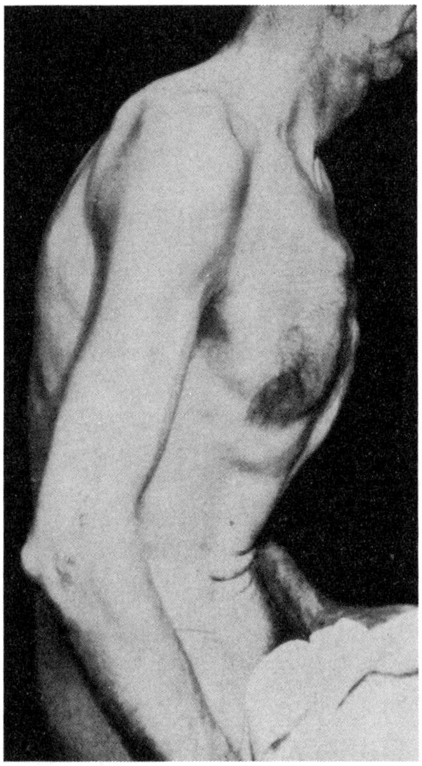

Figure 10-16 Barrel chest of emphysema. Note the increase in anterior-posterior diameter.

When the lower sternum is markedly depressed, with the ribs flared outward, the condition is called *pectus excavatum,* or funnel chest (Fig. 10-17). When the sternum protrudes markedly, the chest takes on the configuration of a pigeon and is thus referred to as a pigeon breast (Fig. 10-18). This is termed *pectus carinatum.*

Asymmetry of the thorax also is common with *scoliosis,* an abnormal condition. The deviation of thoracic shape from these skeletal deformities can be seen as they are super-

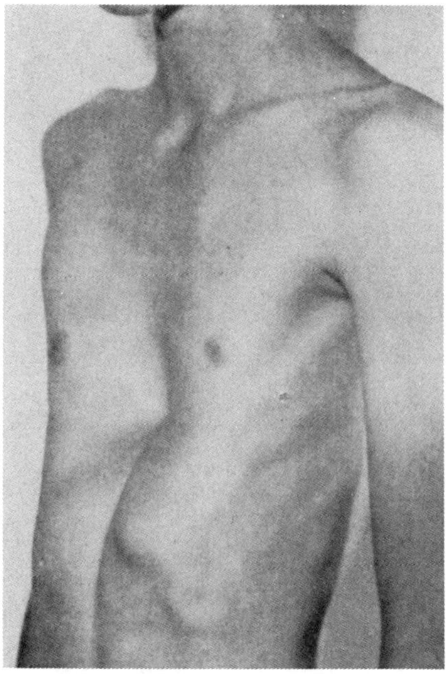

Figure 10-17 Funnel chest. Note the deep depression of the lower sternum and the outward flare of the lower ribs.

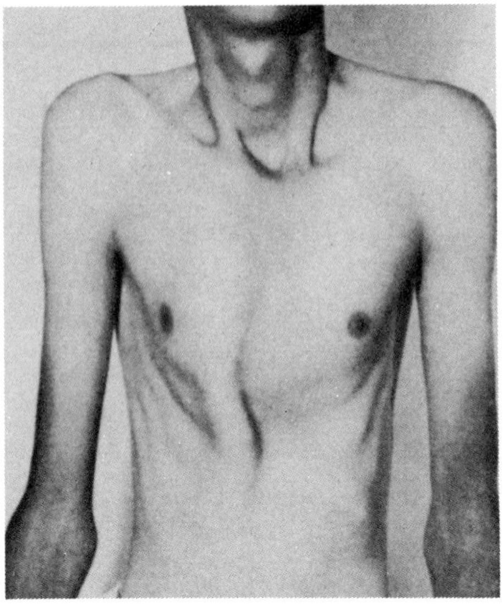

Figure 10-18 Pigeon breast as a result of rickets. Note the bilateral depression of the lower chest portion and the protrusion of the sternum.

imposed on a cross-section of the normally shaped thorax in Fig. 10-19.

Retraction of the ribs and ICSs may indicate a collapsed lung or fractured ribs. Bulging of the chest wall is suggestive of a greatly enlarged heart or of an aortic aneurysm.

Long-standing vitamin deficiencies such as rickets cause prominence of the costochondral junctions. This condition is termed *rachitic rosary* because of the prominent knobs that form at these angles (Fig. 10-20).

The accessory muscles of the neck become strained in such diseases as emphysema and asthma, when the act of breathing becomes an effort.

Palpation

Tracheal deviation to one side may be seen in a mediastinal shift resulting from a pneumonectomy, aortic aneurysm, a mass, or scoliosis. Figure 10-21 shows that pressure from pleural effusion, tension pneumothorax, and a mass causes the trachea to move away from the affected side, whereas

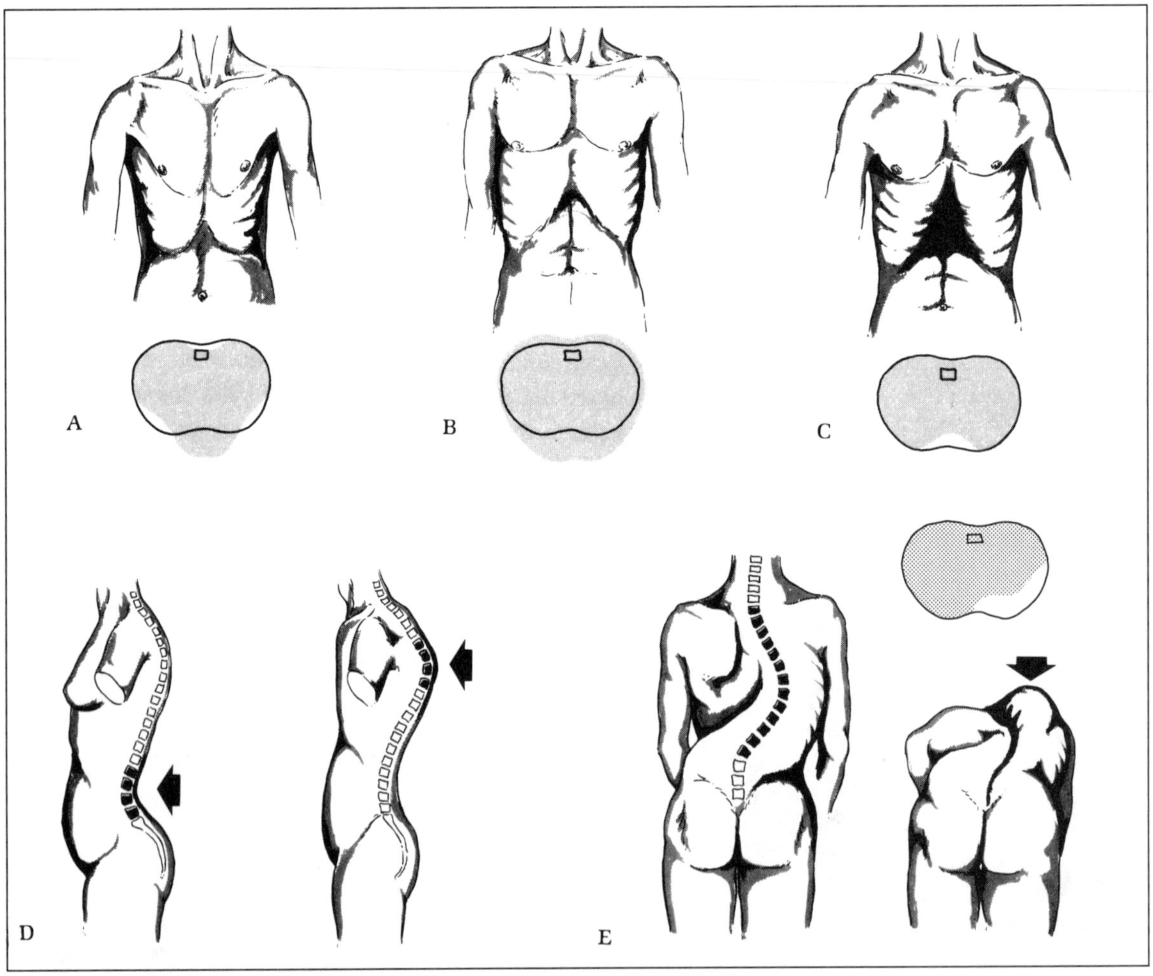

Figure 10-19 Deformities of bony structure of the chest and spine. **(A)** Pigeon breast. **(B)** Barrel chest. **(C)** Funnel chest. **(D)** Lordosis and xyphosis. **(E)** Scoliosis. (From Sana, J.M. and Judge, R.D. *Physical Assessment for Nursing Skills* (2nd ed.). Boston: Little, Brown, 1982, p. 202.)

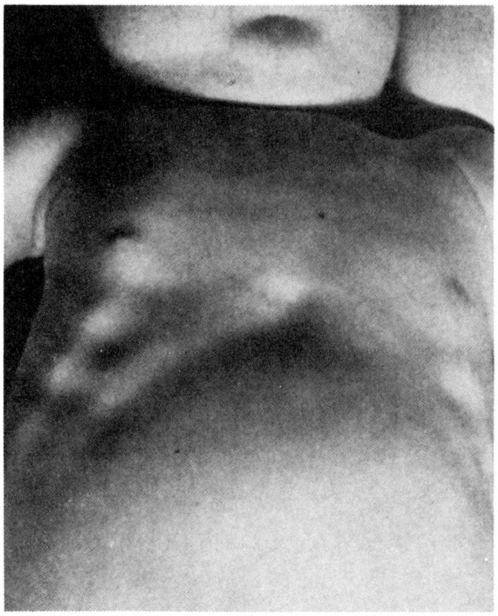

Figure 10-20 Rachitic rosary. Note the series of prominences corresponding to the costochondral junctions.

scar tissue, scoliosis, and atelectasis (collapse) will pull the trachea toward the affected side.

Pain, swelling, or abnormal movement may be indicative of fractured ribs or pleurisy. With pleurisy the pain becomes distinctively more severe on deep inspiration. Pain in the ICSs may be caused by a neuritis of the intercostal nerves and by myositis (irritation of a muscle).

Crepitation, a coarse, crackling sensation of the skin that results from air escaping from the respiratory system and entering the subcutaneous tissues, may be observed in pneumothorax and sometimes in the tissues surrounding a tracheostomy.

Fractured ribs, pleurisy, pulmonary fibrosis, and arthritis of the spine can produce uneven or reduced chest expansion. In severe emphysema, there is little expansion because air is trapped in the lungs, leaving them more or less always expanded, with little room for additional movement.

Increased vocal fremitus occurs when there is consolidation of the lung, as in pneumonia. Decreased or absent fremitus may be found in the obstruction of a bronchus or in pneumothorax.

Percussion

The client with pneumonia will exhibit dullness over the affected lung. Pleural fluid, pleural thickening, fibrosis, tumors, and an area of atelectasis (collapsed lung tissue) will sound dull in relation to surrounding normal lung tissue.

Diaphragmatic excursion is decreased in the hyperinflated condition of emphysema. Upward displacement of the diaphragm is associated with atelectasis, intraabdominal masses, pregnancy, severe obesity, and ascites. Diaphragmatic excursion may be decreased if there is pneumonia, pleural effusion, or pneumothorax. Phrenic nerve paralysis causes the diaphragm to move upward, and its motion may be paradoxical during breathing respiration.

Auscultation

Adventitious sounds are signs and symptoms of a variety of lung disorders, as shown in Table 10-5. Pleural friction rub may be heard in such conditions as pneumonia, pulmonary embolus, emphysema, neoplasm, lung abscess, and tuberculosis.

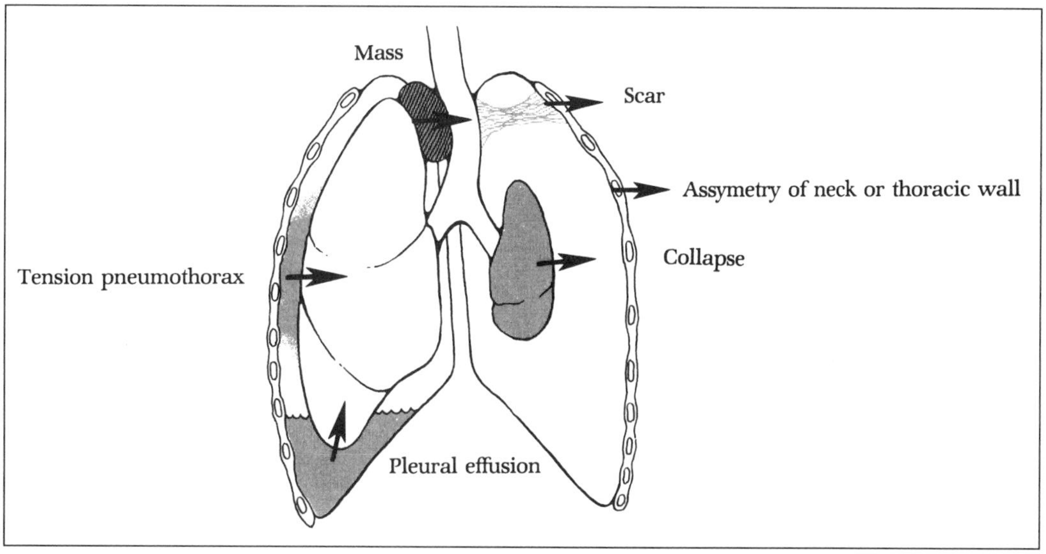

Figure 10-21 Causes of tracheal deviation. (From Sana, J.M. and Judge, R.D. *Physical Assessment for Nursing Skills* (2nd ed.). Boston: Little, Brown, 1982, p. 193.)

RECORDING OF FINDINGS

Normal findings are presented in the left column. The right column contains findings for an individual who has been medically diagnosed as having chronic obstructive lung disease.

Lungs
Inspection: Symmetrical expansion; AP diameter less than transverse diameter.

Palpation: No tenderness, pulsations, or crepitus; expansion equal bilaterally; fremitus present.

Percussion: Lung fields resonant; diaphragmatic excursion 4 cm bilaterally.

Auscultation: Vesicular breath sounds present; no crackles, wheezes, or rubs.

Lungs
Inspection: Increased AP diameter; sits forward with hands on knees; marked retraction of ICS; dyspnea at rest; use of accessory muscles.

Palpation: Expansion decreased, fremitus present; palpable rhonchi over base of left lung.

Percussion: Right lung and left upper lobe hyperresonant; dullness over left lower lobe; diaphragmatic excursion 1 cm bilaterally.

Auscultation: Normal vesicular sounds in right lung and left upper lobe; tracheal breath sounds noted in left lower lobe; inspiratory and expiratory wheezing; egophony in left lower lobe.

Table 10-5 Signs and Symptoms of Lung Disorders

Process	Inspection	Palpation	Percussion	Auscultation
Pneumonia	Coryza symptoms; pyrexia, chills; productive cough; rapid, shallow, grunting respirations (dyspnea); pleuritic pain (splinting of chest); occasional cyanosis	Limited motion of chest on affected side; increased fremitus when consolidation fully established	Dullness; decreased diaphragmatic excursion	Early: decreased breath sounds Later: bronchial sounds; bronchophony; whispered pectoriloquy; fine crackles (crepitant rales); occasional pleural friction rub
Chronic obstructive lung disease	Increased respiratory rate; pursed lip breathing; increased AP diameter (barrel chest); use of accessory muscles and intercostal retraction; leaning forward to assist breathing; cyanosis or hyperemia (depends on type); increased JVP	Decreased fremitus; diminished chest expansion; possible crepitus; rhonchal fremitus	Decreased diaphragmatic excursion; hyperresonance; lowered hepatic dullness	Decreased breath sounds; prolonged expirations; crackles, wheezes, or rhonchi; in some instances, no adventitious sounds present
Bronchitis	Cough with sputum production; sore throat; fever; malaise; occasional dyspnea with use of accessory muscles	Normal fremitus	Resonance	May have prolonged expirations with vesicular breath sounds; wheezes, crackles, and rhonchi may be heard.
Pleural effusion	Pain; dyspnea; pallor	Prominence of interspaces; tracheal deviation from side of effusion; decreased fremitus	Increasing dullness with the increase in amount of fluid	Decreased breath sounds; egophony and whispered pectoriloquy; possible pleural friction rub

Table 10-5 **Continued**

Process	Inspection	Palpation	Percussion	Auscultation
Neoplasm	Asymptomatic or mild cough; fever; chills; sputum	Mass may be palpated if on chest wall; absent fremitus. If site is upper lobes near the trachea, possible trachea deviation away from tumor.	Dull over area of lesion	Decreased breath sounds if airway is occluded; egophony and whispered pectoriloquy if airway is not occluded; often fine crackles and localized wheezes; occasional pleural friction rub
Atelectasis	Increased respiratory rate; increased pulse; often cyanosis	Tracheal shift to side of involvement; decreased fremitus; decreased chest expansion on affected side	Dullness	Diminished breath sounds; occasional rales
Pulmonary edema	Increased respiratory rate; cyanosis; sitting upright; use of accessory muscles; apprehension	Increased fremitus	Dullness	Bronchovesicular breath sounds, often obscured later by crackles, rhonchi, and wheezing
Pneumothorax	Pain; dyspnea and cyanosis; apprehension; increased respiratory rate	Possible tracheal shift away from side of pneumothorax; absent fremitus on affected side	Hyperresonance; decreased diaphragmatic excursion on affected side	Absent breath sounds on affected side
Emphysema	Dyspnea; wheezing; cough with sputum; increased use of accessory muscles of the neck; exhaustion	Normal fremitus or decreased; occasional palpable rhonchi	Hyperresonance; decreased diaphragmatic excursion	Vesicular or bronchovesicular sounds; wheezes/rhonchi throughout chest

BIOLOGIC AND CULTURAL VARIATIONS

Tuberculosis Among African-Americans and Native Americans

Tuberculosis is an infectious disease caused by the bacillus *Mycobacterium tuberculosis.* As a communicable disease, it is usually contracted through inhaling airborne respiratory droplets from an individual with an active case. Because the tubercle bacilli are usually contacted in this way, pulmonary tuberculosis is the most frequent form of the infection, as opposed to renal, intestinal, or bone and joint forms of the disease.

At the beginning of the twentieth century, tuberculosis was the second leading cause of death in the United States, accounting for 11.3% of all deaths. By 1972, however, it was no longer ranked among the twenty leading causes of death. In that year, the age-adjusted death rate from tuberculosis among white Americans was 1.7 per 100,000. The decline in morbidity and mortality rates from tuberculosis is attributed to a number of changes, including improvements in public health and sanitation measures after the turn of the century, and general improvement in the economic status and lifestyle of most Americans, and the onset of specific chemotherapy measures in 1946.

However, there are some population groups in the United States that continue to suffer from relatively high rates of tuberculosis morbidity and mortality. Most notable are Native Americans and African-Americans. In 1972, records from Native American health service agencies and hospitals showed the age-adjusted death rate from tuberculosis among Native Americans to be 9.1 per 100,000, which is more than five times the death rate of white Americans (U.S. Congress American Indian Policy

BIOLOGIC AND CULTURAL VARIATIONS

Tuberculosis Among African-Americans and Native Americans (continued)

Review Commission 1976). Alaskan Natives appear to be particularly at risk. In the same year, the tuberculosis mortality rate for African-Americans was also much higher than that of white Americans. The rate for nonwhite Americans (of which more than 90% are African-Americans) was 5.9 per 100,000 (U.S. Congress American Indian Policy Review Commission 1976). Tuberculosis morbidity rates were also remarkably higher among Native Americans and African-Americans. The proportion of individuals with active cases of tuberculosis in these population groups was 94.3 per 100,000 Native Americans, 151.4 per 100,000 Alaskan Natives, 50.3 per 100,000 nonwhite Americans, and 10.8 per 100,000 white Americans.

Environmental differences appear to be the cause of these higher tuberculosis rates. Native Americans and African-Americans have lower average income and socioeconomic status than white Americans and thus have less adequate medical care, housing, sanitation facilities, and nutritious food. There is a greater probability that individuals from these population groups will live in crowded, poorly ventilated homes with poor sanitation facilities, such as on reservations or in ghettoes in urban centers. Ghettoes and slum areas have long been high-risk environments that allow the rapid spread of tuberculosis. For example, in 1945 the tuberculosis death rate for African-Americans in cities of more than a million people was almost twice that of African-Americans in cities of 100,000 to 200,000 people (Pettigrew & Pettigrew 1974). The poor also tend to have inadequate diets and poor nutritional status, which leads to decreased disease resistance and increased rates of infection. For example, vitamin deficiencies, anemia, and protein deficiencies continue to be major health problems among Native Americans (U.S. Congress American Indian Policy Review Commission 1976).

It had long been hypothesized that African-Americans and Native Americans had decreased resistance to tuberculosis because of genetic and constitutional differences. It is true that African-Americans have a high incidence of a disease type that tends to present as acute tuberculosis pneumonia or to involve the mid-lung (Williams 1975). However, it is now clear that environmental differences offer the real explanation. If economic opportunities and living conditions continue to improve among African-Americans and Native Americans, tuberculosis rates will probably continue to decrease and approach the rate for white Americans.

SUMMARY

This chapter provided information about the structure and function of the thorax and lungs. The chest has certain landmarks that are helpful in describing physical findings. The thorax and lungs were examined, beginning with inspection, then palpation, followed by percussion and auscultation. Percussion should be performed in a systematic manner on the anterior, lateral, and posterior walls of the chest. Auscultation involves listening to breath sounds; all variations, both normal and abnormal, were discussed, as were a number of additional techniques not performed routinely in a screening examination.

DISCUSSION QUESTIONS/ ACTIVITIES

1. Compare the adult thoracic cage with that of the young child.
2. Discuss some possible causes for unequal expansion of the lungs.
3. Describe what is meant by the term *fremitus.* How is fremitus detected?
4. Describe various percussion notes that can be heard over the thorax and why.
5. What is meant by the term *diaphragmatic excursion?* Demonstrate the procedure for determining the degree of diaphragmatic excursion.
6. Describe the three variations of normal breath sounds heard over the lung fields.
7. Name and describe the three categories of sounds heard in the lungs due to pathology and/or fluid.

REFERENCES

Pettigrew, A. H., and Pettigrew, T. F. 1974. Race, disease and desegregation: a new look. In *Ethnic groups of America: their morbidity, mortality and behavior disorders,* vol. II., ed. A. Shiloh and I. C. Selevan. Springfield, Ill.: Charles C Thomas.

U.S. Congress American Indian Policy Review Commission. 1976. *Task force six: Indian health.* Washington, D.C.: U.S. Government Printing Office.

Williams, R. A. 1975. *Textbook of black-related diseases.* New York: McGraw-Hill.

CHAPTER

11

Assessment of the Cardiovascular System

Learning Objectives

1. State the characteristics of inspection and palpation of the extremities in relation to peripheral cardiovascular assessment.
2. Identify the locations for palpation of the peripheral pulses.
3. State the various categories of pulse amplitude.
4. Review the structure and function of the heart.
5. Identify the areas on the anterior chest that are inspected and palpated in assessing heart function.
6. Describe the techniques of percussion and auscultation of the heart.
7. Explain the normal heart sounds.
8. Describe the technique for measuring jugular venous distention.

In this chapter the necessary techniques to assess the cardiovascular system are described in detail, as are the basic structures of the cardiovascular system. Assessment of the cardiovascular system requires mastery of a number of special abilities and techniques. Assessment begins at the periphery and progresses toward the center of the circulatory system, the heart.

ASSESSMENT OF PERIPHERAL PULSES

Palpation of the peripheral pulses is an ancient and time-honored practice. The pulses are an index of the heart's action. With each ventricular contraction, the blood is ejected into the aorta, and the pressure of this is transmitted as a wave. This wave causes expansion and elongation of the arteries, which results in palpable and visible pulses.

- Inspect the skin and nails of the arms and legs.
- Check capillary refill.
- Observe venous pattern and venous circulation. Hand veins will normally fill when in the dependent position. When the hands are raised to the level of the heart, the veins normally will empty within 3 to 5 seconds (Fig. 11-1).
- Palpate the epitrochlear nodes. Normally, they are nonpalpable (Fig. 11-2). Adenopathy may be present with ulnar hand and forearm infections as well as with non-Hodgkin's lymphomas.
- Palpate the popliteal nodes on the medial aspect of the popliteal space. Normally, they are nonpalpable. Adenopathy may be associated with repeated injury, inflammation, and infection of the leg.

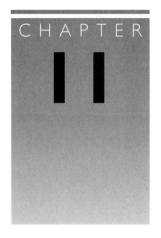

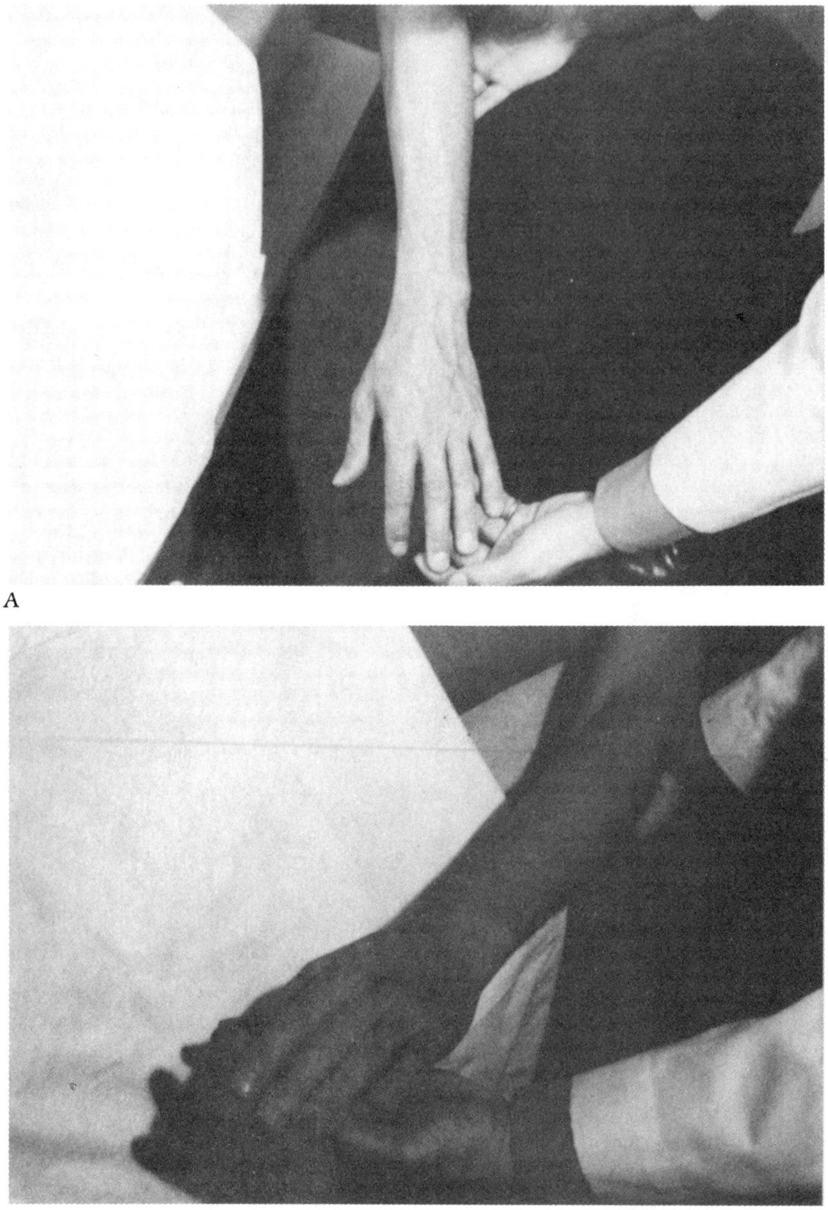

A

B

Figure 11-1 Normal venous distention of the extremities. **(A)** Upper extremity in dependent position: Note apparent distention. **(B)** Upper extremity at heart level: Note absence of venous distention. (From Sana, J.M. and Judge, R.D. *Physical Assessment for Nursing Skills* (2nd ed.). Boston: Little, Brown, 1982, p. 253.)

- The peripheral pulses (temporal, carotid, brachial, radial, femoral, popliteal, posterior tibial, and dorsal pedal) are routinely assessed during the physical examination.
- The peripheral pulses **always** are assessed in clients with peripheral vascular disease (atherosclerosis, arteriosclerosis, diabetes mellitus, alcoholism, Raynaud's disease [Fig. 11-3], Buerger's disease, aneurysm), femoral bypass surgery, and vein ligations.
- With peripheral vascular signs and symptoms of the upper extremities, perform Allen's test on both hands to assess patency of the ulnar and radial arteries. Normally, there is immediate flow to the hand, with pink color return to the skin of the palm.
- Test the legs for calf tenderness and Homan's sign. Normally, there is no tenderness with either testing.

Figure 11-4 illustrates a record of peripheral pulse amplitudes using the standardized 3+ scale. In a normal re-

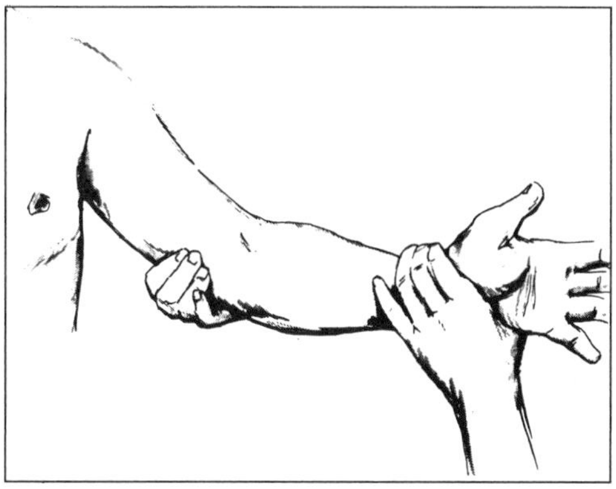

Figure 11-2 Site for assessing the epitrochlear lymph nodes. (From Sana, J.M. and Judge, R.D. *Physical Assessment for Nursing Skills* (2nd ed.). Boston: Little, Brown, 1982, p. 122.)

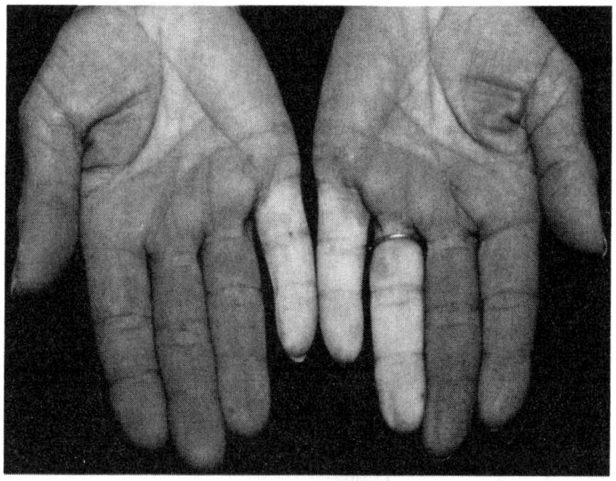

Figure 11-3 Marked pallor of digits due to vasospasm (Raynaud's phenomenon).

A Standardized Scale Used To Categorize Pulse Amplitude

0	Absent pulse
1+	Weak, thready pulse; may fade in and out and is obliterated with light pressure
2+	Normal; easily palpable; not easily obliterated by pressure
3+	Bounding; easily palpable; not obliterated by pressure

cording, 2+/3+, the numerator 2+ indicates normal pulse on a scale, with 3+ as the maximum pulse amplitude.

- The *carotids* should be palpated **one** at a time and **low** in the neck far away from the bifurcation of the carotid artery into the external and internal carotid branches because

Pulses		L	R
Carotid	C	2+/3+	2+/3+
Brachial	B	2+/3+	2+/3+
Radial	R	2+/3+	2+/3+
Femoral	F	2+/3+	1+/3+
Popliteal	P	2+/3+	0/3+
Posterior tibial	PT	2+/3+	0/3+
Dorsal pedal	DP	2+/3+	0/3+

Figure 11-4 Peripheral pulse amplitudes for a client diagnosed for right femoral partial occlusion.

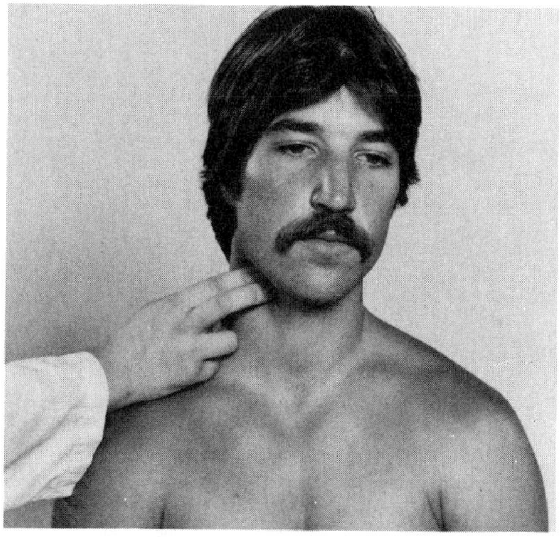

Figure 11-5 Location of the carotid sinus.

1. pressure on both carotids simultaneously may produce vertigo or syncope as a result of cerebral hypoxia (this is especially true in the elderly and in those clients with generalized vascular disease or local carotid artery pathology); and
2. the carotid sinus is located in the neck just above the bifurcation of the common carotid artery, pressure on or massage of this area can slow the heart rate. In certain situations, this slowing of the heart action **could be dangerous** (e.g., in a client with bradycardia or on digoxin).

In Figure 11-5, the examiner indicates the location of the carotid **sinus** high in the neck.

Figures 11-6 through 11-11 illustrate the location of the peripheral pulses that are palpated to detect the existence

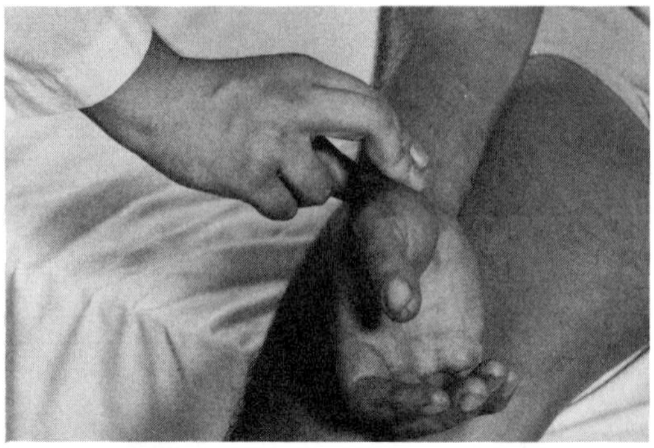

A

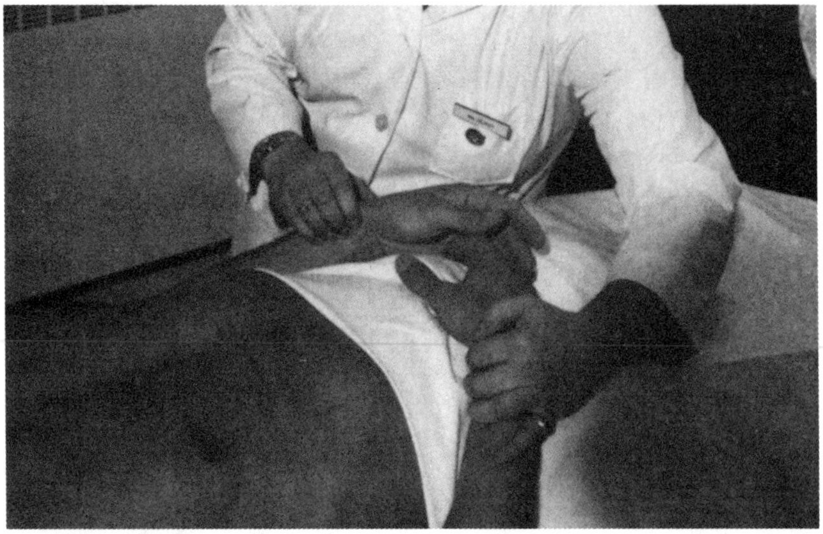

B

Figure 11-6 **(A)** Palpation of the radial artery. **(B)** Technique to assess radial arteries simultaneously. (From Sana, J.M. and Judge, R.D. *Physical Assessment for Nursing Skills* (2nd ed.). Boston: Little, Brown, 1982, p. 236.)

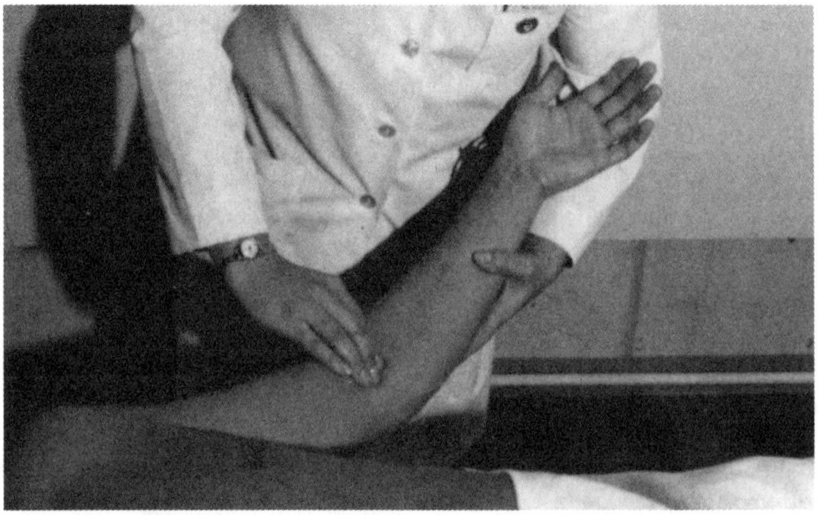

Figure 11-7 Palpation of the brachial artery. (From Sana J.M. and Judge, R.D. *Physical Assessment for Nursing Skills* (2nd ed.). Boston: Little, Brown, 1982, p. 253.)

Figure 11-8 Palpation of the femoral artery.

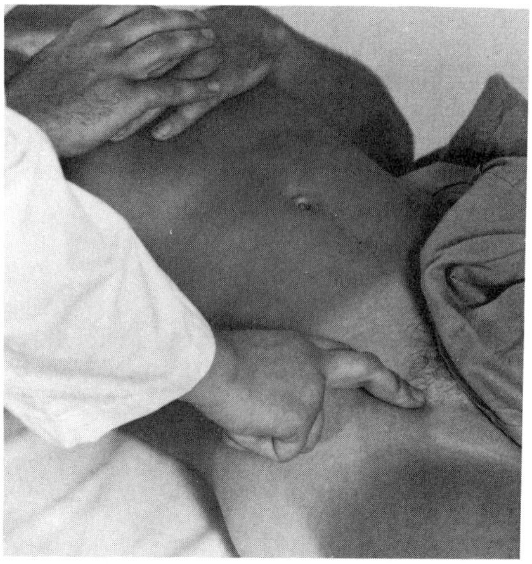

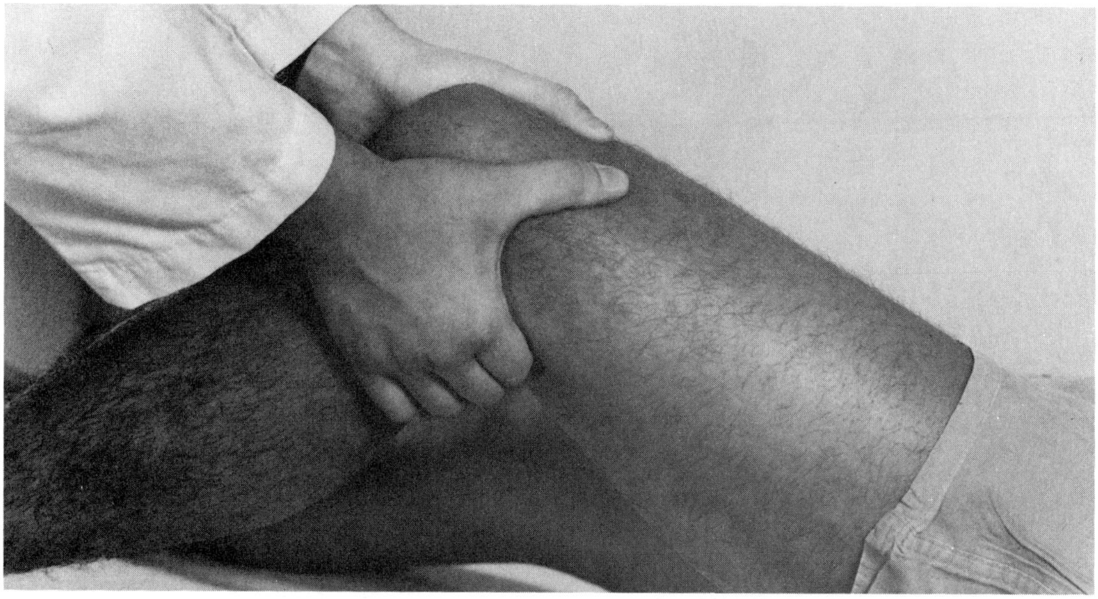

Figure 11-9 Palpation of the popliteal artery.

Figure 11-10 Palpation of the posterior tibial artery.

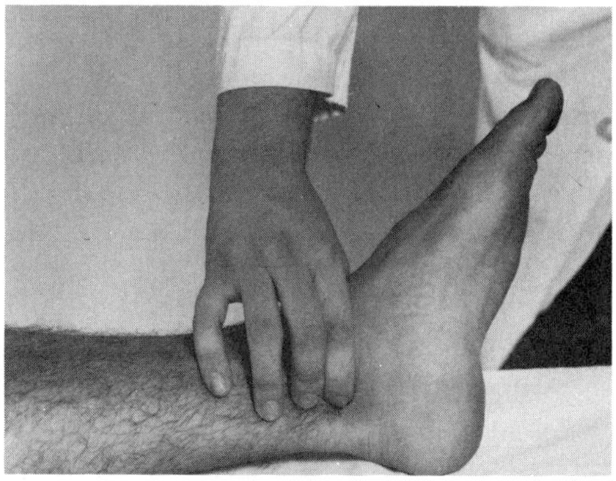

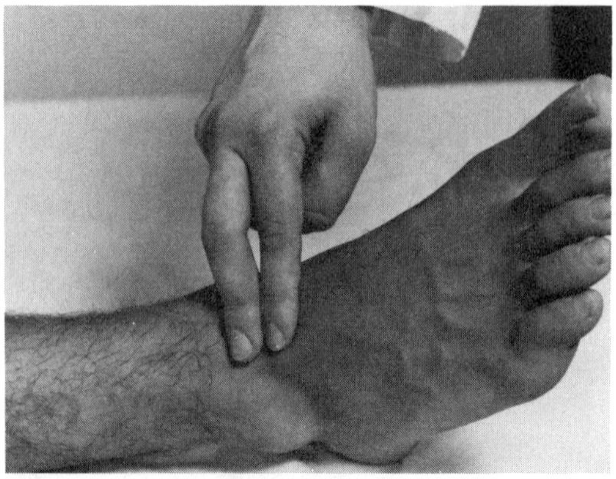

A

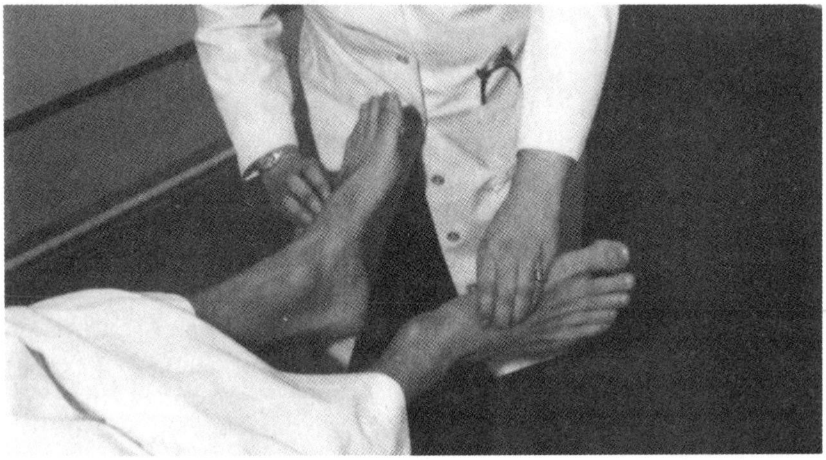

B

Figure 11-11 Palpation of the dorsal pedal artery. Technique for bilateral assessment of pedal pulses. (From Sana, J.M. and Judge, R.D. *Physical Assessment for Nursing Skills* (2nd ed.). Boston: Little, Brown, 1982, p. 234.)

of arterial insufficiency. Particularly in the elderly, the absence of a posterior tibial pulse (Fig. 11-10) or of a dorsal pedal pulse (Fig. 11-11) may be normal, but it can also indicate arterial obstructive disease. It is not uncommon to find a 1+ posterior tibial and/or dorsalis pedis pulse(s) in a normal person. Common abnormalities of rate, rhythm, and intensity in the arterial pulses are noted in Table 11-1.

Allen's test is performed by using your right and left thumbs to occlude the radial and ulnar arteries on both lateral and medial sides of the wrist of one of the client's supine-positioned hands. Have the client pump his hand a few times until it becomes pale and then open it palm up. Then release one thumb to assess the patency of the ulnar or radial artery, whichever artery you release. If patent, the blood will rush to the hand within 3 to 5 seconds; the palm will return to a normal pink color. Repeat the procedure on the same hand, but this time release pressure on the opposite artery to assess its patency. Repeat the two-step process on the client's other hand.

Homan's sign is pain in an extended leg on dorsiflexion of the foot. It is suggestive of inflammation (e.g., thrombophlebitis).

STRUCTURE AND FUNCTION OF THE HEART

The heart is a hollow muscular organ located in the mediastinum (Fig. 11-12). Approximately two thirds of the heart lies to the left of the midline of the body and one third to the right. The *apex* is located close to the diaphragm and points to the left. The apical heart rate can be determined by placing the stethoscope directly over the heart at its apex, which is normally at the 5th or 6th intercostal space (ICS), close to the left midclavicular line. The *base* of the heart lies below the second rib on either side of the sternum.

The strong fibrous sac encasing and protecting the heart is called the *pericardium*. Between the pericardium and the

Table 11-1 Common Abnormalities of the Arterial Pulses

Terminology	Characteristics	Comment
Weak pulse	Slow rise and prolonged peak, diminished pulse pressure	Congestive heart failure, aortic stenosis, shock
Bounding pulse	Pulse reaches higher in intensity than normal, then disappears quickly	Best detected when arm held aloft; may be due to anxiety, exercise, fever, anemia, hyperthyroidism; aortic regurgitation
Pulsus alternans	Regular rhythm with alternating weak and strong pulsations	Left-sided heart failure
Bigeminy	Two regular beats followed by a longer pause	Myocarditis, valvular disease; premature ventricular contractions
Pulsus paradoxus	Abnormal fall (8 mm Hg) in systolic blood pressure on inspiration	Obstructive lung disease, adherent pericarditis
Diminished femoral pulse	Determined in relation to radial pulse	Blood takes longer to reach lower extremities due to obstructed flow through aorta (i.e., coarctation of aorta, occlusive aortic disease)
Posterior tibial or dorsal pedal	Weak or absent	Can be normal, but may indicate arterial obstructive disease

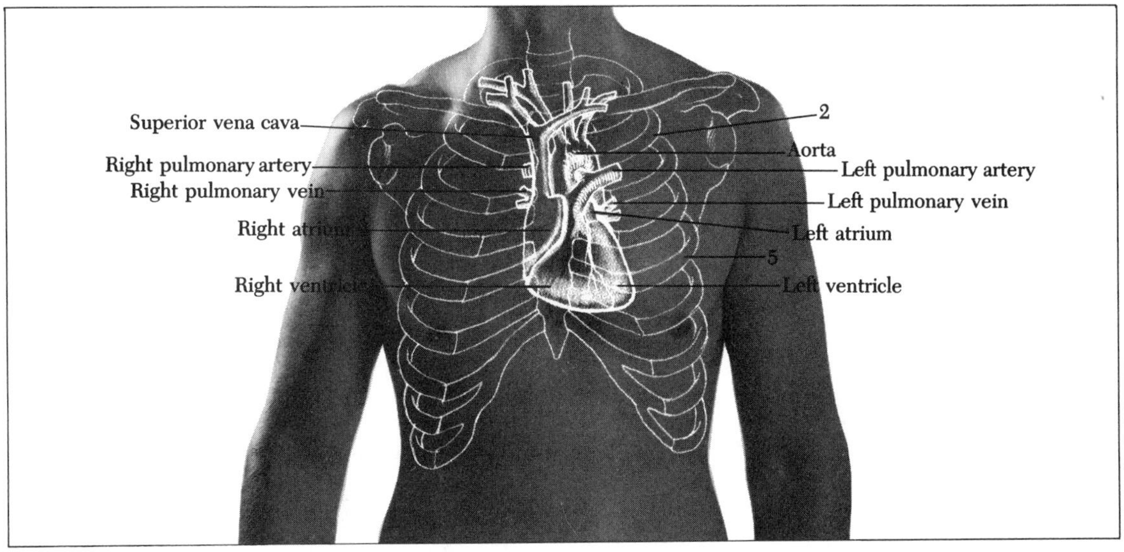

Figure 11-12 Location of the heart and great vessels.

heart is a small amount of serous fluid, which provides for easy, low-friction movement. The pericardium is secured to the diaphragm, sternum, pleura, esophagus, and aorta. The heart is composed of three layers. The *epicardium* is a thin, smooth lining that covers the outside of the myocardium and interfaces with the pericardium. The *myocardium* is a specialized muscular layer of the heart. The *endocardium* is a thin, delicate lining that lines the chambers of the heart and the heart valves.

Due to the way the heart is positioned sideways in the thorax, most of its anterior surface consists of the *right ventricle.* The *left ventricle* lies to the left and behind the right ventricle and forms the *left cardiac border.* The *left atrium* is situated posteriorly except for a small atrial appendage that makes up the left cardiac border. This appendage is located between the *left pulmonary artery* and the left ventricle and cannot usually be identified on physical examination. The right margin of the heart is formed by the right atrium; this portion of the heart is also not usually identifiable on physical examination.

The *superior and inferior vena cavas* carry venous blood from the upper and lower parts of the body and empty into the *right atrium.* The pulmonary artery is located in the superior portion of the right ventricle. It bifurcates into the right and left branches and carries blood to the lungs. Oxygenated blood is returned through the pulmonary veins, which empty into the left atrium. The *aorta* curves upward from the left ventricle to the level of the sternal angle and then arches back and down behind the heart.

The heart valves (Fig. 11-13) are devices that permit flow of blood through the heart in only one direction. The *tricuspid valve,* between the right atrium and the right ventricle, consists of three flaps of endocardium and is anchored to the right ventricle by cordlike structures called *chordae tendinae.* The *mitral valve,* between the left atrium and the left ventricle, is similar to the tricuspid valve in structure except that it has only two flaps and is sometimes referred to as the *bicuspid valve* because of this. The construction of both of these valves is such that blood is allowed to flow into the ventricles but is prevented from flowing back out of them into the atria.

The *aortic valve* and the *pulmonary valve* are located in the left and right ventricles, respectively, and allow the blood to flow from the ventricles into the aorta and the pulmonary artery. The aortic and pulmonary valves are called the *semilunar valves* because they consist of half-moon-shaped flaps growing from the pulmonary artery and the aorta. The valves prevent the blood from retrograde flow back into the ventricles.

The Conduction System

The heart has a specialized system for generating impulses that cause contraction of the heart and for conducting these impulses throughout the heart muscle (Fig. 11-14). The adult human heart generally beats about 70 to 80 beats/min. The impulse for these contractions begins in the *sinoatrial (SA) node,* which is located in the posterior part of the right atrium below the opening of the superior vena cava. The SA node is called the pacemaker of the heart because, under normal circumstances, it initiates each heartbeat. The excitation waves generated by the SA node cause the atria to contract. The impulse is then sent to the *atrioventricular (AV) node,* which is located at the lower part of the right atrium just above the tricuspid valve. At the AV node, the impulse is delayed slightly. From there, the impulse passes through the *Bundle of His* and the *Purkinje fibers* to the ventricles, causing them to contract. These impulses generate electrical currents that can be recorded by the electrocardiograph (ECG).

The following terms are used to describe the ECG waves illustrated in Fig. 11-15:

- P wave—represents electrical activity of the impulse from the SA node and its spread through the atria.

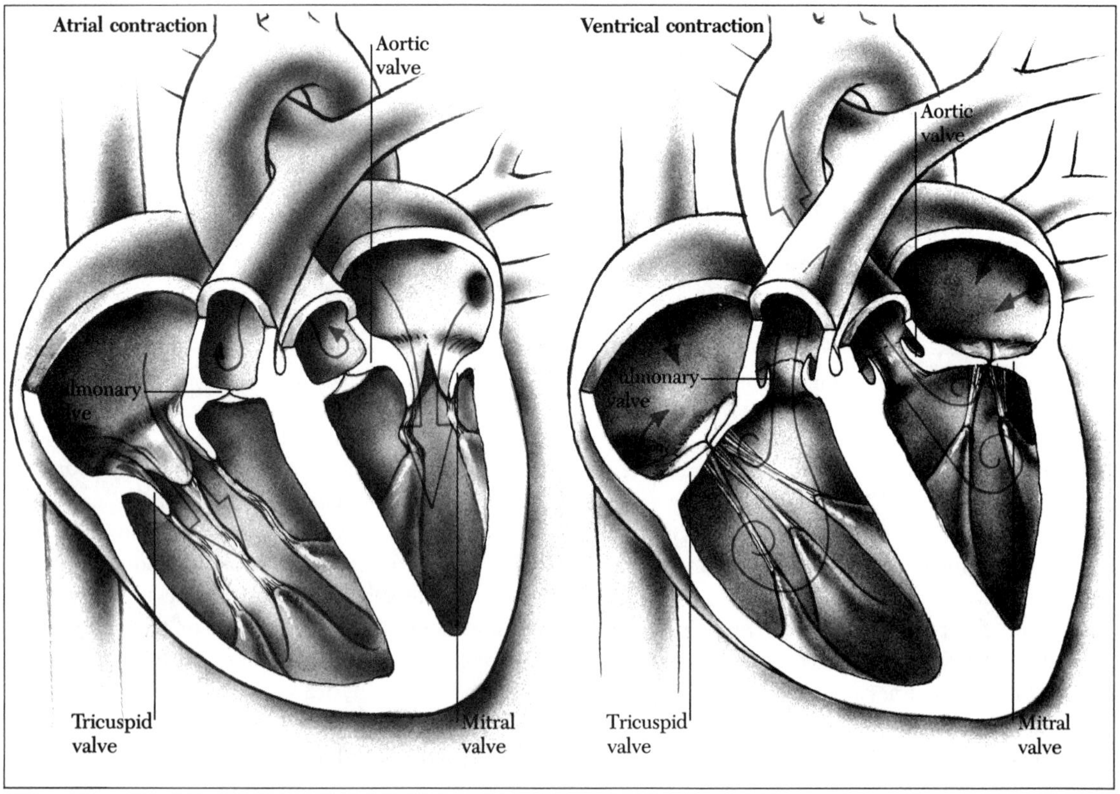

Figure 11-13 Schematic diagram of the heart.

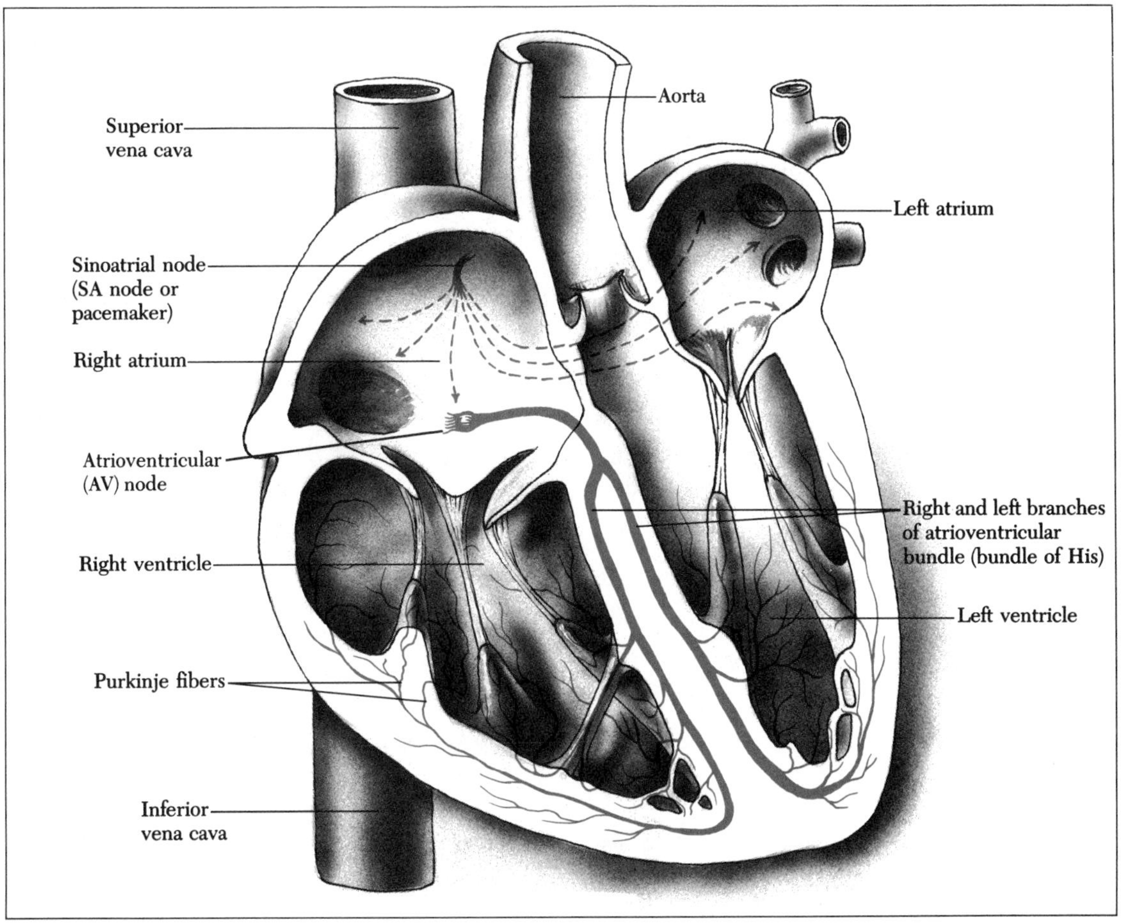

Figure 11-14 Conduction system of the heart.

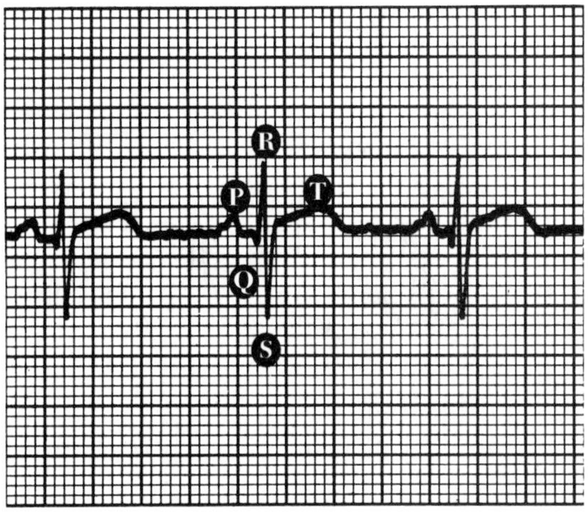

Figure 11-15 The ECG.

- PR interval—represents the time for the original impulse to pass from the SA node through the atria and the AV node to the ventricles.
- QRS complex—represents the spread of the impulses through the Bundle of His and the Purkinje fibers and the ventricular contraction.
- ST segment—represents the period between completion of the ventricular contraction and the recovery of the ventricular muscle.
- T wave—represents the recovery phase of the ventricular muscle.

The Cardiac Cycle

The *cardiac cycle,* or complete heartbeat, has two phases: systole and diastole. *Systole* is the working phase in which blood is ejected from the contracting ventricles of the heart out through the aorta and the pulmonary artery. It is the shortest phase of the two and constitutes one third of the cardiac cycle. At the beginning of systole, the AV valves (tricuspid and mitral valves) close concomitantly with a pressure build-up in the ventricular walls. When this pressure exceeds the pressure in the aorta, the semilunar valves open. At the end of ventricular contraction, the blood flows backward, closing the semilunar valves.

It is during *diastole,* the resting phase of the cardiac cycle, that repolarization of the ventricular muscle and cycle occurs. There is a rapid decrease in ventricular pressure, causing it to be less than the atrial pressure. The AV valves open, and the increased pressure of the atria causes blood to rush into the ventricles. At the closing of this ventricular filling phase, atrial contraction causes the last bit of blood to be emptied into the ventricles. The semilunar valves are closed during this phase. Diastole is longer than systole and constitutes two thirds of the cardiac cycle.

Heart Sounds

The heart makes typical sounds during the cardiac cycle; their relationship to the ECG is illustrated in Fig. 11-16. When heard through a stethoscope, they sound like "lub-dub" (S_1-S_2). The first heart sound occurs at the beginning of ventricular systole and reflects the closing of the mitral and tricuspid valves (M_1 and T_1). This sound is referred to as S_1 (the first heart sound). The second heart sound (S_2) represents the beginning of ventricular diastole and is caused by the closure of the aortic and pulmonary valves (A_2 and P_2). A third sound, S_3, may occur soon after the second sound, and a fourth heart sound, S_4, may be heard immediately preceding S_1. These third and fourth heart sounds represent ventricular filling and are so spaced that they resemble the sound of a galloping horse when they are present.

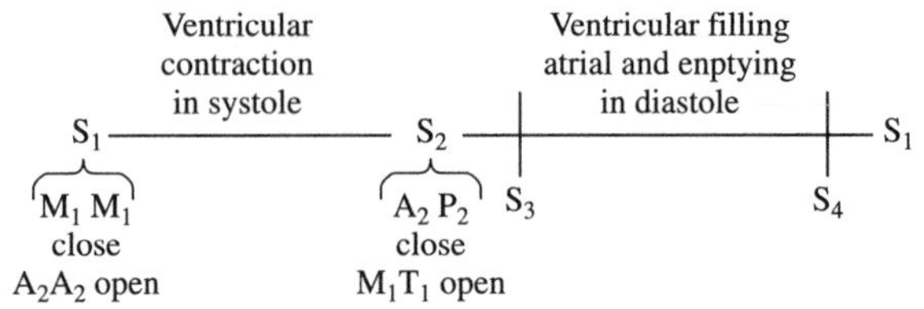

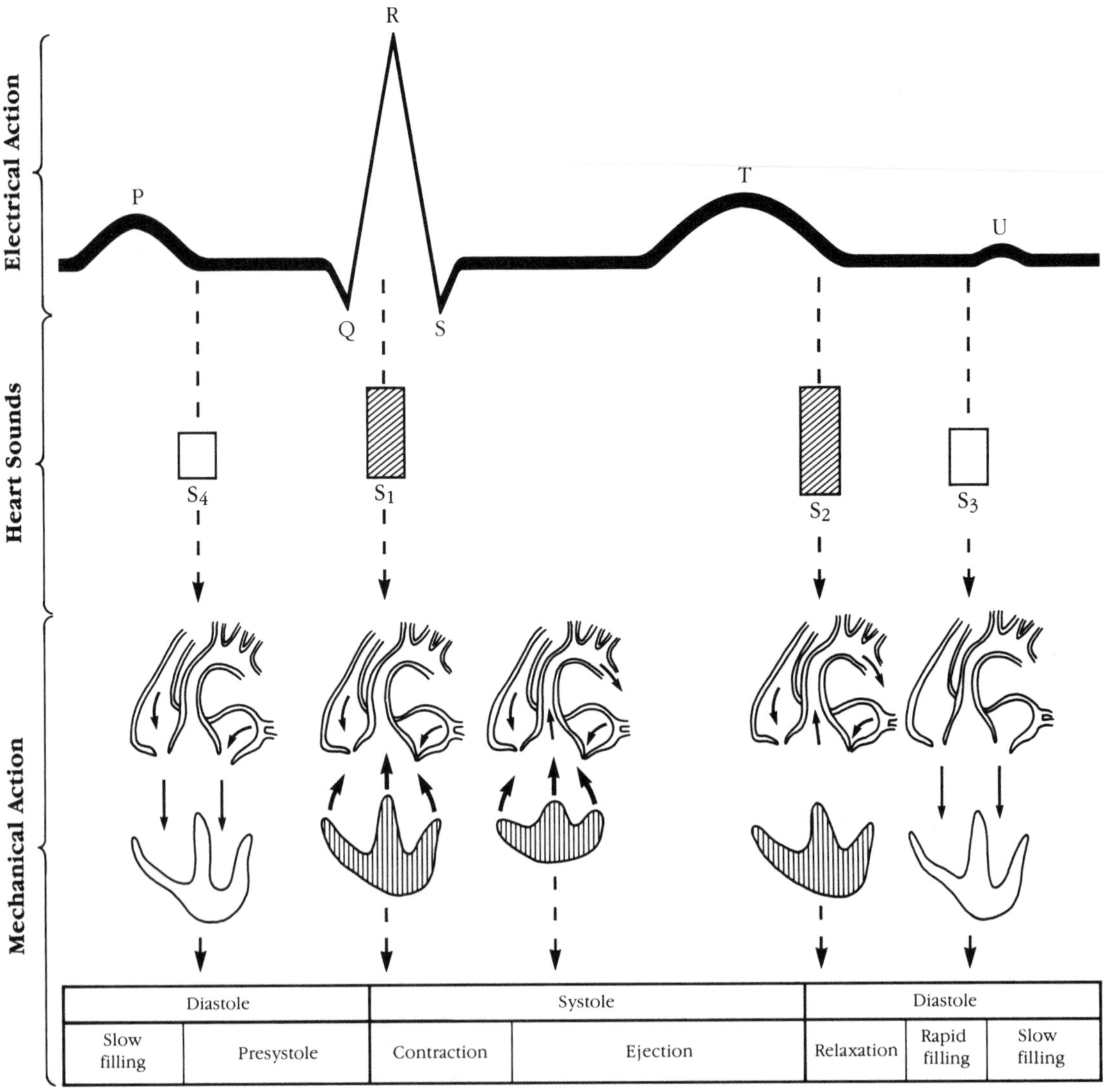

Figure 11-16 The electrical sequence of heart activation and contraction. (From Servonsky, J and Opas, S: *Nursing Management of Children.* © 1987 Boston: Jones and Bartlett Publishers. Reprinted with permission.)

A pathologic S_3 heart sound will be accompanied by a poor or barely audible S_1 heart sound.

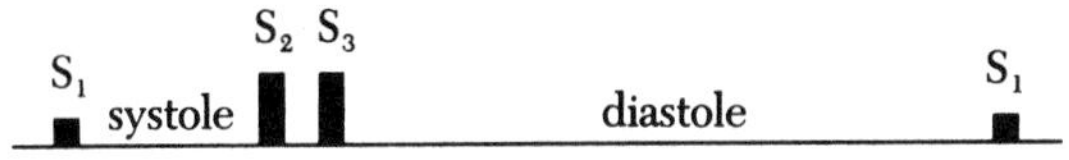

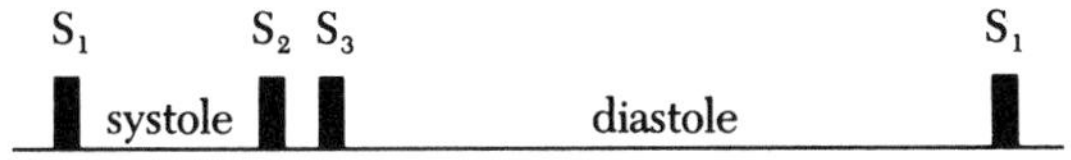

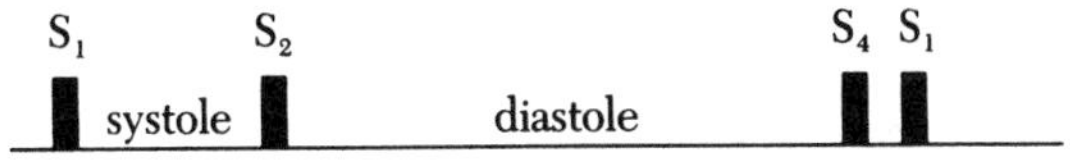

Although the ventricular filling is occurring, S_3 and S_4 heart sounds normally are not heard in adults due to increased breast, adipose, and muscular tissue, as compared with that of the child.

A quadruple rhythm of the heart sounds occurs when both S_1 and S_2 are heard along with protodiastolic and presystolic sounds (S_3 and S_4). This pattern is called a *summation gallop.* Summation gallop is a normal finding in children, in thin people, and in young adults. It is not normal in people over 30 years of age.

Splitting of Heart Sounds

The heart valves do not close simultaneously. During auscultation, physiologic splitting of the heart sounds is often heard, particularly the splitting of S_2. The mitral valve (M_1) closes before the tricuspid valve (T_1) and the aortic valve (A_2) closes before the pulmonary valve (P_2). Thus, there are actually two components to each of the S_1 and S_2 heart sounds, but they are so close together that they are difficult to hear individually. Hearing the normal physiologic splitting takes concentration, time, and practice in listening.

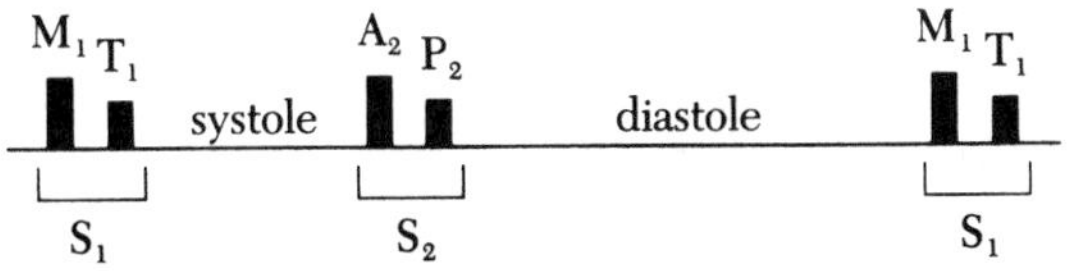

Splitting of the first heart sound is usually faint; if it can be heard at all, it is best heard somewhere between the apex and the sternum. When the split is heard, the mitral component (M_1) is usually louder than the tricuspid component (T_1). The widening of the S_1 split can be heard at the end of expiration.

Splitting of the second heart sound is best heard at the end of inspiration, over the pulmonary valve area or around the third (Erb's point) or fourth left ICS *near* the sternum. In the adult, the aortic valve closure (A_2) is louder than the pulmonary valve closure (P_2) because there is greater backflow pressure from the large aortic artery when the left ventricle is empty, compared with the backflow pressure in the smaller pulmonary artery leading from the right ventricle. Therefore, the relationship of A_2 to P_2 (intensity/loudness of valvular closing) in the adult is $A_2 > P_2$. But $A_2 > P_2$ in the child is indicative of hypertension. In healthy children and young adults, the intensity of the aortic and pulmonary valve closure are usually of equal intensity ($A_2 = P_2$).

CHARACTERISTICS AND TECHNIQUES OF EXAMINATION

Inspection and Palpation

Inspection and palpation are best accomplished with the client lying supine or with the head of the bed elevated approximately 45 degrees. The entire precordium should be observed for symmetry and pulsations and palpated for pulsations and the presence of a *thrill.* A thrill is a murmur so loud that it vibrates, and the vibration can be palpated; it feels something like the sensation of placing your hand on the throat of a purring cat. The palmar surface of the hand is most sensitive to vibrations, and the fingertips are most sensitive to pulsations. If a thrill is palpated, note whether it radiates into the neck area or the left axillary region.

Tangential lighting helps in detecting pulsations. If a pulsation is detected, determine its size; measure its diameter. Also document the location and time it pulsates within the

Technique for Inspection and Palpation of Extremities

1. Inspect skin and nails.
2. Check capillary refill.
3. Observe venous circulation, JVD, hands, and legs.
4. Palpate epitrochlear nodes and pulses:
   temporal
   carotid
   brachial
   radial
   femoral
   popliteal
   posterior tibial
   pedal
5. Determine need for the Allen test.
6. Test calf tenderness and for Homan's sign.

cardiac cycle (systole, diastole, or both). If you see and/or feel the pulsation simultaneously with the carotid pulse or first heart sound, it is a systolic pulsation. If the pulsation occurs after the second heart sound, it is a diastolic pulsation.

Inspect *and* palpate the following areas on the anterior chest (Fig. 11-17):

- *Sternoclavicular area.* Few or no pulsations are normally visualized in this area.
- *Aortic area* (2nd ICS to the right of the sternum). No pulsations should be seen, and no thrills should be palpable.
- *Pulmonary area* (2nd ICS to the left of the sternum). A slight thrill may be palpated in normal children and thin, nervous adults.
- *Right ventricular area* (anterior precordium). This area encompasses the lower half of the sternum and the ICSs to the left and the right of the sternum. No pulsations normally are visualized, and no thrills are felt.
- *Apical area.* Observe and palpate for the apical impulse. This is sometimes referred to as the point of maximum impulse or of maximum intensity (PMI).
  - Prior to age 7, because of the small size of the heart, the PMI is at the 3rd or 4th left ICS just to the left of the midclavicular line.
  - By age 7 and in adults, the apical impulse is normally located at the 5th or 6th left ICS at the midclavicular line or slightly medial to it (Fig. 11-18).
  - The PMI is felt as a slight tap and is normally 2 cm or less in diameter. It begins about the time of the first heart sound and lasts through the first third of systole.
  - If you cannot find the PMI, ask the client to turn to the left side or to sit up and lean forward (see Fig. 11-18C).
  - Occasionally, the apical impulse may be increased in amplitude and duration from noncardiac causes. This situation may be observed in pregnant women or in clients who are thin or have anemia or hyperthyroidism in which the blood flow is dynamic.
- *Epigastric area* (at the end of the xiphoid process in the mid anterior costal margin area). Pulsations in this area occur occasionally in normal individuals, usually following strenuous exercise.
  - It may be difficult to view pulsations in the epigastric area in a client with an emphysemic chest. In such a case, place your hand on the epigastric area and slide your fingers up under the rib cage. Pulsations of right ventricular hypertrophy will be felt on your fingertips, and aortic events will be reflected on the palm of your hand.

Techniques for Inspection and Palpation of Anterior Chest

1. Adequate lighting, warm room, privacy
2. Client exposed to the waist
3. Client in supine or semifowler position
4. Use of tangential lighting best to detect pulsations
5. Inspect and palpate the following areas on the anterior chest with palmar surfaces and then the fingertips of your hand:
   sternoclavicular area
   aortic area
   pulmonary area
   right ventricular area
   apical area
   epigastric area
   ectopic area
6. Identify location of the PMI.
7. Note abnormalities.

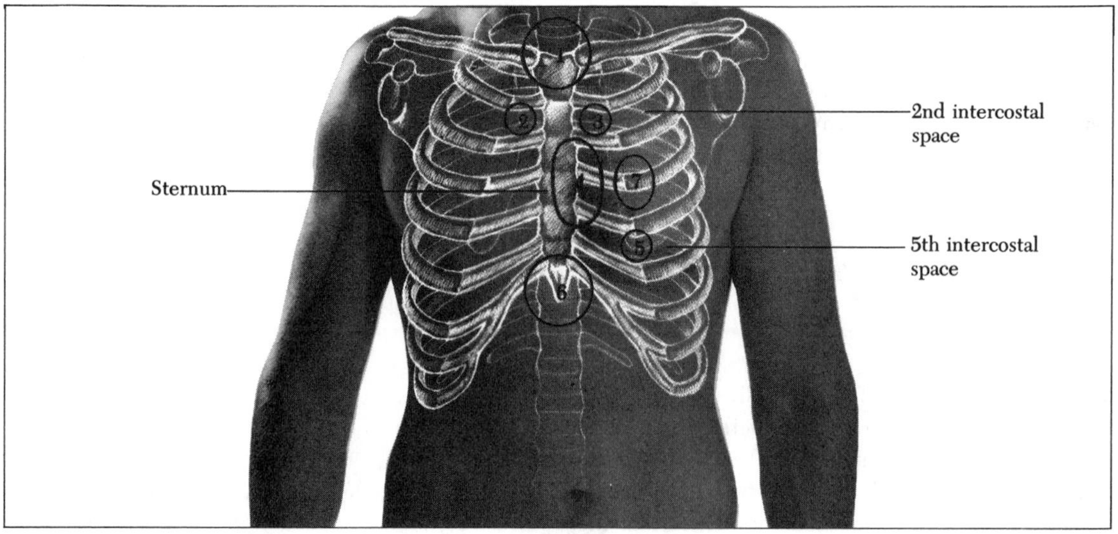

Figure 11-17 Specific areas for inspection and palpation of the anterior chest.

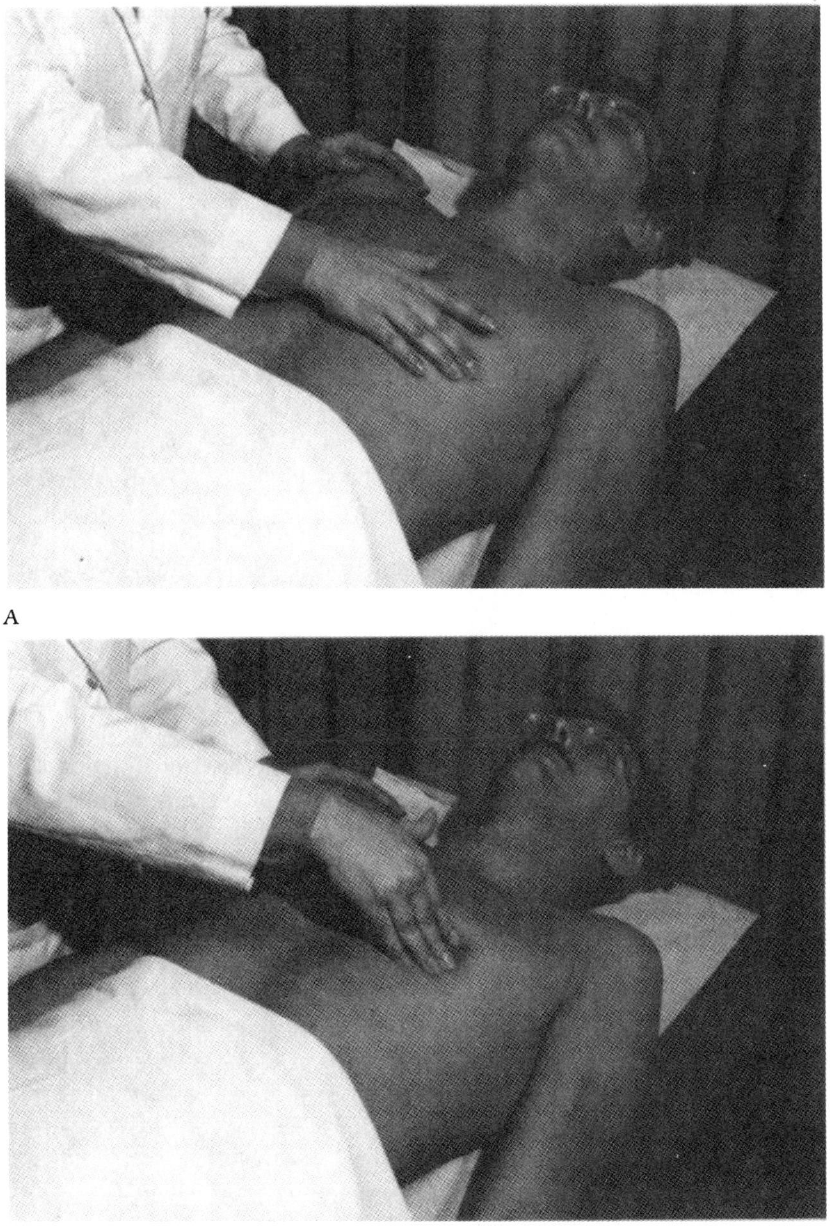

A

B

Figure 11-18 Palpation of the precordium. **(A)** Palmar surface hand position. Note extension of index finger to facilitate curve of palpating hand. **(B)** Correct fingertip-hand position.

- *Ectopic area.* This is located in the left midclavicular line between the pulmonic and apical areas.

Percussion

X-ray and fluoroscopy are much more accurate in determining the size of the heart; however, percussion can provide a gross estimate of the size and contour of the left cardiac border. The right cardiac border lies underneath the sternum, and under normal conditions it is difficult to detect.

Technique for Percussion of Anterior Chest

1. Client preferably in supine position
2. Percuss from the left MAL toward the MSL in the 4th or 5th ICS.
3. Measure from point of first detection of dull percussion note (LCBD) to the MSL.

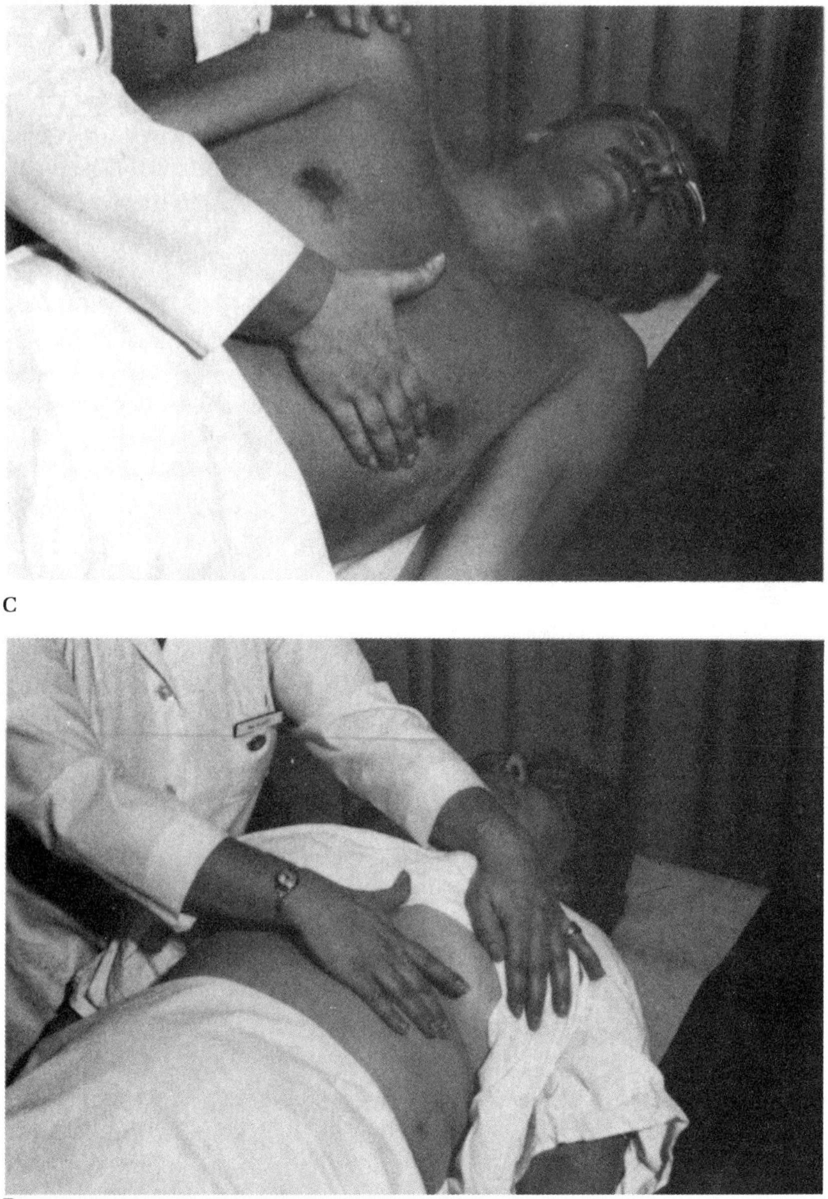

C

D

Figure 11-18 Continued **(C)** Hand position for palpating chest with client in left lateral position. **(D)** Upward pressure exterted on breast during precordial palpation of female client. (From Sana, J.M. and Judge, R. D. *Physical Assesment for Nursing Skills* (2nd ed.). Boston: Little, Brown, 1982, p. 240.)

The use of percussion is not diagnostic in itself but is helpful because results can be correlated immediately with other clinical findings at the time of the examination.

- Percuss the left cardiac border, beginning laterally with the pleximeter finger, either parallel or perpendicular to the ICSs.
- Percuss toward the midline in the 5th, 4th, and 3rd ICS, as shown in Fig. 11-19.
- The left cardiac border dullness (LCBD) usually will be detected about the midclavicular line or slightly medial to it.
- If the LCBD occurs prior to reaching the left midclavicular line, the distance from the midclavicular line should be measured and recorded (Fig. 11-20A).
- Another technique is to measure from the LCBD to the midsternal line. In the adult, the distance ranges from approximately 9 to 12 cm. A sample recording of this type measurement is shown in Fig. 11-20B.

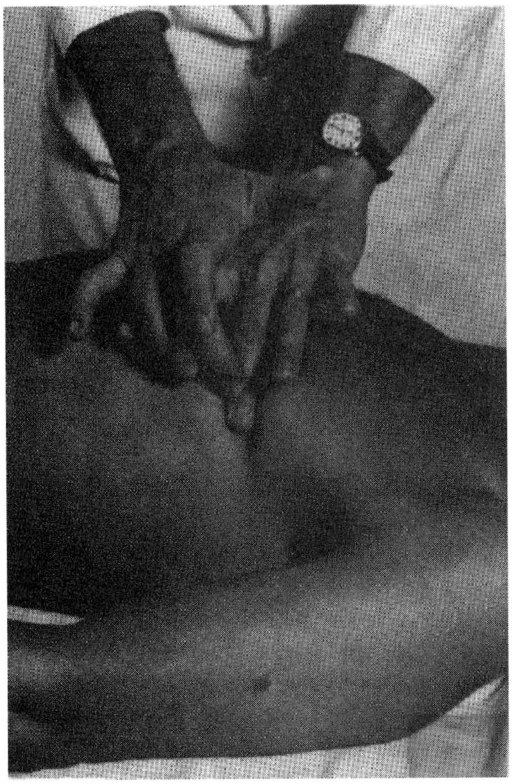

Figure 11-19 Percussing the contour of the left cardiac border.

1. LCBD 2 cm lateral to left of MCL @ 5th ICS.
2. LCBD ⟶ MSL @ L 6th ICS = 11 cm

Figure 11-20 Sample recordings of LCBD.

- Lateral displacement of the left cardiac border can sometimes be detected in such conditions as pregnancy, left ventricular hypertrophy, pericardial effusion (Fig. 11-21), and cirrhosis.
- Absence or decrease in cardiac dullness suggests emphysema.

Auscultation

To become proficient in the technique of auscultation, you will need years of practice and a thorough knowledge of the origins of normal and abnormal cardiac sounds. Because heart sounds are generally low pitched, you must perform auscultation in a quiet room to improve your ability to hear the sounds. Practice listening to your own heart while lying in bed in a quiet, dark room to decrease distractions. You must perform auscultation in an unhurried manner, concentrating on what you hear.

Examine the heart in each of the four valve areas and over the precordial area (Fig. 11-22). Listening should be done systematically. Begin at the apex and inch the stethoscope over to and up the left sternal border to the pulmonary area and the aortic area, or begin in the aortic area and **inch the stethoscope** across to the pulmonary area, then down the left sternum and across to the apex of the heart (Fig. 11-23). Whichever system you choose, stick to it to maintain thoroughness; do not hopscotch the stethoscope about the chest.

Technique for Auscultation of Heart

1. Quiet, warm room
2. Client's chest exposed
3. Client in supine position
4. If hairy chest, wet hair with a washcloth.
5. Warm stethoscope with hands.
6. Place diaphragm of stethoscope firmly at apex.
7. Inch stethoscope toward sternum.
8. Proceed up left sternal border to pulmonary area.
9. Inch across at 2nd ICS level to aortic area on client's right side.
10. Next, place the bell on the aortic area so all sides of the bell rim are lightly touching the skin.
11. Inch across to the pulmonic area.
12. Inch down the left sternal border.
13. Inch over to the apical area.
14. At each area assess the following: S_1, S_2, splitting, A_2:P_2 relationship, presence of extra heart sounds and/or adventitious sounds.
15. Repeat process with client in the left lateral position.
16. Repeat process with the client leaning forward in a sitting position.

- First examine the client in the *supine* position, then in the *left lateral* position, and finally leaning forward in the *sitting* position.
- Auscultate the heart first with the diaphragm (picks up high-pitched sounds) and then with the bell of the stethoscope (detects low-pitched sounds).
- The diaphragm should be held firmly against the skin.
- If the client has a hairy chest, wet the chest with a washcloth to make the hair lie more smoothly. Otherwise, hair under the diaphragm may sound like fine rales of the lungs.
- The bell should be placed lightly on the chest; firm placement will stretch the skin tight, causing the skin to act as a diaphragm, in which case low pitches may go undetected.

Auscultation is performed for the following assessments:

- Evaluation of the rate and rhythm of the heart
- Identification of previously undetected arrhythmias and act as a supplement to what is learned from an ECG.

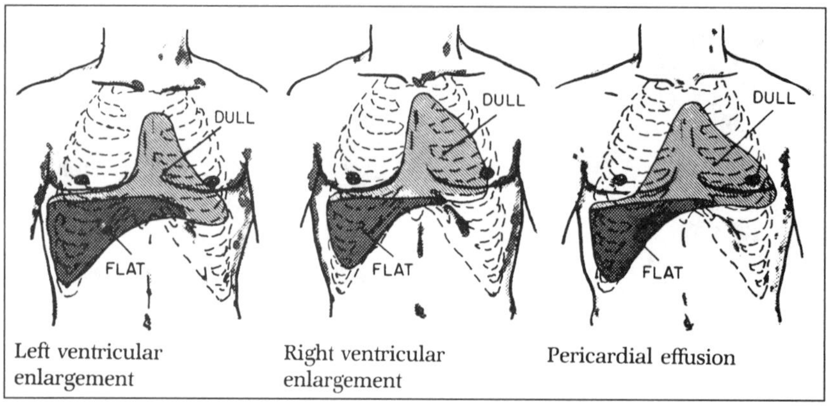

Figure 11-21 Characteristic configuration of the areas of cardiac dullness in left ventricular enlargement, and pericardial effusion. (From Sana, J.M. and Judge, R.D. *Physical Assessment for Nursing Skills* (2nd ed.). Boston: Little, Brown, 1982, p. 268.)

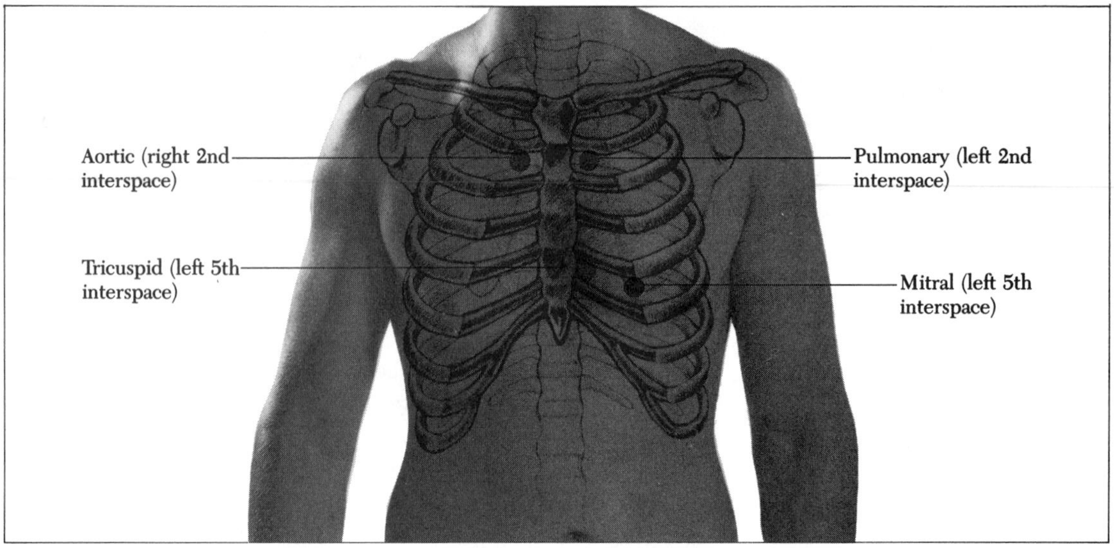

Figure 11-22 Palpatory and auscultatory projections of the heart valves.

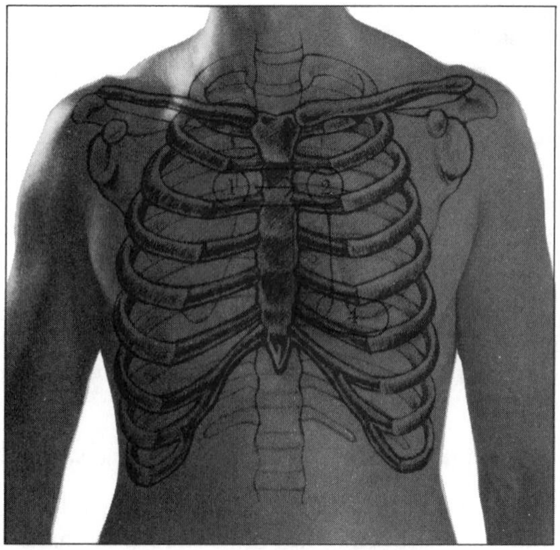

Figure 11-23 Method of cardiac auscultation.

Arrhythmias are classified according to heart rate and the type of rhythm, as illustrated in Table 11-2.

- Determination of whether S_1 and S_2 are normal. Normally, S_1 is of loudest intensity at the apex (as this is where the closure of the M_1 and T_1 valves are nearest), and S_2 is heard loudest at the base of the heart (the site of A_2 and P_2 valve closure at the 2nd ICS level).
- Determination of intensity, variations in intensity, and splitting of S_1, and auscultating S_2 for assessment of these same components.
- Detection of splitting and its relationship to inspiration and expiration, systolic clicks, third or fourth heart sounds, diastolic opening snaps, and murmurs.

Figure 11-24 depicts normal heart sounds relative to the valvular area at which they are best heard.

Table 11-2 Classification of Arrhythmias

Heart rate	Rhythm: Regular	Rhythm: Rhythmically or accidentally irregular	Rhythm: Absolutely irregular
	A.	D.	G.
200	Supraventricular tachycardias	Supraventricular tachycardias with ventricular premature contractions	Atrial fibrillation untreated
175	1. Sinus tachycardia 2. Atrial tachycardia 3. Atrial flutter 4. Atrial tachycardia with block		
150	5. Nodal tachycardia	Atrial flutter	Atrial flutter
125	Ventricular tachycardias		
	B.	E.	H.
100	Sinus rhythm Atrial flutter with 3:1 or 4:1 block	Sinus arrhythmia Ventricular premature contractions	Atrial fibrillation with partial block (digitalis, sclerosis)
75	Sinus or atrial tachycardia with 2:1 block	Atrial premature contraction Partial heart block (Wenckenbach's phenomenon)	Atrial flutter Sinus arrhythmia of the aged
50			
	C.	F.	I.
25	Sinus bradycardia Complete heart block Partial heart block with 2:1 or 3:1 block	Partial or complete heart block with ventricular premature contractions	Partial or complete heart block with ventricular premature contractions

Source: From Abe Ravin, *Auscultation of the Heart,* 2nd ed. Chicago: Yearbook Medical Publishers, Inc., 1967.

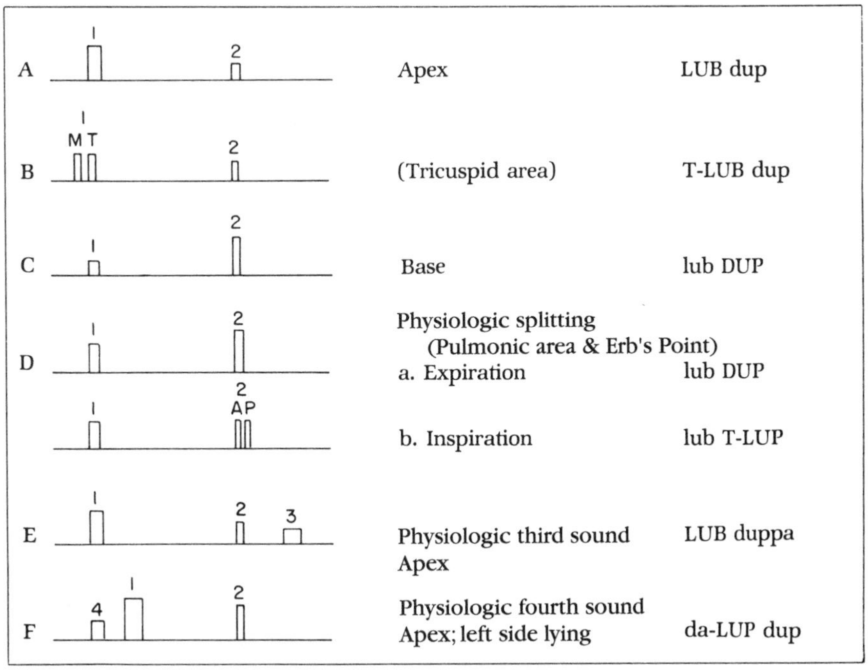

Figure 11-24 Normal heart sounds in respect to valve area and phonetic representation. (From Sana, J.M. and Judge, R.D. *Physical Assessment for Nursing Skills* (2nd ed.). Boston: Little, Brown, 1982, p. 271.)

If you have difficulty differentiating the first from the second heart sound, palpate the carotid pulse. The first heart sound and the beat of the carotid pulse will be simultaneous. Another technique is to listen to the length of the systole and diastole. Systole is normally shorter than diastole; thus, there is only a short pause between S_1 and S_2. The pause following S_2 will be longer (diastole) before S_1 reappears. A third heart sound is usually best detected when the client is in the left lateral position.

Heart Murmurs

Listen for murmurs, during both systole and diastole. Because murmurs often radiate to other areas, listen up into the neck region and over into the left axillary region.

- Murmurs in the aortic area may radiate to the neck and down the left sternal border.
- Murmurs in the mitral area often are heard best after exercise, when the client is in the left lateral position.
- Murmurs in the aortic area are best heard when the client is sitting and on expiration.
- The detection of a heart murmur warrants consultation with a physician for further evaluation. In particular, a murmur that radiates or occurs during diastole is considered indicative of heart disease until otherwise disproved.

It is difficult to determine significant murmurs in a child. Children may have murmurs without having organic pathology, or they may not demonstrate murmurs despite the existence of severe heart disease.

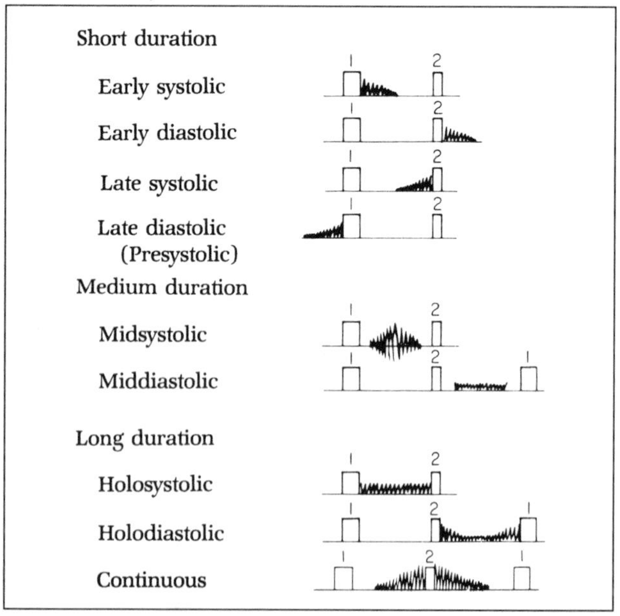

Figure 11-25 Timing and duration of heart murmurs. (From Sana, J.M. and Judge, R.D. *Physical Assessment for Nursing Skills* (2nd ed.). Boston: Little, Brown, 1982, p. 274.)

The features that must be carefully studied and used to describe a murmur are location, timing, quality/pitch, and intensity.

Location

The exact location of the murmur should be described according to the specific anatomic landmarks. Some murmurs may be confined to a small area and may be heard directly over the valve area. Others may be more diffuse and heard over the entire precordium. Certain ones can also be heard radiating to the neck region or axillary region.

Timing

Murmurs are described as either systolic or diastolic. *Systolic* murmurs are referred to as being early, middle, or late. Some murmurs may persist throughout the entire systolic period, in which case they are termed *pansystolic* or *holosystolic* murmurs. *Diastolic* murmurs may occur in various parts of diastole and are described as being early diastolic, mid-diastolic, or late diastolic (presystolic). Early diastolic murmurs start with the second sound. In mid-diastolic murmurs, there is a short pause after the second sound. A murmur is described as continuous if it is heard both in systole and diastole and is of the same quality during both phases (Fig. 11-25).

Quality and Pitch

The quality of a murmur may be described as blowing, harsh, musical, or rumbling. The pitch of a murmur is dependent on the velocity of blood flow. When the velocity is great, the pitch is high; when the velocity is slow, the pitch is low.

Intensity

A six-point grading system is used to describe the loudness of a murmur (see Table 11-3). Grade I murmurs are frequently encountered in persons who do not have organic heart disease. Low-grade murmurs are commonly heard in the elderly, who have valves with ragged edges or that are stiff to open merely from the wear and tear of aging. If a low-grade murmur remains as such for years, it is probably of little or no significance. A summary of normal and abnormal heart sounds is presented in Table 11-4.

Pericardial Friction Rub

- A pericardial friction rub can be differentiated from a pleural friction rub in that it is unaffected by respirations. If the client is instructed to hold her breath, a pericardial friction rub will continue to be heard, whereas a pleural friction rub will cease.
- The intensity of the pericardial friction rub varies with position and is often best heard when the client is sitting upright and leaning forward.

Table 11-3 Grading System of Heart Murmurs

Grade	Loudness of murmur
I	Is difficult to hear; experienced examiner and quiet environment are needed
II	Is not readily heard on laying stethoscope on chest; examiner must listen closely to hear
III	Requires no effort to hear and is readily heard when stethoscope is placed on chest
IV	Is accompanied by a thrill; loud enough that there is no question of its presence
V	Can be heard with stethoscope held an inch away from chest; thrill present
VI	Does not require use of stethoscope to hear; thrill present

- Often, pressure over the liver or right upper quadrant of the abdomen will accentuate the rub, as will pressure from the stethoscope on the chest wall.

Measurement of Jugular Venous Pulse

It is important to inspect the jugular veins, because alterations in pressure or pulse waves indicate the presence of pathology. The internal and external jugular veins terminate at the subclavian vein and return blood from the head to the right atrium. The internal jugular vein is situated deep in the sternocleidomastoid muscle and can be traced as arising from the supraclavicular fossa. The external jugular arises from beneath the clavicle lateral to the internal jugular and crosses it diagonally over the sternocleidomastoid (Fig. 11-26). The jugular venous pulse and pressure reflect the blood volume of the area; thus, they are an indirect indication of the ability of the right atrium to receive blood, as well as of left ventricular contractility.

The internal jugular vein provides the **more accurate data,** as the external jugular may be abnormal because of obstruction or kinking at the base of the neck. If the internal jugular cannot be visualized, use the external jugular to measure the pulse, with the understanding that it will not be as accurate.

Two facets of the pulse must be considered: the venous pressure and the venous pulsations.

Jugular Venous Pressure (Distention) Measurement

- The external jugular veins are often distended with the client in the supine position; they will collapse with inspiration and fill with expiration. In the healthy individual, this distention disappears when the head of the bed is elevated 45 degrees (Fig. 11-27).

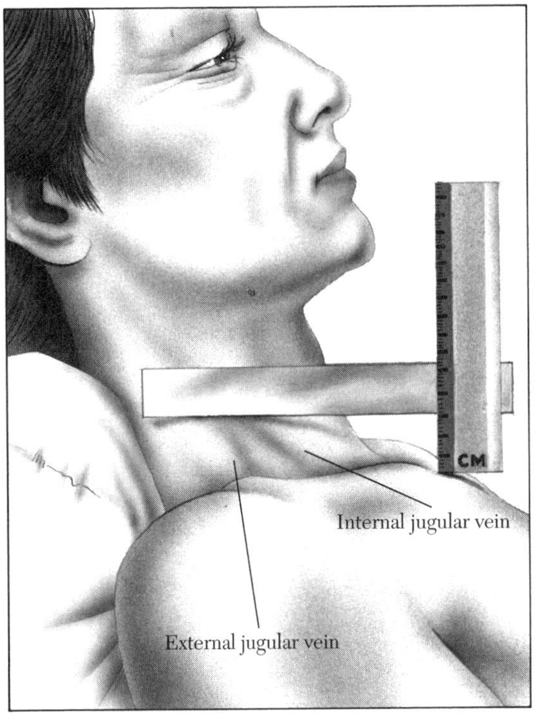

Figure 11-26 Technique for measuring jugular venous distention (JVD = 3 cm).

- Measurement of jugular venous distention (JVD) is made with the client in a semifowler position, because veins that are distended more than 3 to 4 cm at this angle (45 degrees) are a sign of pathology. Figure 11-26 illustrates the technique for measuring JVD.
- Note the highest point of oscillation of the internal jugular venous blood or the level of the external JVD.
- Place your ruler vertically at the sternal junction, and measure (in centimeters) up to the the site where a parallel line placed at the top of venous distention crosses your ruler. This is the venous pressure.

Venous Pulsations

Venous pulsations are described in terms of *a*, *c*, and *v* waves and *x* and *y* troughs (Fig. 11-28). Analysis of these waves reveals important information about the cardiac cycle and the function of the right atrium.

- In most normal adults in the supine position, venous pulsations can be seen at the base of the neck.
- The *a* wave is caused by right atrial contraction, which occurs just before the first heart sound. Identify it by palpating the carotid artery. The *a* wave will immediately precede the carotid pulsation.
- The *c* wave is very small and is rarely seen. It begins at the end of the first heart sound and is sometimes said to be a reflected wave from the carotid artery.

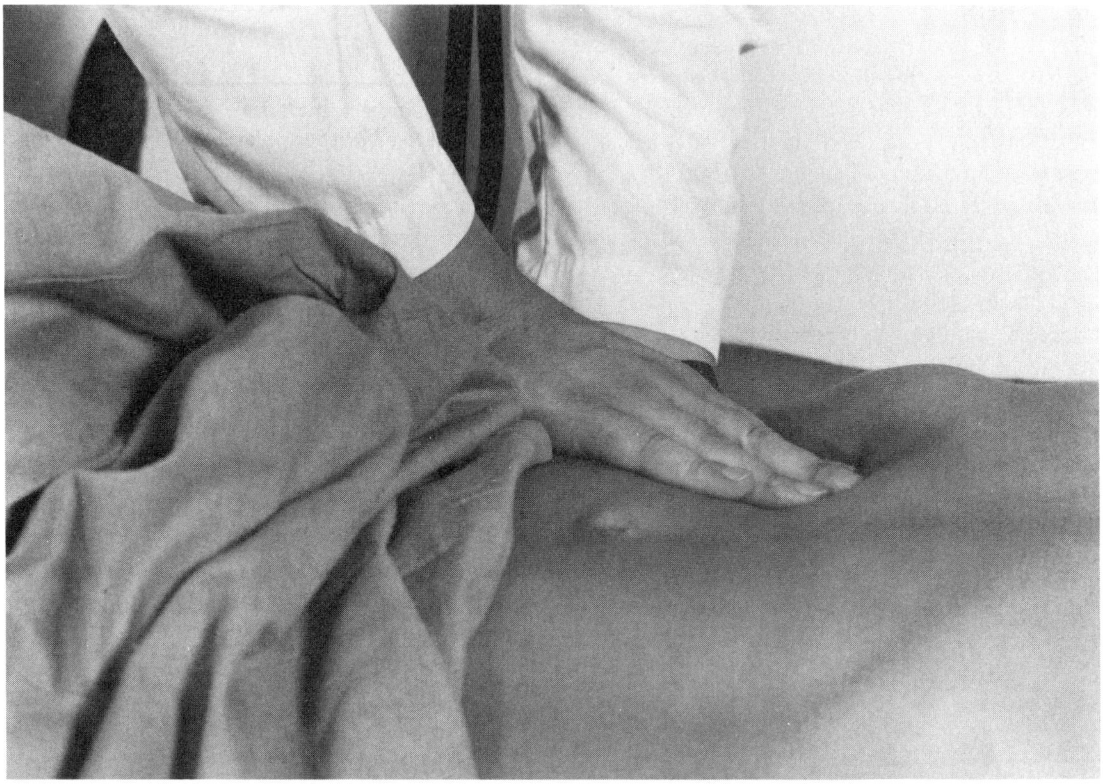

Figure 13-15 Palpation of the right kidney.

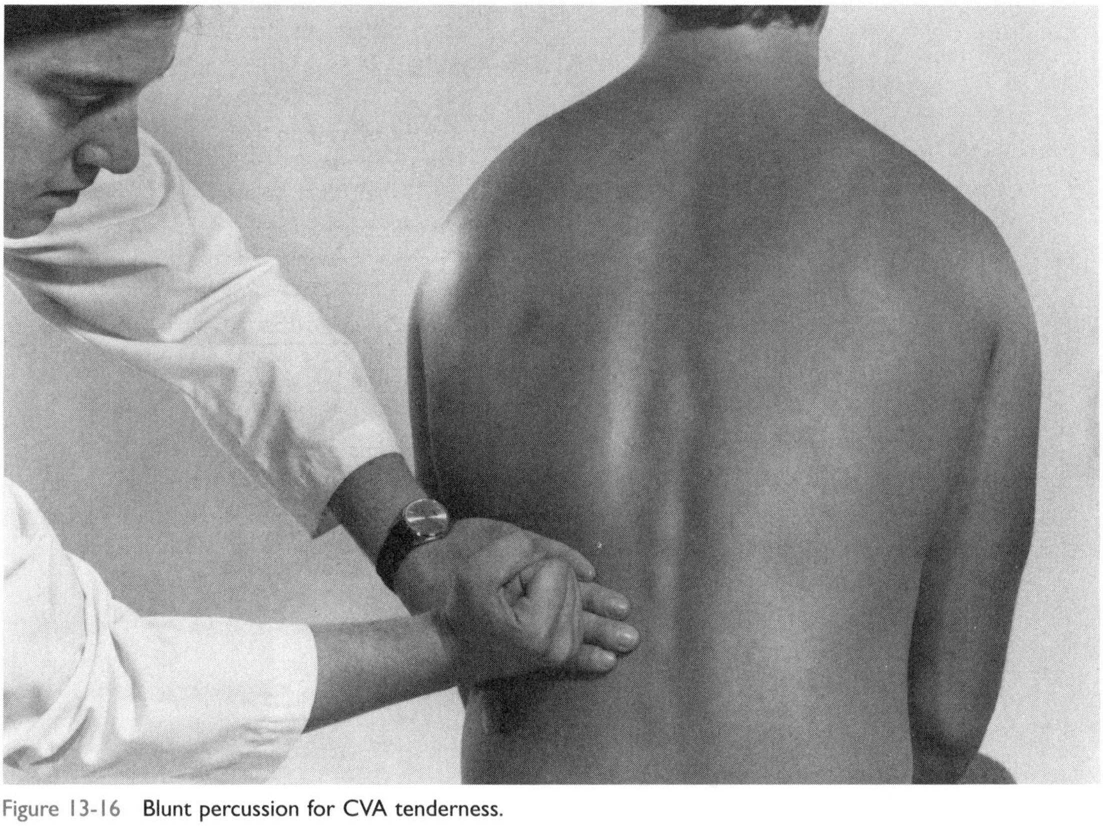

Figure 13-16 Blunt percussion for CVA tenderness.

Abdominal Aorta

Palpate *deeply* in the midline above the umbilicus with your thumb and index finger straddling the aorta. Tenderness on palpation is frequently experienced by the normal client. An aneurysm may be felt as a pulsating mass, and the client may present with complaints of abdominal pain.

If a mass or nodule is palpated, describe to the consulting physician the location, approximate size, consistency, and degree of tenderness. Occasionally, feces may be mistaken for a tumor on abdominal palpation. Every mass in the abdomen must be verified before the client can be deemed free of disease.

Hernias

Next, palpate the abdomen for the presence of hernias. The three most common types of hernias are ventral, umbilical, and inguinal.

Ventral hernias occur at points on the abdomen other than the umbilicus or groin. An incisional hernia is a ventral hernia that occurs at the site of a surgical incision that has not healed properly or where scar tissue is not as strong as normal tissue. This type of hernia often can be seen as well as palpated. It usually appears as a soft mass on the abdominal wall. Coughing generally causes it to bulge outward (Fig. 13-17A).

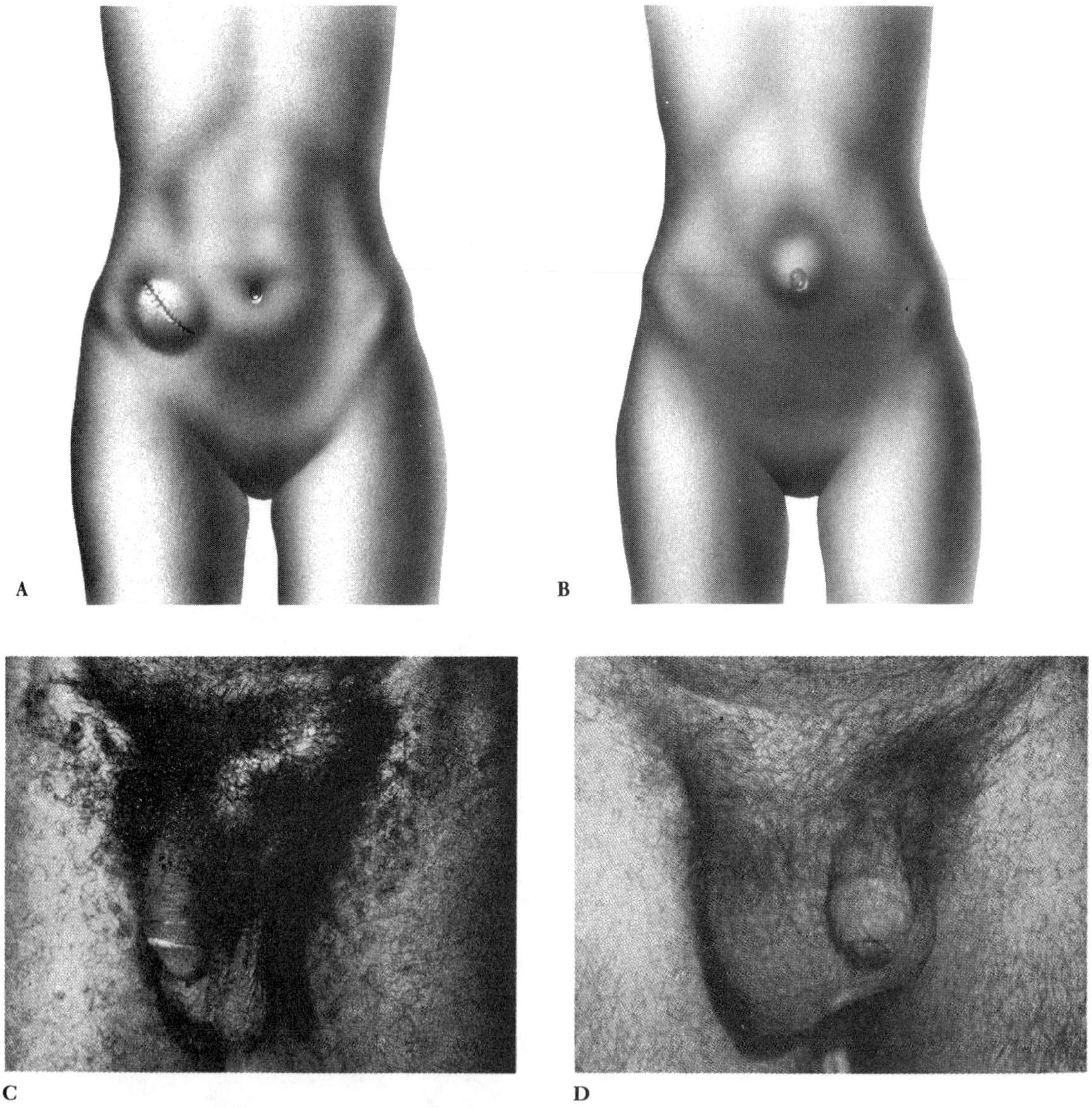

Figure 13-17 Hernias. **(A)** Ventral incisional hernia. **(B)** Umbilical hernia. Periumbilical bulging is seen in a child with umbilical hernia. In an adult, bulging radiates upward from the umbilicus. **(C)** Direct inguinal hernia. **(D)** Indirect inguinal hernia.

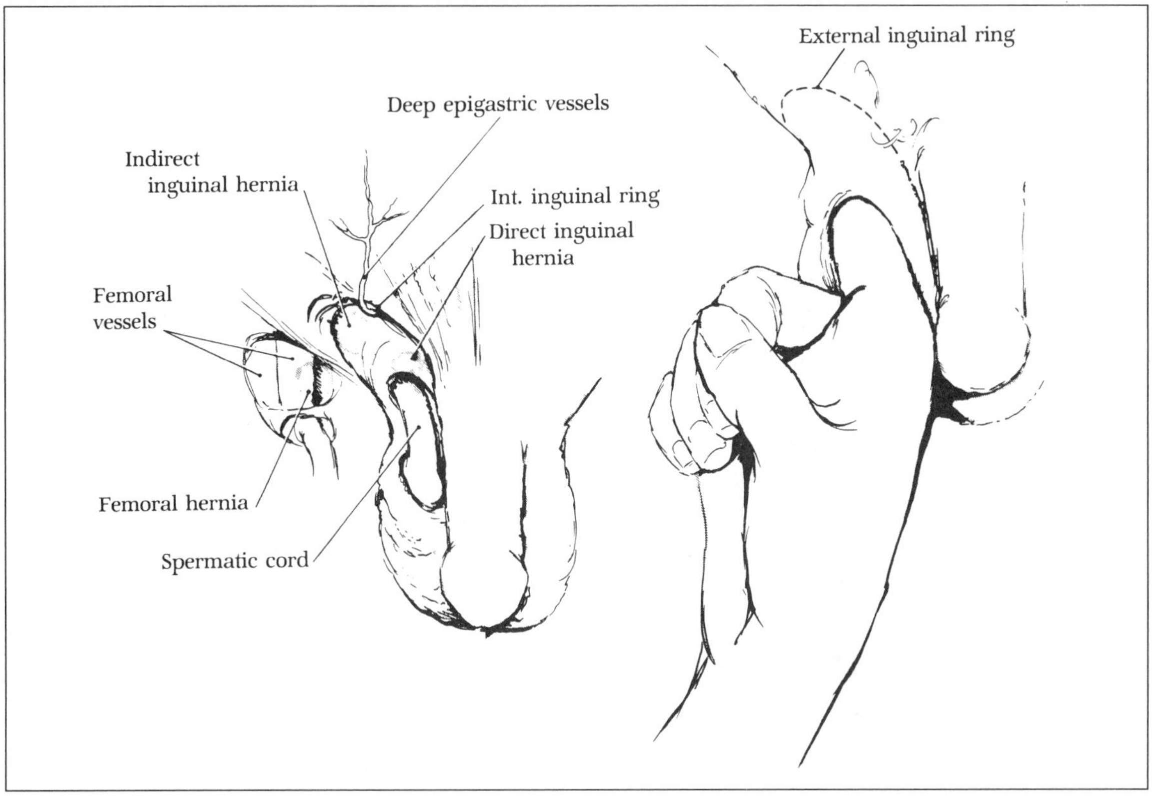

Figure 13-18 Inguinal hernias.

Umbilical hernias are most generally congenital and are best visualized when the client coughs. When you push your index finger into the navel, a ring of fascia will be detected around a soft center. They may occur with pregnancy, ascites, and obesity (Fig. 13-17B).

Inguinal hernias, most often seen in males, may be direct (Fig. 13-17C) or indirect. An indirect hernia follows the spermatic cord through both the internal and external rings and through the inguinal canal. Occasionally, one becomes very large and descends into the scrotum (Fig. 13-17D).

To palpate an indirect inguinal hernia (Figs. 13-18 and 13-19), do the following:

- Have the client stand with his ipsilateral (same side as being examined) leg slightly flexed.
- Place an index finger into the loose skin low on the side of the scrotum and advance it up to the external inguinal ring. If possible, advance the finger through the inguinal ring.
- Instruct the client to strain or "bear down." An indirect hernia will be felt as a small soft mass that presses against the fingertip.

A direct hernia passes through the weak muscular wall and into the external inguinal ring; it may be visualized. To palpate a direct hernia, follow this procedure:

- Press the palmar aspects of the hand over the inguinal area.
- Instruct the client to cough or bear down.

Lymph Nodes and Pulses

Figure 13-20 illustrates the position of the inguinal lymph nodes, which drain the lower abdomen, buttocks, and genital area. The femoral lymph nodes, also shown in Fig. 13-21, drain the lower extremities.

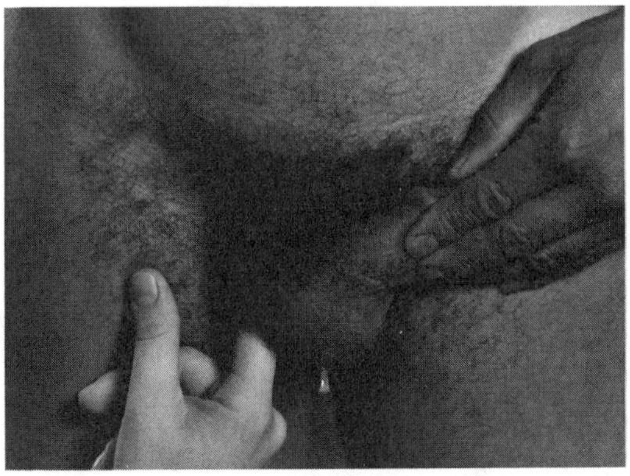

Figure 13-19 Examination technique for indirect inguinal hernia.

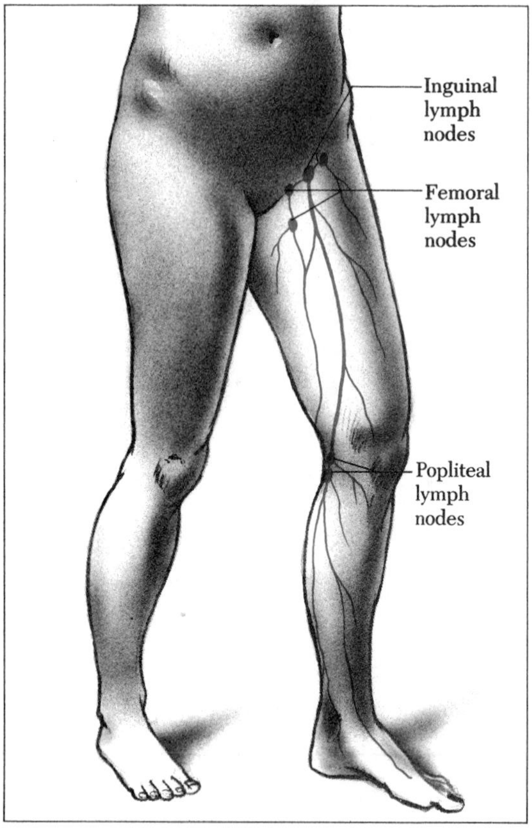

Figure 13-20 Location of inguinal and femoral lymph nodes.

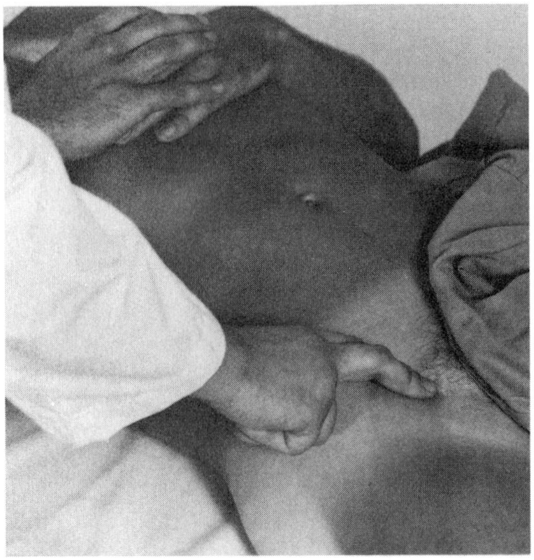

Figure 13-21 Palpation of the femoral artery.

It is not uncommon to find nontender lymph enlargement in the groin; if not accompanied by other signs and symptoms, such enlargement is not significant. This is a common finding in the elderly.

- Use a rotary motion of the fingertips to palpate the lymph nodes.
- Palpate the groin areas to determine the status of the lymph nodes and the femoral pulses.

The femoral pulse is located bilaterally with the tips of several fingers as shown in Figure 13-21.

CLINICAL CORRELATIONS

Inspection

Little or no respiratory movement may be observed in the abdomen when severe abdominal pain is present (e.g., perforated ulcer, peritonitis). Decreased respirations accompany muscle rigidity and severe abdominal distention. Abdominal retraction on inspiration is termed *Czerny's sign;* it usually is associated with a central nervous system disorder.

Relative to size and symmetry of the abdomen, that of children under age 4 is always large, but an increase may be due to tumor, ascites, or congenital defect. Babies who cry a lot often swallow air, which causes distention. The scaphoid abdomen is seen in very thin individuals of any age. In a child, a scaphoid abdomen is not normal and is usually the result of severe malnutrition and dehydration.

Asymmetry of the abdomen can result from a variety of causes. It may be due to a hernia, organomegaly, bowel obstruction, tumor, cysts, or spinal curvature. In the upper abdomen, changes may represent involvement of such structures as the liver, pancreas, spleen, stomach, or transverse colon. A tumor of the liver may be seen as a mass in the right upper quadrant that moves with respirations. Asymmetry of the lower abdomen may result from bladder distention, pregnancy, or masses in the ovaries, uterus, or colon.

Generalized symmetrical fullness can be caused by ascites, obesity, or gas distention. The characteristic picture of ascites is of a tense, distended abdomen with tightly stretched skin and bulging flanks. If the ascites is extreme, the umbilicus becomes everted. When the abdomen has the shape of a dome with the intestinal loops displayed as visible ridges, it is usually due to intestinal obstruction or distention. A mass in the epigastrium with left-to-right visible peristalsis may indicate pyloric obstruction (stenosis) and may be accompanied by projectile vomiting.

Visible peristalsis is considered an abnormal sign, and obstruction must be ruled out. In developing intestinal obstruction, the peristalsis above the point of pathology becomes increased. Pain usually accompanies peristalsis in both the hyperactive bowel and the tensely distended bowel of abdominal obstruction. It is therefore important to note whether the client presents any manifestations of pain.

Illness not involving the GI system can be detected during the abdominal examination. For instance, lesions of tinea

RECORDING OF FINDINGS

Normal findings are presented in the first column. Findings for a client complaining of being "constantly tired" are presented in the second column.

Normal findings	Client findings
Abdomen	**Abdomen**
Inspection: Abdomen flat; no scars; no venous engorgement; no lesions; no visible pulsations; symmetrical; no flank fullness	*Inspection:* Abdomen round, asymmetrical—right upper quadrant; flank fullness with some pitting edema; 3 cm McBurney's scar in right lower quadrant; no lesions, no visible pulsations.
Auscultation: Bowel sounds present in all four quadrants; no bruits	*Auscultation:* Bowel sounds present in all four quadrants; no bruits; friction rub at ® costal margin
Percussion: Tympany in all four quadrants; gastric air bubble; liver 9 cm at right MCL; lower edge of liver dullness at costal margin; splenic dullness 6 cm at left MAL	*Percussion:* Decreased tympany in all four quadrants; liver 15 cm at right MCL; gastric air bubble; spleen 7 cm; 2-cm shifting dullness present
Palpation: No masses; no tenderness; liver, spleen, kidneys nonpalpable	*Palpation:* Liver palpated at 5 cm below RCM—smooth contour; spleen and kidneys nonpalpable; no tenderness or masses

corporis and scabies are often found on the abdomen. Characteristic pigmented striae on the abdominal wall are observed in clients with Cushing's disease.

Scars or burns are easily observed. Overgrowth of scar tissue (keloid) may be seen. Dotted scars over the abdomen and the thighs may reflect insulin injection sites in clients with diabetes mellitus. Scars can reflect previous injury and illness requiring surgery. Common surgical scars can be seen in Fig. 13-22.

Many GI disorders are manifested by changes in the skin. Multiple small nodules may be the first indicator of carcinoma. Cutaneous angiomas (spider nevi) can be seen on the upper abdomen and chest of clients with cirrhosis; clients with ulcerative colitis may exhibit erythema nodosum (tender nodules in or under the skin). Localized ecchymosis in the flank may reflect abdominal or retroperitoneal hemorrhage.

Failure of the newborn's umbilical cord to heal creates the potential for the development of ventral and umbilical hernias or defects in the abdominal wall, such as extrophy of the bladder or diastasis recti. Inguinal hernias are most often detected as a mass in the scrotum in males but occasionally can be observed as a mass in the groin.

Note the presence of distended or dilated abdominal veins, which may indicate obstruction of the portal circulation or of the inferior vena cava. In adults, observable veins accompany portal hypertension, ascites, and portal or hepatic obstruction.

Sparse pubic hair and associated thin, smooth skin may be reflective of deficient pituitary function. Cirrhosis in the male client generally shows a female pubic hair pattern due to the inability of the diseased liver to conjugate estrogenic substances.

Auscultation

Bowel Sounds

Lack of bowel sounds occurs in such serious conditions as inflammation, paralytic ileus, late obstruction, gangrene, intraabdominal bleeding, and peritonitis. Weak and infrequent sounds often indicate that the bowel is becoming increasingly immobile as a result of these conditions. Absent or decreased bowel sounds may exist 1 to 3 days after abdominal surgery.

High-pitched tinkling sounds are indicative of bowel obstruction. When obstructed, the bowel fills with air, and the peristalsis occurring in the tensely distended bowel produces high-pitched tinkling sounds called borborygmus. Other conditions in which the bowel is hyperactive are gastroenteritis, severe diarrhea, and intestinal hemorrhage; borborygmi sounds are present also in these conditions. Sometimes, esophageal bleeding may cause hyperperistalsis.

Blood Flow

Bruits of hyperdynamic circulation or an aneurysm may be heard in the abdomen, as well as those occurring from stenosed arteries. A venous sound, the venous hum, represents portal obstruction; it may be heard with hepatic or splenic disease.

Friction Rub

Peritoneal friction rubs usually occur when there is an abscess or tumor of the liver or spleen.

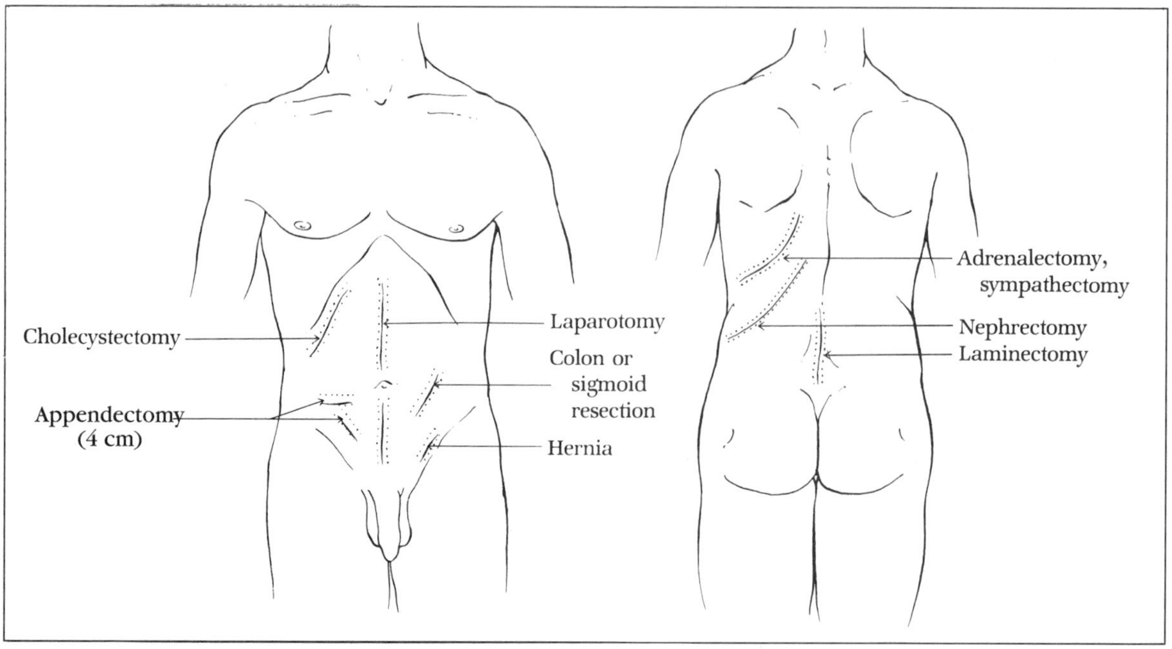

Figure 13-22 Common surgical scars. (From Sana, J.M. and Judge, R.D. *Physical Assessment for Nursing Skills* (2nd ed.). Boston: Little, Brown, 1982, p. 287.)

Percussion

In the alcoholic with cirrhosis, the liver can be enlarged, but in an advanced stage of cirrhosis, the liver becomes necrotic and atrophied. In severe hepatitis, the liver also decreases in size after initial hepatomegaly.

Size of the gastric bubble is variable. Abdominal distention and increase in the size of the gastric bubble may be due to gastric dilatation. Dullness in the area where the gastric bubble normally exists may also indicate enlargement of the left lobe of the liver. Dullness over other areas of the abdomen suggests the presence of tumor masses or fluid.

Palpation

An inflamed appendix (as well as inflammation of the peritoneal lining) will cause rebound tenderness. Table 13-3 lists

Table 13-3 Common Disease Conditions of the Abdomen

Terminology	Characteristics	Comments
Appendicitis	Low-grade fever, malaise, sometimes nausea or vomiting, abdominal pain and either constipation or diarrhea. Discomfort begins in periumbilical area. Pain localizes in RLQ at McBurney's point; as well as the sharp, stabbing pain of *rebound tenderness.* If appendix retrocecal, pain may be in flank or pelvic area.	Can occur at any age, although characteristically a disease of the young. Cause of abdominal sepsis in the elderly. If appendix perforates into free peritoneal space, peritonitis will occur with symptoms of pallor, a *quiet* abdomen, and shock.
Pyloric obstruction (stenosis)	Excessive projectile vomiting of sour and fermented undigested food. Obstinate constipation. Bulging of epigastric area. Left-to-right visible peristalsis. Palpation splashing fremitus. Percussion—(↑) area of gastric bubble. Auscultation—splashing sounds often audible at some distance.	May be due to narrowing of pyloric orifice or hypertrophy and hyperplasia of mucosa and submucosa.
Paralytic ileus	Weak, infrequent tinkling sound as ileus progresses. Silent abdomen when ileus becomes adynamic. Abdomen tense.	Acute intestinal obstruction—failure of progression of intestinal contents due to inadequacy of intestinal muscular activity.

Table 13-3 Continued

Terminology	Characteristics	Comments
Gastroenteritis	Abdominal cramps, vomiting, diarrhea. Bowel sounds—high-pitched and tinkling. Borborygmi sounds may be present.	Inflammation of the stomach and intestinal tract affect the small bowel predominantly.
Acute peritonitis	Chills, fever, abdominal pain. Severe abdominal tenderness, resulting in difficulty with respiration and body position. Vomiting, constipation. Bowel sounds—weak, infrequent, and then absent.	Rupture of an intraabdominal viscus, such as appendix or stomach. Infection from an inflamed adjacent organ or septicemia.
Acute cholecystitis	Tenderness of a palpably enlarged gallbladder on inspiration (Murphy's sign). Client unable to take full, deep breath when examiner's fingers are deep beneath right costal arch below hepatic margin.	Almost always caused by gallstones. Other causes may be bacteria or chemical irritants. RUQ or epigastric pain may be referred to the right subscapular area.
Acute pancreatitis	Sudden, intense, boring epigastric or left upper quadrant pain, with nausea, vomiting, and severe prostration. Paralytic ileus develops, characterized by abdominal distention, absence of bowel sounds. There is a rigid boardlike abdomen with rebound tenderness if peritoneal contamination occurs.	Most common pathologic factor is excessive alcohol consumption.
Acute diverticulitis	Similar to appendicitis but involving lower left quadrant, cramping pain, and dyschezia (painful defecation). May have flatulence and diarrhea.	Diverticula of bowel develop over time. If they become inflamed or obstructed, diverticulitis results.

characteristics of common disease conditions of the abdomen.

Inflammation and venous congestion can cause hepatomegaly that reveals a smooth, tender edge on palpation. The hepatomegaly associated with cirrhosis may have a firm, nontender edge. A firm or hard irregular edge of an enlarged liver suggests malignancy. The liver edge in chronic cirrhosis may feel nodular.

The spleen enlarges in several contagious diseases, systemic infections, and blood dyscrasias. These include infectious mononucleosis, septicemia, sickle cell anemia, and hemolytic jaundice. Bacterial endocarditis is an infection that is accompanied by splenic enlargement. Although not often seen in this country, malaria and schistosomiasis, endemic in other countries, lead to splenic enlargement. Extremely large spleens are encountered in leukemia, Hodgkin's disease, and lymphosarcoma.

Enlarged kidneys may be palpated in hydronephrosis. Large kidneys with palpable cysts are found in polycystic kidney disease. In children with Wilms' tumor, a rapidly developing sarcoma of the kidneys presents as a large abdominal mass. In hypernephroma, the most common neoplasm in adults, a large abdominal mass may be felt. CVA tenderness is often due to kidney infection.

Lymph Nodes and Pulses

Lymphadenopathy accompanies acute infections and systemic diseases. Enlarged, tender nodes may be present with inflammation of the thighs, legs, or feet. A weak, delayed, or absent femoral pulse is found with coarctation of the aorta; this warrants that the blood pressure be taken in the leg as well as the arm. With coarctation of the aorta, the leg blood pressure will be lower than the arm pressure reading. Weak or absent femoral pulse may also be detected in vascular insufficiency of the lower extremities due to advanced atherosclerosis. Enlarged, tender ingunal nodes may indicate lower abdominal inflammation.

BIOLOGIC AND CULTURAL VARIATIONS

Diabetes and Gallbladder Disease Among Native Americans

Epidemiologists and physicians have noted an alarming rise in the frequency of diabetes among various Native American tribes in the United States (West 1974). Whereas prior to 1940 diabetes seemed to be extremely rare or nonexistent among Native Americans in the Midwest, Southwest, and Alaska, in more recent years diabetes rates have equalled or surpassed those of white Americans. For example, in 1954 there were 94 known cases of diabetes among a Pima population of about 6,000. By 1961, the number of diabetics had risen to 283 out of a population of approximately 7,000.

Between 1963 and 1967, the records of 46 Public Health Service hospitals serving Native American communities and reservations showed the percentage of admissions due to diabetes to be 2.2%. The comparable figure for non-Native American hospitals throughout the United States was between 1.0% and 1.5% (Niswander 1968). The 2.2% admission rate was, of course, an average of a range of values for different tribes. In some Native American groups, the occurrence of diabetes is extremely high. Among the Cherokees of North Carolina, for example, the admission rate for diabetes was 10%. It is estimated that the prevalence rate for diabetes among Cherokees over age 30 in 1964 exceeded 25%, which is the highest rate for any population group reported up to that time.

The reason for this epidemic of diabetes is not clear. As is the case in many chronic diseases, the etiology is probably a combination of genetic and environmental factors. There is probably an underlying genetic propensity for the disease among Native Americans that has been triggered by changing dietary practices and increasing rates of obesity. Neel (1967) proposed the "thrifty gene" hypothesis, which points to the aboriginal lifestyle of Native Americans. He hypothesized that during the many centuries in which Native American groups lived a migrating, hunting-and-gathering way of life, marked by periods of feast and famine, a thrifty gene rose in frequency in many population groups. This gene might have affected carbohydrate metabolism and storage so that in times of feast carbohydrates would have been efficiently stored to serve energy needs in times of famine. In modern times, marked by an excessive supply of carbohydrates and calories, the thrifty gene leads to problems in carbohydrate metabolism, which in turn lead to diabetes (Niswander 1968). The thrifty gene hypothesis has never been proven, nor has the exact physiological mechanism been precisely stated. There are, of course, problems with generalizing the varied experiences and cultures of Native Americans. However, it may be that the high incidence rates of diabetes are due to some combination of genetic factors and modern dietary patterns and practices.

Another metabolic disease that exists in high frequency in many Native American population groups is gallbladder disease. For example, among Pimas the prevalence rate of gallbladder disease among adult males is 37.5% and among adult females is 67.6% (Burch, Comess, & Bennett 1968). Again, the factors contributing to these high rates are not known. Burch, Comess, and Bennett point to the potential contribution of diet, obesity, and diabetes. The rates of gallbladder disease are highly correlated with the diabetes incidence rates. Tribes that had high admission rates for diabetes also had high rates of gallbladder disease (Niswander 1968). It can be concluded that diabetes and gallbladder disease among Native Americans are important health problems for which mechanisms and contributing factors are very possibly related.

SUMMARY

This chapter discussed the structure and location of the various organs in the abdomen and the various techniques used in assessment of the organs. Assessment of the abdomen is best accomplished with the client in a supine or side-lying position. In contrast to the other areas of the body, initial inspection is not followed by palpation but by auscultation and percussion. The sounds listened for on auscultation are those of peristalsis and of vascular abnormalities. Percussion is performed to determine whether there is enlargement of an organ, presence of masses, or abdominal distention. Specific sounds heard at differing locations were described in the chapter. Palpation, the last technique performed in assessment of the abdomen, is performed to examine the liver, spleen, kidneys, hernias, and lymph nodes. Emphasis is placed on the importance of making the client as comfortable and as relaxed as possible.

DISCUSSION QUESTIONS/ ACTIVITIES

1. List the abdominal contents within each of the four abdominal quadrants and the midline area of the lower abdomen.

2. Give the rationale for the following sequence of approaches to the assessment of the abdomen: inspection, auscultation, percussion, palpation.
3. State the criterion for documenting "absence of bowel sounds."
4. What areas of the abdomen would be auscultated to assess whether bruits, venous hums, and peritoneal friction rubs are present?
5. Demonstrate the techniques for palpating the liver, spleen, and kidneys.
6. Demonstrate the method for determining the size of the liver and spleen by the percussion technique.
7. Describe the techniques used for detecting the various hernias.

REFERENCES

Burch, T. A.; Comess, L. J.; and Bennett, P. H. 1968. The problem of gallbladder disease among Pima Indians. In *Biomedical challenges presented by the American Indian,* Pan American Health Organization scientific publication no. 165. Washington, D.C.: World Health Organization.

McElroy, A., and Townsend, P. K. 1979. *Medical anthropology in perspective.* Boston: Duxbury Press.

Neel, J. V. 1967. Current concepts of the genetic basis of diabetes mellitus and the biological significance of the diabetic predisposition. *Excerpta Medica Internat. Congr.* Series no. 1725.

Niswander, J. D. 1968. In *Biomedical challenges presented by the American Indian,* Pan American Health Organization scientific publication no. 165. Washington, D.C.: World Health Organization.

West, K. M. 1974. Diabetes in American Indians and other native populations in the new world. *Diabetes* 23:841–855.

CHAPTER

14 Assessment of the Musculoskeletal System

Learning Objectives

1. Review the structure and function of the musculoskeletal system.
2. Recognize the characteristics noted in inspection and palpation of the muscles, bones, and joints.
3. Interpret muscle movement in order to categorize the grade of muscle strength.
4. Define the abnormal curvatures of the spine, such as kyphosis, lordosis, and lateral scoliosis.
5. List the joints that are routinely inspected and palpated.
6. Describe range of motion of the various joints of the body.
7. Describe the technique for detecting effusion of the knee.

In assessing the musculoskeletal system, three specific structures should be examined: the muscles, bones, and joints. It is important that the anatomic area being examined be fully exposed and free from any kind of restriction of movement from clothing or appliances. Merely rolling up a pant leg is not sufficient for thoroughly examining the leg. The anatomic area being assessed must be accessible to the main techniques to be used, inspection and palpation.

The comprehensiveness of the examination of the musculoskeletal system varies from client to client. A client with questionable musculoskeletal history would warrant a detailed, systematic physical assessment of this system. You would need to proceed carefully, placing emphasis on identifying existing deformities and on determining the status of specific muscles and joints. The most valuable adjunct assessment modality for evaluating the musculoskeletal system is x-ray. Certain observations of the musculoskeletal system are mentioned elsewhere in this text. For example, inspection of the cranium is more appropriately performed during the assessment of the head. Similarly, a cursory inspection of spinal curvature is easily accomplished during examination of the posterior thorax.

STRUCTURE AND FUNCTION OF THE MUSCULOSKELETAL SYSTEM

Muscles, Tendons, and Ligaments

Muscle fibers are grouped together to form fascicular bundles, which in turn are surrounded by connective tissue. The muscle mass consists of groups of these bundles. The skeletal muscles, which are characteristically composed of cross-striated muscle fibers, move parts of the body and are

BIOLOGIC AND CULTURAL VARIATIONS

Bone Density and Disorders Among White Americans

Certain differences in body constitution among population groups are associated with different disease rates. It has been shown, for example, that African-Americans have greater body density than white Americans. This difference is due to a number of differences in body constitution between the two population groups. African-Americans have less average subcutaneous fat than whites and smaller fatfold thicknesses at various sites on the body, such as the arms, legs, and torso. Because fat is less dense than muscle mass, this difference contributes to the lesser body density of white Americans. African-Americans also have longer leg length in relation to sitting height, which includes length of the head and torso. A third reason for the greater body density of African-Americans is that they have denser bones. African-Americans have a greater skeletal mass than white Americans and also tend to lose less bone in the later decades of life, when bone resorption becomes a significant problem for other population groups.

The increased bone density of African-Americans may account for their remarkably low frequency of certain bone disorders that present health problems for white Americans. The rate of occurrence of congenital dislocation of the hip during infancy and Legg-Calvé-Perthes disease during childhood is 50 times greater for whites than for African-Americans (Damon 1977). There are also significant differences in bone disease patterns during old age. Among elderly women, the rate of traumatic fractures is 50 times greater among white Americans than among African-Americans, and osteoporosis affects 5 times as many elderly white women as African-American.

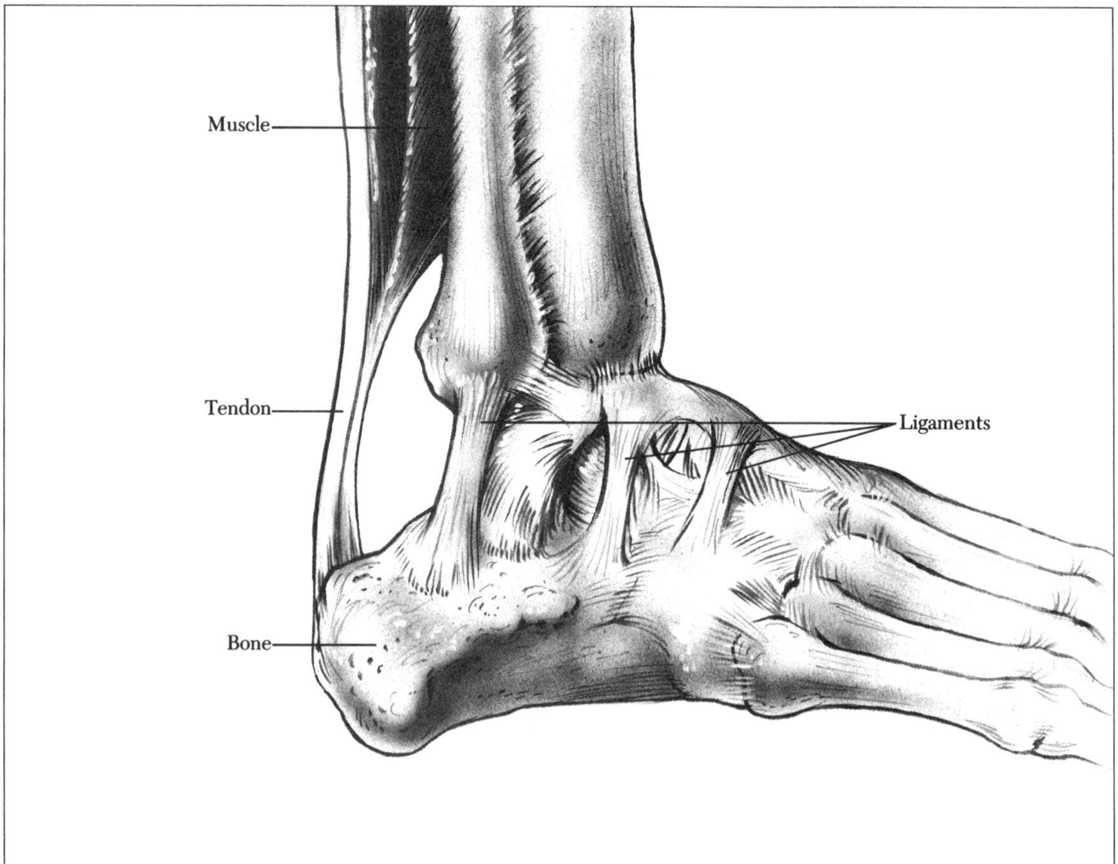

Figure 14-1 The relation of muscle to bones, tendons, and ligaments.

used in voluntary and reflex movements. They are the major focus in this chapter.

Muscular tissue is specialized for contractility. The point of attachment of the muscle to the bone is called the *origin.* The freely movable end is called the *insertion. Tendons* are fibrous connective tissues that attach muscles to the skeletal structure. *Ligaments* are bands of strong fibrous connective tissue that connect cartilage together, that connect the articular ends of the bones, and that serve as support or attachment for fascia or muscles (Fig. 14-1).

Bones

The skeletal system forms the solid structure around which the body is built. The bones provide surfaces for the attachment of muscles, tendons, and ligaments. Some of the bones form cage-like configurations to house and protect internal structures and organs. Examples are the cranium, which contains the brain, and the vertebral column, which protects the spinal cord. Many bones act as passive levers for moving various parts of the body.

Bone growth occurs in circumference and in length. Growth in diameter is due primarily to the activity of the osteoblastic cells. Longitudinal growth results from activity of the epiphyseal cartilage cells, at the end of the long bone shafts, which are eventually replaced by osteoblasts. Growth in bone length continues until the epiphyses are closed; this happens at about 18 to 20 years of age.

Joints

The articulation or point of juncture between two bones is called a *joint.* Joints are classified as synarthrodial, or immovable (as in cranial sutures); amphiarthrodial, or slightly movable (symphysis pubis); and diarthrodial, or freely movable, which provides the greatest range of movement (wrist, elbow, hip).

Bursae, closed sacs lined by synovial membrane, are found in some regions. The synovial membrane secretes fluid that prevents friction between the surfaces that glide over each other within the bursa. The most important bursae are located at the shoulder, elbow, knee, hip, and heel.

CHARACTERISTICS AND TECHNIQUES OF EXAMINATION

Muscles

The muscular portion of the musculoskeletal system is examined by assessing symmetry, muscle size, muscle tone, and muscular strength. As these components are assessed systematically, the corresponding muscles on each side of the body should be compared. Each individual has his own normal range of muscle strength; thus, he serves as his own scale by self-comparison. The muscle strength of an elderly client or that of a child cannot be compared with that of an athlete, nor is it easily compared with a scale of norm.

Inspection

- Compare right and left muscle size of the arms, thighs, and calves.
- Note any signs of contractures, muscular atrophy or hypertrophy.
- If there appears to be a discrepancy, measure and compare sizes.
- Inspect all muscles for signs of tremors or fasciculations. Fasciculations are involuntary twitchings of isolated bundles of muscle fibers and often occur with damage to neurons in the spinal cord (lower motor neuron damage).
- Examine the fine muscles of each hand for wasting.
- Observe the hands for tremors by asking the client to stretch his arms out in front of him.
- Fine tremors can be made more easily visible by placing a sheet of paper on top of the client's hands.
- If tremors do exist, determine whether they are resting tremors or intention tremors. A resting tremor is accentuated by rest and diminishes on movement. An intention tremor is accentuated by voluntary movement.
- Note any tics or other involuntary muscle movements.

Palpation

The tone and consistency of the muscles should be documented as normal, flaccid, or spastic.

- Palpate the muscles at rest to determine muscle tone.
- Assess the muscle tone during active and passive ranges of motion (ROM).
- Evaluate muscle strength or power by having the client squeeze your index finger with each hand; compare the pressure of the two grasps.
- When testing strength of hand grip, cross your arms so that the client grasps your left index finger with her left hand, and vice versa. In this way you can easily identify which hand grasp may be weaker by associating the weakness with your own body side. Otherwise, it is easy to mix up the client's left and right sides, as they are opposite of your own left and right sides.
- Ask the client to flex and extend the major joints actively without resistance.
- Ask the client to move her limbs horizontally without the influence of gravity; that is, she should move her arms while they are resting on a table and abduct her legs while supine.
- Compare the distal strength of each limb with the proximal strength.
- Have the client move the following major joints against applied resistance to test muscle strength:
  - Neck flexion, extension, and rotation
  - Shoulder abduction and adduction

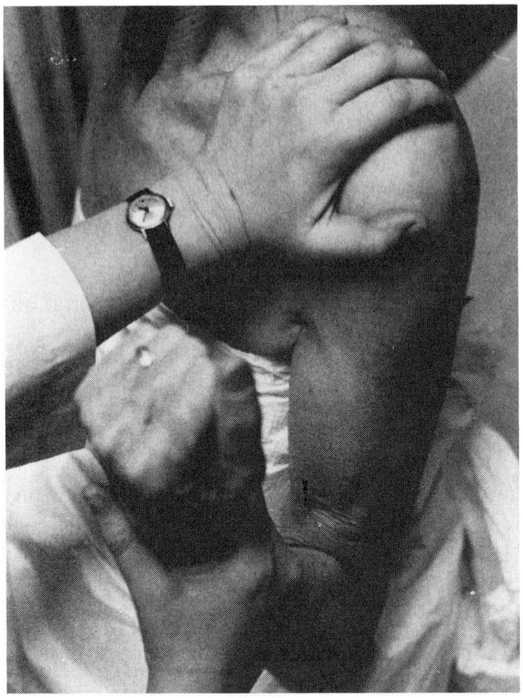

Figure 14-2 Testing muscle strength, left biceps. Ask the client to bend her elbow and resist attempts to straighten it. Place your left hand on the client's shoulder. With your right hand, grasp the client's wrist and attempt to straighten the arm. The degree of resistance is then assessed. If you release the client's wrist suddenly, her fist should not strike the hand on her shoulder. Such an overshooting response occurs in cerebellar disease.

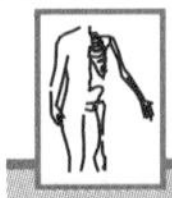

Technique for Inspection and Palpation of the Bones

1. Observe client from front, side, and back.
2. Ask client to straighten and hold back shoulders.
3. Ask client to bend over at the waist.
4. Palpate all bones for tenderness, pain.

- Elbow flexion and extension
- Wrist flexion and extension
- Hip flexion and extension
- Knee flexion and extension
- Ankle plantar flexion and dorsiflexion.

For examples of measuring strength against resistance, see Figs. 14-2 and 14-3. The normal individual has equal strength in all areas—on both sides and on the proximal and distal portions of the body. Table 14-1 presents the various scales used to document the grading of muscle strength.

Bones

Inspection

In gross examination of the skeletal system, keep in mind not only the normal structure and form of the body but also the deformities that can occur as well. The normal

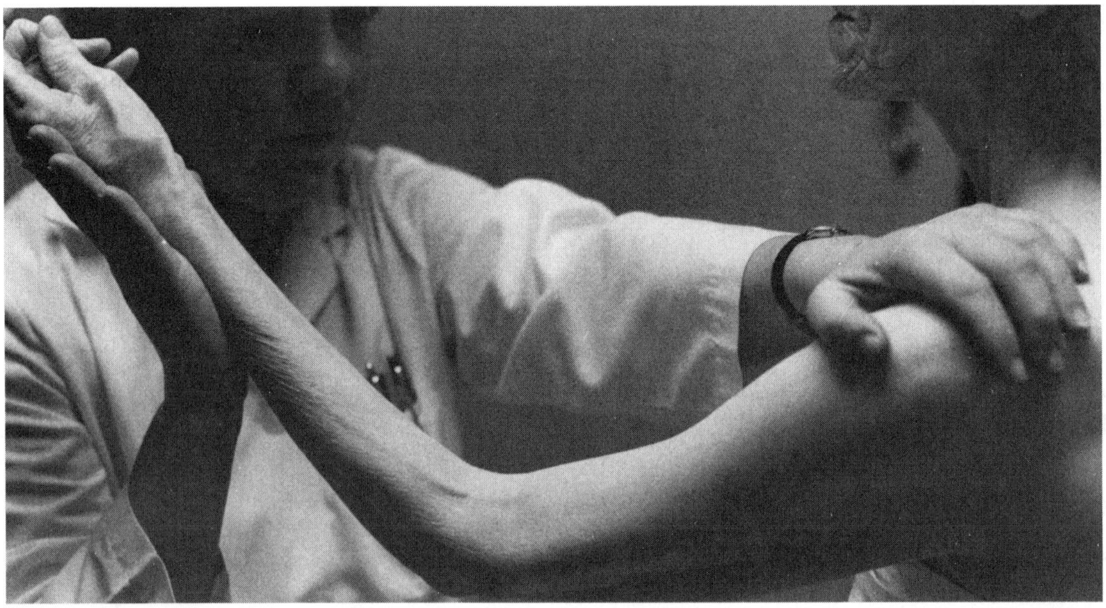

Figure 14-3 Testing muscle strength, left triceps. Ask the client to hold her left arm bent at the elbow. Place your left hand on the client's shoulder. Support the client's wrist with your right hand and ask the client to straighten her elbow against the resistance of your right hand.

Table 14-1 Scales for Grading Muscle Strength

Letter scale	Percent scale	Number scale	Interpretation
Normal (N)	100	5	Normal power
Good (G)	75	4	Muscle can make full normal movement but not against resistance.
Fair (F)	50	3	Muscle cannot move against resistance nor make full normal movement but can make normal movement against gravity.
Poor (P)	25	2	Full muscle movement possible with force of gravity eliminated.
Trace (T)	10	1	No movement of limb or joint, but contraction is visible or palpable.
Zero (0)	0	0	Total paralysis

spinal column is curved posteriorly in the thoracic region and anteriorly in the cervical and lumbar regions. From a posterior view, the normal spinal column is straight.

- Observe the client from the side to note any abnormality in the cervical, thoracic, or lumbar curvature.
- Observe the client from behind for any abnormality in lateral curvature. Occasionally, posture will simulate a mild scoliosis, so instruct the client to straighten up and hold back his shoulders.
- Observe the spinal curvature as the client bends over from the waist. Scoliosis that occurs from unequal leg length will disappear in this position. Structural scoliosis will be exaggerated in this position.
- Movements that will tend to exaggerate spinal deformities and aid in their detection are
  1. twisting the shoulder side to side
  2. bending to each side
  3. bending backward

The common spinal curvature abnormalities (Fig. 14-4) are kyphosis (humpback), lordosis (swayback), and scoliosis (lateral S curve).

Palpation

- Palpate all bones for tenderness as you examine each anatomic area. Bone pain is often the only symptom of osseous disease.
- Be alert, when examining the musculoskeletal system, to the signs and symptoms of fractures, including pain with acute tenderness over the site of the fracture, edema and bruising, deformity and possible shortening of a part, and limitation of movement.
- The elderly, whose bones tend to become more porous and brittle with decreasing circulatory nutrition, are particularly prone to fractures.
- The tumbling preschooler is also prone to fractures, especially of the clavicle, as are school-age and college students who are active in sports.

Technique for Inspection and Palpation of the Joints

1. Inspect and palpate:
   Temporomandibular joints
   Neck
   Interphalangeal, intermetacarpal, carpal bones and joints
   Elbows
   Shoulders
   Hips
   Patellar areas
   Ankles and feet
   Vertebral column and thoracic cage
2. Range of motion:
   Active
   Passive

Joints

Disease within or outside of a joint can cause limitation of joint movement.

- If joint movement is uniformly restricted in all directions, the disease process is within the joint.
- Limitation of movement in only one direction is usually the result of bony or soft tissue block outside the joint.
- A joint is considered unstable if motion can be carried through a greater than normal range.
- Excessive motion ordinarily occurs in only one direction and results from injury to a specific ligament or ligaments, as in a sprain.
- Carefully palpate joints at the points of attachment of the various ligaments to pinpoint identification of the injured ligament; the point of maximum tenderness indicates the site of injury.

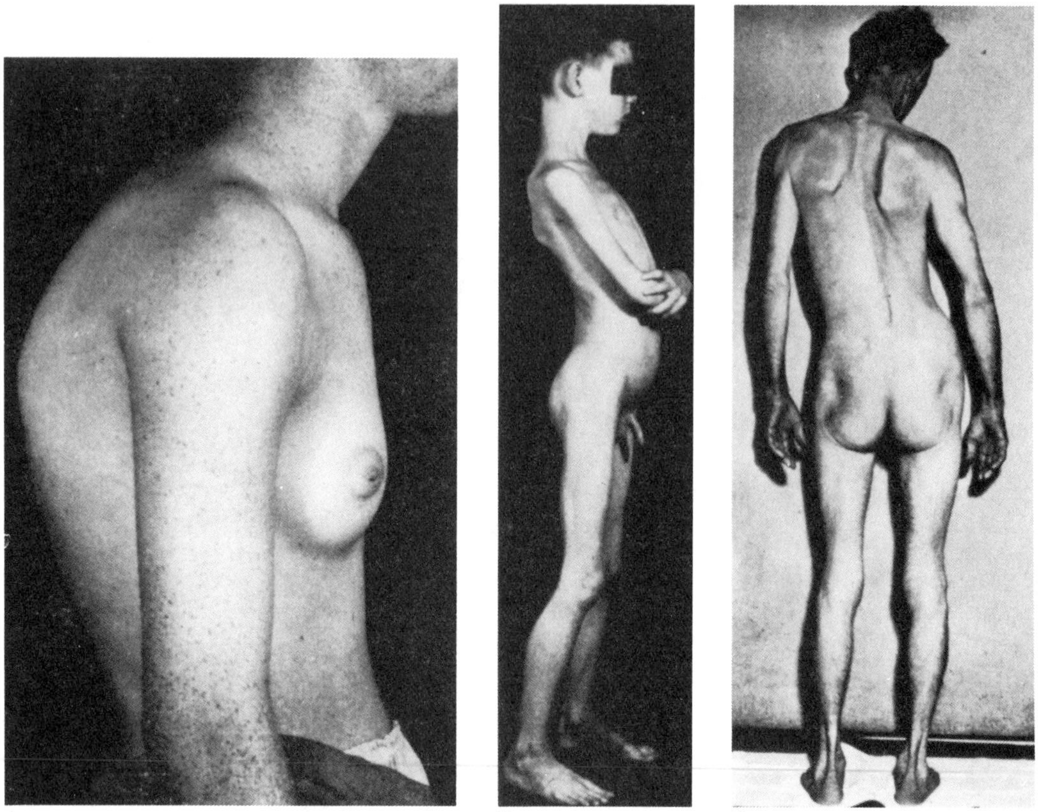

A B C

Figure 14-4 Spinal deviations. **(A)** Kyphoses. **(B)** Lordosis. **(C)** Scoliosis.

- Hyperflexibility of joints is a hereditary trait, and people with this condition are referred to as double-jointed or loose-jointed.
- Listen and palpate for crepitus. Crepitus is an audible crackling, or it may be palpated as a grating sensation, or both, as the joint is moved through its ROM.
- Swelling of a joint may be caused by fluid within the joint or within an overlying bursa.
  - Swelling is palpated over the entire joint area when the fluid exists within the joint.
  - Palpation reveals a smaller sharply localized area of swelling when the fluid is in a bursa.

Inspection and Palpation

All joints should be assessed for symmetry, tenderness, bogginess, swelling, thickening, crepitation, and nodules. The following joints (Fig. 14-5) are routinely inspected and palpated:

1. *Temporomandibular (TMJ) joints:* Inspect, palpate, and listen for crepitation as client opens and closes his mouth (Fig. 14-6). Place index fingers over the joints and have client open and close jaw slowly. TMJ symptoms consist of pain on one or both sides of the jaw which is aggravated by chewing and may be accompanied by "clicking" of the jaw.
2. *Neck:* Inspect and note suppleness of movement.
3. *Interphalangeal, intermetacarpal, and carpal bones and joints:* Inspect and palpate (Fig. 14-7). Repetitive movement may irritate the medial nerve running through the carpal tunnel under the carpal bones of the wrist, or it may be entrapped by inflammatory edema; the client complains of pain, numbness, and tingling in the area and will have increased symptoms when asked to hold the wrist in full palmar flexion for 2 minutes (Fig. 14-8).
4. *Elbows:* Inspect and, with the elbow mildly flexed, palpate the groove on either side of the olecranon process, paying close attention to the epitrochlear lymph nodes at the medial, inner aspects of the elbow. With tennis elbow, it is very painful when the dorsiflexed wrist is forced into plantar flexion position.
5. *Shoulders:* Inspect and palpate the sternoclavicular joint, the acromioclavicular joint, and the head of the humerus. Commonly, shoulder pain is due to muscular problems rather than bone. Also, consider health problems that

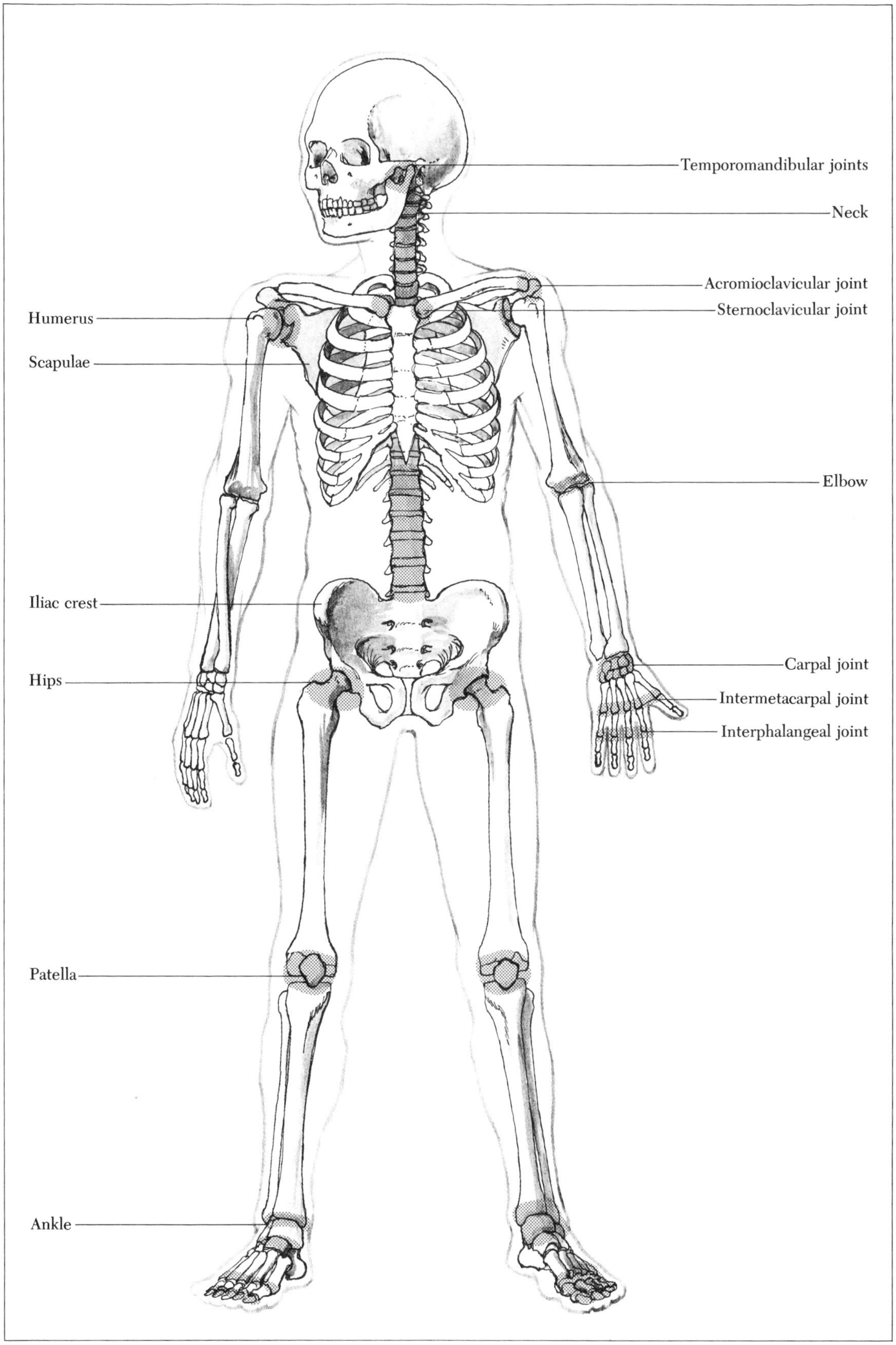

Figure 14-5 The major joints of the body.

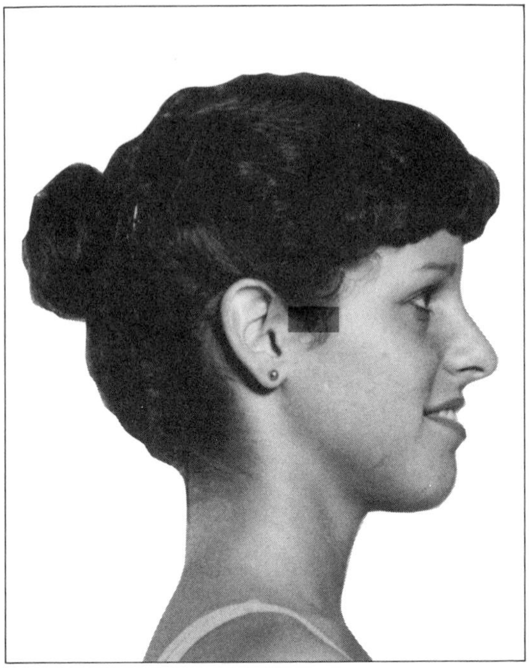

Figure 14-6 Location of the temporomandibular joint.

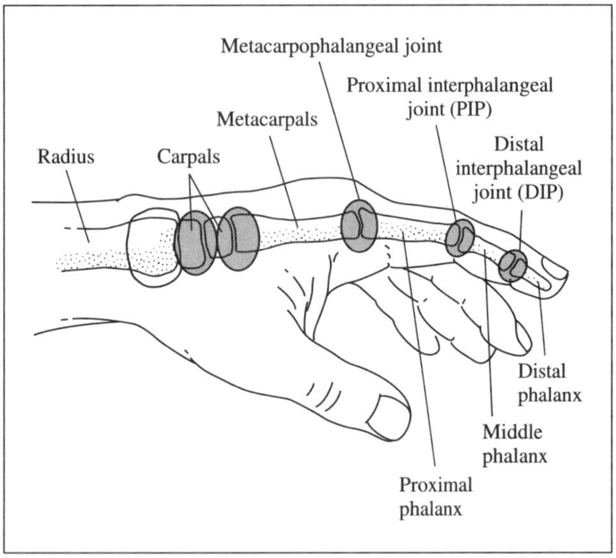

Figure 14-7 Bones and joints of the hands.

have referred pain to the shoulder (e.g., gallbladder and heart disease and lung tumors).

6. *Hips:* Inspect length of legs as well as alignment, and palpate areas for tenderness.

7. *Patellar areas:* Inspect and palpate the popliteal space, and then have the client sit to palpate both sides of each patella and the suprapatellar pouch (Fig. 14-9). When fluid exists, it is "milked" to the knee by using your thumb to compress the area above the knee with your left hand, and

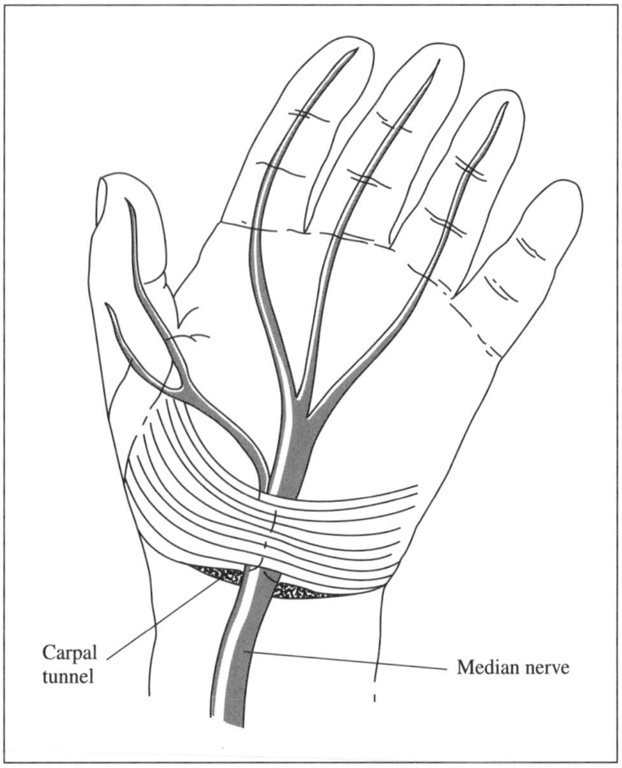

Figure 14-8 Carpal tunnel and medial nerve.

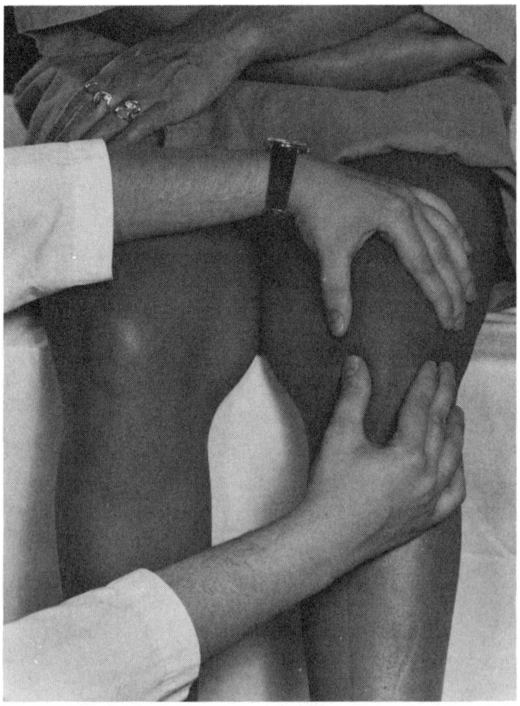

Figure 14-9 Palpation of the knee. With the client seated and her leg allowed to hang loosely, palpate the articulation between the thumb and index finger of your right hand. To test for effusion, apply compression above the patella with your left hand. If fluid is present, it is forced down and causes a bulge below and on either side of the patella.

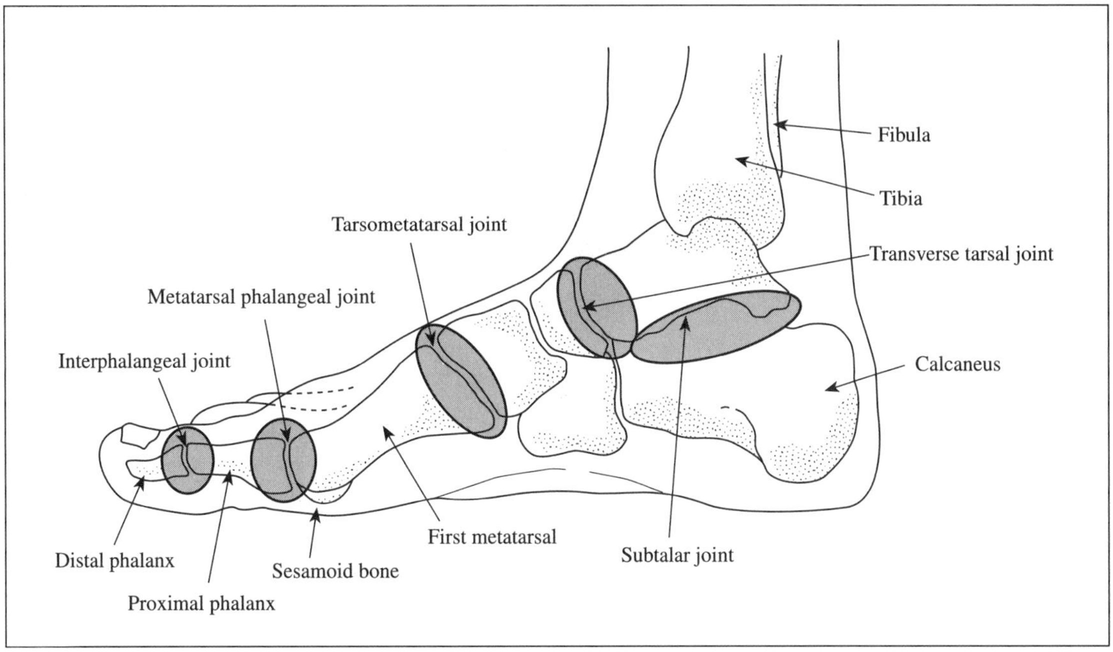

Figure 14-10 Bones and joints of the foot.

with your opposite hand tap the patella while the knee is extended on the examining table. *Ballottement* will result in a fluid-pressure pulsation against the fingertips on either side of the patella when edema is present.

8. *Ankles and feet:* Inspect and palpate for tenderness. Hold the leg with one hand and rotate the heel and foot into eversion and inversion. An early sign of rheumatoid arthritis is pain on squeezing the metatarsalphalangeal joints between your thumb and index finger (thumb and index finger on either side of the foot at the level of the base of the toes.) Figure 14-10 illustrates the bones and joints of the foot.
9. Vertebral column and thoracic cage:
   - Inspect, noting any difference in the height of the scapulae and the iliac crests.
   - Inspect for straightness of the spine from the back as the client bends forward to touch her toes.
   - Palpate the spinous processes and ribs for tenderness or muscle spasm.

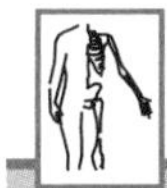

Technique for Inspection and Palpation of the Muscles

1. Examine both sides of the body.
2. Compare muscle size of arms, thighs, and calves. Measure with tape if discrepancy noted.
3. Examine for tremors: Have client stretch arms in front. To detect fine tremors, place sheet of paper on top of client's hands.
4. Palpate muscles at rest.
5. Note condition of muscles when client does active and passive range of motion.
6. Assess client's muscle strength.

Range of Joint Motion

- Ask the client to *actively move* his body through various movements.
- Note the extent of movement and the smoothness and ease of performance.
- Normally you should observe smoothness and little effort exerted on the part of the client.

Figures 14-11 through 14-18 show the normal ROM for each joint.

- *Passively* move the client's joints through ROM.
- Record any resistance or limitation in movement.
- There are several means of measuring joint motion:
  - Noting the comparison between the corresponding joints of the client (the easiest way)
  - Using your own range of movement as a gauge if you have no limitations
  - Using a standard method based on the neutral position of a joint (when extremity is extended) being zero degrees (0°)
  - Using a goniometer, a device that incorporates a protractor

Tables that list degrees of range of joint motion are useful; however, you need to realize that there are differences between individuals and between age groups.

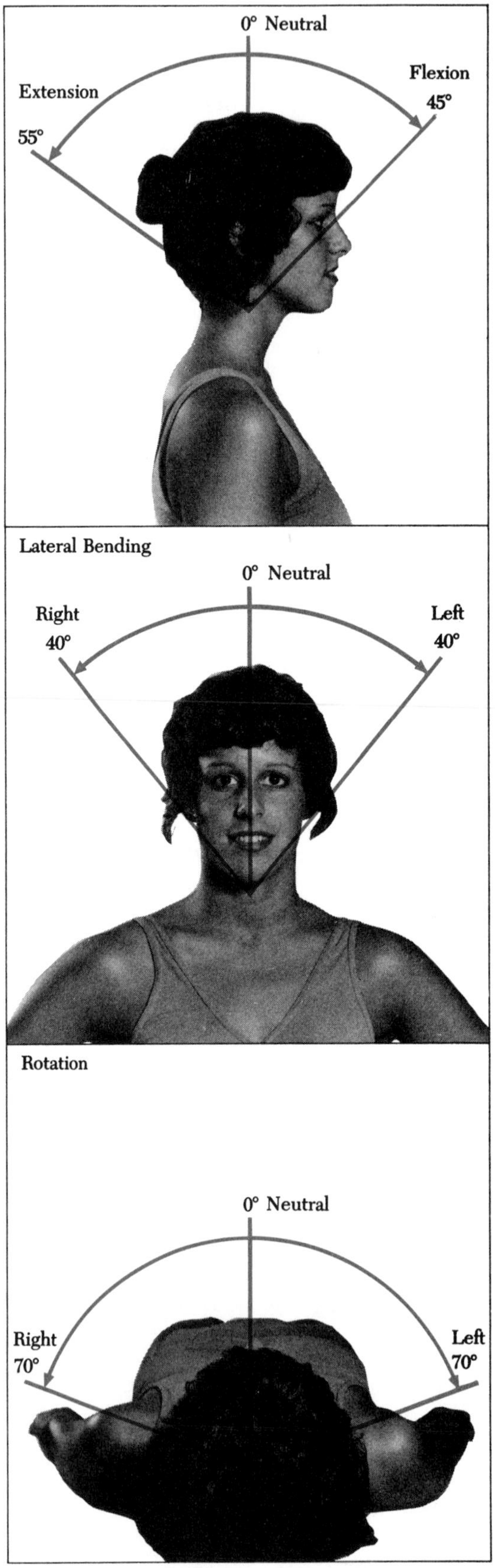

Figure 14-11 Range of motion of the neck.

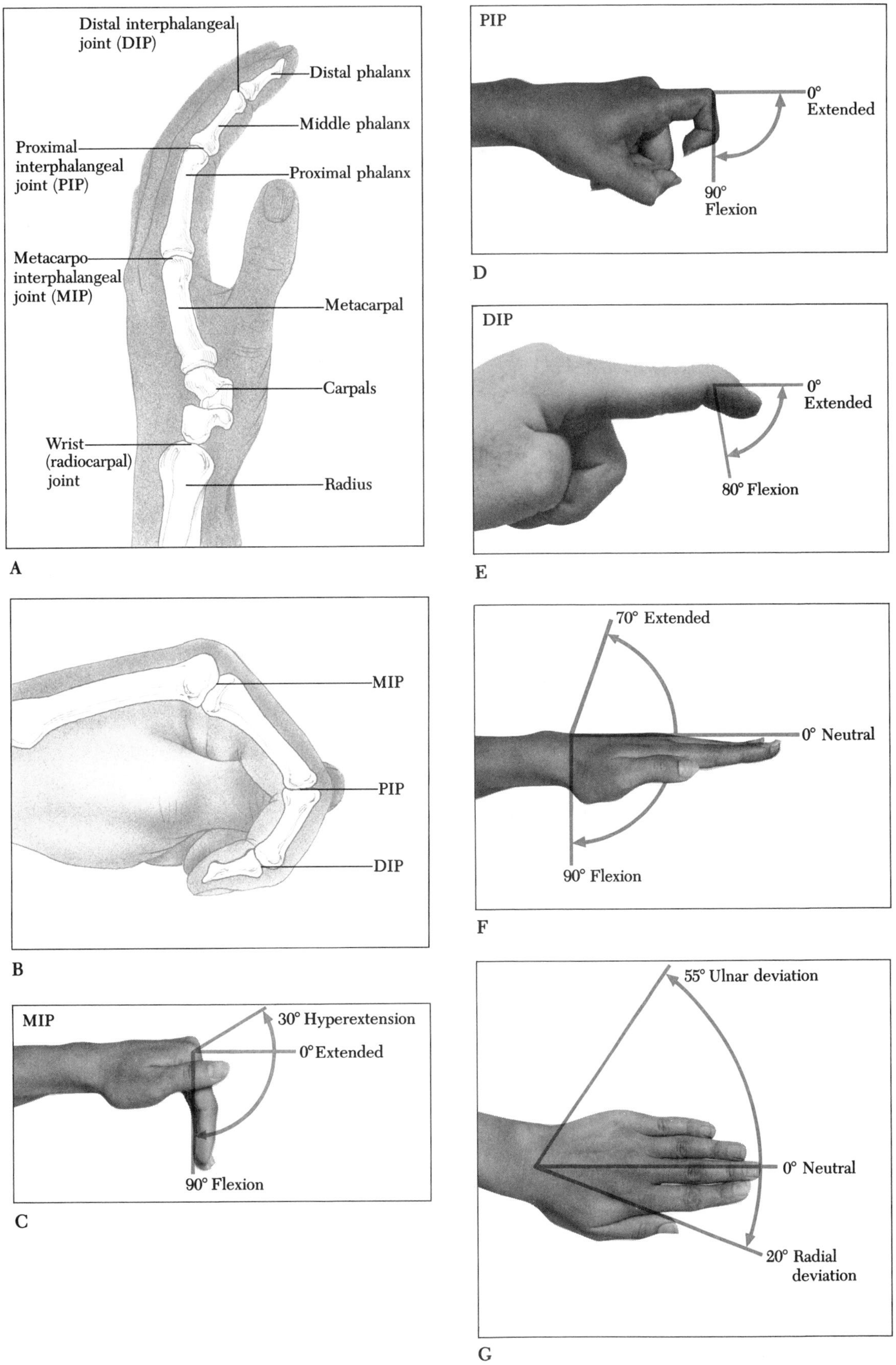

Figure 14-12 Location and range of motion of the interphalangeal, intermetacarpal, and carpal joints and bones. **(A)** Basic joints of the hand. **(B)** Normal fist. **(C, D, E)** Range of movement of finger joints. **(F, G)** Range of wrist motion.

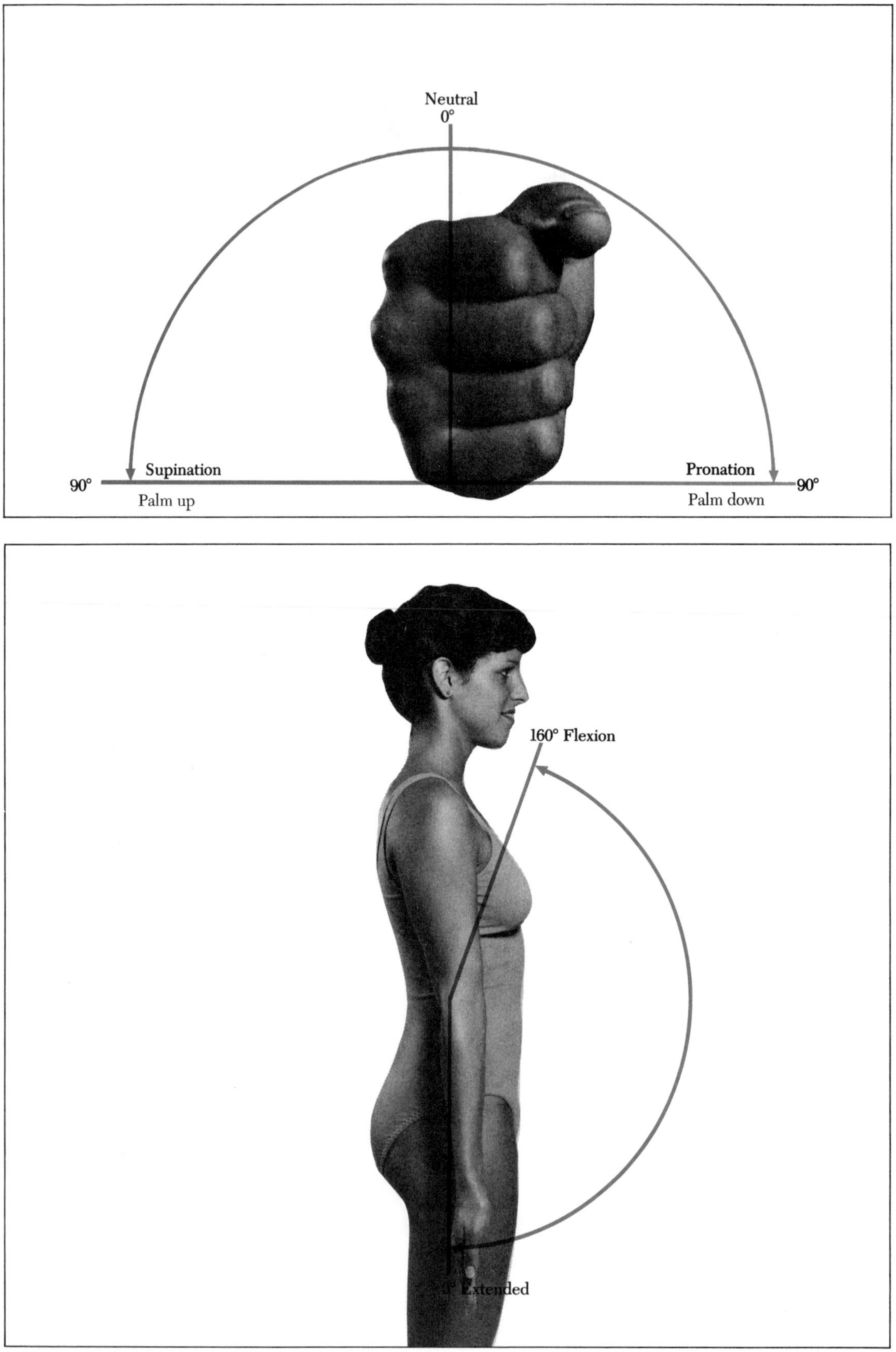

Figure 14-13 Range of motion of the elbow.

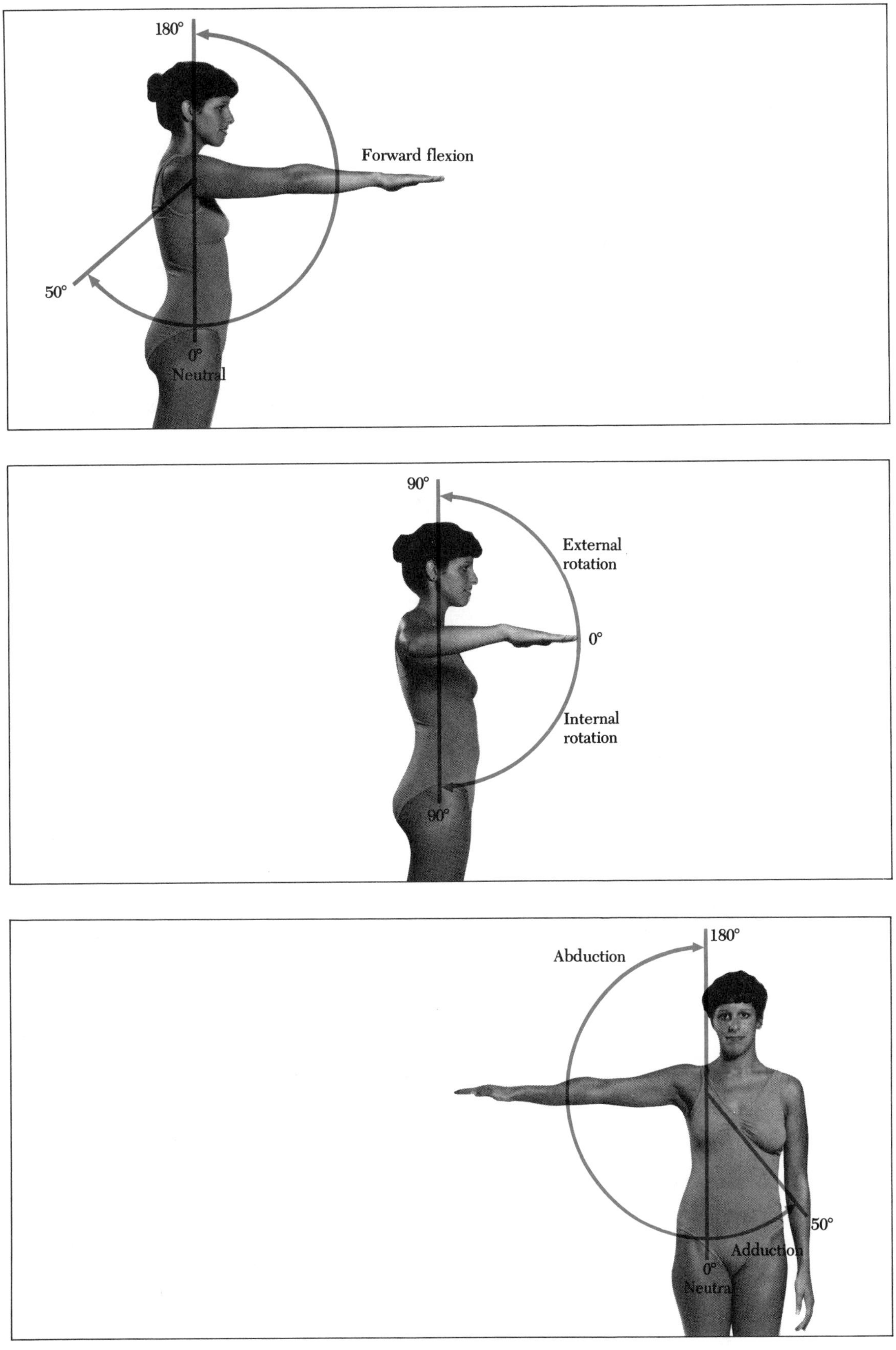

Figure 14-14 Range of motion of the shoulder.

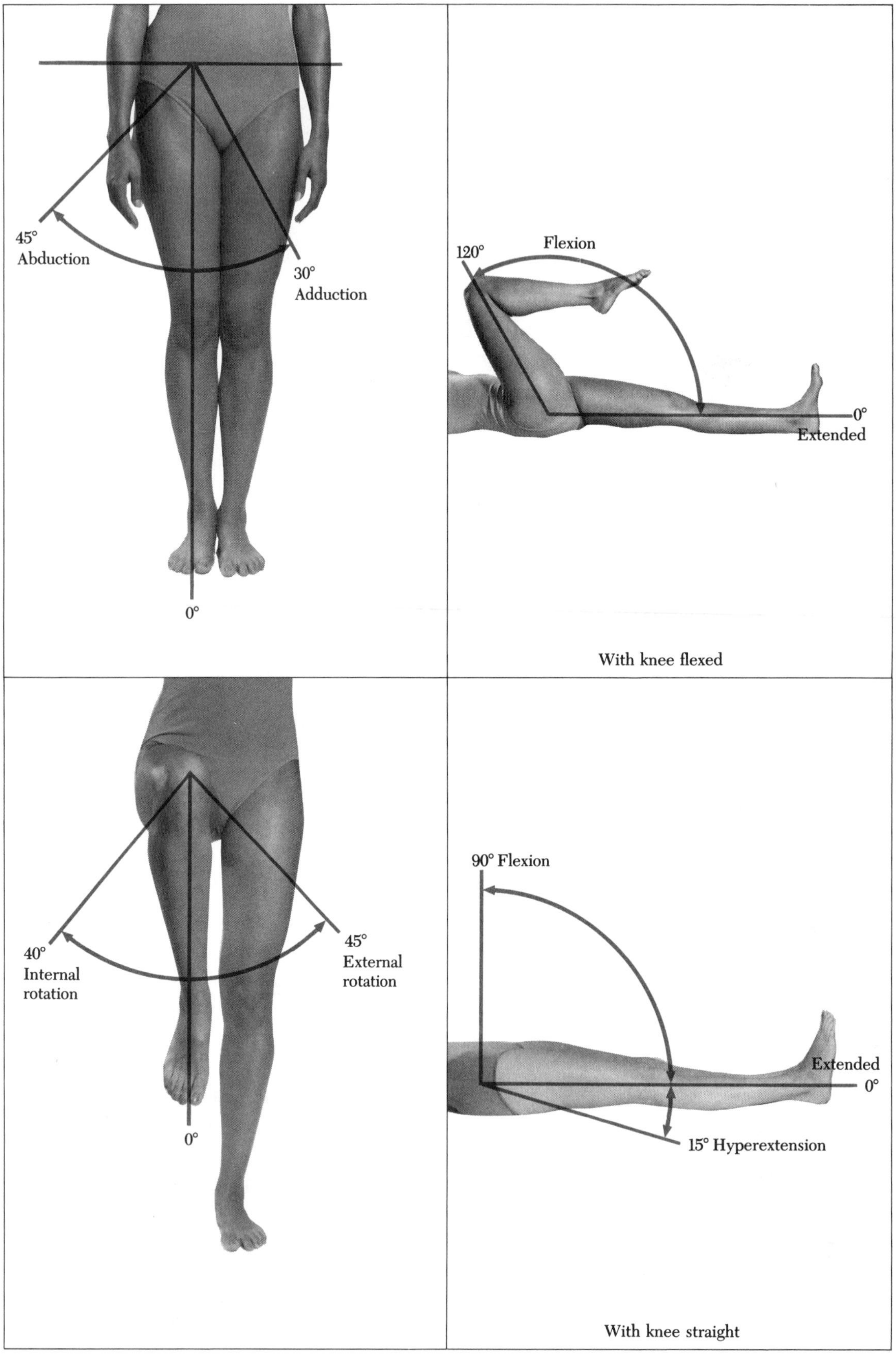

Figure 14-15 Range of motion of the hip.

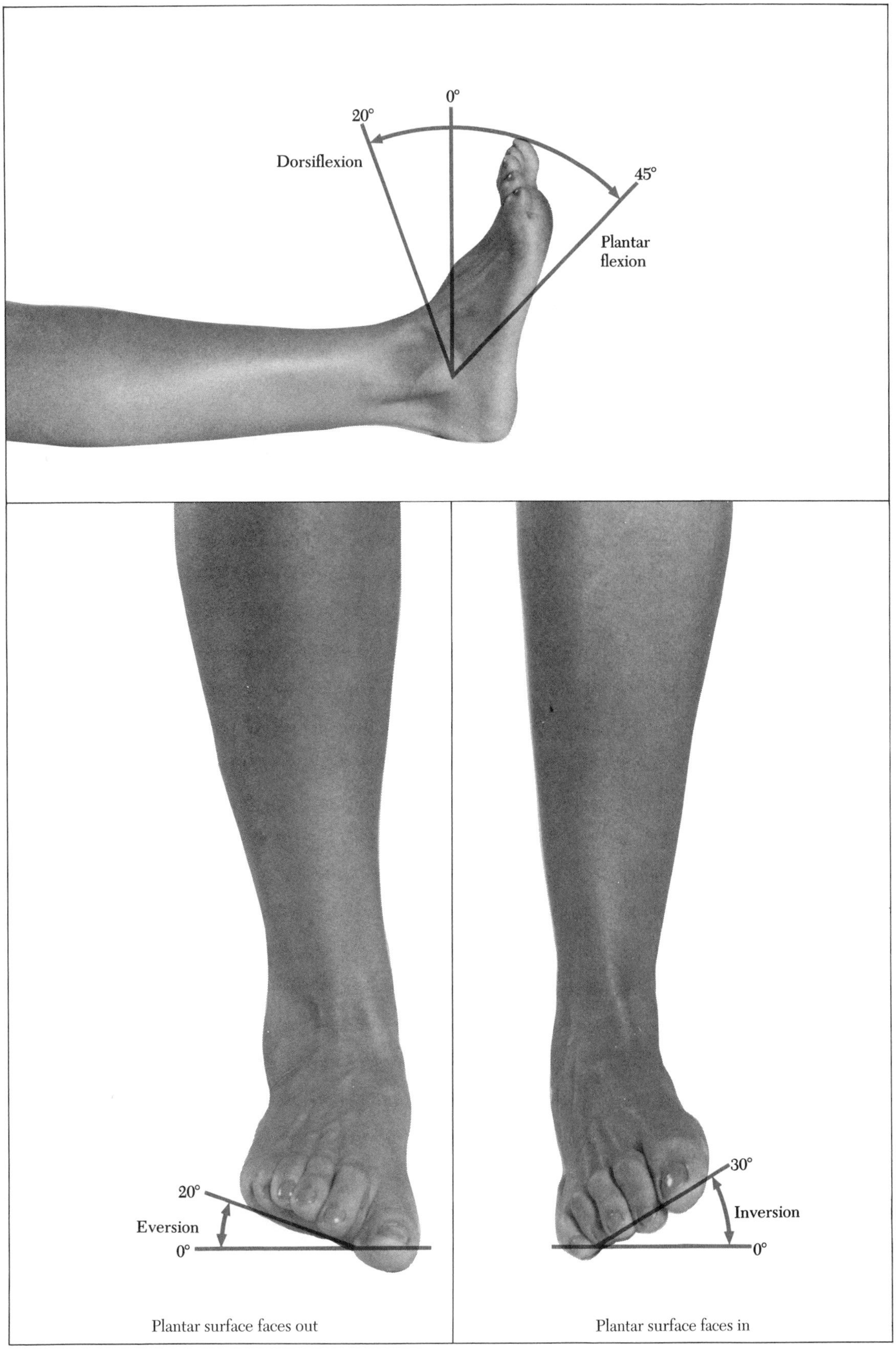

Figure 14-16 Range of motion of the ankle and foot.

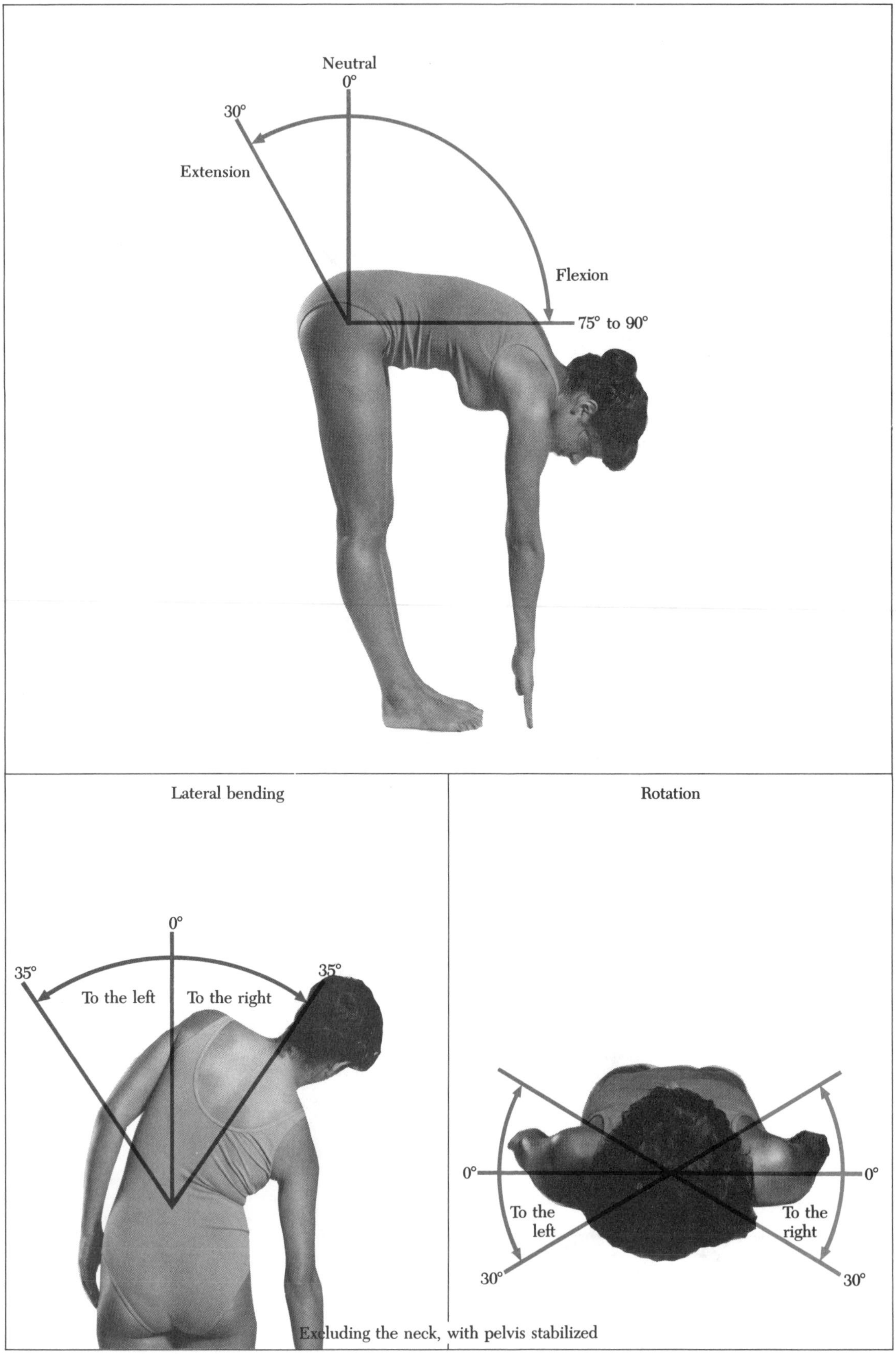

Figure 14-17 Range of motion of the spine.

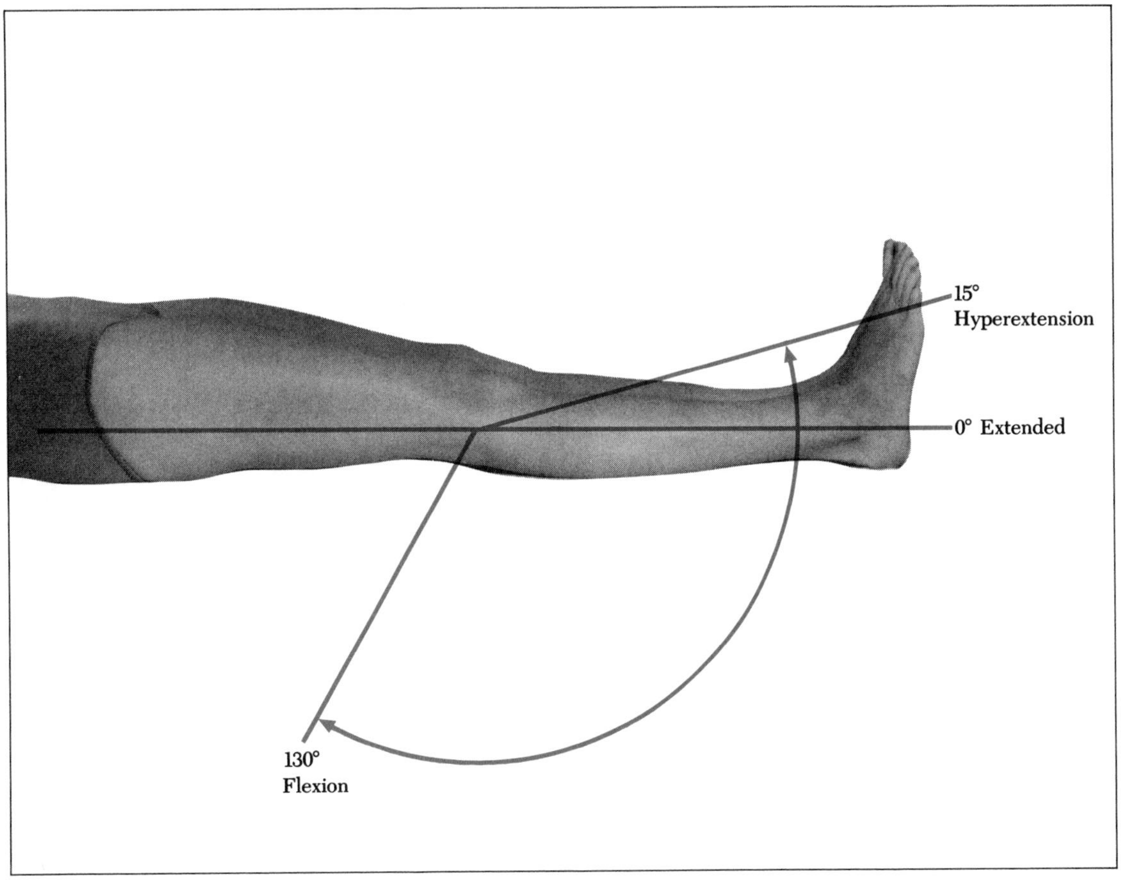

Figure 14-18 Range of motion of the knee.

CLINICAL CORRELATIONS

Muscles

Contractures or shortening of muscles and tendons may result in skeletal atrophy or deformity. Diminished muscle mass can be associated with disuse or can be the result of neuromuscular disease such as poliomyelitis, diseases of the brain or spinal cord, peripheral neuropathy, or peripheral nerve injury. Atrophy of the muscle may also be due to primary muscle disease such as muscular dystrophies and myotonia. Muscular dystrophies manifest as muscular weakness, yet there is the appearance of hypertrophied muscles. This is because muscle tissue has been replaced by fibrous tissue.

The small tender nodules often palpated in the periscapular, back, and gluteal muscles are called fibrocytic nodules. Tumors of the muscle are rare.

Myositis ossificans, found in the quadriceps muscles and in back and arm muscles, is so typical among football linemen that it is referred to as "blockers' node." Sports injuries and nursing management are delineated in Table 14-2.

Congenital anomalies of muscles occur most frequently in the sternocleidomastoid and the pectoralis major muscles. Portions of these muscles may be absent.

Enlargement of muscles or groups of muscles is found in congenital hypertrophy and in pseudohypertrophic muscular dystrophy.

A resting tremor is the characteristic tremor of Parkinson's disease. An intention tremor is found in cerebellar disease and multiple sclerosis. Tics and certain other gross involuntary muscle movements become exaggerated when the client is under stress and usually disappear when the client is sleeping. These movements suggest disturbance of the extrapyramidal motor areas, in particular the basal ganglia. Some involuntary movements may be of an emotional origin or may be due to muscle fatigue.

Flaccid, easily movable muscles are present in lower motor neuron disease, whereas spastic muscles (which demonstrate initial resistance and then suddenly give) are found in pyramidal disease, for example, upper motor neuron damage in the motor strip of the cerebrum or brain stem (cerebrovascular accident). Typically, with pyramidal disease, the tone in the flexor muscles of the arms increases, whereas in the legs, the tone of the extensors increases.

Table 14-2 **Sports Injuries**

Injury	Etiology	Behavioral assessment	Medical therapy	Nursing management
		Acute Injuries		
Knee				
Contusion	Blunt force to soft tissue; common in gymnastics, hockey	Ecchymosis, edema, tenderness *Mild*—full ROM 24 hr later *Moderate*—½ ROM 24 hr later *Severe*—⅓ ROM 24 hr later	Ice Compression wrap ankle to thigh Elevation Crutch or cane in hand opposite side of injury	Demonstrate correct application of compression wrap.
Sprain	Force is exerted that exceeds normal range of motion: *Mild*—few fibers of ligaments torn *Moderate*—ligament torn, some functional loss *Severe*—fibers completely torn	*Mild*—pain, swelling; joint stable with no locking *Moderate*—pain, swelling, limitation of movement; joint stable but may lock *Severe*—pain, immediate swelling; joint unstable and may lock	*Mild*—ice for 24–48 hr, aspirin, activity limited as necessary *Moderate*—knee immobilizer splint 2–3 weeks; exercises: 10 straight leg lifts per hour while awake, quad sets, ROM; resume sports 6–8 weeks *Severe*—surgical repair of ligaments; cast 3–4 weeks; no weight bearing; may be 6–10 months before resuming sports	Assess neurovascular status of affected leg. Apply ice and elevate leg. Reinforce explanations regarding purpose of knee immobilizers, compression wraps, casts. Demonstrate correct application of immobilizers, compression wrap. Explain cast care. Demonstrate crutch walking, if needed. Demonstrate leg lifts, isometric exercises. Give specific explanations regarding limitations of movement.
Cruciate ligaments	Hyperextension or excessive external rotation on anterior ligament, especially with abrupt stops Fall on flexed knee injures posterior ligament	"Pop" as knee gives way		
Collateral ligaments	Valgus stress to knee injures medial collateral ligament Varus stress injuries lateral collateral ligament	Tearing, ripping sound		
Meniscal tears	Vigorous rotation of femur on tibia Internal rotation injures medial meniscus	Sudden and severe pain Click heard when rotating tibia on femur when knee is flexed	*Conservative*—evacuate joint of intraarticular fluid; ice 24–36 hr followed by heat; avoidance of weight bearing; quadriceps exercises	

	External rotation injures lateral meniscus	Inability to extend joint fully Swelling Knee locks occasionally Buckling during walking	*Surgical*—Removal of meniscus surgically; ice, compression dressing, elevation of affected leg; quadriceps setting exercises beginning on 2nd day postoperatively, done 10–15 min 3–4 times daily; progress to straight leg raising; return to sports within 10 weeks Immobilization in extension for 4–6 weeks May require surgery to repair Quadriceps exercises	Demonstrate exercises. Teach crutch walking or use of cane. Postoperatively, apply ice; elevate extremity; assess neurovascular status.
Patellar dislocation	Lateral (valgus) rotation stress or direct blow to medial aspect of knee	Buckling Pain in medial aspect of knee Can feel knee "go out of place" but return to normal when leg is extended Excessive movement of patella possible in lateral direction Crepitation between patella and femoral groove Reports having heard sound "like canvas ripping" at time of injury	Immobilization in extension for 4–6 weeks May require surgery to repair Quadriceps exercises	
Shoulder dislocation	Force causing excessive abduction, extension, and external rotation Humerus displaced anteriorly and inferiorly	Pain Humeral head palpable in anterior axilla	With child lying prone on examination table and arm suspended over side, sustained anterior traction (toward floor) is manually applied.	Assess for injury of axillary nerve by testing for sensation where deltoid inserts on humerus and by asking child to attempt to abduct arm. Assess for ulnar nerve injury by asking child to abduct and adduct the four medial digits. Administer analgesic prior to reduction procedure.
Ankle sprain	Violent force at high speed exceeding normal range of motion: *Mild*—ligament stretched but not torn *Moderate*—ligament partially torn *Severe*—ligament(s) completely torn	"Pop" or "snap" heard with injury Obvious deformity Swelling Pain when moved through range of motion Discoloration at joint	Ice or cold water applied during acute phase Compression bandages or tape strapping Crutches After 48 hr, contrast baths or whirlpool	Apply ice and elevate leg. Apply compression bandage. Demonstrate both non-weight-bearing and weight-bearing gaits on crutches. Demonstrate ROM exercises.

Continued

Table 14-2 Continued

Injury	Etiology	Behavioral assessment	Medical therapy	Nursing management
Acute Injuries, continued				
Leg Quadriceps contusion	Excessive force applied, usually to anterior or anterolateral portion of muscle	Decreased ability to bend knee Occasionally, a palpable hematoma present; discoloration after 48 hr	Ice Compression bandage Crutches or bedrest Rehabilitation exercises: quadriceps contractions, ROM exercises	Apply ice. Apply compression bandage. Demonstrate crutch walking. Demonstrate exercises.
Overuse Injuries				
Achilles tendinitis	Repeated forcible stretching of short Achilles' tendon	Pain usually around tendon itself when exercising or when plantar flexing the foot	*For all overuse injuries:* Rest, decreased training activities, alternate exercise such as cycling instead of running, crutches or casting for 4–5 days	*For all overuse injuries:* Stress the need to change those activities that brought on the pain of the injury. Teach stretching exercises: 1. Stretch affected muscle for 15–20 sec almost to where pain occurs. 2. Relax 15–20 sec. 3. Repeat 5–6 times at least 3 times daily or as ordered. Teach restrengthening exercises: *Isometric* 1. Tighten involved muscle for 8–10 sec. 2. Relax briefly. 3. Repeat 8–10 times at least 3 times daily or as ordered. *Isotonic* 1. Lift prescribed weight with affected muscle through range of motion for 3 sec. 2. Relax briefly. 3. Repeat 10 times at least 3 times daily or as ordered. Apply ice. Teach patient to check condition of skin beneath splints, braces daily. Review purpose and side effects of aspirin.
Stress fractures	Repeated stress, usually in tibia	Swelling in area of fracture Limp Pain may be sharp and persistent or dull and aching Tenderness over a specific point	Stretching exercises Restrengthening exercises Ice for 30–40 min over injury Whirlpool at 10°–20°C Alternate cold with heat Ultrasound	
Plantar fascitis	Repeated stretching of plantar fascia	Pain in arch or heel Limp Walks on lateral aspect of foot	Tape strapping, splints, braces High-intensity galvanic stimulation Aspirin 2–3 tablets 4 times daily	
Anterior leg pain ("shin splints")	Repeated traction on anterior or posterior tibialis muscles	Pain and tenderness along middle or distal portions of tibia		

Source: From J. Servonsky and S. Opas: *Nursing Management of Children.* Boston: Little, Brown, 1987.

RECORDING OF FINDINGS

Normal findings are recorded in the first column. Findings for a client diagnosed as having suffered a right cerebrovascular accident are recorded in the second column.

Muscles
Inspection: Symmetrical; no hypertropy or atrophy noted; no tremors; no fasciculations; no abnormal muscle movements

Palpation: No tenderness; proximal and distal strength equal; good muscle tone on palpation

Bones
Inspection: Body and limb symmetry; no increase in normal spinal curvatures; no deformities

Palpation: No tenderness

Joints
Inspection: Full range of movement—smooth without limitations; no swelling

Palpation: No tenderness; no crepitation

Muscles
Inspection: Atrophied fine muscles of left hand; left hemiplegia

Palpation: Strength good on right side with equal proximal and distal strength; muscle tone rigid on left side

Bones
Inspection: Body and limb symmetry; no increase in normal spinal curvatures; no deformities

Palpation: No tenderness

Joints
Inspection: Full active range of movement on right side; left-sided, marked reduction and pain of shoulder and hip abduction and extension, elbow extension and dorsiflexion of foot with passive movement pressure; no swelling.

Palpation: No tenderness; no crepitation

A pattern of weakness may aid in determining whether there is dysfunction of a single peripheral nerve or of an entire nerve root. Muscle weakness or paralysis indicates neurologic disturbance or a lesion along the pyramidal pathway in the cerebrum, within the brain stem and spinal cord, in the peripheral nerves, at the neuromuscular junctions, or in the muscle tissues themselves.

Bones

Limb deformities include such conditions as clubfoot (talipes varus and valgus), toe-walking deformities (talipes equinus) (Fig. 14-19), flatfoot (pes planus), abnormal hollowness of the sole of the foot (pes cavus), and congenital amputation (the absence of a limb or portion thereof). Knee deformities include genu varum (bowlegs) and genu valgum (knock knees). Another deformity of the skeletal system is Sprengel's deformity, a congenital elevation of the scapula (Fig. 14-20). A skeletal deformity that follows a Colles' fracture of the wrist is sometimes referred to as a "silver fork" deformity.

Two common hip deformities are those of dislocation and fracture. Adduction of the leg and internal rotation with hip and knee flexion are characteristic on the side of hip dislocation. A fractured hip results in external rotation and leg abduction of the affected side (Figs. 14-21). Arthritis causes skeletal deformity of the joints (Figs. 14-22 through 14-25 and Table 14-3).

Nutritional deficiencies can influence skeletal structure. The disease of rickets (Fig. 14-26), caused by vitamin D deficiency or by renal insufficiency, is manifested in skeletal malformation.

Legg-Calvé-Perthes disease also causes skeletal disorders. This condition generally has its onset in children between the age of 3 and 12. It occurs 4 times more often in boys than in girls. The signs of this skeletal problem are intermittent and include a protective limp, limited movement of the hip joint, and atrophy of the thigh muscles due to disuse. Any child who displays such signs should be referred to a physician.

Acute pain accompanies fractures and osteomyelitis. Chronic bone pain is present in such conditions as osteoporosis, neoplasms, hyperparathyroidism, Legg-Calvé-Perthes disease, and Paget's disease of the bone.

Massive instability of a joint, permitting grotesque motion, is characteristic of neurologic diseases. This type of condition can be seen in the Charcot's joints associated with tabes dorsalis and occasionally with diabetic neuropathy. Note the unusual alignment (Fig. 14-27) as the client supports himself on such joints. Ehlers-Danlos syndrome is a rare condition in which clients exhibit generalized hyperflexibility.

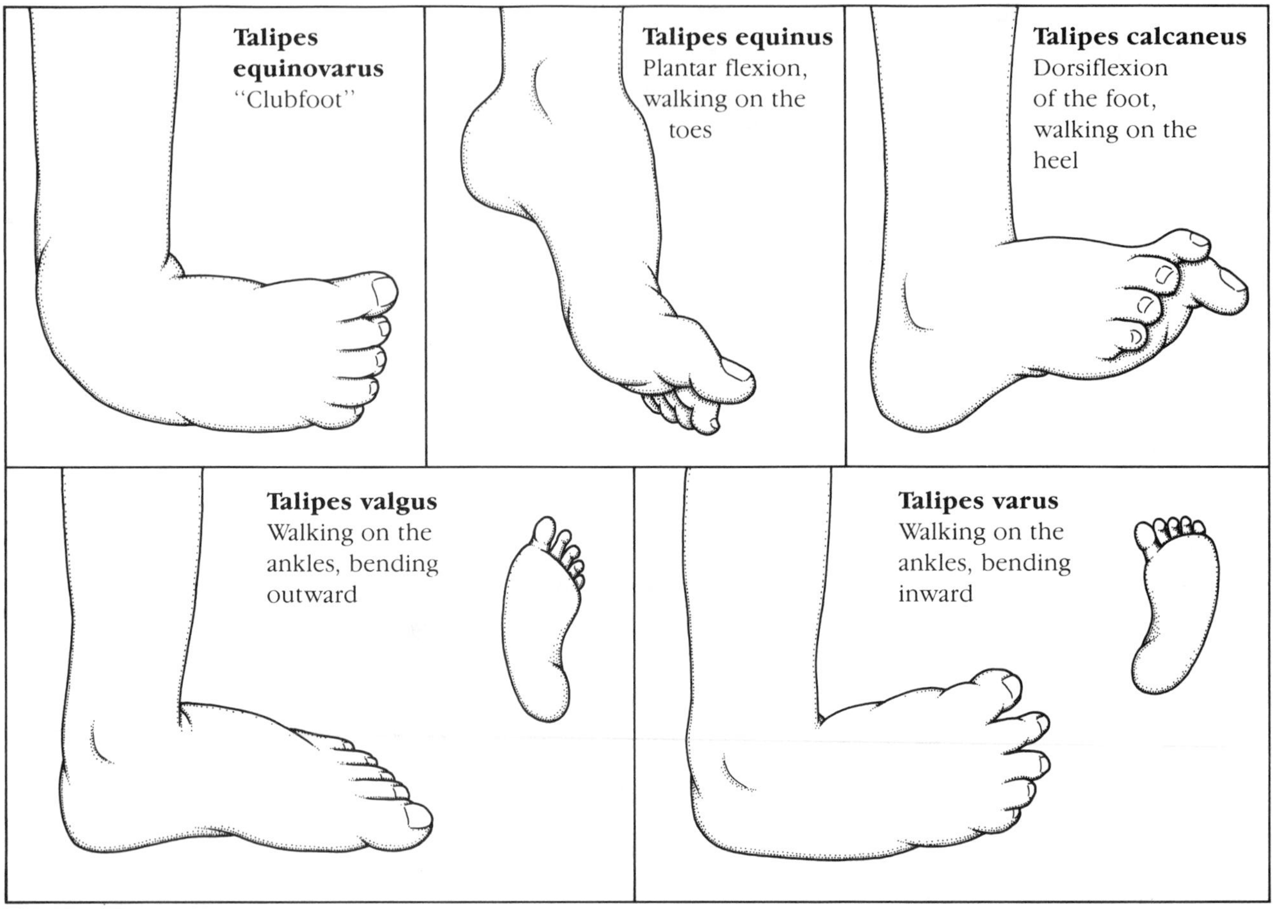

Figure 14-19 Variations of congenital clubfoot. (From Servonsky, J. and Opas, S. *Nursing Management of Children.* Boston: Little, Brown, 1987.

Table 14-3 Juvenile Rheumatoid Arthritis

Subgroup	Behavioral assessment	Diagnostic criteria
Polyarticular: seropositive	Large and small joints affected—warm, tender, and swollen; morning stiffness; may have mild fever, anemia, malaise; progression to severe, crippling arthritis common; 80% female	Positive RF Positive ANAs HLA DR4
Polyarticular: seronegative	Large and small joints affected—warm, tender, and swollen; morning stiffness; progression to severe arthritis unusual; 90% female	Negative RF Negative ANA
Pauciarticular: type I	Large joints, such as knees, ankles, and elbows, commonly affected; iridocyclitis common; crippling arthritis rare; young age of onset; 80% female	Negative RF Positive ANAs HLA DR5 HLA DR8
Pauciarticular: type II	Large joints commonly affected as in type I, plus sacroiliac and hip; iridocyclitis rare; may develop ankylosing spondilitis or bowel disease; onset late childhood; 90% male	Negative RF Negative ANAs HLA B27
Systemic-onset	High fever; fleeting macular rash; hepatosplenomegaly; lymphadenopathy; pericarditis; pleuritis, abdominal pain; multiple small and large joints affected; outlook variable, with severe arthritis in 25%	Negative RF Negative ANAs

RF, rheumatoid factor; ANAs, antinuclear antibodies; HLA, human lymphocyte antigen.

Source: From J. Servonsky and S. Opas: *Nursing Management of Children.* Boston: Little, Brown, 1987.

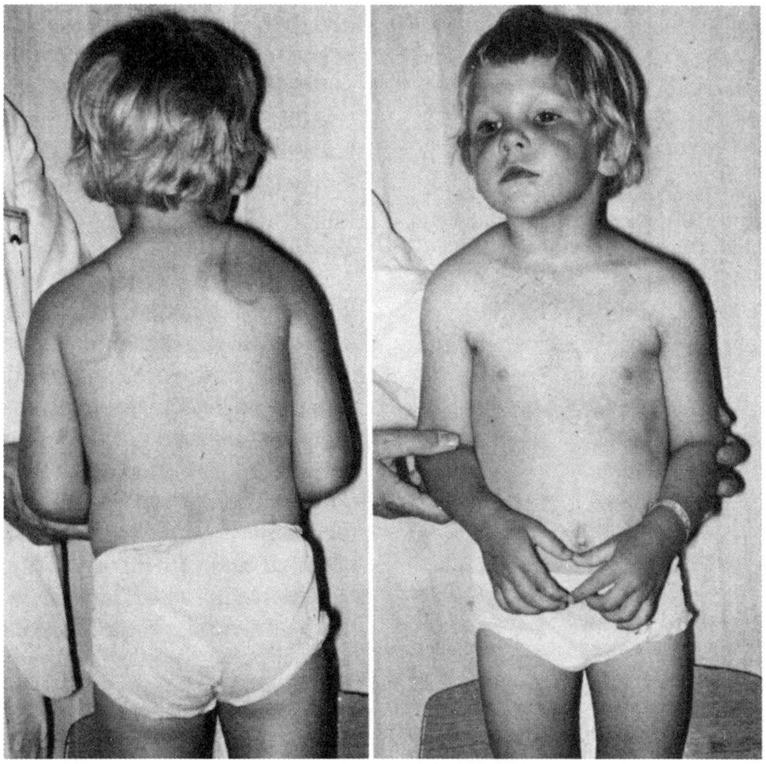

A B

Figure 14-20 **(A)** Congenital elevation of the scapula (Sprengel's deformity). **(B)** Same patient from front demonstrating asymmetry of the shoulder girdles and short neck.

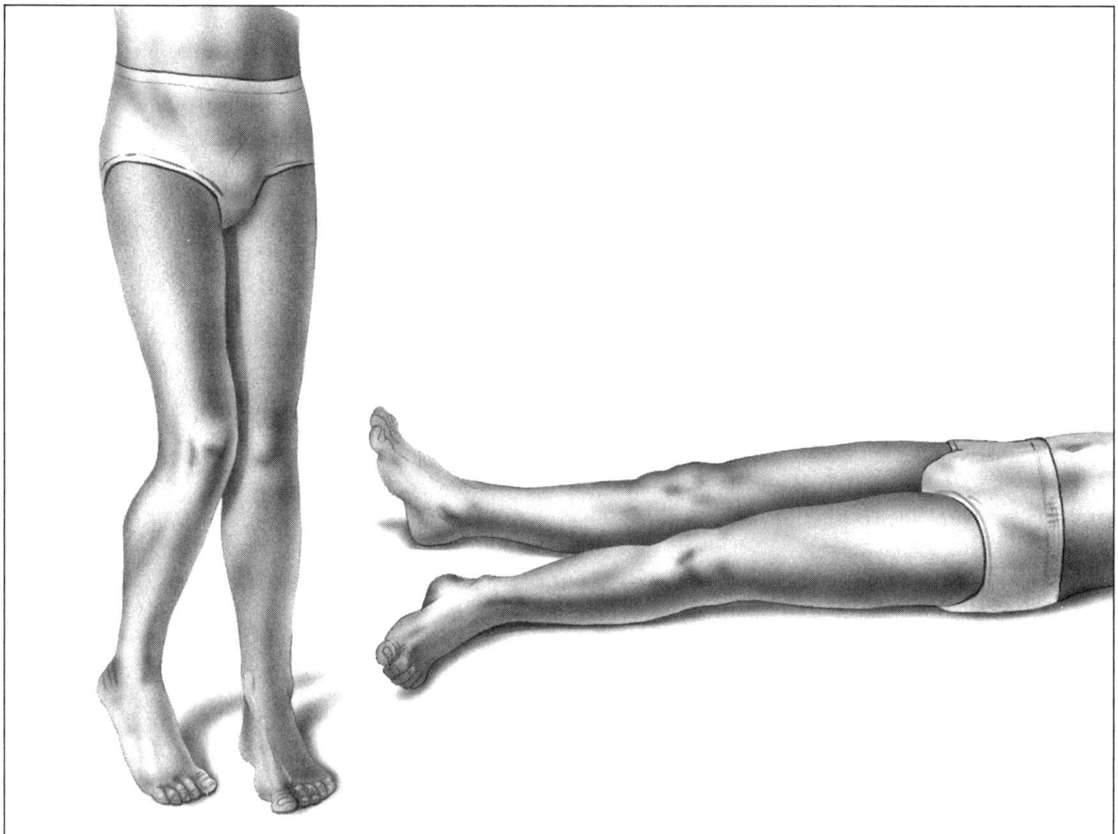

A B

Figure 14-21 Hip deformities. **(A)** Characteristic position of traumatic dislocation of the hip. **(B)** Typical position assumed in fracture of the left hip.

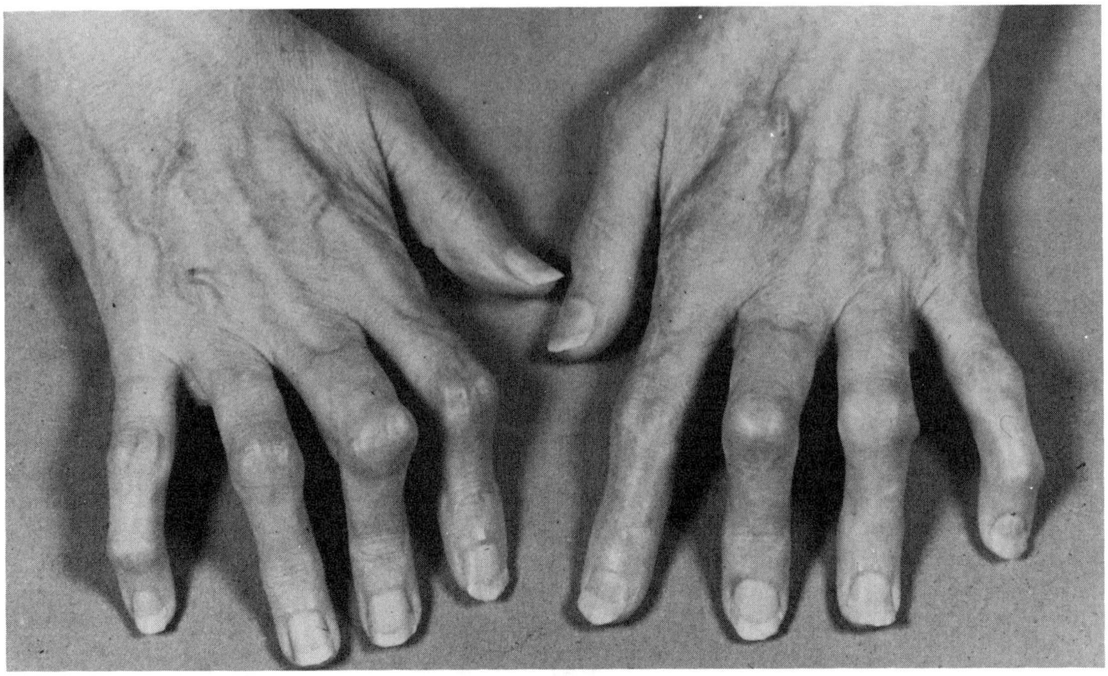

Figure 14-22 Arthritic hands. Note distortion and swelling, particularly the proximal interphalangeal joints.

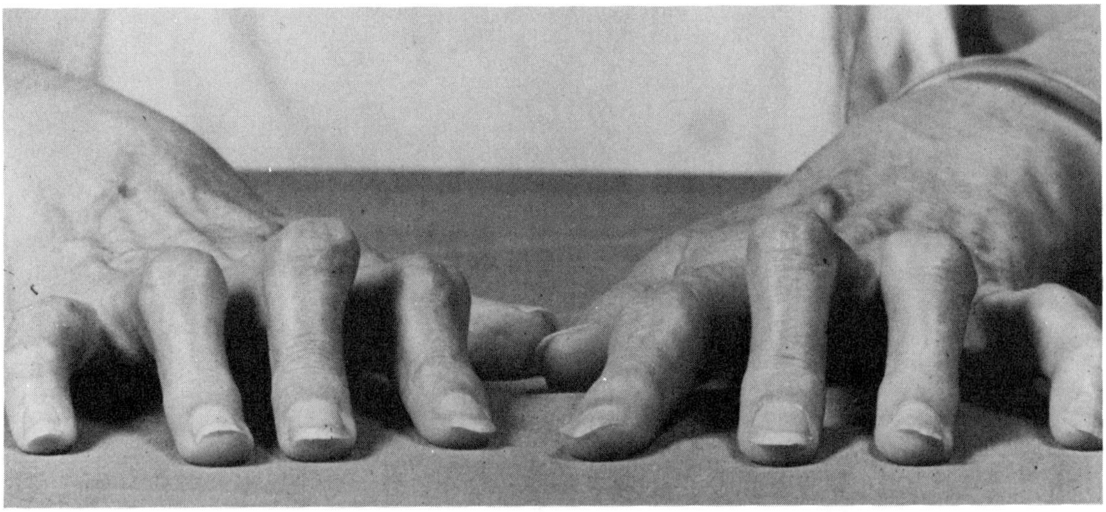

Figure 14-23 Arthritic hands. Note retraction of fingers.

Joints

A rise in the local skin temperature about a joint suggests inflammation. Crepitus occurs with roughening of the articular surfaces and also is found in stenosing tenosynovitis. Crepitation may be heard on movement of a complete fracture in which the bone is completely severed; it is heard on movement of the ends of the broken bone at the fracture site.

The knee joint is a site of frequent traumatic and medical disorders throughout life because it is vulnerable, particularly for athletes. Swelling of the knee within several hours following an injury usually implies inflammatory effusion. Swelling minutes after trauma suggests a laceration of tissues with blood in the joint. The client with a locked knee (limitation of complete extension) usually relates a history of something slipping in the knee, accompanied by pain in the lateral or medial region and the inability to extend the joint. Also

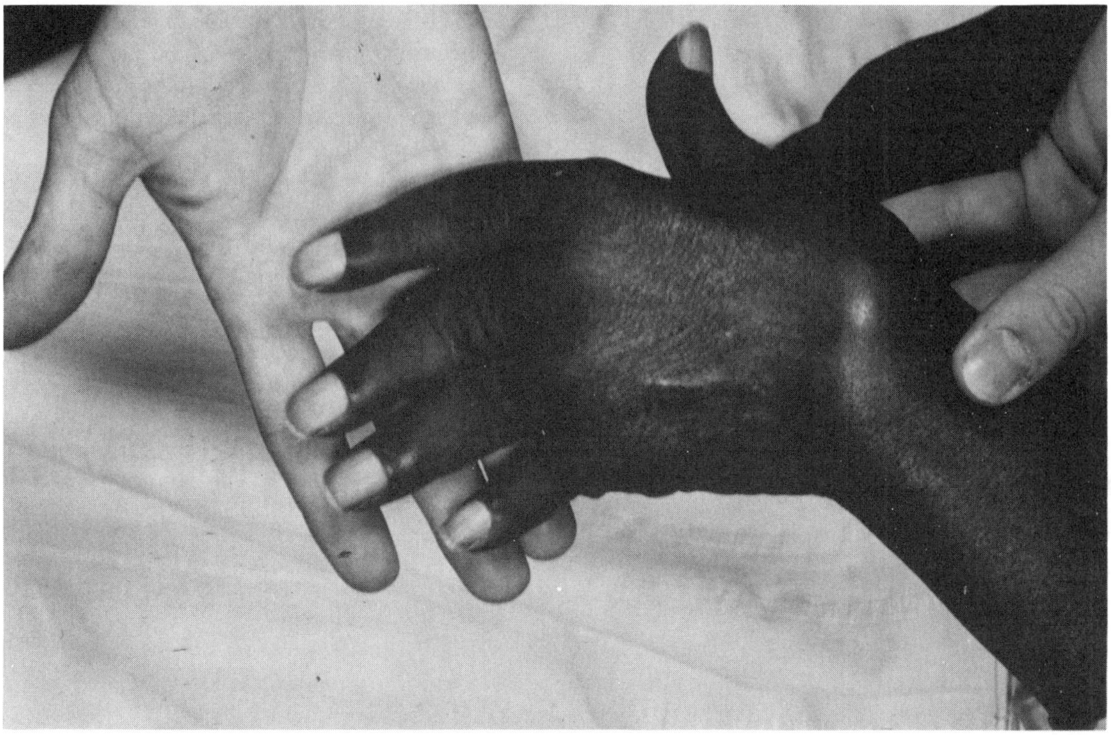

Figure 14-24 Arthritic hand. Note the characteristic ulnar deviation.

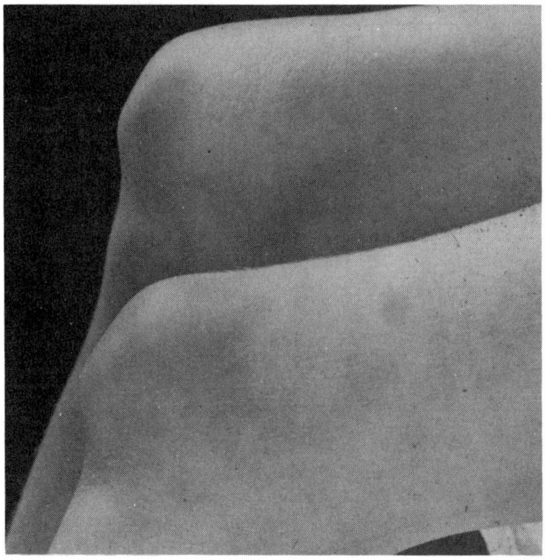

Figure 14-25 Nodular appearance of arthritic knees.

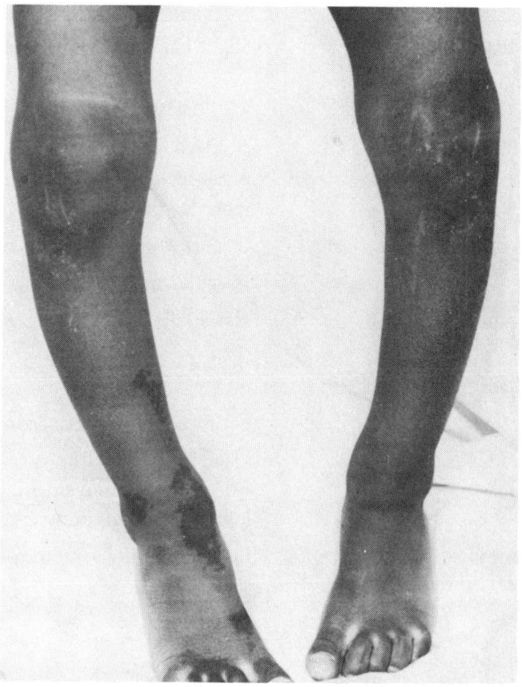

Figure 14-26 Rickets disease. Note bowing of legs.

in the area of the knee, three types of discrete masses can be noted:

1. Popliteal cysts, found in the posterolateral and posteromedial aspect. These cysts occur in children and adults and are often termed *Baker's cyst.*
2. Cysts of the lateral semilunar cartilage, which are in close proximity to the lateral joint compartment
3. Synoviomata, which are neoplasmas arising from normal or abnormal synovial elements

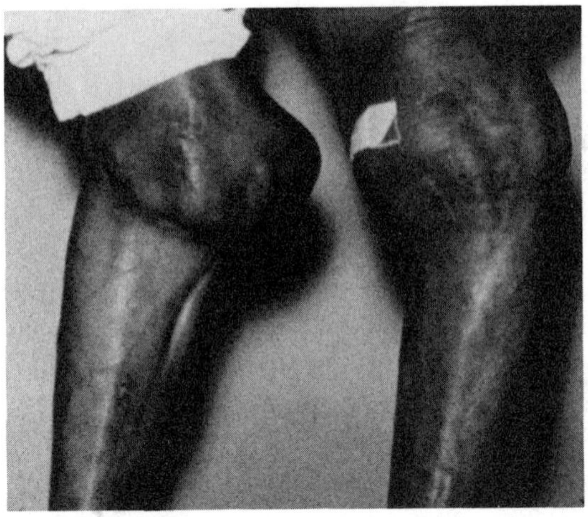

Figure 14-27 Charcot's joints in a patient with tabes dorsalis.

- Range of joint motion may be disrupted by joint damage or deformity, or muscular or neurologic problems.
- Common signs and symptoms of musculoskeletal involvement are fasciculation, tremors, and acute and chronic bone pain.

Characteristics and comments regarding these signs and symptoms, deformities, and disease states affecting the musculoskeletal system are listed in Table 14-4.

Table 14-4 Common Abnormalities of the Musculoskeletal System

Terminology	Characteristics	Comments
Fasciculations	Slight twitching in a resting muscle	Frequently occurs; associated with strain, muscle weakness, and atrophy; may be due to denervation of muscle fibers
Tremors		
Resting tremor	Accentuated by rest; diminishes on movement; more rhythmic	Seen in Parkinson's disease; usually indicates basal ganglia disease
Intention tremor	Increases with voluntary movement Irregular movement	Seen in multiple sclerosis; could suggest cerebellar disease
Flapping tremor	Hand falls momentarily, only to raise again	Transient loss of extensor tone at the wrist; seen in hepatic failure, hypercapnia, uremia
Bone pain		
Acute	Localized tenderness; redness, swelling, increased warmth Intensified by movement, abnormal mobility, loss of function, bony crepitus	Associated with trauma
Chronic	Bone pain only symptom—no other physical signs	Especially occurs in vertebrae and pelvic bones; incidence increases with age, due to disuse, inadequate nutrition, and excessive loss of minerals
Pain of multiple myeloma	Pain localized or general; on x-ray punched-out areas in bone; anemia and high globulin levels in blood	Invasion and destruction of bone and bone marrow by malignant cells; most common malignant bone tumor; more frequent in men and in the sixth decade
Osteoporosis	Back pain, loss of stature, "dowager's hump" from vertebral compression; increase of fractures, particularly of hip	Common in women past menopause; results from inadequate calcium intake, insufficient exercise, and unknown effects of reduced steroid levels

Table 14-4 **Continued**

Terminology	Characteristics	Comments
Abnormal spinal curvatures		
Arthritis		
Osteoarthritis	Stiffness after periods of rest; exacerbation of symptoms with changes in barometric pressure; signs include joint crepitation and pain, limitation of motion, changes in shape of affected joints; signs of inflammation minimal	Increases in prevalence with age.
Rheumatoid arthritis	Morning stiffness, pain and swelling of joints, subcutaneous nodules, positive rheumatoid factor, typical x-ray joint changes	Adult form develops insidiously. Specific cause unknown but generally believed that joint changes are related to antibody reaction.
Kyphosis	Excessive rounding of the back due to an increase in the posterior curvature of the thoracic spinal column	Frequently associated with osteoporosis; ankylosing spondylitis. Senile kyphosis of osteoporosis caused by collapse and anterior wedging of thoracic vertebrae. Adolescent round back or juvenile kyphosis caused by epiphysitis of lower thoracic vertebrae or Scheuermann's disease. Occupationally induced.
Lordosis	Abnormal anterior convexity of lumbar spinal column	Increased lordosis found in clients with spondylolysis, those with tight hamstring muscle. Also seen in clients with hip disease, especially congenital dislocation of hips, and in persons with flexion contractions of the hips who hyperextend lumbar spine to stand erect.
Scoliosis	Lateral curvature of spine	Usually consists of two curves, the original abnormal curve and a compensatory curve in the opposite direction; most commonly idiopathic and occurs most frequently in adolescent girls.
Vitamin D deficiency	Defective mineralization of bone resulting in sides of thorax flattening, sternum protruding; knobs on end of ribs (rachitic rosary); may have lordosis, kyphosis, scoliosis, liver and spleen enlargement, curvature of long bone	Rickets (children); osteomalacia (adults); renal insufficiency.
Paget's disease	Chronic inflammation of bones, resulting in thickening, softening, and bowing of long bones.	Also called osteitis deformans. Among most common of chronic skeletal diseases of elderly.
Legg-Calvé-Perthes disease	Protective limp, limited movement of hip joint; atrophy of thigh muscle.	Occurs in children, onset between ages 3 and 12. Occurs more often in boys.
Ankylosing spondylitis (Marie-Strümpell disease)	Stiff back, gradual ankylosis with kyphosis, involvement of sacroiliac and spinal apophyseal joints; decreased chest expansion.	Affects young men, familial. Measure chest expansion at nipple line (4ICS level). Normal expansion for young adults is at least 5 cm.
Osteogenesis imperfecta	Blue sclera, early deafness, multiple fractures—"loose" joints in some forms, backache	Inherited disorder—autosomal dominant trait. Tendency to fracture decreases and often disappears later in life.
Gout	Podagra (of the foot or great toe) and weight-bearing joints affected; involves more joints as progresses; tophi with joint destruction; acute attacks, severe pain	Occurs more frequently in males; increased serum uric acid level.

Continued

Table 14-4 Continued

Terminology	Characteristics	Comments
Sickle-cell disease	Acute crisis with bone and abdominal pain, fever, and shortness of breath; edema of hands and feet; tenderness of joints and limited range of motion	Hereditary, chronic form of anemia. Frequency of gene that causes disease high in Mediterraneans and African-Americans. Physical and emotional stress can precipitate a crisis.
Acromegaly	Hypertrophy of articular cartilage and joint enlargement, particularly in fingers and knees; elongation and enlargement of bones of extremities and certain head bones, especially frontal bones and jaws	A chronic disease of middle age. First sign may be that client needs to buy a larger hat and gloves.

SUMMARY

This chapter discussed the basic structure and function of the musculoskeletal system and described the characteristics and techniques used in the examination of the muscles, bones, and joints. Muscles must be examined for strength, and joints examined for range of motion. The client should be checked for fasciculations, tremors, muscle tone, skeletal deformities, and bone tenderness.

DISCUSSION QUESTIONS/ ACTIVITIES

1. What are the three specific structures of the musculoskeletal system that are examined during a routine physical assessment?
2. What areas of the body would you assess in regard to muscle strength? Perform this assessment step by step.
3. What other aspects of the muscular system would you assess in addition to muscle strength?
4. Demonstrate the technique used to assess whether fluid is present in the knee joint.
5. What characteristics are observed in range of joint motion?
6. Demonstrate how you would assess the nine major joint areas of the body.
7. Describe some of the signs and symptoms of musculoskeletal assessment that you have observed in clients.

REFERENCE

Damon, A. 1977. *Human biology and ecology.* New York: W. W. Norton.

CHAPTER

15 Assessment of the Neurologic System

Learning Objectives

1. State the primary functions of the frontal, parietal, occipital, and temporal lobes.
2. State the various sensory modalities and explain how to test for them.
3. Describe the difference between expressive and receptive aphasia.
4. Describe tests used to evaluate balance and coordination.
5. Name the 12 cranial nerves and explain how each is evaluated.
6. Identify the site for percussion of each of the deep tendon reflexes.
7. Interpret reflex findings and categorize into an appropriate grading scale.
8. Name the superficial reflexes and the normal response for each.
9. Recognize common pathologic reflexes.
10. Compare the findings of upper motor neuron damage to those of lower motor neuron damage.

The extent of physical assessment of the neurologic system depends on the presence and type of signs and symptoms elicited during the health history. A health history that is negative for signs of dysfunction shortens the assessment procedure considerably, as you will better understand after reading about the assessment of the neurologic system.

A detailed neurologic assessment may take from 2 to 3 hours. Such a long and tedious in-depth assessment may anger, frustrate, or fatigue the client. Therefore, you need to be aware of this and proceed in a tactful, kind, and understanding manner, because it is imperative to have the client's full attention and cooperation.

The techniques of examining the neurologic system are relatively simple. It is the complexity of the functioning of the neurologic system that is difficult to understand; therefore, a brief, simple, and clear explanation of the structure and physiologic functioning of the various parts of the neurologic system is provided to aid you in understanding the scientific rationale for, in many cases, one simple observation. Once you understand the basic functioning, the techniques for testing are easily learned.

The areas assessed are the cerebrum, the cerebellum, the cranial nerves, and the neurologic reflexes. The assessment technique primarily employed in evaluating the neurologic system is inspection, that is, observation of behavior and body movement.

BRIEF OVERVIEW OF THE NEUROLOGIC SYSTEM

The *cerebrum* is the major portion of the human brain; it is responsible for sensations, voluntary actions, thoughts, and personality. The *cerebellum* is located at the posterior aspect and inferior to the cerebrum. It controls coordination and equilibrium. Within the *brain stem* are the respiratory and vasomotor centers, which regulate respirations and heart rate and blood pressure, respectively. These functions are generally evaluated during assessment of the respiratory and cardiovascular systems. The majority of the cranial nerve nuclei are housed in the brain stem; it is during neurologic assessment that these are tested and evaluated. The *spinal cord* is the communication line through which impulses and messages are transmitted to and from the brain. When assessing this area, you will become aware of the functioning of the sensory and motor tracts, the reflex arc, and the end areas in the cerebrum.

STRUCTURE AND FUNCTION OF THE CEREBRUM

The four distinct areas of the cerebrum are the frontal, parietal, occipital, and temporal lobes.

Frontal Lobes

The frontal lobes are responsible for higher thought functions and for regulating personality and behavior (Fig. 15-1). The key function of the frontal lobe is to regulate cortical tone—in other words, the state of consciousness.

A motor tract area is located in the posterior portion of the frontal lobe. Each part of the body is represented by

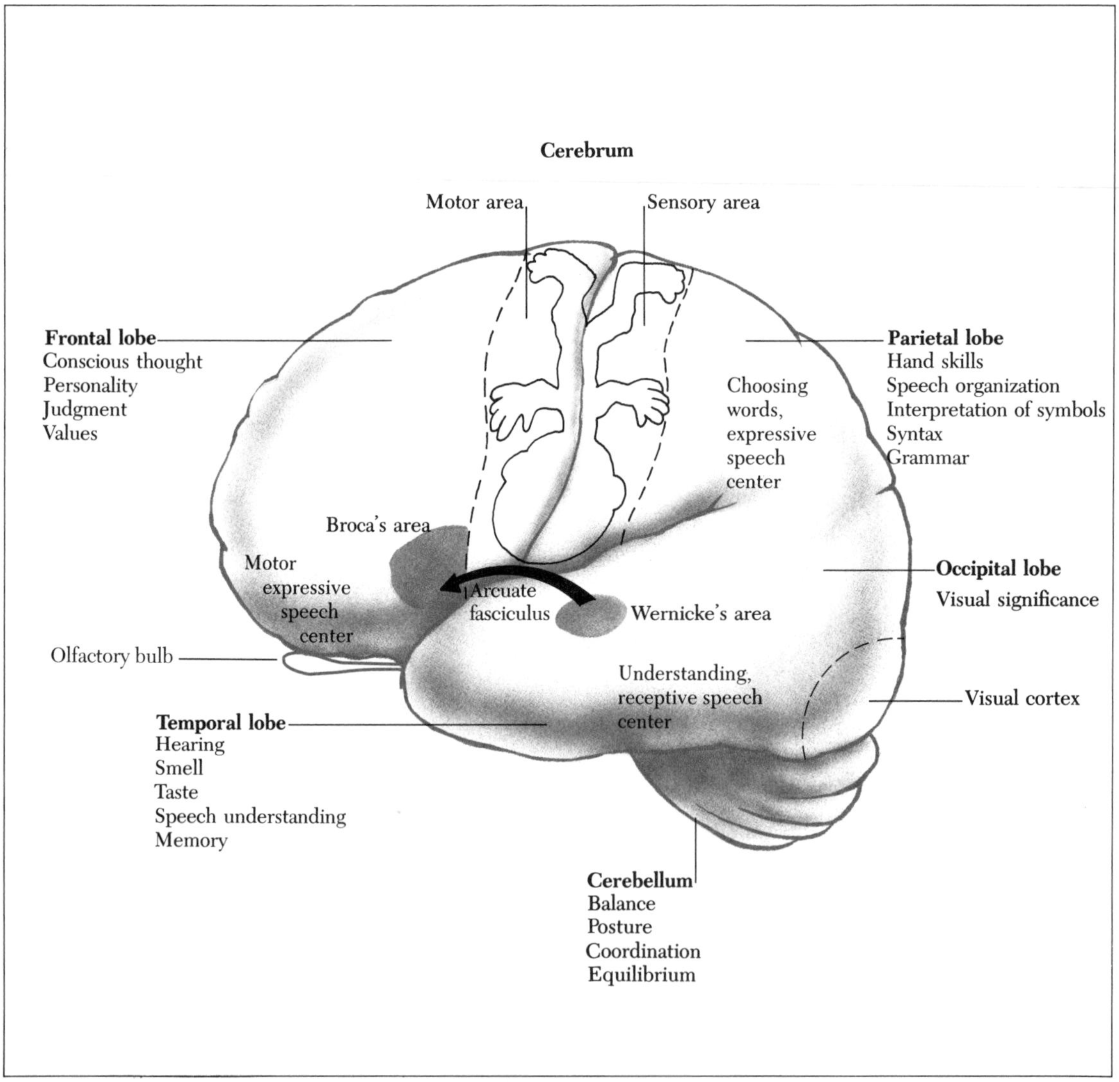

Figure 15-1 Functions of the cerebrum and cerebellum, including three major speech centers in the frontal, parietal, and temporal lobes.

Techniques for Assessing Frontal Lobe Areas

1. *Mental status:* Refer to Chapter 3.
2. *Motor status:* Refer to Chapter 14.
3. *Motor speech:* Note ability to speak and articulate words.
4. *Sense of smell:* Client closes eyes; press one naris closed with your index finger; ask client to identify common scent (e.g., soap, mint, tobacco); repeat with opposite naris.

large pyramidal cells (motor neurons) in this tract. These neurons initiate voluntary movement of the skeletal muscles on the body side opposite of the cerebral hemisphere. Figure 15-1 shows that the arrangement of these representative cells resembles an upside-down person, with the head and face areas just superior to the temporal lobes and constituting more than half of the motor tract; the remainder of the body is represented in the superior portion of the tract.

Figure 15-2 illustrates how nerve fibers from the motor cortex tracts converge and descend through the internal capsule. Some motor nerve fibers project down the corticobulbar tract directly without crossing and end in the various cranial nerve nuclei in the brain stem; others continue down the corticospinal tract, cross over in the lower medulla, and descend in the spinal cord, eventually terminating in the anterior gray motor horn of the spinal cord at all of the correlating levels from the cervical cord area through the sacral.

As Figure 15-3 illustrates, the extent and location of a lesion within the cerebral motor area determine the degree of paresis or paralysis experienced. A localized lesion of an isolated represented area of the cerebral motor tract confines the paresis or paralysis to that contralateral portion of the body (e.g., arm or leg weakness).

A lesion involving the internal capsule disrupts all of the neural fibers of the motor tract and results in ipsilateral paresis or paralysis of the face and contralateral hemiparesis. Thus, you should make a note of any weakness or lack of ability to move a body part in your assessment of frontal lobe function.

Sets of left and right cranial nerve nuclei I (olfactory) and II (optic) are contained in the cerebral cortex; III (oculomotor) and IV (trochlear) in the midbrain; V through VIII (trigeminal, abducens, facial, auditory/acoustic) in the pons; and IX through XII (glossopharyngeal, vagus, spinal accessory, hypoglossal) in the medulla (Fig. 15-4). The cranial nerves do not cross but branch out from the brain stem on their respective sides.

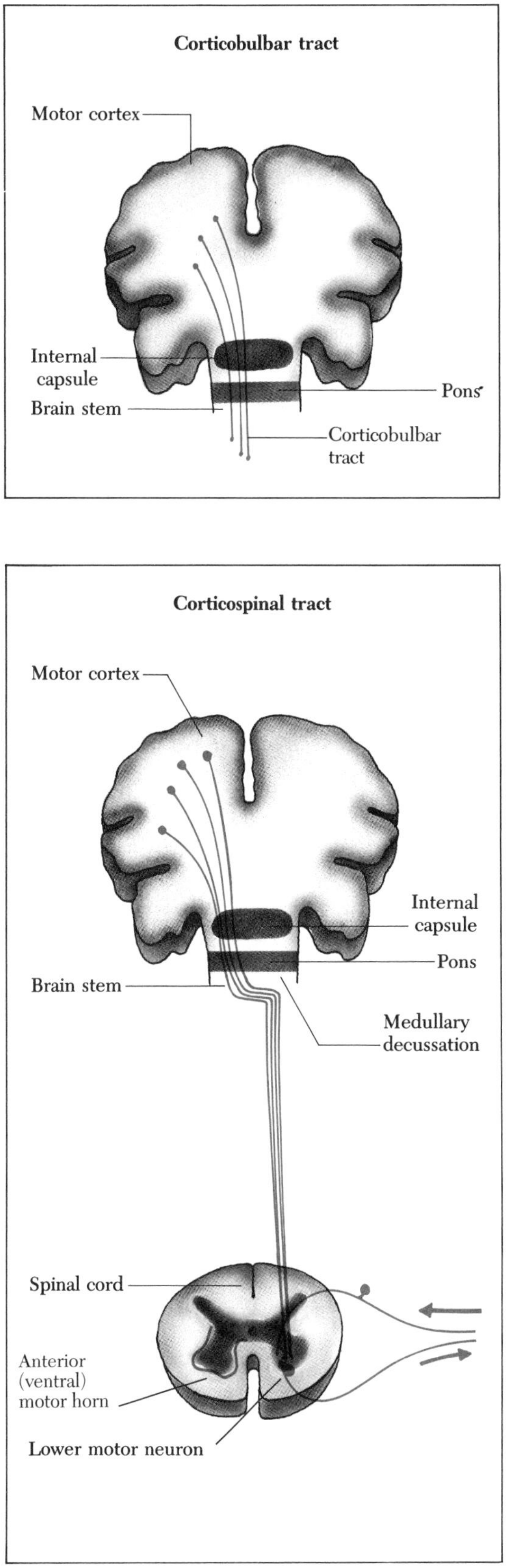

Figure 15-2 The corticobulbar tract and the corticospinal tract.

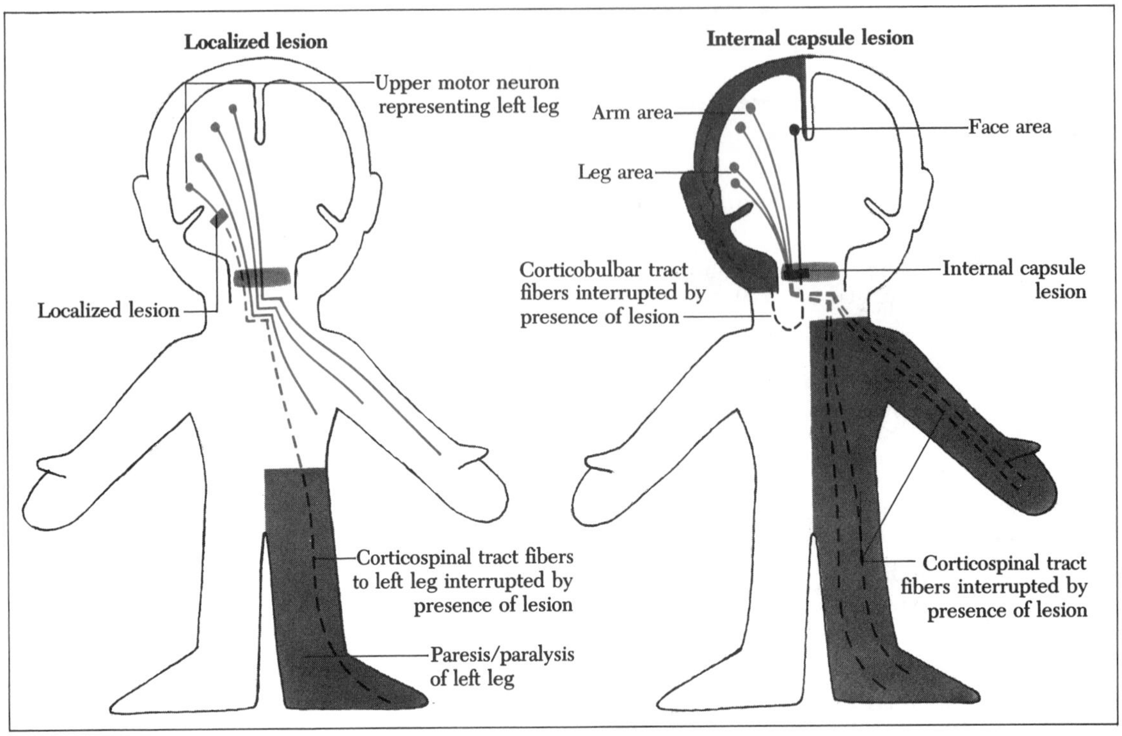

Figure 15-3 Localized and internal capsule lesion with corresponding paresis/paralysis areas of the body.

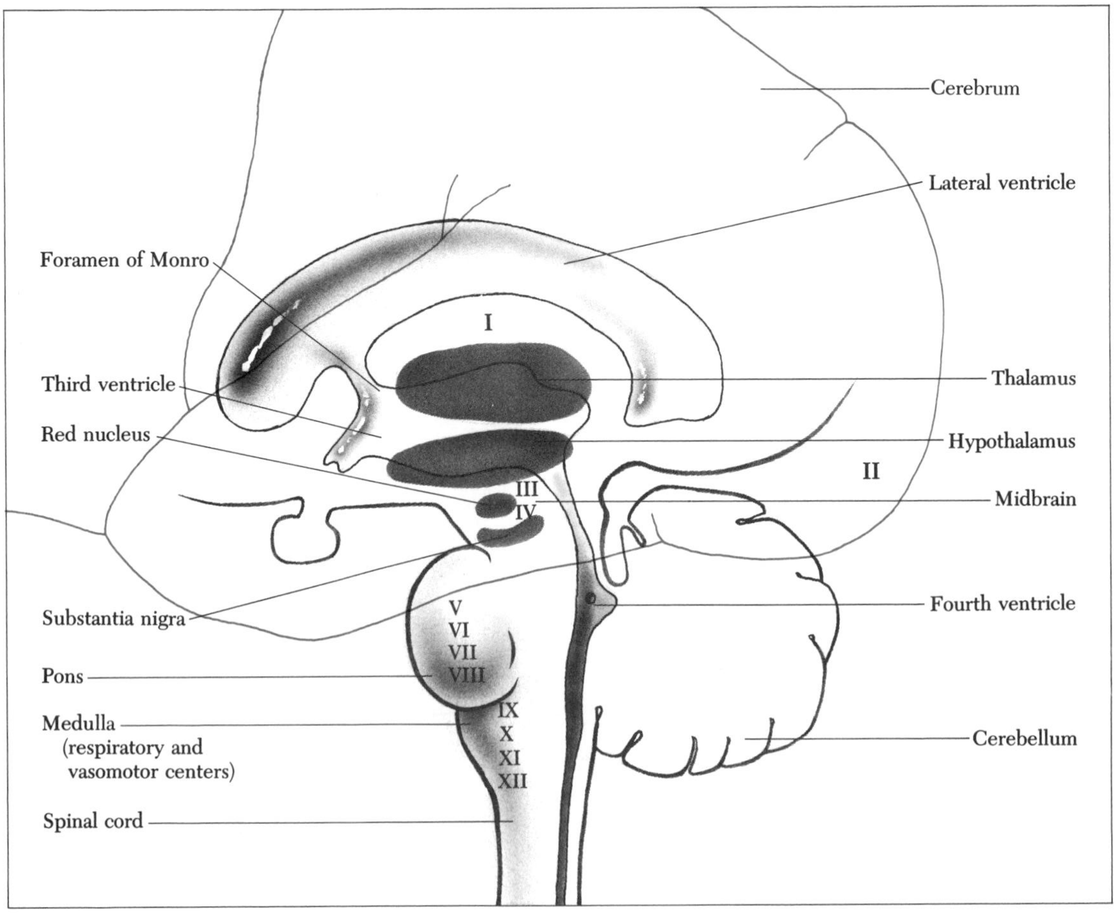

Figure 15-4 Location of cranial nerve nuclei.

Techniques for Assessing Parietal Lobe Areas

Client's eyes should be closed for all testing of parietal lobe areas.

1. *Sensory status:* Stimuli applied in dermatomal areas of the body; ask client to identify whether sensation is "dull" or "sharp" and hot or cold, and to point to areas of body where touched by cotton wisp.
   a. Pain (pinprick)
   b. Temperature (test tubes of hot and cold water)
   c. Light touch (cotton wisp applied to body)
2. *Vibration:* Place vibrating tuning fork on major bony prominences—toes, ankles, knees, iliac crests, knuckles, wrists, elbows, shoulder; ask client to identify presence of vibration and when it stops; place your hand on upper end of tuning fork to stop vibration to detect if client senses cessation of vibration.
3. *Proprioception:* Hold digit with your index and thumb on either side; move in up and down direction; ask client to identify direction of movement; test each extremity.
4. *Stereognosis:* Place two objects in succession in each hand; ask client to identify the shape, and to compare the size and weight of the two objects; this tests both left and right parietal lobes.
5. *Decision making:* If a neurologic problem is suspected, perform additional special techniques for assessing parietal lobe function.

The lower motor neuron system is located within the ventral (anterior motor) horn of the spinal cord (see Fig. 15-2; see also Fig. 15-12). In the evaluation of clinical signs and symptoms, a distinction can be made between upper motor neuron damage and lower motor neuron damage by the motor system findings and those of the deep tendon reflexes (DTRs). These distinctions are discussed later in this chapter, at the end of the section on reflexes.

Broca's area is located in the left frontal lobe in the lower prefrontal area (see Fig. 15-1). This is a motor expressive speech center that is used in appropriately moving the muscles of speech to articulate words (e.g., the lips, tongue, cheeks, pharynx). The client may know what he wants to say but cannot coordinate the muscle movements necessary to form the words.

The olfactory bulbs, fiber tracts, are situated just under the anterior portion of the frontal lobes (see Fig. 15-1). The bulbs transmit the sense of smell from the receptive nerve endings in the nose to the temporal lobe on the ipsilateral side.

Social behavior and personality are molded through learning. The frontal lobes are the seat of intellectual functioning and decision making (see Chapter 3 for more detail).

Parietal Lobes

A tract similar to the motor tract of the frontal lobes lies in the anterior portion of the parietal lobes and deals with body sensation. In this sensory tract, as in the motor tract, each part of the body is represented by cortical cells.

Within the spinal cord are pathways for transporting the various sensations to the thalamus for awareness and on to the cerebrum for location and intensity. In assessing the sensory system, it is important to have a basic understanding of the spinal tracts and their routes. Of particular importance are (1) the posterior (dorsal) columns tract, (2) the lateral spinothalamic tract, and (3) the ventral spinothalamic tract. Figure 15-5 shows the location of these various tracts on the right; the functions of these ascending tracts are indicated on the left.

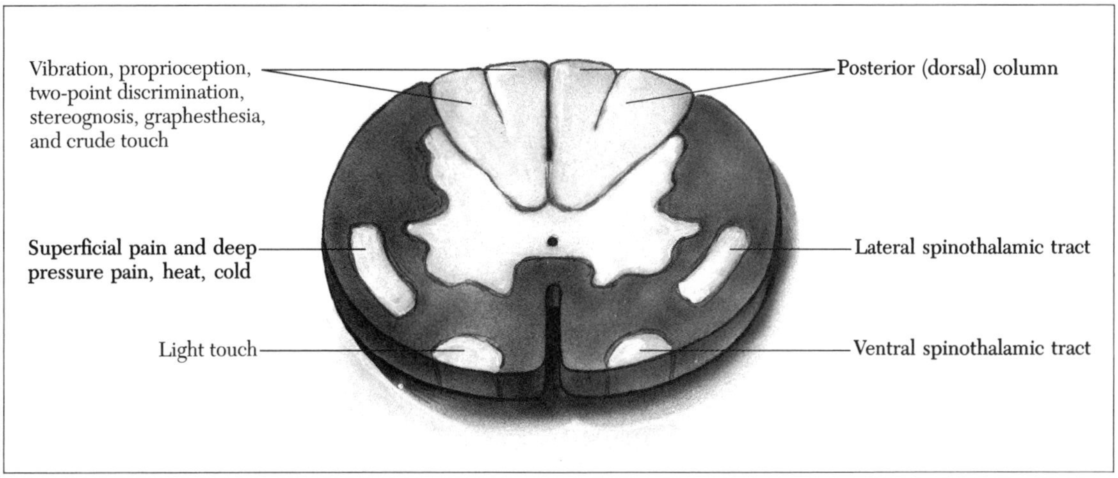

Figure 15-5 Cross-section of the spinal cord.

Sensory impulses are picked up by the receptors in the skin, mucous membranes, muscles, and body organs. Figure 15-6 illustrates how afferent nerves transmit these impulses from the receptors to the cell body in the ganglion on the posterior root of a spinal nerve and on the posterior or dorsal horn (gray matter of the cord). From the sensory or dorsal horn, the impulses ascend, according to the type of sensation, up either the dorsal column (solid color), the lateral spinothalamic tract (broken color), or the ventral spinothalamic tract (solid black).

The *dorsal column* transmits the impulse sensations of *vibration, proprioception, two-point discrimination, stereognosis,* and *graphesthesia* up to the thalamus; from there, the impulses proceed to the parietal cortex (see Fig. 15-5).

The sensory impulses of *superficial and deep pain* and of *temperature (hot and cold)* enter the dorsal horn of the spinal cord, ascend a segment or two, and then decussate to the *lateral spinothalamic tract* to continue to ascend to the thalamus and on to the sensory cortical tract of the anterior parietal lobe (see Figs. 15-5 and 15-7).

Both *crossed* and *uncrossed peripheral fibers* carry the sensation of touch. Some enter the dorsal ipsilateral (same) side of the spinal cord via the thalamus to the parietal lobe on the same side. Others travel the ventral spinothalamic tract, which ascends and decussates at the medullary level (see Fig. 15-5). Thus, the *touch sensation is rarely absent,* except in cases of severe damage to the spinal cord or cerebrum.

Occipital Lobes

The cortical functions of vision and visual significance (interpretation) are located in the occipital lobes. The visual center is assessed during testing of visual acuity and visual field. A lesion involving the whole of the visual center of both occipital lobes would result in total "cortical blindness" in spite of normal eyes and optic tract. Destruction of the visual center in only one lobe would result in contralateral homonymous hemianopia (see discussion of cranial nerve II, optic nerve, and Fig. 15-9).

Techniques for Assessing Occipital Lobe Areas

1. *Visual object recognition:* Ask client to identify familiar objects.
2. *Visual-verbal comprehension:* Ask client to read a sentence from newspaper or magazine and explain it.
3. *Visual acuity and visual fields:* Refer to Chapter 8.

Temporal Lobes

A receptive speech center, Wernicke's area (see Fig. 15-1), is central in the left temporal lobe and is joined to Broca's area by a nerve bundle called the *arcuate fasciculus.* Its function is to make sense and meaning out of spoken words, that is, to understand speech.

Also within the temporal lobes are centers of sensory interpretation for hearing, smell, and taste. Much of recent memory is stored in the temporal lobes. Remote memory is more diffusely stored throughout the cerebrum.

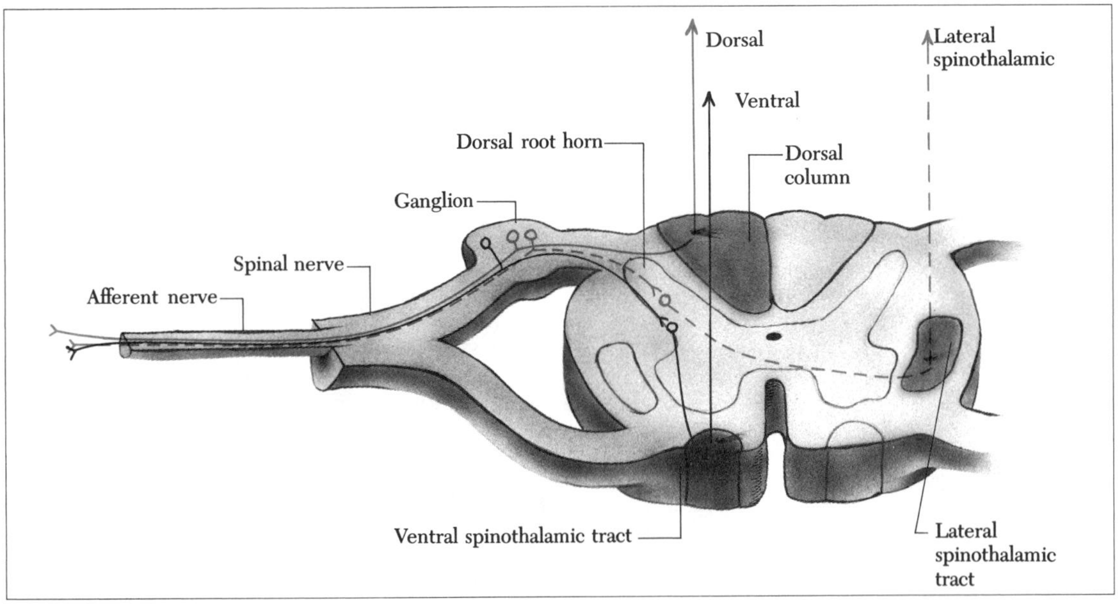

Figure 15-6 Sensory impulse transmission from receptor site to the appropriate tract according to type of sensation.

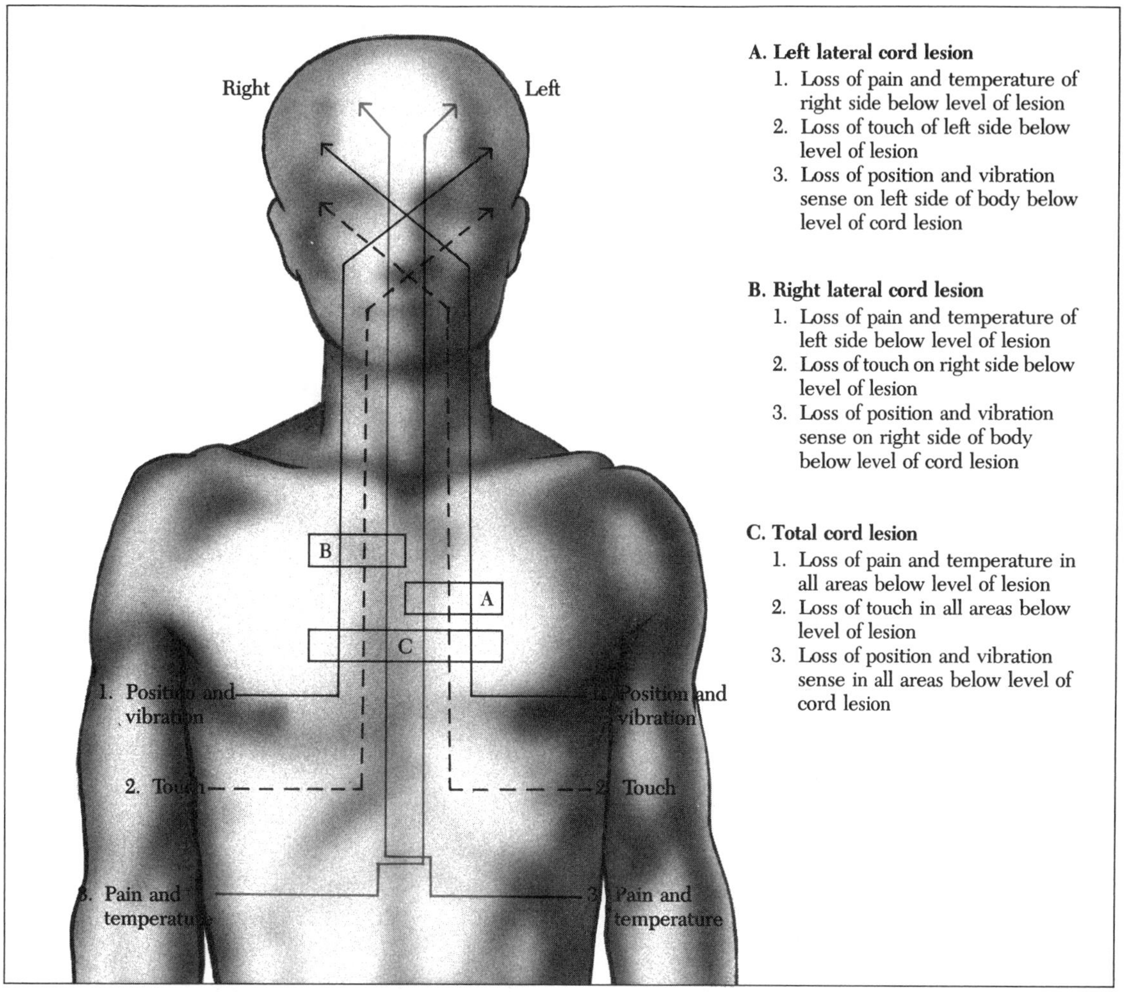
Right
Left
B
A
C
2. Touch
Touch
A. Left lateral cord lesion
1. Loss of pain and temperature of right side below level of lesion
2. Loss of touch of left side below level of lesion
3. Loss of position and vibration sense on left side of body below level of cord lesion
B. Right lateral cord lesion
1. Loss of pain and temperature of left side below level of lesion
2. Loss of touch on right side below level of lesion
3. Loss of position and vibration sense on right side of body below level of cord lesion
C. Total cord lesion
1. Loss of pain and temperature in all areas below level of lesion
2. Loss of touch in all areas below level of lesion
3. Loss of position and vibration sense in all areas below level of cord lesion

Figure 15-7 Cord lesions and sensory loss.

Techniques for Assessing Temporal Lobe Areas

1. *Visual fields:* Refer to Chapter 8.
2. *Speech understanding:* Receptive aphasia. Check if client can follow command and if client can repeat command verbally.
3. *Recent memory:* Refer to Chapter 3.

ASSESSMENT OF THE CEREBRUM

Frontal Lobe Function

If you suspect cerebral dysfunction, you should conduct a meticulous mental status assessment employing the tests of cerebral function discussed in Chapter 3. It is noteworthy to comment that generalized convulsions occur in 50% of the clinical cases involving frontal lobe lesions. Therefore, precaution is taken not to examine a client under artificial lighting that may be going bad. Lighting that tends to flicker may trigger convulsive seizures.

Parietal Lobe Function

The parietal lobe does not become fully functional until 7 to 8 years of age. This is why young children can easily get lost—they are unable to find their spatial bearings. The parietal lobe also is necessary for understanding grammatically complex instructions. Therefore, an adult client with a parietal lesion, or a young child, will respond better when instructions are short and simple. For example, do not give them three instructions in one command. Give each command separately and pause for response before continuing to the next command. The expressive speech center in the parietal lobes enables the individual to select the appropriate words to communicate thoughts.

Cortical sensory tract and discriminatory sensations *are not routinely tested;* however, when warranted, evaluate sensory system status by testing the perception of the following modalities: touch, pain, temperature, proprioception (position sense), and vibration.

Obviously, you cannot test the entire body surface, but you are guided by the client's history and other neurologic findings in determining the areas that need to be closely scrutinized. Testing is difficult to evaluate and depends on the cooperation of the client.

- The client's eyes should be **closed** during the testing.
- Compare sensitivity of each modality with the opposite side of the body or with corresponding extremities, as well as the difference between sensitivity of proximal and distal parts of the extremity.
- Normally, all sensations are perceived equally.
- Construct sketches to show areas of sensory disturbances, such as on one side, dermatomal or peripheral confinement.

Figure 15-8 indicates the body surface areas (dermatomes) associated with the major nerves.

Posterior (Dorsal) Columns Assessment

Vibration

- Place a vibrating tuning fork on the bony prominences of the body (finger joints, wrists, elbows, shoulders, hips, knees, shins, ankles, and toes).
- Note the ability of the client to determine the presence of the vibrations and when they stop.
- You can grossly countercheck the client's responses by comparing them with your own sensations, providing you have no sensory deficit. When the client states that the vibration sensation has stopped, place the tuning fork on your own wrist to see if it *has* stopped.
- Sensitivity to vibration is compared from one side of the body to the other and between the proximal and distal areas of the extremities.

Joint Position Sense: Proprioception

Every extremity should be evaluated for proprioception (awareness of body position and joint motion sense). It is not necessary to test position sense of proximal joints if the perception of the distal (finger and toe) joints is normal, as position sense is always lacking distally in organic lesions.

- The client's eyes should be **closed.**
- Passively move the client's fingers and toes upward and downward; mix the movements (e.g., up, up, down, up, down, down).
- It is important to hold the **sides** of the finger or toe being tested and not the top (nail) and bottom of the finger, because upward or downward *pressure* on the client's skin may reveal the direction of the movement; thus, you would be testing crude touch rather than joint position (proprioception).
- Ask the client to state whether the movement is upward or downward.

Stereognosis

Stereognosis is the ability to identify shape, weight, and size of an object.

- Client's eyes should be **closed.**
- Place two objects in succession in the client's *left* hand.
- First place an object (e.g., golf ball) in the client's left hand.
- Ask her to identify the form and approximate size.
- Next place another object (e.g., coin) in the same hand and ask about its size and shape.
- Then ask the client which object weighs more.

You have just tested *right* parietal lobe functioning.

- To test *left* parietal lobe stereognosis, repeat the procedure by placing two different objects in succession (e.g., pencil, matchbook, drinking glass, paperweight) in the *right* hand.

Inability to discriminate between objects is abnormal and is termed *astereognosis.*

Other discriminatory tests performed in an *extensive* neurologic assessment are two-point discrimination, point localization, texture discrimination, the extinction phenomenon, and graphesthesia. These tests are *not* ordinarily performed during a routine screening of health assessment.

Two-point Discrimination

- Touch various parts of the body with two closely approximated sharp points, while the client keeps his eyes **closed.**

Special Techniques for Extensive Neurologic Assessment

1. *Two-point discrimination:* Touch various areas with two closely approximated points. Ask client to identify if touched by one or two points.
2. *Point localization:* Touch various body areas. Ask client to name and point to the area where he is being touched.
3. *Texture discrimination:* Place such materials as sandpaper, silk, and velvet in client's hand to identify rough, smooth, and soft textures.
4. *Extinction phenomenon:* Simultaneously touch the same areas of the body on both left and right sides. Ask client to identify whether he feels the touch on one or both sides.
5. *Graphesthesia:* With your fingertip, write letters or numbers on the client's palm or other body part. Ask client to identify the letters or numbers.

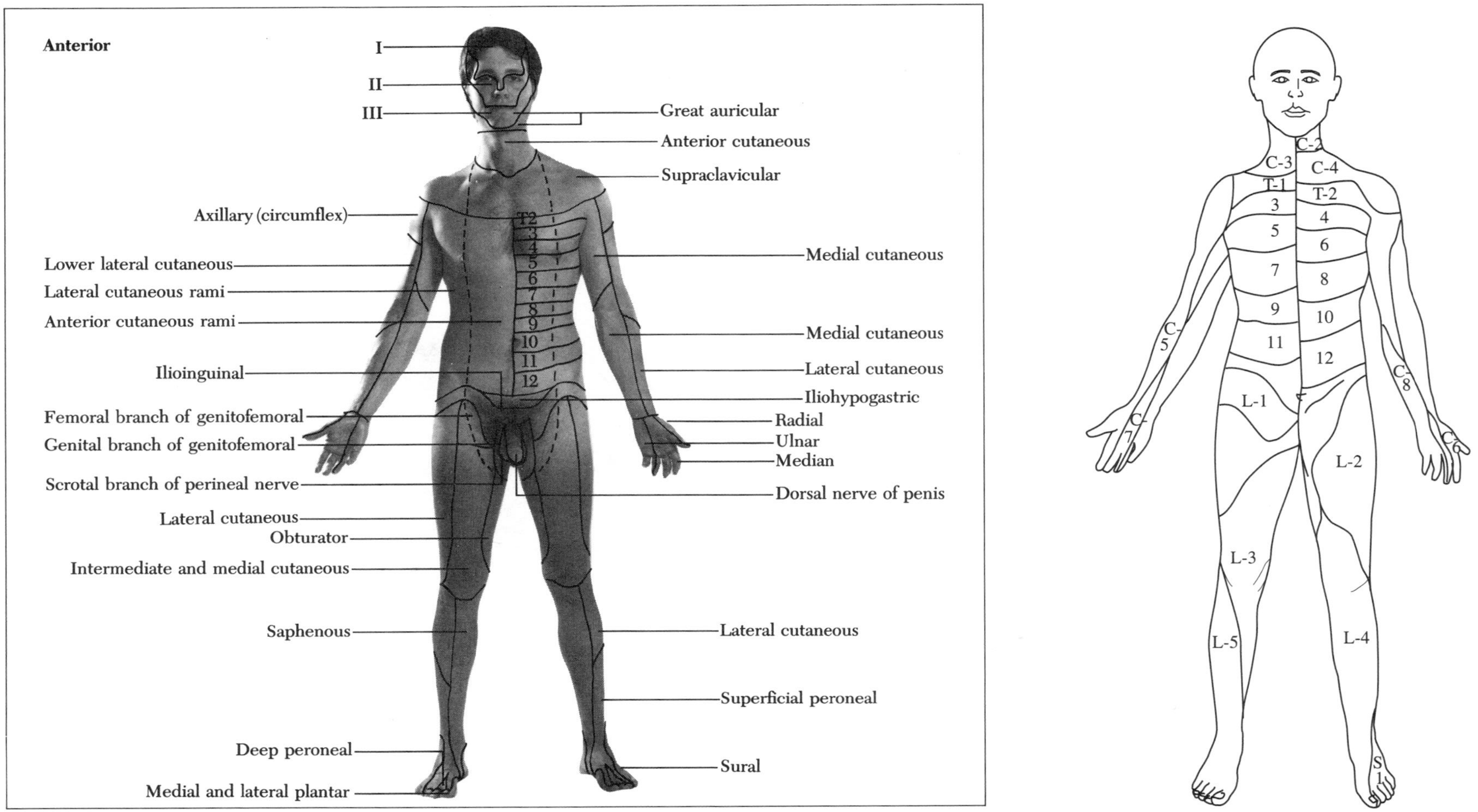

A

Figure 15-8 **(A)** Dermatomal areas of the major nerves, anterior view. **(B)** Dermatomal areas of the major nerves, posterior view. (From Westmoreland. *Medical Neurosciences.* Boston: Little, Brown, 1994, p. 373.)

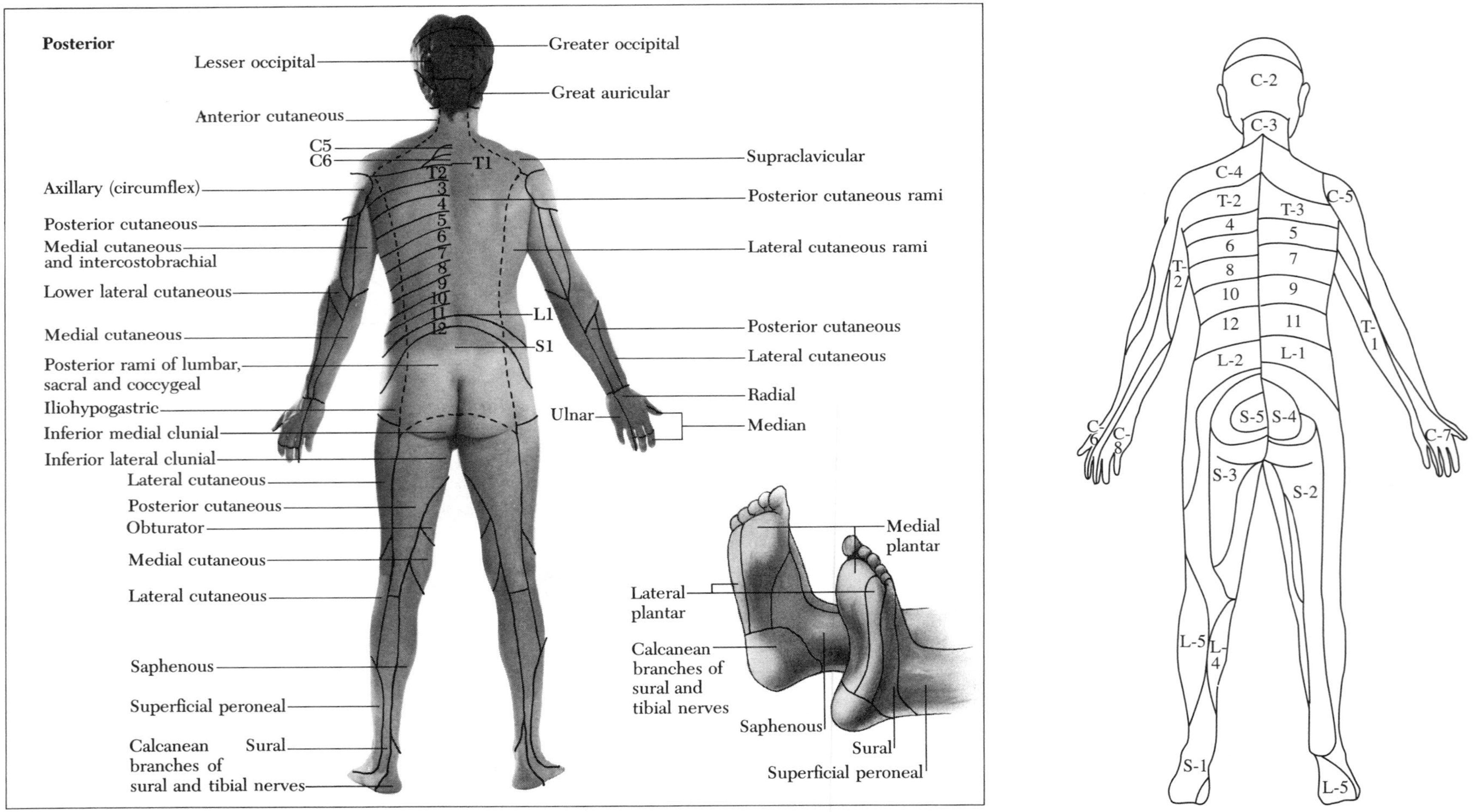

B

Figure 15-8 Continued

- The normal individual is able to identify that he is being touched by two points.

With cortical pathology, the client cannot discriminate two sharp points placed close together. The distances that a client can detect two points varies on different parts of the body. However, a minimal distance of 2 to 3 mm can be found on the fingertips of the normal client.

Point Localization
- Ask the client to keep her eyes **closed** and name and point to the area where she is being touched.

Texture Discrimination
- Ask client, with his eyes **closed,** to identify the feel (rough, smooth, soft) of materials (e.g., sandpaper, silk, velvet).

The Extinction Phenomenon
- With the client's eyes **closed,** touch the same area on both sides of the body **simultaneously** (e.g., the shoulders, forearms, hands, thighs, lower legs, feet).
- Ask the client to name where she feels you touching her and to point to the area(s). Does she feel it on one side or on both sides?
- With a parietal cortical lesion, the client will be inattentive to the diseased side.

In addition to not noticing the touch on the side with parietal lobe damage, the client will also have difficulty identifying left from right body parts, for example, when you ask her to raise her right hand.

Graphesthesia
- Ask the client, with his eyes **closed,** to name the letters, numbers, or shapes (e.g., circle, square, triangle) that you write with your finger on his palms or on other parts of his body. Inability to do this is called *agraphesthesia.*

The normal individual is able to discriminate point localization, texture, left from right body parts, and letters or numbers written on a portion of his body while his eyes remain closed.

Lateral Spinothalamic Tract Assessment
Test *both* superficial and deep pain perception, as only one may be deficient.

- With the client's eyes closed, randomly alternate use of the blunt and sharp ends of a safety pin to test *superficial* pain.
- Ask the client to identify whether the sensation is "sharp" or "dull."
- Squeeze the intrinsic muscles of the hands, forearm muscles, Achilles' tendon, or calf muscles to check perception of *deep pressure* pain.

Because temperature sensations travel over the same spinal tract as those of pain, temperature perception is not routinely tested if pain testing demonstrates the tract to be functioning. However, if you suspect a lesion of the lateral spinothalamic tract, if there are doubtful findings regarding pain perception, or if the client complains of a lack of perception of temperature, evaluate temperature perception by placing test tubes containing hot and cold water against the client's skin for identification.

Ventral Spinothalamic Tract Assessment
Light Touch
- With the client's eyes **closed,** have her point to the areas of her body where she has been touched lightly with a wisp of cotton.

A summary of the assessment of tactile perception is seen in Table 15-1.

Table 15-1 Summary Assessment of Tactile Perception

Sensation	Assessment technique	Behaviors: Normal	Behaviors: Abnormal
Primary Sensation			
Light touch	A wisp of cotton is touched to each of the designated areas bilaterally to elicit sensation.	Perceives and identifies the area lightly touched	Anesthesia, hyperesthesia
Pain/temperature			
Superficial	Superficial sharp and dull points tested using a hypodermic needle and the hub. Each area is tested bilaterally for sharp and dull.	Easily and bilaterally distinguishes sharp and dull	Hypoesthesia, hyperesthesia, paresthesia, anesthesia
Deep	Achilles tendon or biceps is squeezed.	States pain is felt	

Continued

Table 15-1 Continued

Sensation	Assessment technique	Behaviors: Normal	Behaviors: Abnormal
	Primary Sensation, continued		
Pain/temperature, continued			
Temperature	Hot or cold temperature is tested bilaterally in all designated areas (if pain tests abnormal)	Easily and bilaterally differentiates heat and cold	
Vibration	Vibrating tuning fork is applied over bony prominences (ankle or wrist) to elicit sensation.	Easily identifies when vibrations felt and when they stop	Hypoesthesia, anesthesia
Kinesthesia/ Proprioception			
Position sense	With client's finger or toe in a neutral position, examiner gently elevates or depresses digit to elicit position sense.	Easily distinguishes whether digit is elevated or depressed	Inability to correctly identify position
Romberg test	Client stands with feet together, arms down, eyes open. If normal, retest with eyes closed.	Slight swaying but maintains balance and upright posture	Loses balance
Alternating motion	Client rapidly alternates pronation and supination of both hands.	Rate and rhythm bilaterally equal	Lacks coordination
Finger-to-nose test	Client, the eyes closed, touches forefinger to nose.	Touches nose easily	Unable to directly locate nose
	Secondary Sensation		
Graphesthesia	A blunt object is used to draw a number or letter on client's hand, arm, or back.	Easily identifies number or letter bilaterally	Unable to identify or identifies incorrectly
Stereognosis	A familiar object is placed in client's hand, and after feeling it, client is asked to identify the object (paper clip, button, coin).	Easily, correctly, and bilaterally identifies object	Unable to identify or identifies incorrectly
Two-point discrimination	Using a compass or two sharp objects, examiner touches client simultaneously with both points and asks if one or two points are felt.	Two points can be discriminated at the following separations: fingertips 2.8 mm; toes 3–8 mm; chest and forearm 40 mm; back 40–70 mm	

Source: Adapted from J. P. Bellack and P. Bamford, *Nursing assessment: A multidimensional approach.* Boston: Little, Brown, 1987, pp. 333–334.

Occipital Lobe Function

When neurologic difficulties exist, the functions of the occipital lobes should be examined carefully.

- To assess visual object recognition, ask the client to identify familiar objects, such as a glass or wristwatch.
- Evaluate visual-verbal comprehension by asking the client to read a sentence from a newspaper or magazine and explain its meaning.

If the client is unable to follow this verbal command, print the instructions and evaluate whether the client can follow the written command.

Temporal Lobe Function

Assessing temporal functioning is done throughout the history-taking process in regard to the following:

- Recent memory
- Ability to understand the spoken word and to articulate understandable words
- Interpretation of odor, sound, and taste. These are assessed with the appropriate cranial nerves (CN I olfactory, CN VIII, auditory, and CN VII facial and IX glossopharyngeal, respectively) associated with the smelling, hearing, and gustatory centers in the temporal lobe.
- Monitoring emotional stability; attention to behavior is warranted. With dysfunction, the client is extremely emotionally labile, for example, rapidly shifts from apathy to anger and rage.

STRUCTURE AND FUNCTION OF THE CEREBELLUM

The cerebellum, or hindbrain, which consists of two hemispheres, is located posteriorly and inferiorly to the cerebrum (see Fig. 15-1). It is connected to the cerebrum, pons, and medulla oblongata by three fiber bundles: the superior peduncles, middle peduncles, and inferior peduncles, respectively. Thus, some of the nerve fibers from the cerebrum, pons, and medulla pass through the cerebellum.

Of particular importance are the impulses received from the cortical motor tract (muscle movement) and the semicircular canals of the inner ear, as these structures play a major role in *body position* (posture, balance) and *movement* (coordination, tone). The cerebellum receives, sorts, and synergizes these impulses, after which they are sent out to maintain posture, balance, muscle coordination, and the tone of the voluntary muscles.

ASSESSMENT OF THE CEREBELLUM

Cerebellar assessment procedures focus on balance and coordination.

- Observe closely for any abnormalities in rhythm and smoothness in body movements.
- Note any tremors or impairment in rhythm and coordination in speech.
- Observe the equilibrial position of the eyes.

Nystagmus may be present with inner ear difficulties, but it, too, may indicate cerebellar involvement. With cerebellar involvement, the nystagmus is most marked when the client gazes toward the side with the lesion.

Balance Assessment

Gait

- Observe the client's gait by having the her walk barefoot across the room away from you and back.
- Observe the movements of the extremities. The arms normally swing smoothly in opposition to the advancement of the foot.
- Note width of stance and size and speed of steps.
- The client should be able to start and stop locomotion easily.

Romberg's Sign

Romberg's sign, the inability to stand with feet together and eyes closed, may indicate cerebellar disease.

- Stand nearby to catch the client if necessary. With cerebellar dysfunction, the client will fall toward the affected side.
- Ask the client to stand with his feet together and eyes closed.
- A small amount of swaying during this test is normal.

If you discover difficulty, you may ask the client to perform several other tests to verify the suspected finding of loss of balance:

- *Tandem walking*—the familiar heel to toe along a straight line—frequently associated with the testing of balance control when inebriation is suspected.
- Have the client *hop on one leg* or perform a shallow knee bend, first one leg and then the other.

Taking the client's age and general status into consideration, these maneuvers are normally accomplished with little difficulty.

Coordination Assessment

Test **both** upper and lower extremities, one limb at a time.

Techniques for Assessing Balance

1. *Observe gait:* Have client walk barefooted away from you and toward you. Characteristics: movement of extremities, position of torso, size and speed of steps, width of stance.
2. *Romberg's sign:* Stand close to the client. Ask the client to place feet together and close eyes.
3. *Tandem walking:* Have client walk in a straight line alternating the placement of the heel of one foot in front of the toe of the opposite foot.
   Have the client hop or do a shallow knee bend on one leg and then on the other.

Techniques for Assessing Coordination

1. Upper Extremities:
   a. *Finger-to-nose tests:* Have client touch index finger of each hand to nose. Have client touch nose and then your moving finger with her index finger.
   b. *Rapid alternating movements:* Have client rapidly move hands to and from supination to pronation positions. Tap fingers of each hand on a table surface; rapidly oppose each finger of each hand to the thumb.
2. Lower Extremities:
   a. *Heel to shin:* Have client place the heel of one foot at the knee of the opposite leg and run the heel down the shin to the ankle level. Perform with eyes both opened and closed.
   b. *Figure "8":* Have client write an imaginary "8" in the air with each foot.
   c. *Toe to finger:* Have the client point her great toe to your finger as you move it in different left/right/up/down directions.
   d. *Tapping toes:* Have client rapidly tap toes of both feet on the floor.

Upper Extremities

Use the finger-to-nose tests.

- Test one hand at a time.
- Ask the client to do such things as button and unbutton a button, write her name, or rapidly tap her fingers on a table.
- Ask the client to touch each finger of her hands to the thumb in rapid succession (finger-to-thumb opposition).
- Ask the client to rapidly alternate her hands from the prone to the supine position. An easy instruction to the client is, "Slap your thighs with the palm of your hands and then with the top of your hands as fast as possible." Demonstrate this for the client.
- Ask the client to touch her nose and then your finger; change the position of your finger and have the client continue to touch your finger with each move. Repeat this action with increasing rapidity.
- Ask the client to close her eyes and hold her arms straight out from her sides. Ask her to touch her nose, first with one hand and then the other.

With pathology, *past pointing* will occur on the diseased side. Fine coordination does not develop until age 5 or 6; therefore, if a younger child can point to 2 inches away from her nose, this is within normal limits.

Lower Extremities

- Ask the client to place the heel of one foot on the knee of the opposite leg and move it down the shin (the heel-to-shin test).
- This is normally performed without difficulty, both with the eyes open and then closed.
- Ask the client to "write" a figure 8 in the air with each foot or to point to your hand with each big toe while lying down.
- Normally, these feats are easily and smoothly accomplished.
- Ask the client to rapidly tap his toes on the floor; this should be done easily and smoothly.

ASSESSMENT OF THE CRANIAL NERVES

The routine assessment of each of the cranial nerves has been discussed throughout the text in the appropriate anatomic section. Generally, the first cranial nerve, the olfactory, is not routinely tested. However, when there is suspicion of neurologic disorder, each of the cranial nerves is meticulously assessed.

To ensure assessment of all 12 cranial nerves, the first hurdle is to memorize their sequence and names. This may be facilitated by the use of the following mnemonic device: "On Old Olympus' Towering Tops A Finn and German Viewed Some Hops."

Another mnemonic that helps to remember whether the cranial nerve is sensory, motor, or both sensory and motor is "Some Say Marry Money But My Brother Says Bad Business Marrying Money." Sensory is designated by words beginning with the letter *S*, motor by *M*, and both motor and sensory by *B* words (see box on page 351).

Concepts in Assessing the Cranial Nerves

Olfactory (I)

- A familiar odor is used to assess smell (e.g., coffee, tobacco, lemon, peppermint); avoid such volatile substances as ammonia.
- Most important is whether the client can make a distinction between odors, not whether she is able to identify precisely the given substances.
- Loss of smell (anosmia) can be affected by many factors, including a cold, aging, sinusitis, heavy cigarette smoking, and nasal obstruction.
- It is important to assess the function of smell in clients who have
  - head trauma
  - meningitis
  - subarachnoid hemorrhage
  - visual failure
  - progressive intellectual deterioration

Mnemonics for Remembering Cranial Nerves

On	I Olfactory	Some—Sensory
Old	II Optic	Say—Sensory
Olympus'	III Oculomotor	Marry—Motor
Towering	IV Trochlear	Money—Motor
Tops	V Trigeminal	But—Motor and Sensory
A	VI Abducens	My—Motor
Finn	VII Facial	Brother—Motor and Sensory
And	VIII Auditory or Acoustic	Says—Sensory
German	IX Glossopharyngeal	Bad—Motor and Sensory
Viewed	X Vagus	Business—Motor and Sensory
Some	XI Spinal accessory	Marrying—Motor
Hops	XII Hypoglossal	Money—Motor

Optic (II)

- Test vision for accuracy by means of a Snellen chart.
- Assess the visual fields with a perimeter and tangent screen.
- Do an ophthalmoscope examination of the retina and the optic nerve head. Chapter 8 provides a more detailed discussion of the procedures used to assess the eyes.

Figure 15-9 illustrates how the optic nerve receives visual images from the retina of the eye. At the optic chiasm, the temporal portion of each visual field crosses over, and both temporal and nasal impulses are transported to the occipital lobe of the cerebral cortex. Here the images are recognized and interpreted. If the visual cortex of the occipital lobe is damaged, "cortical blindness" results.

Disturbances in vision are better understood and detected if you possess knowledge of the anatomy of this system. Figure 15-9 (the color portions represent areas of no vision) helps you to visualize the bases for the various hemianopias. *Hemianopia* refers to visual defects that involve half of the visual field. The term is generally used to refer to bilateral defects resulting from a single lesion. It can be seen with visual field defect number *(1)* that the occurrence of a lesion anterior to the optic chiasm could cause a totally blind eye. A lateral lesion at the optic chiasm *(2)* would cause a unilateral medial defect. Observe *(3)* that the medial aspect of each retina is served by optic nerve fibers that decussate (cross) at the optic chiasm before continuing to the contralateral occipital lobe. A lesion at this point may involve only those medial tracts and would therefore result in a bitemporal hemianopia because of the inversion of the field of vision on the retinas. When the optic tract between the chiasm and the geniculate body in the temporal and occipital lobes is interrupted *(6)*, a homonymous (same) hemianopia occurs, wherein the field of vision is obliterated on the same side of both eyes. Generally, homonymous hemianopia is accompanied by pupillary abnormalities. A lesion of only a portion of the optic tract fibers may cause a homonymous

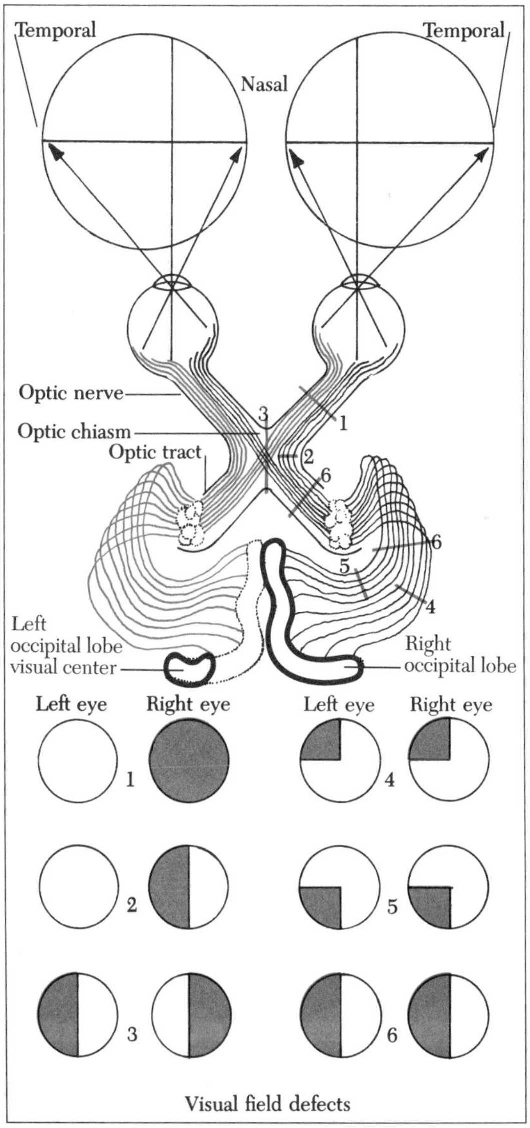

Figure 15-9 Lesions of the optic tract and resultant visual field defects.

quadratic defect (*4* and *5*). In this situation, the field of vision is lost in a similar quadrant of both eyes.

Detection of visual defects not only is important for detection of client problems and for diagnostic purposes but also is extremely pertinent for the planning of nursing care.

Oculomotor (III), Trochlear (IV), and Abducens (VI)

The oculomotor, trochlear, and abducens nerves innervate the extraocular muscles of the eyes. Additionally, the oculomotor nerve serves to contract the iris muscles, constrict the pupils, and elevate the eyelid.

- Observe the client following through the six cardinal gaze positions.
- Note whether the eyes are symmetrical at rest.

In Adie's syndrome, the pupil is dilated and sluggish in reacting to light. However, on sustained accommodation, the pupil may actually become smaller than the normal pupil. This syndrome usually occurs in young women and is an idiopathic, benign condition (see Fig. 8-9).

Trigeminal (V)

The trigeminal nerve is a mixed nerve; that is, it contains both sensory and motor fibers. Its sensory distribution evolves in three branches (Fig. 15-10): (1) ophthalmic, (2) maxillary, and (3) mandibular. These divisions consist of superficial sensory nerves of the cornea, the oral and nasal mucosa, and the skin of the face. These anatomic areas are normally sensitive to pain, temperature, and light touch. In addition, the motor fibers of the trigeminal nerve innervate the masseter and temporalis muscles.

- Lightly touch the cornea with a wisp of cotton; be sure to touch the cornea and not just the sclera of the eye when assessing the ophthalmic tract. The eye normally will blink; this is called the *corneal reflex.*
- Testing of the three branches for temperature sensation is generally done only when there appears to be a loss or a questionable finding regarding pain perception, as temperature and pain are carried on the same nerve tract.
- If an area of sensory loss is identified, determine its outermost margins by proceeding outwardly from the center of loss until sensation is felt.
- A loss of sensation should be documented by a sketch of the area of sensory loss in the context of the anatomic part involved.

The motor portion of the mandibular branch normally maintains the jaw in midalignment. The masseter muscles (chewing muscles) of both cheeks normally will contract as the client clenches his teeth. This aids in the detection of any muscle atrophy, paresis, or paralysis.

Facial (VII)

The facial nerve is also a mixed nerve, with motor fibers to the facial muscles and sensory fibers mediating taste perception of sweet and salty on the anterior two thirds of the tongue. Therefore, the normal client displays facial symmetry and the ability to identify sweet and salty tastes. (The taste sensations of bitter and sour are involved with the glossopharyngeal nerve.) The facial nerve also innervates the lacrimal glands and certain salivary glands.

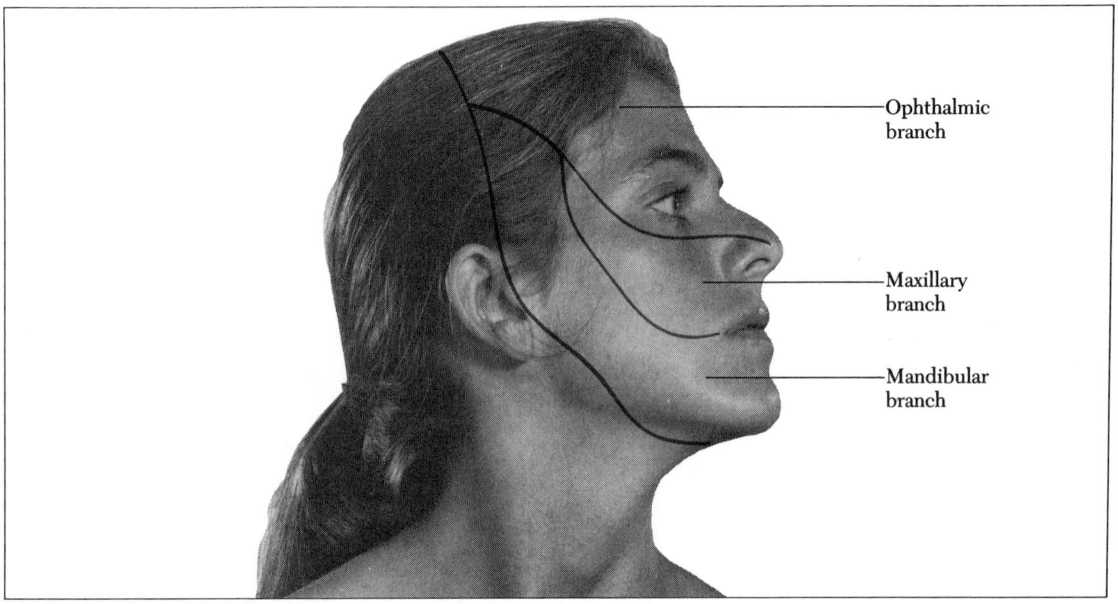

Figure 15-10 Sensory divisions of the trigeminal nerve.

The taste sensation ability of the sensory component of the facial nerve is *not* assessed during a routine health screening. It is pursued only if the client complains of an abnormality regarding taste or if facial nerve damage or a brain stem lesion is suspected. Figure 15-11 identifies the various taste regions of the tongue.

- It is important that the client keep his tongue out until the taste is identified—the material will spread to all areas of the tongue if he retracts it before identifying the taste.
- Test each side of the tongue separately and in succession with the various solutions for salty (salt solution), sweet (sugar water), bitter (quinine water), and sour (vinegar solution) tastes.
- After each application to the tongue and identification of the solution by the client, have him rinse her mouth well with water.

Auditory or Acoustic (VIII)

The auditory nerve has two divisions: the cochlear branch and the vestibular branch. The cochlear portion is concerned with hearing and is routinely assessed on health screening. The gross assessment procedures are described in Chapter 9. When difficulties arise with this portion of the auditory nerve, an audiometry examination must be conducted for a more accurate evaluation.

The vestibular portion of the auditory nerve is concerned with equilibrium. Unless there is suspicion of disease of the vestibular system, evaluative tests of its function are *not* performed. However, symptoms of vertigo, ataxia, nausea, and vomiting warrant investigation of the vestibular system, and you should observe closely for signs of nystagmus and past pointing.

A specific test for evaluating vestibular function is the *caloric test:*

- Place the client in a supine position with his head elevated approximately 30 degrees. (This is done to place the horizontal semicircular canals in a vertical position.)
- Instill 5 mL of ice water or very warm water into the ear under gentle pressure with a syringe and a soft-tipped rubber catheter.
- In the normal individual, this will produce vertigo, nystagmus, nausea, and often vomiting, because the vestibular branch is functioning. These symptoms occur because the vestibular nuclei are connected to the cranial nerves governing the extraocular muscles and to the visceral organs of the abdomen and thorax.
- Test both ears.
- If there is no reaction to the caloric test, the vestibular branch on that side is affected.

Glossopharyngeal (IX) and Vagus (X)

The glossopharyngeal and vagus nerves are discussed under a single heading to emphasize their close anatomic and functional relationship. The glossopharyngeal nerve innervates the pharynx, palate, and posterior third of the tongue. Its motor function to the stylopharyngeus muscle is minimal;

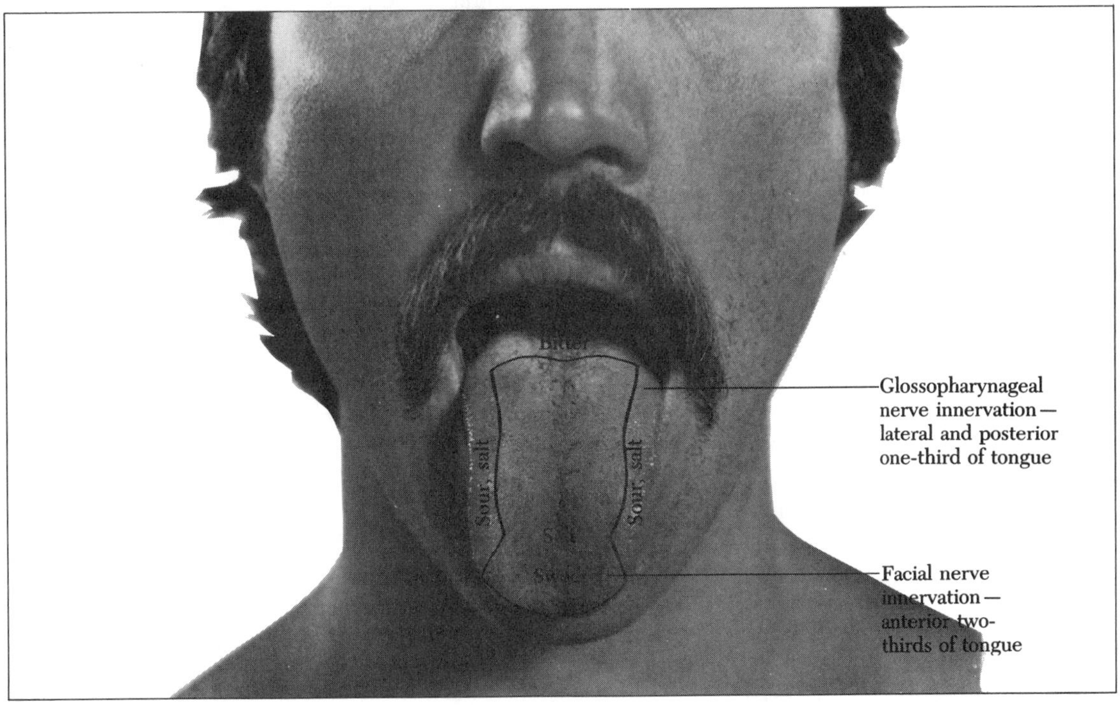

Figure 15-11 Taste regions of the tongue.

this muscle widens the pharynx during the process of swallowing, and its impairment is not usually recognized clinically.

- Check the presence of sensation and gag reflex by touching the sides of the pharynx lightly. The gag reflex is often brisk in heavy smokers and nervous individuals.
- The gag reflex is *not* routinely tested because it is an unpleasant experience. It is checked, however, when a neural disorder is suspected.

In light of neurologic complaints or signs, the taste sensation of the posterior third of the tongue, which is for bitter and sour, is tested to evaluate the glossopharyngeal nerve (see Fig. 15-11). The normal individual has no difficulty with swallowing or identifying bitter and sour tastes.

The vagus nerve has motor fibers supplying the larynx, pharynx, and palate (external laryngeal, recurrent laryngeal, and pharyngeal nerves, respectively); visceromotor fibers also innervate the heart, lungs, and alimentary tract. The sensory function of the vagus is widespread, as it receives impulses from the pharynx, larynx, epiglottis, trachea, esophagus, heart, lungs, stomach, and small intestine.

Basically, **swallowing and phonation** are the most important functions of the vagus nerve neurologically and **are checked routinely.**

- Have the client swallow water. Note whether the water is regurgitated back through the nose.
- Check the uvula at rest and during phonation to aid in evaluation of the vagus nerve. When the client says "aah," the uvula will normally rise symmetrically in midline.
- With vagus nerve damage, the uvula will deviate away from the affected side. If both sides are affected, movement will be absent.

If a client complains of hoarseness persisting longer than 2 weeks, consult a physician.

Spinal Accessory (XI)

The function of the spinal accessory nerve is clear-cut. It innervates the trapezius and sternocleidomastoid muscles.

- Check for symmetry of the shoulders, neck, and scapulae.
- Observe for drooping of the shoulder as well as difficulty or inability to raise the arm above the head.
- With involvement,
  - the scapula is displaced downward, and there may be a slight winging (outward displacement)
  - atrophy and flatness of the neck may be on the affected side
  - weakness in neck flexion occurs with paralysis of both sternocleidomastoid muscles

This nerve is rarely affected alone but is seen in accompaniment with other cranial nerve palsies.

Hypoglossal (XII)

The hypoglossal is a motor nerve that innervates the tongue. The appearance, movement, and strength of the tongue should be evaluated.

- Observe the tongue inside the mouth and sticking out.
- Atrophy and increased coating may be observed on a paralyzed side.
- In early involvement, atrophy is quite difficult to detect, but scalloping or indentation may be seen along the edge of the tongue.
- Normally, the tongue is symmetrical in shape, protrudes midline, and possesses motor strength.

In summary, if the client displays signs and symptoms, the cranial nerves should be meticulously tested. Table 15-2

Table 15-2 Techniques for Cranial Nerve Assessment

Cranial nerve	Technique	Common problems
I. Olfactory	1. Have client close eyes. 2. Close off client's naris by placing pressure against the side with an index finger. 3. Hold substance—e.g., soap, lemon, coffee—near naris. 4. Ask client to identify substance. 5. Repeat procedure for the remaining naris.	Anosmia
II. Optic	See techniques described in Chapter 8 "Assessment of the Eye," e.g., visual acuity, visual fields, eye grounds.	Decreased or loss of visual acuity, visual field defects, changes in optic nerve disk
III. Oculomotor	1. Inspect eyelids 2. Inspect pupil sizes and reaction to light, accommodation, and convergence (see Chapter 8). 3. Check EOMS. 4. Note whether eyes are symmetrical at rest.	Ptosis of eyelid Dilated pupil

Table 15-2 Continued

Cranial nerve	Technique	Common problems
IV. Trochlear	1. Check EOMS. 2. Note whether eyes are symmetrical at rest.	Unable to gaze in nasally downward direction
V. Trigeminal	1. Check corneal reflex (see Chapter 8) and three sensory divisions (ophthalmic, maxillary, and mandibular) with a cotton wisp, pinprick, and temperature (hot and cold water–filled test tubes). 2. Observe for jaw deviation.	Brain stem lesion, herpes zoster, tic douloureux
	3. Palpate masseter muscle while teeth are clenched and unclenched. 4. Have client open lower jaw against resistance (place your hand under lower jaw to provide resistance).	Masseter and temporalis muscle weakness with myasthenia gravis and amyotrophic lateral sclerosis
VI. Abducens	1. Check EOMS. 2. Note whether eyes are symmetrical at rest.	Unable to gaze in lateral direction
VII. Facial	1. Observe for symmetry at rest and while client smiles, frowns, clenches teeth, blows out cheeks, purses lips.	Bell's palsy
	2. Test for sweet and salty taste sensation on anterior two thirds of tongue.	Change in taste sensation
	3. Dip applicator in saltwater solution. 4. Ask client to extend tongue and identify taste before retracting tongue into mouth. 5. Place applicator on anterior portion of tongue. 6. Rinse mouth with water. 7. Repeat procedure with sugar-water solution.	Decrease in salivation and tearing
VIII. Auditory or acoustic	1. Weber test (see Chapter 9) 2. Rinne test (see Chapter 9) 3. Special tests a. Audiometry examination b. Caloric test	Decreased or loss of hearing; acoustic neuroma
IX. Glossopharyngeal	1. Observe for difficulty swallowing. 2. Check gag reflex. 3. Test for bitter and sour taste sensation on posterior one third of tongue using quinine water and vinegar respectively.	Dysphagia, decreased gag reflex, glossopharyngeal neuralgia, and change in taste sensation
X. Vagus	1. Observe for difficulty swallowing as client drinks water. 2. Check uvular reflex.	Hoarseness or aphonia, regurgitation of water through the nose.
XI. Spinal accessory	1. Have client shrug shoulders against resistance (place your hands on client's shoulders). 2. Observe scapula. 3. Place hand on side of client's forehead. 4. Ask client to flex his head against your hand. 5. Repeat on opposite side of face.	Drooping of shoulder, unable to raise arm above head; scapula displaced downward and maybe slight winging.
XII. Hypoglossal	1. Have client stick out tongue. 2. Have client move tongue against resistance (tongue blades or examiner's finger on outside of cheek). 3. Observe for scalloping or indentation along edge of tongue.	Tongue deviation, weakness, atrophy

EOMS, extraocular muscle movements.

RECORDING OF FINDINGS

The first column contains normal findings; the second column contains recordings of abnormal findings.

Cerebrum
Inspection: Oriented to person, time, and place; recent and remote memory intact; appropriate behavior and speech; alert and cooperative; stereognosis, two-point discrimination, and graphesthesia intact.

Cerebellum
Inspection: Normal gait; Romberg's sign absent; tandem walking, finger to nose, heel to shin smoothly intact; rapid alternating hand movements and fingers intact; thumb opposition without difficulty; no tremors.

Cranial Nerves
Inspection: Grossly intact. I: able to discriminate between soap, tobacco; II: OU 20/20 with corrective lenses; peripheral vision intact; III, IV, VI: PERRLA; no ptosis; EOMs intact without nystagmus; no strabismus; V: corneal reflex present; light touch and pain sensation intact; can open mandible against resistance; VII: facial symmetry; no weakness; sweet and salty taste discrimination; VIII: hearing intact; IX, X: gag reflex present; bitter and sour taste intact; no dysphagia; uvular reflex intact; XI: neck-head movement and shoulder shrug intact; no weakness; scapulae in horizontal plane; XII: tongue protrudes midline; no weakness; no atrophy; no fasciculations.

Reflexes
Inspection: Plantar reflex; no Babinski; no clonus; normal abdominal reflexes.

	B	T	BR	P	A	PR
R	+ +	+ +	+ +	+ +	+ +	↓
L	+ +	+ +	+ +	+ +	+ +	↓

Cerebrum
(Client with cerebral arteriosclerosis)

Inspection: Oriented to person; disoriented to time and place; poor immediate recall and recent memory; remote memory fair at times; slow to respond; short attention span.

Cerebellum
(Client with Parkinson's disease)

Inspection: Forward lunging gait; short shuffling steps; difficulty stopping; arms held stiffly at sides; resting tremors.

Cranial Nerves
(Client with amyotrophic lateral sclerosis)

Inspection: I, II, III, IV, VI, VIII: intact; V: light touch and pain intact; corneal blink; weak masseter muscles; unable to hold eyes closed tightly; IX, X: slurred speech; mild dysphagia with occasional nasal regurgitation of liquids; diminished gag and uvular reflex; XI: decreased shoulder shrug and movement of head from side to side against resistance; XII: decreased strength of tongue, atrophy and fasciculations present.

Reflexes
(Client with right cerebrovascular accident)

Inspection: Right plantar reflex; left clonus; left Babinski present; cremasteric and abdominal reflexes absent on left side.

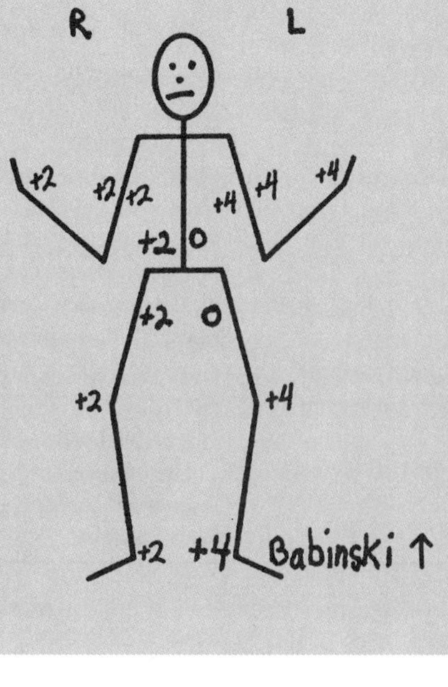

provides a summary of techniques for cranial nerve assessment and common problems of cranial nerve damage.

Note: If time limits are imposed during routine health assessment, the most pertinent evaluations to be performed regarding the cranial nerves are assessment of

- visual fields
- extraocular muscle movements
- pupillary reflexes
- facial innervation
- tongue movement
- swallowing

ASSESSMENT OF NEUROLOGIC REFLEXES

A reflex is elicited by applying a sensory stimulus that initiates the transmission of a muscle-stretch impulse or a cutaneous stimulation through the flex arc in the spinal cord. The reflex arc involves the union of a sensory and a motor nerve fiber (Fig. 15-12). The sensory stimulus creates a sensory impulse that is carried by a sensory nerve fiber within a peripheral nerve to the posterior root horn. It synapses with a motor neuron in the anterior root horn, and the motor nerve fiber carries the impulse back to the muscle, which contracts. If any of the fibers of the reflex arc are interrupted, the reflex is absent (lower motor nerve damage).

The briskness of the intact reflex arc is regulated by the upper motor neurons of the cerebral cortex. Therefore, cortical motor tract damage (motor strip in the cerebrum), characteristically seen in the majority of cerebrovascular accidents, results in exaggerated reflexes or hyperreflexia because the cord reflex arc is still intact, but there is loss of the cerebral "dampening" ability.

It is **extremely important** that the client's muscles be relaxed in order to elicit and accurately evaluate the neurologic reflexes. The stimulus should be applied evenly to corresponding sides of the client's body and the results then compared. For assessment purposes, the reflexes are considered in three basic categories: (1) DTRs, (2) superficial (cutaneous) reflexes, and (3) pathologic reflexes.

Deep Tendon Reflexes

DTRs are unstable in the newborn, so testing results are of little significance at this age. Some individuals normally have been areflexic all of their lives and may not have any demonstrable DTRs.

- With an absence of DTRs or with diminished responses, you should instruct the client to perform isometric muscular contractions elsewhere in the body before drawing your final conclusions regarding his reflex status.
  - Ask the client to lock his fingers together and pull when you test his reflexes in the lower extremities.
  - Ask the client to squeeze his thigh or clench his teeth as you test the reflexes in his upper extremities.
- At the moment of muscle tenseness during these maneuvers, strike the tendon with the percussion hammer.

These reinforcement techniques are thought to either facilitate neural conduction in the reflex arc, if the arc is intact, or distract the client, thus, making his muscles more relaxed.

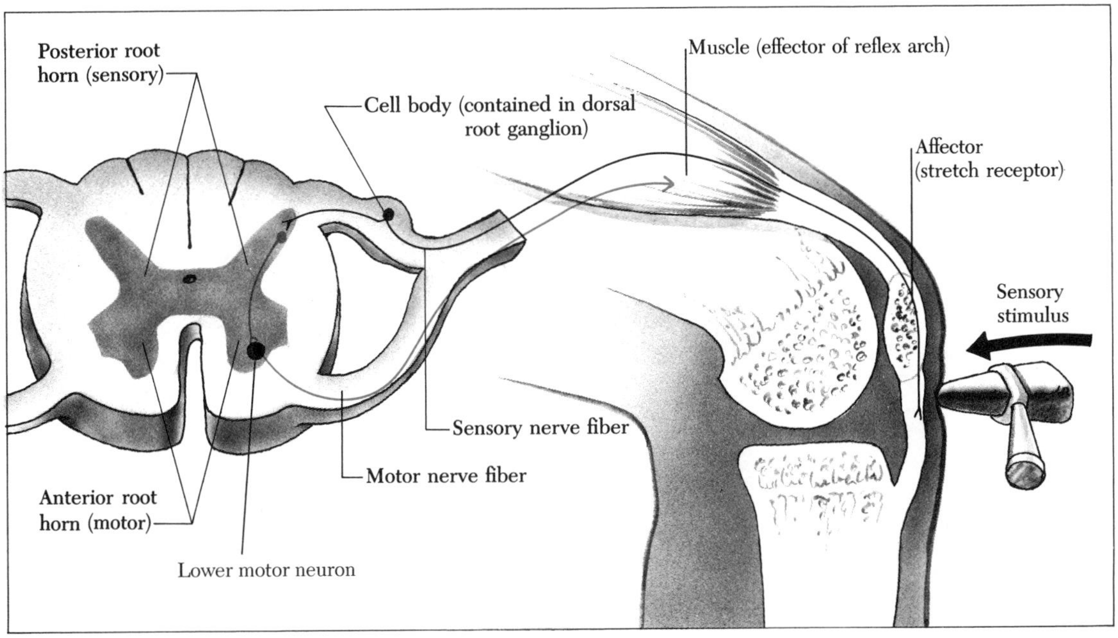

Figure 15-12 The reflex arc.

The most common DTR tests are presented in Table 15-3. The grading system for tendon reflexes (Table 15-4) is an arbitrary method of categorizing DTRs. Figure 15-13 gives examples of how the grading system is implemented for a client with normal tendon reflexes and for a client diagnosed with a right cerebrovascular accident.

Superficial (Cutaneous) Reflexes

The commonly tested superficial reflexes (Table 15-5) are the abdominal, cremasteric, plantar, and anal. These reflexes are present by approximately 6 months of age.

The upper and lower *abdominal reflex* is difficult to elicit if the abdominal muscles are not relaxed.

Table 15-3 Deep Tendon Reflexes

Reflex	Percussion site	Response	CNS dermatomes
Biceps	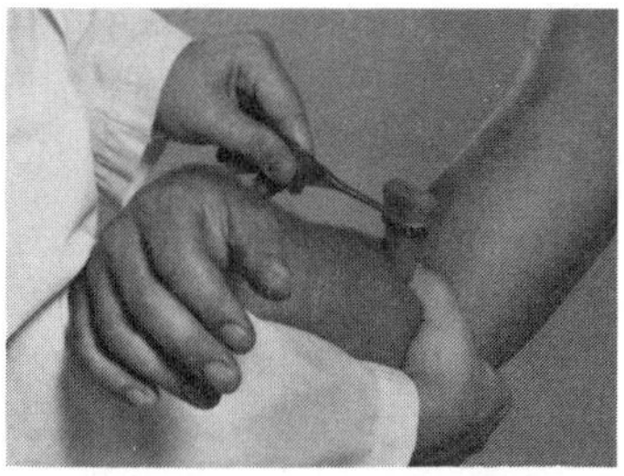	Biceps contraction (Place your thumb on tendon cord in midantecubital space with client's elbow flexed. Strike your thumbnail with percussion hammer.)	Cervical 5 and 6
Triceps	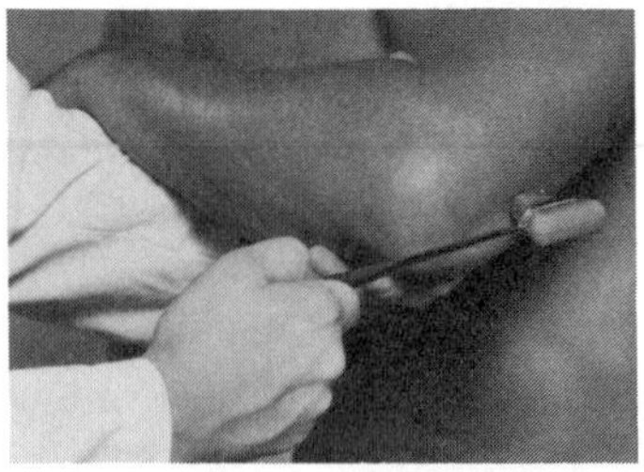	Elbow extension; triceps contraction (Strike tendon with percussion hammer about 1.5 inches above the olecranon process.)	Cervical 6–8
Brachioradialis	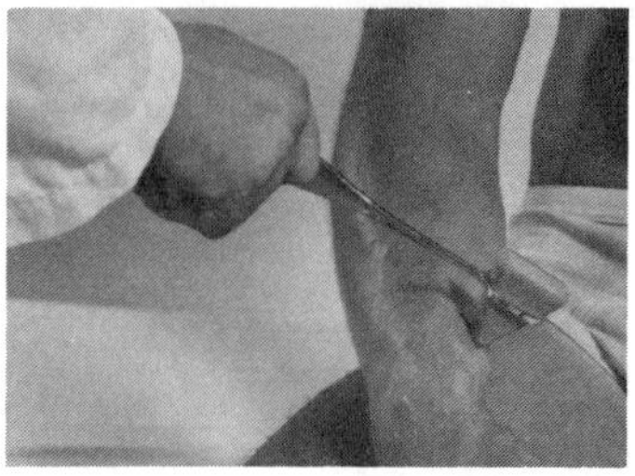	Pronation of forearm and hand (Strike tendon about 2 inches above the wrist on the radial [thumb] side of the arm.)	Cervical 5 and 6
Patellar	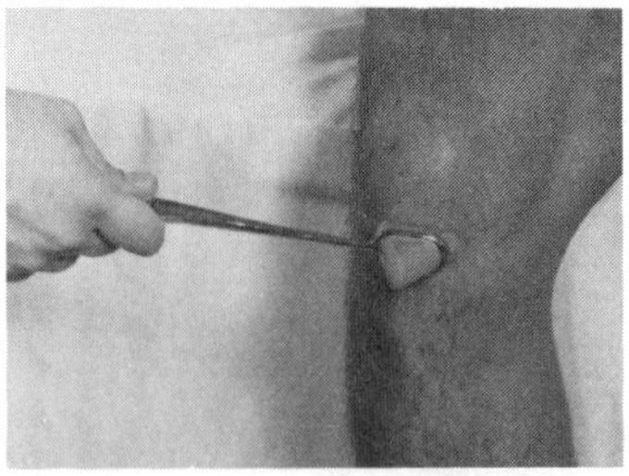	Knee extension (Strike tendon immediately below the patella [knee cap].)	Lumbar 2–4
Achilles	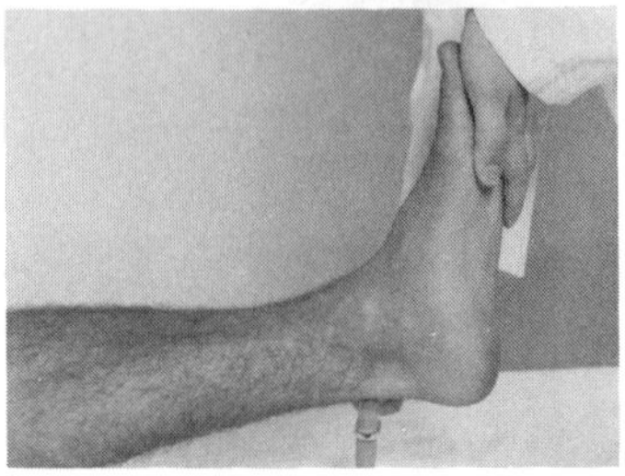	Plantar flexion of foot (Strike heelcord as you gently apply pressure to bottom of foot.)	Sacral 1 and 2

Table 15-4 **Grading System for Tendon Reflexes**

Grade	Symbols	Interpretation
0	0	Absent (indicate whether reinforcement used)
1	+	Diminished but present
2	+ +	Normal; average
3	+ + +	Normal; brisker than average—may or may not indicate pathology
4	+ + + +	Hyperactive; very brisk—most often pathologic

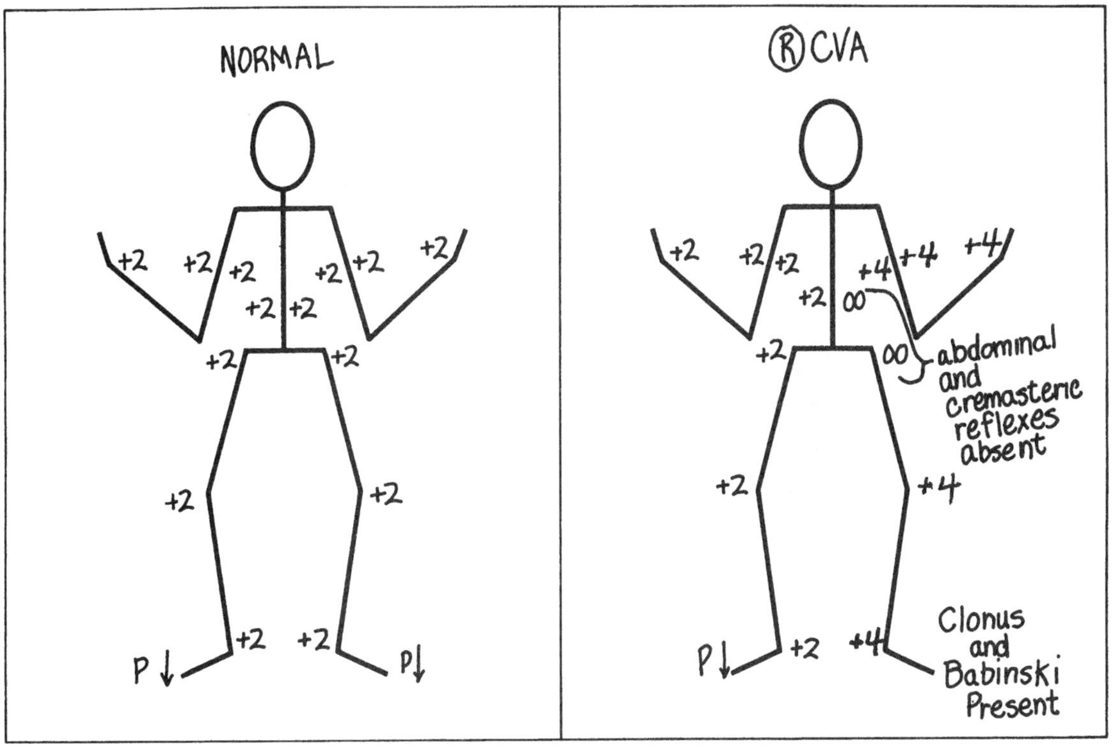

Figure 15-13 **Grading of tendon reflexes.**

- Briskly stroke the skin of the upper abdomen in the four quadrants from periphery to umbilicus with a sharp object (key, tongue blade, end of applicator).
- Normally the umbilicus will move toward the area stimulated.
- The lower abdominal reflex is similarly tested, resulting in a downward movement of the umbilicus.
- The abdominal reflex is generally elicited quite easily in the young. It maybe absent in the elderly, in the obese, or in persons having a history of multiple abdominal surgeries or several pregnancies.
- In the obese client, you may be able to palpate the presence of muscular contraction if you first retract and hold the umbilicus away from the direction being stimulated.

The *cremasteric reflex* is tested in the male client by stroking the inner aspect of each thigh with a sharp object. The normal response is elevation of the scrotum on the side stroked.

Absence of these cutaneous reflexes will be contralateral to damage of the corticospinal tract above the level of the medulla (cortex damage), whereas the absence will be on the same side of a lesion involving the corticospinal tract below the medullary level. Thus, both abdominal and cremasteric reflexes may be absent with both upper and lower motor tract damage.

- Stroke the bottom of the foot to elicit the *plantar reflex,* in which the toes curl under. This normal response is recorded as "plantar," or a downward arrow, or "toes down."
- Insert a gloved finger into the rectum to elicit the *anal reflex* and evaluate the intactness of the sacral neural dermatome. The normal response is contraction of the anal sphincter muscle.

Table 15-5 **Superficial Reflexes**

Reflex	Stimulus site	Response	CNS dermatomes
Abdominal	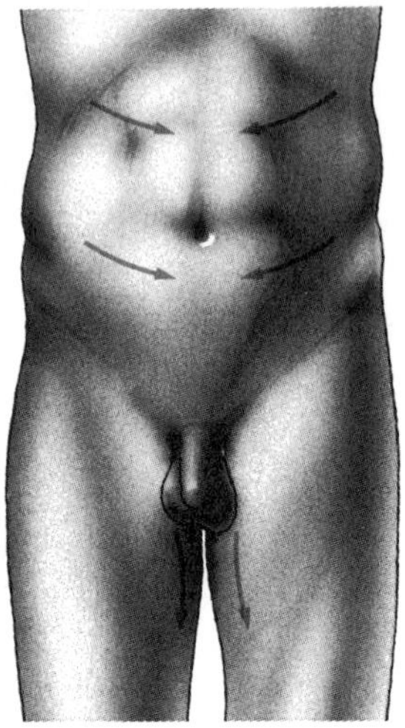	Umbilicus moves toward area stroked	Upper thoracic 7–9
Cremasteric		Scrotum elevates	Thoracic 12 and lumbar 1
Plantar	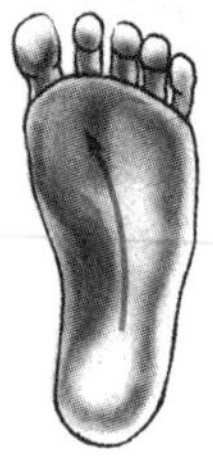	Toes flex	Sacral 1 and 2
Anal	Rectal stimulation by gloved finger	Contraction of anal sphincter	Sacral

Pathologic Reflexes

Pathologic reflexes (Table 15-6) are documented as absent or present. In the healthy individual, they should be absent. However, these reflexes may normally be present at birth and remain up until 2 years of age because of the immaturity of the infant nervous system. Their appearance in individuals over age 2 is a sign of pathology and requires medical consultation and evaluation.

- The *Babinski reflex* is tested during a routine physical assessment, because it is elicited, if present, by the same stimulus used for testing the plantar reflex.
- Ankle clonus is tested if the DTRs or superficial reflexes are hyperactive.
- The pathologic reflexes—Babinski, Chaddock, Oppenheim, Gordon, Hoffmann, and ankle clonus—are significant signs of upper motor neuron (cortex) damage (see Table 15-6).
- Check for Kernig's and Brudzinski's signs when meningeal irritation (meningitis, encephalitis, head trauma, blood in the cerebrospinal fluid) is suspected (see Table 15-6).

Table 15-7 attempts to summarize the findings of upper motor neuron (UMN) damage typically observed in such conditions as cerebrovascular accidents, brain tumors, and cerebral aneurysms, as compared with those findings characteristic of lower motor neuron (LMN) damage, as in clients with paraplegia and quadriplegia.

CLINICAL CORRELATIONS

Frontal Lobe Dysfunction

Dysfunction of the anterior portion of the frontal lobes may produce alternating personality, mood, and attitude changes or may result in difficulties in thought content, learning, decision making, and the ability to generalize or to perform mathematical computations. Thus, interpersonal relationships and the management of one's household or employment are commonly disrupted.

A client with frontal lobe pathology may display behaviors that range from apathy to preoccupation with self to irritability, hostility, suspicion, or grandiose ideation. The indi-

Table 15-6 Pathologic Reflexes

Reflex	How elicited	Response if present
Babinski	Stroke lateral aspect of sole of foot.	Extension of great toe and fanning of the toes
Chaddock	Stroke lateral aspect of foot beneath the lateral malleolus.	Same response as above
Oppenheim	Stroke anteromedial tibial surface.	Same as above
Gordon	Squeeze calf muscles firmly.	Same as above
Hoffmann	Flick terminal phalanx of middle finger downward.	Flexion of thumb and/or fingers (clawing)
Ankle clonus	Sudden, brisk dorsiflexion of foot with knee flexed and applying sustained and moderate pressure	Exaggerated rhythmic up-and-down movements of foot (a rapidly exhaustible clonus may be normal)
Kernig's sign (meningeal irritation)	Straight leg raising or below knee extension with thigh flexed on abdomen	Limitation with pain down posterior thigh
Brudzinski's sign (meningeal irritation)	Flexing chin on chest	Limitation with pain

Table 15-7 Comparison of Findings: Damage to Upper Motor Neurons and Lower Motor Neurons

Signs	UMN damage	LMN damage
Muscle tone	Increased/spastic—greater in flexors in arms and extensors in legs	Flaccid, hypotonus, loss of tone, wasting of muscles (atrophy)
Reflexes	Hyperreflexia; Babinski present; ankle/knee clonus	Areflexic; Babinski absent; clonus absent
Fasciculations	Absent	Present
Paralysis or weakness	Paralysis or weakness in limb(s) according to degree of pressure damage to the pyramidal distribution of lesion; weakness usually in hand grip, arm extensors, and leg flexors	Paralysis or weakness in appropriate muscles, depending on which spinal segment, root, or peripheral nerve is damaged

vidual may become rigid in her beliefs and difficult to deal with because of impaired reasoning. The individual also is not able to adequately assess the emotionality of others in a given situation. For instance, she cannot detect when another person is sad. This places her at a social disadvantage. Emotional stress (anxiety, depression, psychosis) or physical stress (tumor, infarction, abscess, penetrating head wound) may be an etiologic factor underlying such altered behavior.

Irritation of the motor tract, such as by a slow growing meningioma, can initiate a jacksonian seizure beginning on the opposite side of the body. Observation of this type of seizure readily reveals the typical jacksonian march. Characteristically, clonic contractions start in one portion of the body, such as the face or fingers, and can march along to eventually include the entire half of the body and may even spread to the opposite side of the body, culminating in a grand mal seizure and unconsciousness. However, this is not always the case; the seizure motor march may stop at any point.

A lesion in Broca's area, which is in the inferior frontal gyrus just anterior to the motor tract of the left frontal lobe, can cause expressive or nonfluent aphasia (see Fig. 15-1). A lesion of the posterior frontal area produces disturbances in expressive writing.

Anosmia (loss of smell) suggests the possibility of a lesion of the anterior inferior portion of the frontal lobe, where the olfactory fiber tracts are situated.

Parietal Lobe Dysfunction

A lesion interfering with these sensory cells may result in numbness, tingling, or other unusual sensations. Such symptoms would most likely be mentioned during an investigation of a chief complaint or the review of systems while collecting the health history. Episodic bouts of numbness and tingling may occur, as well as a focal seizure followed by a sensory march similar to the motor march. Other sensory disturbances that may be experienced by clients with cortical lesions of the sensory tract are hyperesthesia (increased sensitivity to touch stimuli) and paresthesia (spontaneous sensations such as pins, needles, "crawling" sensations).

Loss of touch perceptions is generally accompanied by absence of other sensations. This is a common finding in peripheral neuropathies. Ordinarily, the feet and legs are more severely involved than the upper extremities, and the loss may manifest as a "glove and stocking" pattern, a sensory loss in which all sensory modalities, including pain, temperature, touch, vibration, and proprioception, are diminished.

Peripheral nerve pathology is often associated with decreased perspiration as well as diminished sensation, because the peripheral nerves also carry sympathetic fibers to the corresponding sensory distribution of the nerve. The peripheral nerves most commonly affected are the medial, ulnar, radial, tibial, and common peroneal.

Peripheral nerves may be affected by such conditions as direct trauma, vascular insufficiency, nutritional deficiencies, and metabolic disease processes. The dorsal root ganglion may be attacked by such diseases as tumors, a herniated intervertebral disk, herpes zoster, or tabes dorsalis. A lesion of the dorsal root ganglion will cause sensation to be lost in the related dermatome distribution. Figure 15-14 illustrates common patterns of sensory loss. Figure 15-7 illustrates how the position of a lesion affects sensory loss.

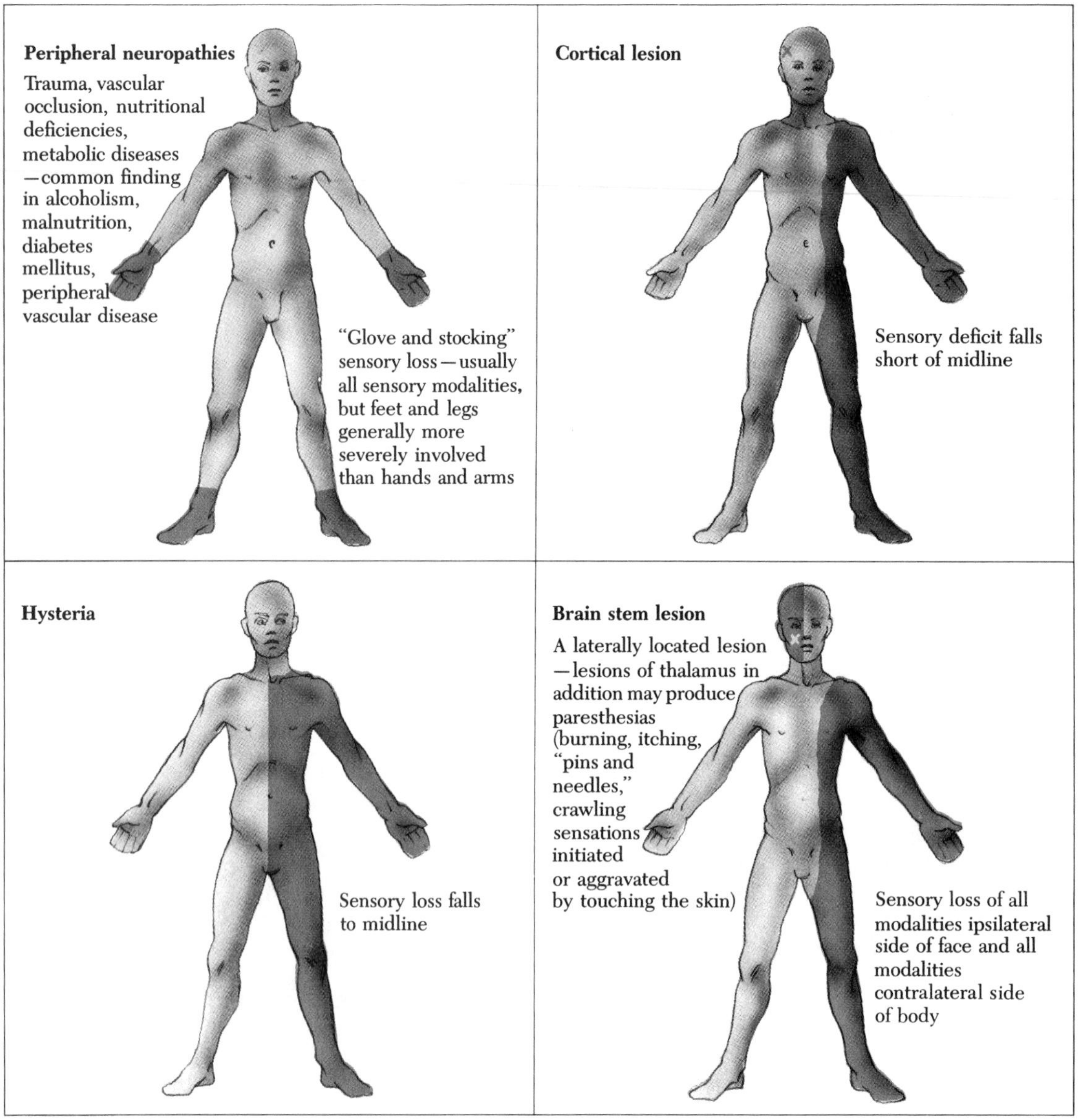

Figure 15-14 Common patterns of sensory loss.

In tabes dorsalis, the client may perceive superficial pinpricks but lack all perception of deep pressure pain, which is why it is important to test both superficial and deep pain perception—only one may be deficient.

An expressive aphasia may occur with a parietal lesion if the speech center responsible for choosing the words for verbal communication is affected. If this speech center is destroyed, the client's speech is gibberish (see Fig. 15-1).

The parietal lobes are also involved in specific sensory interpretations. They are the seat of stereognosis, the ability to recognize the shape, size, and relative weight of objects. A lesion involving this area of the parietal lobes would interfere with this discriminatory ability.

Occipital Lobe Dysfunction

With occipital lobe tumors, visual disturbances and seizures, preceded by an aura of light and visual hallucinations, are common. Headache and papilledema may also exist.

Temporal Lobe Dysfunction

Much of the visual (optic) tract projects through the temporal lobes; therefore, visual defects are also common with temporal lobe lesions. The most common defect is homonymous hemianopia contralateral to the side of the temporal lesion, but if the lesion is small, a homonymous superior quadrant may result (see the discussion of the cranial nerves, particularly the optic nerve, later in this chapter).

Damage to a Wernicke's area, a center for speech understanding, in the temporal lobe results in receptive aphasia, in which the client is unable to interpret the meaning of words. When the nerve bundle (arcuate fasciculus) is disrupted, the client can comprehend words but cannot repeat them. When Wernicke's area per se is damaged, speech is fluent but is wordy and has little substance to its content; comprehension is usually lost—that is, sentences do not make much sense (see Fig. 15-1).

Because the posterior temporal lobes are in close proximity to the visual association areas, visual hallucinations may occur that comprise familiar sights, including people, animals, and places. Some clients with temporal lobe tumors may have distorted vision, such as micropsia (seeing things as smaller than they actually are), macropsia (seeing things as larger), or wavy-deformed vision, or they may experience colors in unusual ways.

Because portions of the auditory, olfactory, and gustatory systems are located in the temporal lobes, lesions of these areas may produce tinnitus, auditory hallucinations (e.g., voices, unusual noises, or music), and olfactory hallucinations, occasionally accompanied by smacking movements of the lips. Singing of a melody all day long may occur with a temporal lesion in a center for musical recall. In addition, auditory agnosia (difficulty in recognition of verbal words) may result. These attacks are similar to behaviors manifested in psychiatric disorders but differ in that temporal lobe attacks are episodic and of brief duration.

Some "psychic" phenomena are related to temporal lobe structures; temporal lobe pathology may result in such experiences as dejà-vu, dreamy states, and psychomotor seizures. Dejà vu is the dreamlike impression that one is in a situation that is an exact repetition of a previous experience. Occasionally, jamais vu occurs, in which a familiar situation suddenly becomes totally strange. In psychomotor seizures, the client suddenly performs inappropriate or, at times, appropriate behavior ranging from nonsignificant movements to states of rage, after which he has no memory of his behavior. The client may "wake up" and find himself in a strange place or may suddenly find himself home with amnesia as to how or why he got there. The duration of psychomotor seizures is generally 20 to 30 minutes. Longer episodes must be differentiated from the fugue states of psychiatric origin.

Cellular Dysfunction

Romberg's sign may indicate cerebellar disease; however it is also observed in clients with vestibular damage.

A cerebellar lesion can be manifested in a characteristic staccato, explosive speech pattern. The common findings in cerebellar disease are disturbances in walking and making alternating movements, and the presence of tremors. The characteristic tremor of cerebellar pathology is the intention tremor, a tremor that is associated with every voluntary movement of the body. However, clients with multiple sclerosis may also demonstrate an intention tremor with voluntary efforts.

Cranial Nerve Dysfunctions

Pathology such as tumors at the base of the frontal lobes, involving the olfactory groove, or trauma of the olfactory bulbs or the ethmoid plate may result in anosmia—complete loss of smell. Olfactory hallucinations may also occur with brain lesions, particularly those of the temporal lobes.

Loss of visual acuity, defects in peripheral vision, and changes in the optic nerve disk characterize optic nerve tract difficulties. Bitemporal hemianopia commonly occurs in the presence of a pituitary tumor, as the pituitary gland is nestled anteriorly in the arms of the optic chiasm (see Fig. 15-9).

All three nerves (III, IV, and VI) pass in close proximity to the internal carotid artery; therefore, it is not uncommon for vascular aneurysms in this area to cause disturbances in visual gaze. Thus, defects of the III nerve may result in the eyeball turning downward and out, a dilated pupil, or ptosis of the eyelid.

With trochlear paralysis, the client is unable to rotate the eyeball nasally downward, and with abducens paralysis, the client is unable to rotate the eyeball outward. However, weakness of the lateral rectus muscle is not always a focal sign but may result indirectly from increased intracranial pressure, which may stretch the abducens nerve as it traverses its long course from the pons within the brain stem to the lateral rectus muscles of the eyes.

Frequently, frontal lobe lesions will cause the eyes to deviate toward the location of the lesion—"the client looks at his lesion." In Parinaud's syndrome, the client is initially unable to gaze upward, and eventually the ability to look downward is also affected, designating increased pressure from an upper midbrain lesion. This phenomenon may be accompanied by dilated pupils.

Strabismus and diplopia can occur in conditions in which the extraocular muscles are rendered weak, such as muscular dystrophies, myasthenia gravis, and occasionally, hyperthyroidism.

Nystagmus may be observed in clients with multiple sclerosis, cerebellar lesions, or inner ear inflammation, as well as in clients who are taking barbiturates and tranquilizers. (These medications interfere with the intricate pathways between the vestibular system and the nuclei of the third, fourth, and sixth cranial nerves.)

With trigeminal damage, all modalities (pain, touch, and temperature) may be affected, or you may find that there is only a loss of pain and temperature sensation on one side of the client's face but that the perception of touch is intact. These variations in findings are relevant to the level of the lesion in the brain stem. A high brain stem lesion will generally obliterate all modalities, whereas a lower brain stem lesion will not impair touch perception. A tumor involving the mandibular branch is rare, but it is helpful to remember that numbness of the chin is the first client complaint.

Two afflictions of the trigeminal nerve are herpes zoster and tic douloureux. Herpes zoster (shingles) is a very painful, acute virus infection that appears as a vesicular eruption along the area of distribution of a sensory nerve. Its symptoms of constant itching and pain render it an exhausting disease, particularly for the elderly client. Herpes zoster of the eye produces a severe conjunctivitis and presents the potential danger of corneal ulceration and scarring if untreated. Tic douloureux (trigeminal neuralgia) is characterized by sharp pain spasms of one side of the face, which may be triggered by brushing the teeth, drinking cold liquids, chewing, talking, blowing the nose, shaving, washing the face, or brushing the hair, or by cold drafts. Surgical treatment is necessary if a medical regimen proves unsuccessful. When surgery is performed, the client has a complete loss of facial sensation on the affected side. Thus, infection of the eye may develop as a result of the loss of the corneal reflex. The client should therefore be instructed to watch for signs of corneal infection and to examine the eye frequently for signs of any foreign particles. Weakness of the masseter and temporal muscles is characteristic in clients with myasthenia gravis and amyotrophic lateral sclerosis (ALS).

Damage to the motor component of the facial nerve results in paralysis of the facial muscles of expression. A change in taste sensation and an increase or decrease in salivation and tearing occurs with damage to the sensory component of the facial nerve. Occasionally, when trauma has severed the facial nerve fibers, they regenerate and heal incorrectly. This has been evidenced by clients who will weep instead of salivate at the sight of food.

The anatomic tract of the facial nerve extends from the nucleus in the lower pons through the temporal bone and the internal auditory meatus to one side of the face. Its close proximity to the middle ear makes it susceptible to trauma by diseases or surgery in that area, such as otitis media, mastoiditis, fractured temporal bone, or parotid gland tumor.

In routine health assessment, the status of the facial muscles should be observed. Peripheral facial nerve and facial nuclei damage (Bell's palsy) are manifested by weakness or paralysis of all the facial musculature on one side of the face. Generalized weakness of the facial muscles is observed in myasthenia gravis and Guillain-Barré syndrome. You will be able to note that the usual wrinkles seen on the forehead are absent on the weak side.

Should the function of the forehead muscles remain intact but weakness or drooping of the mouth exists, a lesion along the tract from the cerebral cortex motor area of the opposite hemisphere to the nucleus of the facial nerve in the pons (brain stem lesion) is suspected. This type of facial involvement is commonly observed in cerebrovascular accidents because the lower facial musculature receives fibers only from the opposite cerebral cortex.

With damage to the vestibular branch of the auditory nerve (CN VIII), nystagmus or vertigo will present when the client is made to perform sudden alterations in head position. With glossopharyngeal nerve damage, the gag reflex may be dampened. Also, a rare disease, glossopharyngeal neuralgia, may result from insult to the glossopharyngeal nerve. This affliction is characterized by severe paroxysms of pain in the throat initiated by swallowing. With a glossopharyngeal lesion, there is a loss of taste over the posterior third of the tongue and decreased sensation in the pharynx and palate.

With vagal dysfunction, regurgitation of the water through the nose indicates weakness of the soft palate and an inability to close off the nasopharynx; this inability is commonly found in hemiplegic clients, but it can occur with other conditions, such as multiple sclerosis, ALS, meningitis, encephalitis, cerebral and aortic aneurysms, enlarged glands, and tumors in the neck and thorax, as well as trauma to the neck or thorax from injury or surgical procedures (particularly thyroid operations).

It is also important to study the timbre of the client's voice. Dysphagia (weakness or paralysis of swallowing), aphonia (loss of voice), or hoarseness may indicate vagal damage, and direct mirror laryngoscopy is advisable.

Spinal accessory nerve involvement is commonly seen in association with other cranial nerve palsies and may be observed in trauma to the neck.

BIOLOGIC AND CULTURAL VARIATIONS

Tay-Sachs Disease in Ashkenazic Jews

The Jewish population is often divided into three major groups based on historical migrations and geographic location (Groen 1973). The Ashkenazic Jews are the descendants of Jews who migrated from Judea and Jerusalem to France and Germany in the first century, and who were later forced to migrate to northern, central, and eastern Europe. The United States Jewish population is largely Ashkenazim. The Sephardic Jews left Palestine and Galilee in the fifth century and settled in Spain and Portugal. After total expulsion in the late fifteenth century, they migrated to all parts of the Mediterranean. The Asian Jews are the descendants of groups that left the Middle East and migrated to the Near and Far East.

A large number of simple inherited genetic disorders occur in relatively high frequencies in the Ashkenazim. These disorders include dystonia musculorum deformans, Riley-Day syndrome (familial autonomic dysfunction), Gaucher's disease (familial splenic anemia), Niemann-Pick disease (lipid histiocytosis), and Tay-Sachs disease (infantile amaurotic idiocy).

Tay-Sachs disease has one of the highest incidence rates of this group of genetic conditions. In the United States the disease occurs in approximately 1 out of 6,000 Jewish births, as opposed to 1 in approximately 500,000 non-Jewish births (Myrianthopoulos & Aronson 1973). It has been shown to be due to the inheritance of a recessive gene from both parents. Thus, symptoms of the disease appear only in recessive homozygotes (who have inherited two Tay-Sachs genes). From the incidence rate of Tay-Sachs disease, the frequency rate of the recessive gene in heterozygotes (those who have inherited one normal gene and one Tay-Sachs gene) can be computed. Thus, it has been estimated that 1 of 40 Jewish persons and one of 380 non-Jewish persons is a heterozygote for the Tay-Sachs gene.

Among Ashkenazic Jews, symptoms of the disease generally appear in infancy. Nerve cell degeneration and muscle weakness occur in the first few months after birth. These symptoms are due to the accumulation of lipid deposits in the cytoplasm of brain neurons. Cerebral function and mental development fail as the brain atrophies. Death usually occurs within the first or second year of life.

Various researchers have addressed the question of how such a gene, which is fatal to recessive homozygotes in infancy, could have risen to such a high frequency in a population. Homozygotes for the Tay-Sachs gene die well before reproductive age and do not pass the gene on to their offspring. In such cases of early mortality from a recessive homozygotic genetic condition, the recessive gene usually falls to a much lower frequency than the 1 heterozygote out of 40 found in Tay-Sachs disease.

The most plausible explanation is that heterozygotes for the Tay-Sachs gene have some advantage over dominant homozygotes (those individuals who have inherited two normal genes and do not carry the Tay-Sachs gene). This advantage might be that they have more children than the dominant homozygotes and that they live longer and thus tend to complete their reproductive years. Greater fertility for the heterozygotes would result in the Tay-Sachs gene remaining in the population from one generation to the next.

Some investigators think that the heterozygotic condition might offer an individual an increased resistance to certain infectious diseases. Such disease resistance would have been a great advantage in the past few centuries, for Ashkenazic Jews tended to live in the cities of northern, eastern, and central Europe, which had continuous epidemics of infectious diseases such as bubonic plague, cholera, smallpox, and diphtheria. If the Tay-Sachs gene offered a selective advantage in the face of these severe infectious diseases, we might expect heterozygous carriers to have greater survival and fertility rates than dominant homozygotes.

This hypothesis has received partial support from the findings of at least one study. Myrianthopoulos and Aronson (1973) compared the fertility of grandparents of a Tay-Sachs child, as measured by completed family size, with the fertility of a control group of grandparents with no Tay-Sachs grandchildren. It was assumed that at least one maternal and one paternal grandparent of an affected child was a heterozygote. Overall, they found that grandparents of Tay-Sachs children had produced 6% more offspring than grandparents who presumably did not carry the gene. The results were most marked for offspring not born in the United States. These findings suggest that there is a selective advantage associated with being a heterozygote for the Tay-Sachs gene. This heterozygote advantage might explain the rather high rate of this lethal homozygotic disease among United States and European Ashkenazic Jewish population groups.

In corticobulbar tract damage, pseudobulbar palsy occurs, displaying severe tongue weakness. Severe tongue weakness also occurs in poliomyelitis and amyotrophic lateral sclerosis, diseases that affect the cranial nerve nuclei and, therefore, are of lower motor neuron damage. Differentiation of lesion origin is possible, because diseases involving lower motor neuron damage will have accompanying signs of muscle atrophy and fasciculation.

Unilateral hypoglossal nucleus damage, which may result from a neck injury, would manifest unilateral weakness, atrophy, and fasciculations of the tongue. In this case, the strong, intact side of the tongue would push and cause the tongue to deviate toward the affected, weak side as it protrudes.

DTRs may be absent during neural shock, which generally lasts from 4 to 7 days following a severe injury. They are also absent in increased intracranial pressure of a high degree, as well as in lower motor neuron damage, such as in poliomyelitis, tumor, or injury to the anterior motor horn of the spinal cord. Peripheral nerve diseases and herniated intervertebral disks can also cause absent DTRs. Diseases of the muscles (muscular dystrophy) may result in decreased or absent DTRs, not because of neural or reflex arc damage but because of the muscle fiber involvement. Gradually diminishing DTRs are observed in myasthenia gravis with successive testing; that is, when the percussion site is struck 3 or 4 times in a row, each response decreases in quality. With myxedema a slowed relaxation phase may be noted.

SUMMARY

Learning the assessment techniques and normal functioning of the neurologic system is facilitated by understanding this system's structure and physiologic functioning. The main areas to be assessed are the cerebrum, cerebellum, cranial nerves, and reflexes.

Assessment of this system begins with initial contact with the client. Data on mental status are recorded during the history taking, and mental status continues to be noted throughout the nursing assessment process. Cerebral assessment includes observation of frontal, parietal, occipital, and temporal lobe functions. Cerebellar assessment includes balance and coordination examination techniques. The functions of the cranial nerves are assessed in sequence. Reflexes to be examined include the deep tendon reflexes, superficial or cutaneous reflexes, and pathologic reflexes.

DISCUSSION QUESTIONS/ ACTIVITIES

1. Draw a diagram of the cerebrum and label the various lobes, indicating the major functions of each.
2. What manifestations would be present with damage to Broca's area? to Wernicke's area? Where are these areas located in the cerebrum?
3. What are some of the signs and symptoms characteristic of a client with a temporal lobe tumor? What would be a differentiating factor between a temporal lobe attack and a psychiatric disorder?
4. What cranial nerve palsies frequently accompany cerebellar dysfunction? What is the structural explanation for this phenomenon?
5. Discuss the factors considered when assessing gait.
6. What are the two categories of cerebellar assessment? Demonstrate the techniques used to test them.
7. Name the cranial nerves; discuss how you would assess each one; state the normal findings for each cranial nerve.
8. Where along the optic tract would you find a lesion causing each of the following conditions: (a) cortical blindness? (b) bitemporal hemianopia? (c) homonymous hemianopia?
9. What two cranial nerves are concerned with taste? In what circumstances and how would you assess the sensation of taste?
10. State the signs and symptoms that would alert you to the need for investigation of the vestibular branch of the auditory system.
11. If you have only a short period of time to test the cranial nerves, what are the most pertinent evaluations that you would perform?
12. Name the DTRs that are routinely assessed and the normal response of each.
13. Discuss how the commonly assessed superficial reflexes are each tested, and state the normal response of each.
14. State the physical responses that you would observe if the following pathological reflexes were present: Babinski, ankle clonus, Hoffmann, Kernig's sign, and Brudzinski's sign. What techniques would you use to attempt to elicit each of these responses?

REFERENCES

Groen, J. J. 1973. Gaucher's disease: hereditary transmission and racial distribution. In *Ethnic groups of America—their morbidity, mortality and behavior disorders,* ed. A. Shiloh and I. C. Selevan. Springfield, Ill.: Charles C. Thomas.

Myrianthopoulos, J. C., and Aronson, S. M. 1973. Population dynamics of Tay-Sachs disease—I. Reproductive fitness and selection. In *Ethnic groups of America—their morbidity, mortality, and behavior disorders,* ed. A. Shiloh and I. C. Selevan. Springfield, Ill.: Charles C. Thomas.

CHAPTER

16 Assessment of the Genitals and Rectum

Learning Objectives

1. Review the structure and function of the genitals.
2. List the characteristics of the genitals that are considered during inspection.
3. Describe the techniques for palpation of the testes and scrotum.
4. Describe the procedure for insertion of a vaginal speculum.
5. State the areas from which smears are obtained for a Papanicolaou test.
6. Describe the bimanual pelvic examination and the reason for doing this procedure.
7. Describe the rectovaginal-abdominal examination and the reason for doing this procedure.
8. Recognize the importance for putting on a new glove when proceeding from the genital exam to the recto-vaginal-abdominal examination.
9. State the characteristics noted in inspection and palpation of the anus and rectum.
10. Describe the technique used in performing a rectal examination.

It is not uncommon to discover in the client's record that the genital and rectal examination has been deferred. In most cases such deferment is due to cultural and sexual attitudes or problems on the part of both clients and health workers. It is important to have a positive attitude geared toward promotion of health and detection of disease, because pathology can occur in the genitals and rectum as well as in any other anatomic region of the body.

- Wear gloves while conducting the examination, as infection is a reality.
- Client preparation and support during the assessment is essential because this particular portion of the physical assessment may be embarrassing and uncomfortable.
- Assemble the equipment and arrange the environment beforehand to provide comfort and privacy for the client.
- Inform the client that the procedures may cause discomfort at moments but that you will proceed as gently as possible.
- Ask the client to tell you immediately if he experiences any pain.
- Explain each step to the client prior to performing it.

STRUCTURE AND FUNCTION OF THE MALE GENITALS

Figure 16-1 identifies the major structures of the male reproductive system. The function of the *testes* is the production of *spermatozoa* (by the seminiferous tubules) and the production of *testosterone* (by the Leydig's cells). The *epididymis* is located posterolateral to the testis. The distal portion of the epididymis, called the *vas deferens,* is part of the

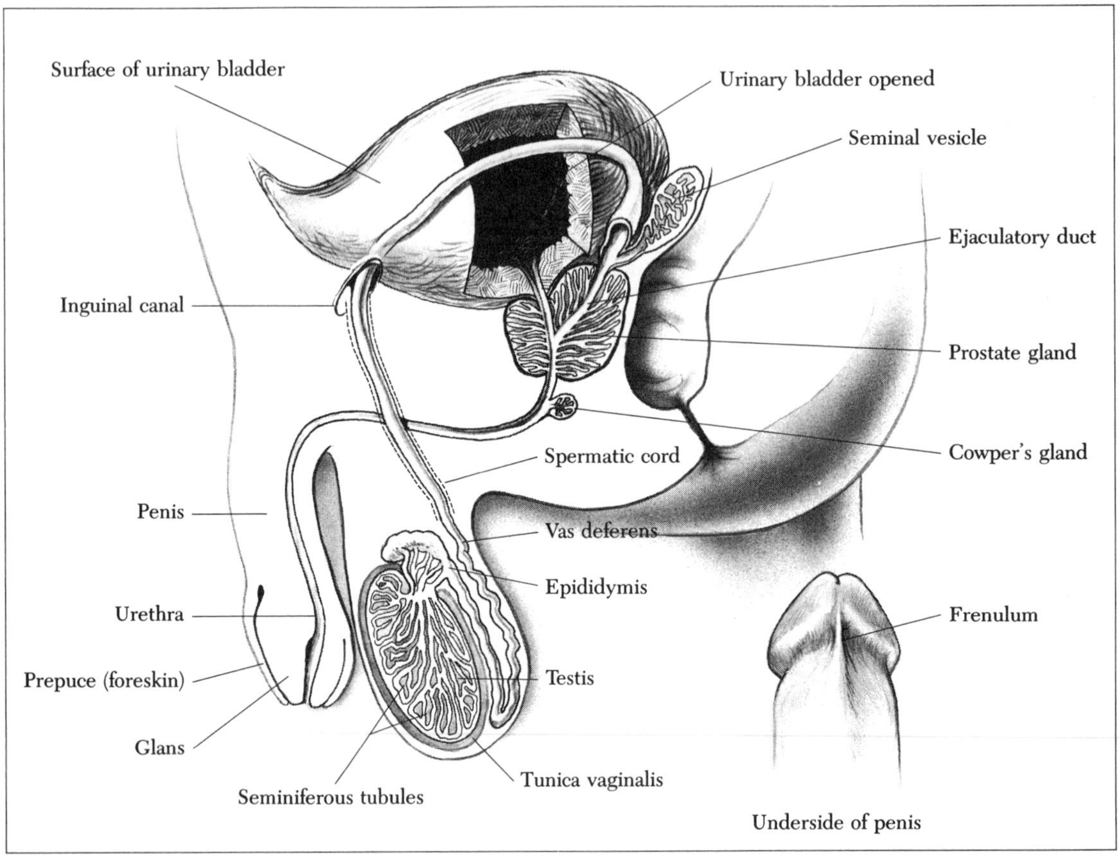

Figure 16-1 The male genitals.

BIOLOGIC AND CULTURAL VARIATIONS

Cancer and Circumcision

Mortality rates for different types of cancer vary by region, degree of urbanization, population group, and religious affiliation. Two interesting associations are those of cancer of the uterine cervix and cancer of the penis in different religious groups. Because cancer of the cervix is extremely rare among Jewish women, it has been hypothesized that this may be linked to the fact that Jewish women often have as sexual partners Jewish men, who are uniformly circumcised after birth. Jewish men also have extremely low rates of cancer of the penis, which is also hypothesized to be associated with circumcision. Moslem men, who are circumcised at puberty, have intermediate cancer rates. Hindus, who are uncircumcised, have rather high rates (Damon 1977).

spermatic cord. Encased within the spermatic fascia and constituting the *spermatic cord* are the vas deferens, arteries, veins, nerves, and lymphatic vessels. The spermatic cord passes through the inguinal canal and enters the abdominal cavity. It continues upward to join the seminal vesicle behind the bladder. The seminal vesicle secretes a nutritious protective fluid for the sperm. Another protective (alkaline) fluid is produced for the sperm by the *Cowper's gland* and serves as a lubricant as well.

CHARACTERISTICS AND TECHNIQUES OF EXAMINATION

Inspection and palpation of the male genitalia is conducted simultaneously.

Hair Pattern

- Check the pubic hair distribution. It may vary somewhat from person to person; only the absence or extreme sparseness of pubic hair in the adult man needs to be reported. Usually, the diamond-shaped pattern is observed (Fig. 6-23).

Penis

- Note the size and shape of the penis. Figure 16-2 shows the normal male penis. Size will vary from person to person. Only wide deviations in size are likely to be of significance.
- Inspect the skin covering the penis for color changes and lesions.
- Observe whether the client is circumcised or uncircumcised.
- Retract the foreskin of the penis back over the glans; this normally is accomplished easily (see Fig. 16-1). A small amount of thick white secretion may be observed between the foreskin and the glans; this is a normal secretion called smegma.
- Palpate the penile shaft from the glans to the base of the penis for any signs of tenderness or induration.
- Note the placement of the urethral meatus; normally it is present at the distal end of the frenulum.
- Inspect the urethra by using your thumbs to separate the meatus (Fig. 16-3).
- A culture should be taken if a thick, purulent discharge is noted, as this suggests gonorrhea.

Scrotum

To best examine and palpate the scrotum, the client should stand and you should sit in front of him.

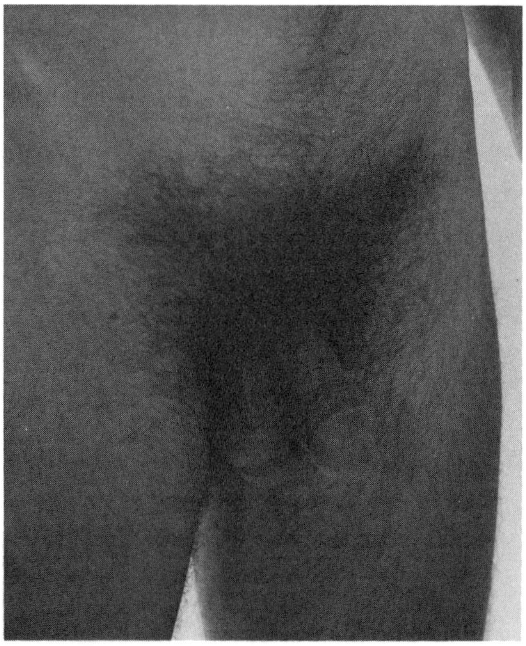

Figure 16-2 Normal male genitals.

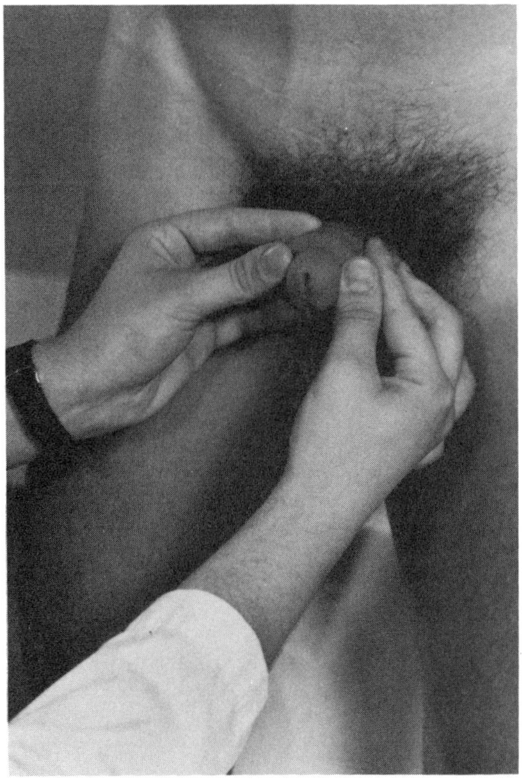

Figure 16-3 Inspection of the urethra.

Techniques for Inspection and Palpation of Penis

1. Arrange for client comfort and privacy.
2. Have adequate lighting.
3. Sit on chair facing standing client.
4. Put on gloves.
5. Explain each step prior to doing it.
6. Characteristics of inspection:
   Hair distribution
   Size and contour
   Skin surfaces
   Position of urethral meatus
   Abnormalities
7. Palpate penile shaft between thumb and first two fingers.
8. Retract foreskin.
9. Separate meatus with thumbs.
10. Decision making: If client complains of dysuria or change in urination stream, observe client voiding.
11. Decision making: If thick, purulent urethral discharge, take culture of discharge.

- Gross inspection of the scrotum generally reveals that the left testis is lower than the right; anatomically, the left spermatic cord is longer than the right (see Fig. 16-2).
- Inspect the skin covering the scrotum to detect the presence of any color changes and lesions. Scrotal edema causes the skin to stretch, causing less wrinkling of the scrotum.
- Palpate the scrotum by using your index and middle fingers like a pair of scissors to separate the testes and divide the scrotum in half (Fig. 16-4).
- Examine the right testis and epididymis with the left hand, and vice versa.
- Gentle palpation is warranted; the testes are normally tender.
- Note the size and consistency of the testes; normally they are 2 × 4 cm and are rubbery (neither hard nor soft). The testes become softer and decrease in size during middle age.
- Palpate the epididymis by using your thumb on the anterior surface of the scrotum and your index finger behind the scrotum.
- The epididymis is palpable on the posterolateral sides of each testis. With epididymitis, there is extreme tenderness, and you should be unable to distinguish the epididymis from the testis.
- Palpate the spermatic cord by using the same thumb and index finger technique. The cord is of a harder consistency

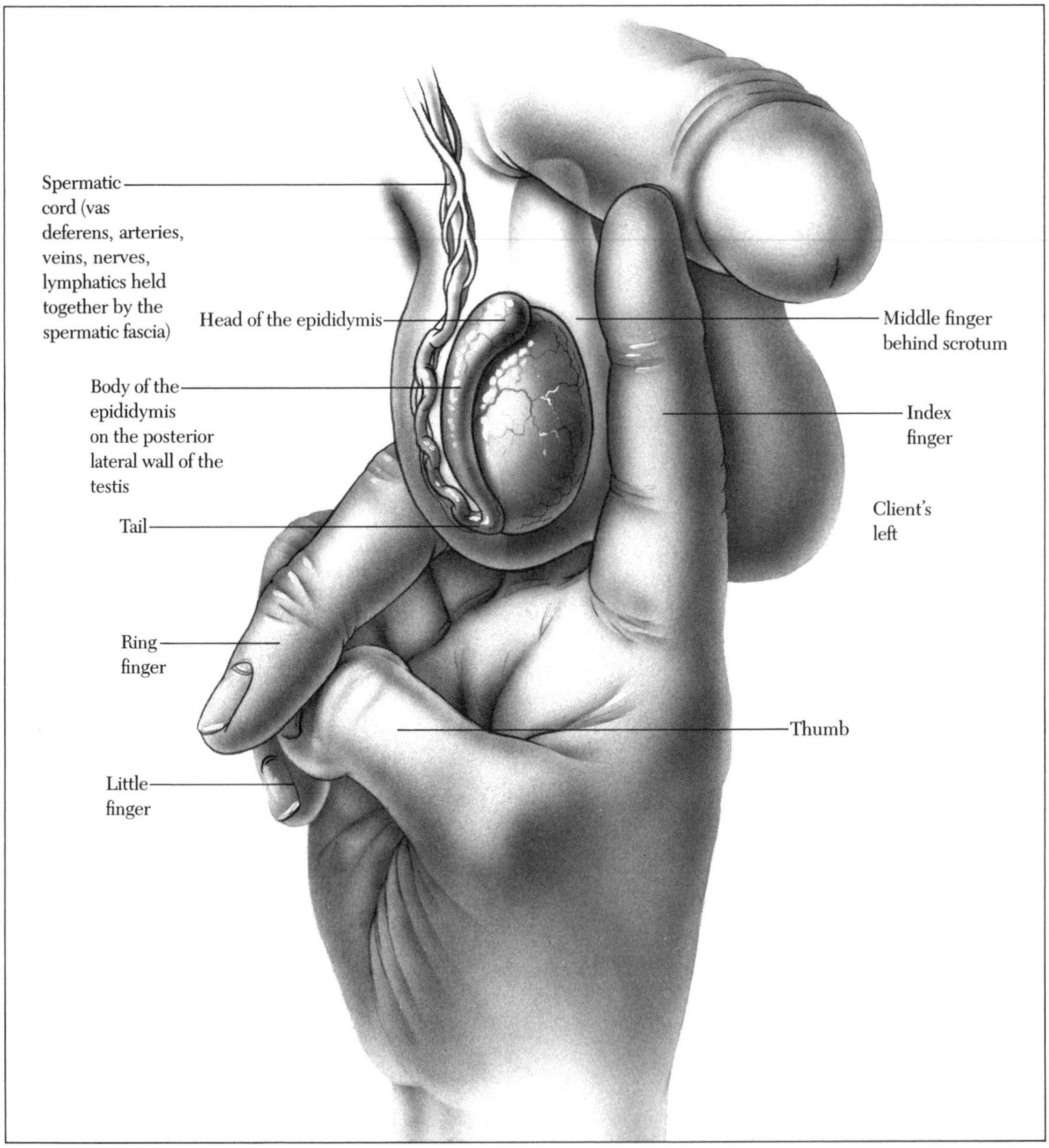

Figure 16-4 Palpation of the scrotum.

Technique for Inspection and Palpation of Scrotum

1. Sit in chair facing standing client.
2. Characteristics of inspection:
   Size and contour
   Skin surfaces
   Abnormalities
3. Decision making: If swelling, use technique of transillumination.
4. Separate scrotal sac into two sides with index and middle finger of right hand.
5. Palpate right testis and epididymis with left thumb and index finger.
6. Continue to palpate upward on lateral aspect for right spermatic cord between right testis and inguinal canal.
7. Separate scrotal sac with left hand and palpate left testis, epididymis, and spermatic cord with right hand.

than the epididymis and is best palpable high in the lateral portion of the scrotum as it ascends toward the inguinal canal.

- This same technique (thumbs on top and index fingers behind the scrotum) is explained to male clients when teaching them how to perform the testicular self-examination (STE) (Fig. 16-5). Also explain that STE is best done in the shower, because the fingers slide more easily over

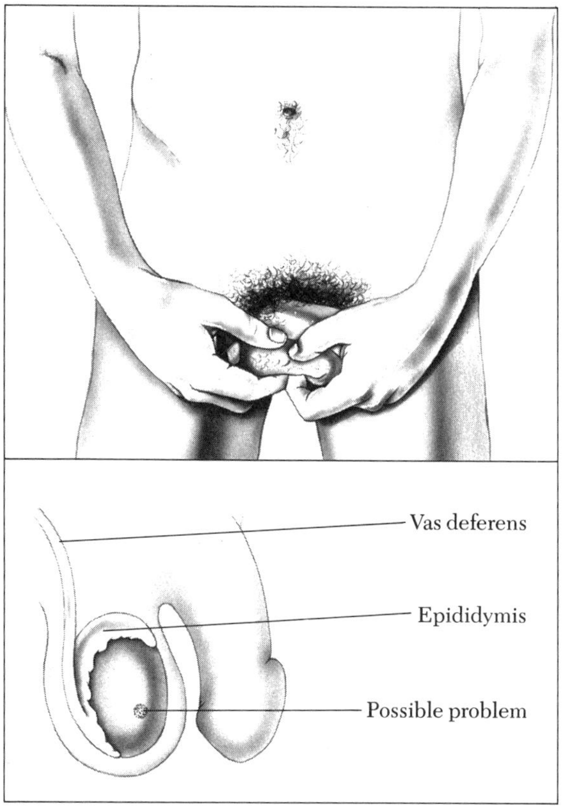

Figure 16-5 Testicular self-examination.

the wet skin. Any nodule found within the testis must be regarded as suspicious and warrants medical referral.

- Transilluminate any evidence of swelling in the scrotal

Technique for Inspection and Palpation of Female External Genitals

1. Have client empty bladder.
2. Provide comfort, privacy, and adequate draping and lighting.
3. Ask client to lie on examining table with buttocks at bottom edge of table.
4. Place client's feet in stirrups.
5. Adjust foot stirrups for comfortable flexion of knees.
6. Use mirror for client to view genitalia (aids health teaching).
7. Explain each step prior to doing it.
8. Put on a pair of gloves.
9. Characteristics of inspection:
   Pubic hair distribution
   Symmetry
   Skin
   Abnormalities
10. Touch inner aspect of thigh and inform client that you are going to separate the labia for further inspection.
11. Inspect surfaces of labia majora and labia minora.
12. Inspect size of clitoris.
13. Inspect vestibule, urethral meatus, Skene's glands, and vaginal introitus.
14. Instruct client to "bear down" and examine fourchette.
15. Inspect Bartholin gland areas on either side of the vaginal introitus.
16. Insert lubricated gloved index finger into vagina with palmar side up.
17. Milk urethra by pressing gently upward and withdrawing your finger from the vagina.
18. Decision making: If a greenish yellow discharge is present or if a discharge is elicited upon milking the urethra, take a culture of the discharge.

area. A hernia or fluid should be suspected with enlargement.
- The normal testis, a tumor, or a hernia that has descended into the scrotal sac will not transilluminate, whereas fluid (hydrocele) will transilluminate. Additionally, a hydrocele will present as a mass above which you are able to palpate.
- An indirect inguinal hernia is palpated as a continuous structure to the external inguinal canal.
- Hydroceles are commonly found in toddlers and are nontender.

If the client has complained of dysuria or a change in urination stream, try to observe him voiding, if possible.

STRUCTURE AND FUNCTION OF THE FEMALE GENITALS

The mons pubis (Fig. 16-6) is an eminent fatty pad that lies over the symphysis pubis and is covered by pubic hair. Lip-shaped structures, the *labia majora* and *labia minora,* straddle the more delicate structures of the external genitals and provide protection. The labia majora are composed of adipose tissue, while the labia minora are constructed of thin, pink-appearing stratified squamous epithelium. The elongated oval area between the labia minora is termed the *vestibule.* The *clitoris,* located at the anterior angle of the vestibule, is the site of concentrated sensory nerve endings and is homologous to the glans penis in the male. Below the clitoris is the *urethral meatus,* which displays the openings of the paraurethral glands, or *Skene's glands,* on either side. In the posterior portion of the vestibule is the *vaginal introitus.* Nearby (occasionally on the inferior surface of the vaginal introitus) are the ducts of the *Bartholin's glands.* These ducts are not generally visible. The *fourchette* is the posterior boundary of the vestibule.

The internal genitals include the *vagina,* a flexible channel that leads to the *uterus;* the *cervix,* which connects the vagina and uterus; the uterus, which is the site for development and nourishment of a growing fetus; the *ovaries,* which produce ova and estrogenic hormones; and the *fallopian tubes,* through which ova travel from the ovaries to the uterus.

CHARACTERISTICS AND TECHNIQUES OF EXAMINATION

Your approach, in addition to establishing nurse-client rapport, is important for promoting cooperation. Relaxation

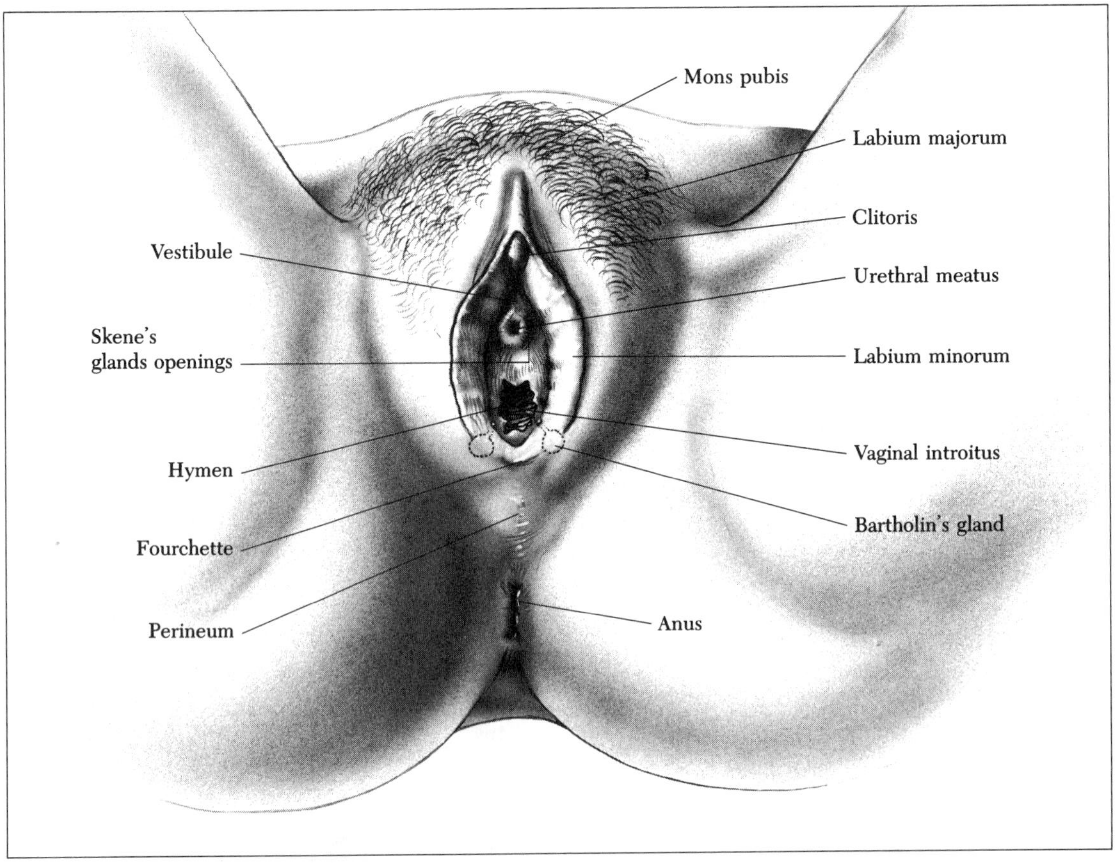

Figure 16-6 The female external genitals.

of the client is necessary to ensure a good examination and to avoid unnecessary discomfort. Good lighting is needed. Adequate draping should be used so that the client will not be overexposed. A mirror may be used for the client to view her own genital area; this technique facilitates health teaching and client learning.

The female client should be instructed not to douche 24 hours prior to a pelvic examination, as douching may interfere with smears, cultures, and cytology. Immediately before the examination takes place, have the client empty her bladder. The urine specimen should be collected, because in most cases a routine urinalysis is performed.

- Position the client with her buttocks down to the bottom edge of the table.
- Adjust the foot stirrups for comfortable flexion of the knees. The legs should be relaxed, with the knees apart.
- The client's head should be elevated sufficiently to use the viewing mirror.

Inspection and Palpation

External Genitalia

- Observe the mons pubis for amount and pattern of pubic hair. The pubic hair pattern of the female presents as an inverted triangle (Fig. 6-23).
- Absence of pubic hair by age 16 is abnormal.
- Inspect the labia majora. The perineum should be inspected for lesions, fissures, excoriations, erythema, edema, and leukoplakia (white, thick precancerous patches).
- Before **each** step, explain what you are going to do.
- Inform the client you are going to touch her leg; then touch the inner aspect of the client's thigh with the back of your hand before proceeding to touch the labia. This aids in the prevention of tenseness.
- Inform the client that you now are going to separate the labia.
- Separate the labia, inspect the interior of the labia majora and the surfaces of the labia minora.
- Inspect the clitoris. It should be 0.5 cm or less in diameter.
- Note any erythema, ulcerations, or other lesions of the vestibule because this is the most common site of venereal lesions and malignant changes.
- Inspect the urethral meatus and the vaginal introitus for discharge, edema, and lesions.
- The Skene's glands, or paraurethral glands, on either side of the urethral meatus should be barely distinguishable unless infected.
- Observe the fourchette, where the labial folds join together posteriorly, for the strength of the walls as the client "strains" and for the presence of an anterior or posterior bulging of the vaginal wall, suggesting a cystocele or a rectocele, respectively (Figs. 16-7 and 16-8).
- Inspect the Bartholin's gland area. Bartholin's glands, which open into either side of the vagina just outside the hymen, cannot be visualized.

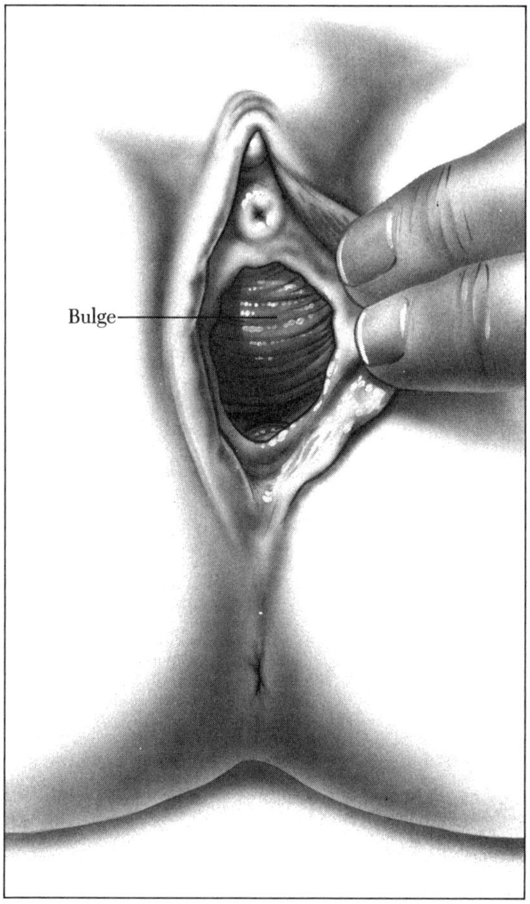

Figure 16-7 Cystocele: a bladder hernia that protrudes into the anterior wall of the vagina. Inspect for bulging of the anterior vaginal wall as the client strains down. Occasionally, the bulging may extend out of the introitus.

- The Bartholin's gland area is carefully checked for inflammation, erythema, tenderness, and swelling. If any of these signs are present, and if the client has a history of labial swelling, palpate this area on each side by using the index finger on the inside surface and the thumb on the outside surface.
- Culture any discharge from the ductal area to validate diagnosis. Infection of the Skene's glands and Bartholin's glands and endocervicitis are common with gonorrhea (greenish yellow discharge).
- Untreated gonorrhea can lead to pelvic inflammatory disease (PID) as well as arthritis and endocarditis.
- Gently insert a gloved index finger (with the palmar surface up) into the vagina. The urethra should be "milked" by withdrawing the finger while exerting gentle pressure on the anterior wall of the vagina. Figure 16-9 illustrates the technique for "milking."
- Normally, there is no discharge from the urethra or pain

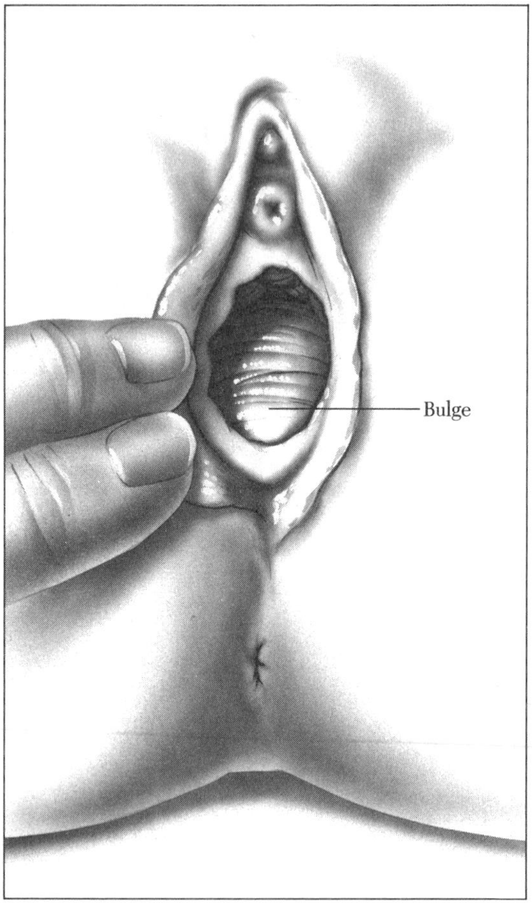

Figure 16-8 Rectocele: herniation of the posterior vaginal wall and the anterior rectal wall into the vagina. Inspect vaginal wall as client strains down.

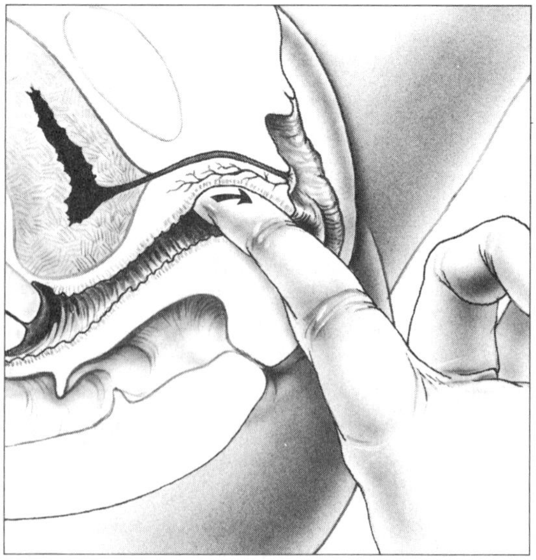

Figure 16-9 "Milking" the urethra.

Technique for Speculum Examination

1. Decision making: If client is a virgin or elderly woman with vaginal atrophy, use small vaginal speculum or nasal speculum as warranted.
2. Lubricate vaginal speculum with warm water.
3. Spread labia apart with thumb and index finger cupping the pubic hair back from the vaginal area.
4. Insert the vaginal speculum gently downward at a 45-degree angle, with the blades in a vertical position.
5. When blades are within the vagina, rotate them horizontally.
6. Locate the cervix and lock the speculum blades in open position.
7. Characteristics of cervical inspection:
   Color
   Surface
   Os
   Abnormalities

during this maneuver. If a discharge is elicited, a culture should be done to identify the causative organism and to establish a diagnosis.

Internal Genitalia

Speculum Examination

To examine the internal genitalia, use a speculum (Fig. 16-10). The vaginal speculum should be lubricated with warm water, because jelly lubricant interferes with cytologic studies. After all smears and cultures have been collected, a jelly lubricant may be used to facilitate further examination.

- The labia should always be widely separated, and the pubic hair should be cupped away from the vaginal area to avoid pulling the pubic hair with the speculum or examining fingers.
- Insert the speculum into the introitus with the blades held in a vertical position.
- Once the speculum blades are within the vagina, rotate them to a horizontal position and continue insertion as a downward 45-degree angle is maintained to avoid trauma to the sensitive anterior tissue over the urethral area (Fig. 16-11).
- Lock open the blades of the speculum when the cervix is located (Fig. 16-12). You may not be able to visualize the cervix if the speculum blades are too short or if the blades have been inadvertently opened anteriorly or posteriorly to the cervix.
- Observance of rugae suggests that the blades have been opened anterior to the cervix, whereas a smooth surface

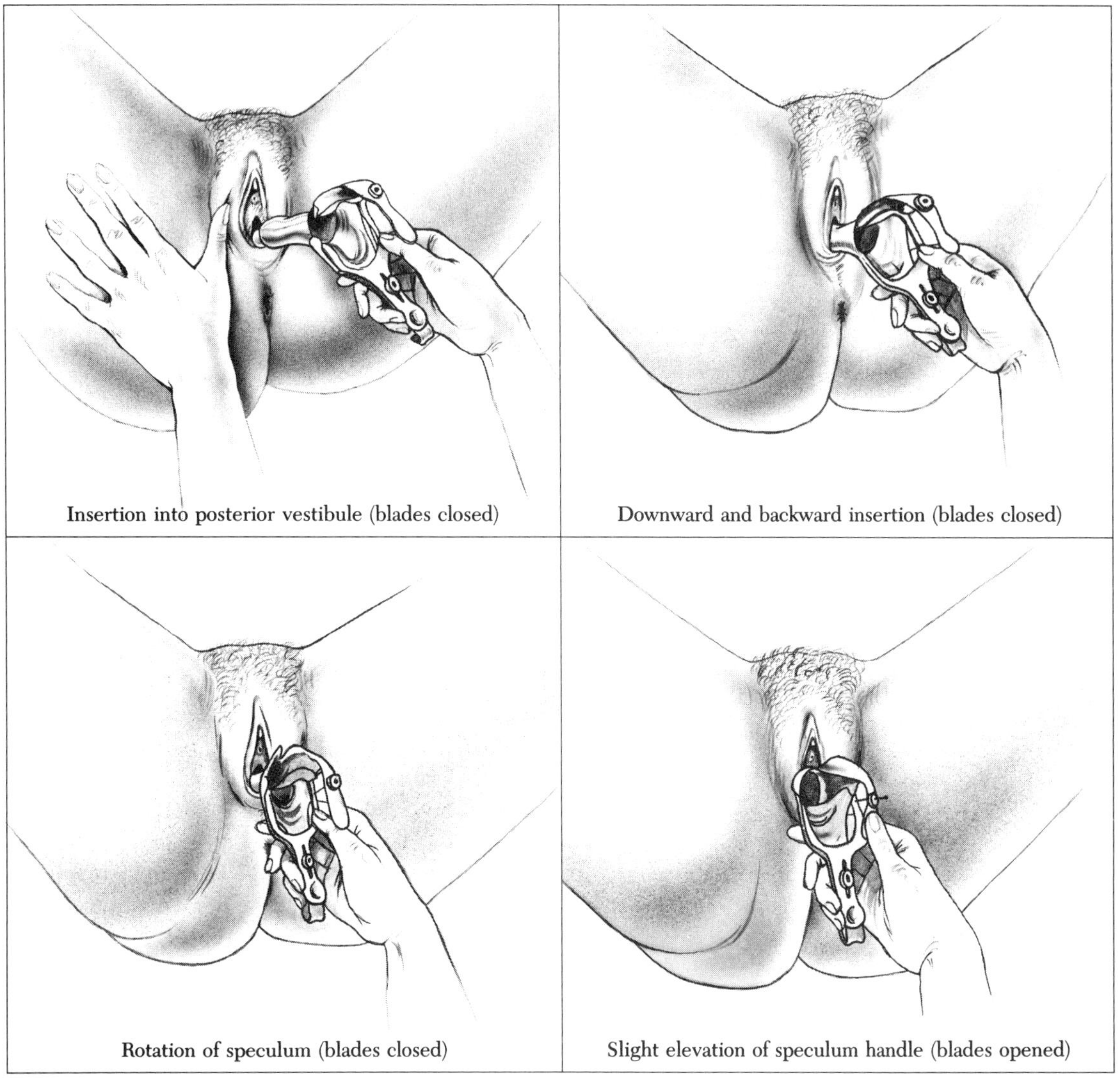

Insertion into posterior vestibule (blades closed)
Downward and backward insertion (blades closed)
Rotation of speculum (blades closed)
Slight elevation of speculum handle (blades opened)

Figure 16-10 Speculum insertion.

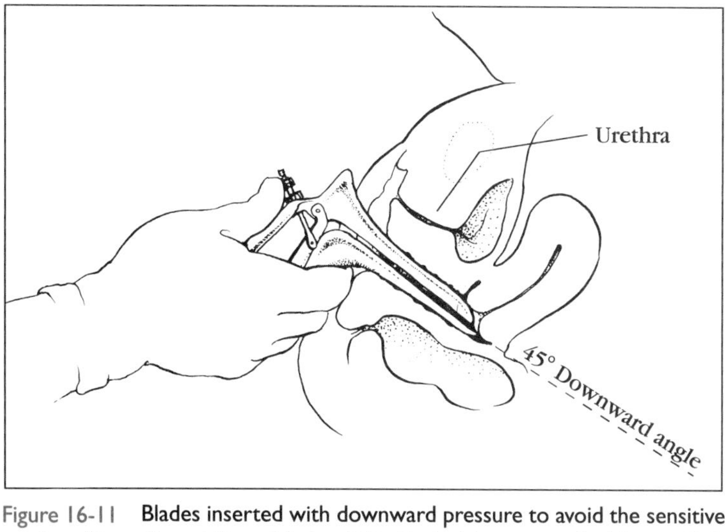

Figure 16-11 Blades inserted with downward pressure to avoid the sensitive urethra. (From Sana, J.M. and Judge, R.D. *Physical Assessment for Nursing Skills* (2nd ed.). Boston: Little, Brown, 1982, p. 327.)

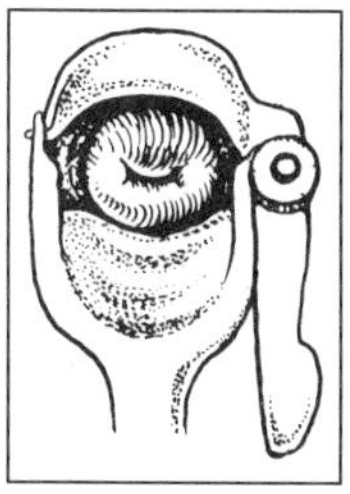

Figure 16-12 Blades separated and locked in place. (From Sana, J.M. and Judge, R.D. *Physical Assessment for Nursing Skills* (2nd ed.). Boston: Little, Brown, 1982, p. 327.)

Technique for Papanicolaou Smears

1. Moisten cotton applicator in saline.
2. Insert applicator into cervical os.
3. Rotate applicator clockwise and then counterclockwise and remove.
4. Roll applicator on a glass slide.
5. Spray glass slide with fixative or place it in a container of fixative.
6. Label slide "E" (endocervical specimen).
7. Place the longer side of the tip of an Ayre spatula into the cervical os.
8. Rotate the spatula in a full circle, scraping the surface of the cervix.
9. Place scrapings on glass slide; fix and label "C" (cervix specimen).
10. Roll applicator wet with saline in cul-de-sac area between inferior aspect of cervix and posterior vaginal wall or aspirate specimen from this area with soft aspiration syringe.
11. Place smear on glass slide; fix and label "V" (vaginal specimen).
12. Release lock on speculum blades.
13. Hold blades in comfortable open position and withdraw slowly, inspecting the vaginal mucosa.

suggests the position to be posterior to the cervix. If this occurs, withdraw the speculum a short distance and attempt to better position the distal ends of the blades.

- The normal cervix is pink, about 2 to 3 cm in diameter, and free from lacerations, erosions, and growths.
- The normal cervical os of a nulliparous female (Fig. 16-13) is small and either round or oval; the os of the normal parous female (Fig. 16-14) has a slit-like appearance.

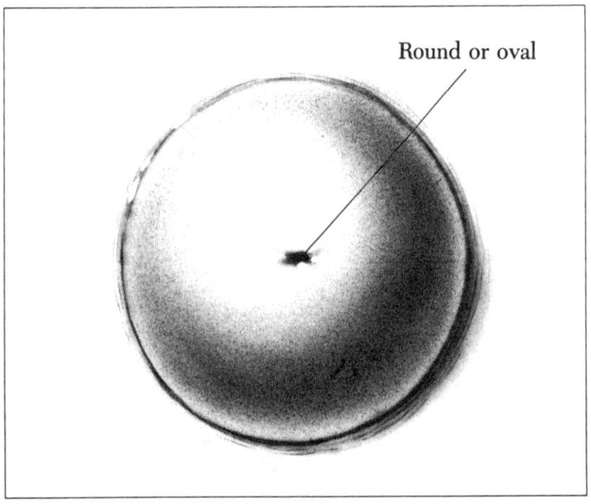

Figure 16-13 Normal nulliparous cervical os.

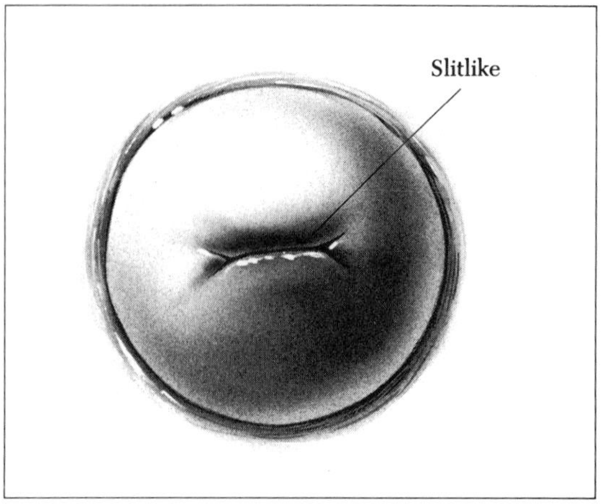

Figure 16-14 Normal parous cervical os.

- Transverse or stellate lacerations of the cervix (Fig. 16-15) may occur with difficult deliveries.
- The normal color of the cervix changes from a pink to purplish during pregnancy.

Papanicolaou Test

When performing a Papanicolaou (Pap) test, it is best to secure *three* specimens for cytology, as shown in Fig. 16-16:

1. The *endocervical* smear from the cervical os
   - Insert into the os a cotton applicator that has been moistened with normal saline.
   - Rotate the applicator both clockwise and counterclockwise before removal.
   - Roll the applicator on a glass slide lettered "E", and either fix with fixative spray or place in a bottle of fixative solution. If specimens are placed in a bottle, place paper clips on the slides to prevent the surfaces from rubbing together.
2. The *cervical* scrape from the cervical surface
   - Place the longer arm of the Ayre spatula in the cervical os and rotate it in a full circle.
   - Place the scraping on the "C" slide, and fix it.
3. The *vaginal* smear from the vaginal pool
   - Roll a wet applicator over the vaginal wall beneath the cervix or use an aspiration technique to collect the specimen from the vaginal pool.
   - Place the specimen on the "V" slide, and fix it.

After the cervix and cervical os have been inspected and the Pap smear specimens have been collected, slowly remove the vaginal speculum as you inspect the vaginal mucosa.

Bimanual Examination

The bimanual pelvic examination is performed to attempt palpation of the uterus and ovaries.

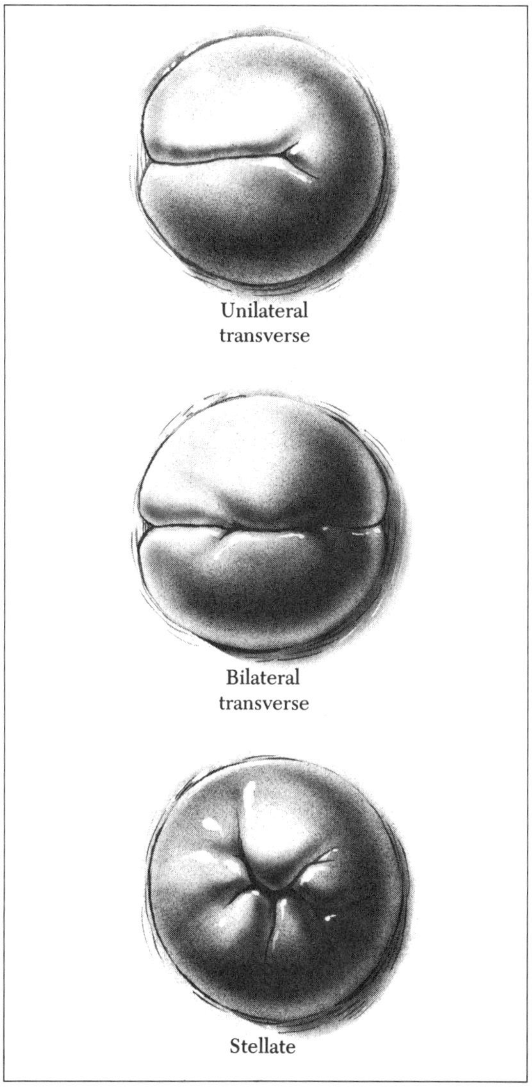

Figure 16-15 Cervical lacerations.

Palpation of the Cervix

- The examining finger is well lubricated before insertion into the vagina.
- After insertion of your finger, place your other hand between the umbilicus and pubic symphysis to steady the uterine body as your vaginal finger palpates the entire surface of the cervix. Figure 16-17 illustrates the bimanual palpation technique.
- Normally the *cervix* is smooth and firm; it is freely movable 2 to 3 cm in all directions, and the movement is painless.

Palpation of the Uterus

- With the palm upward, position a finger of the vaginal hand on either side of the cervix to stabilize the uterus in midline position.

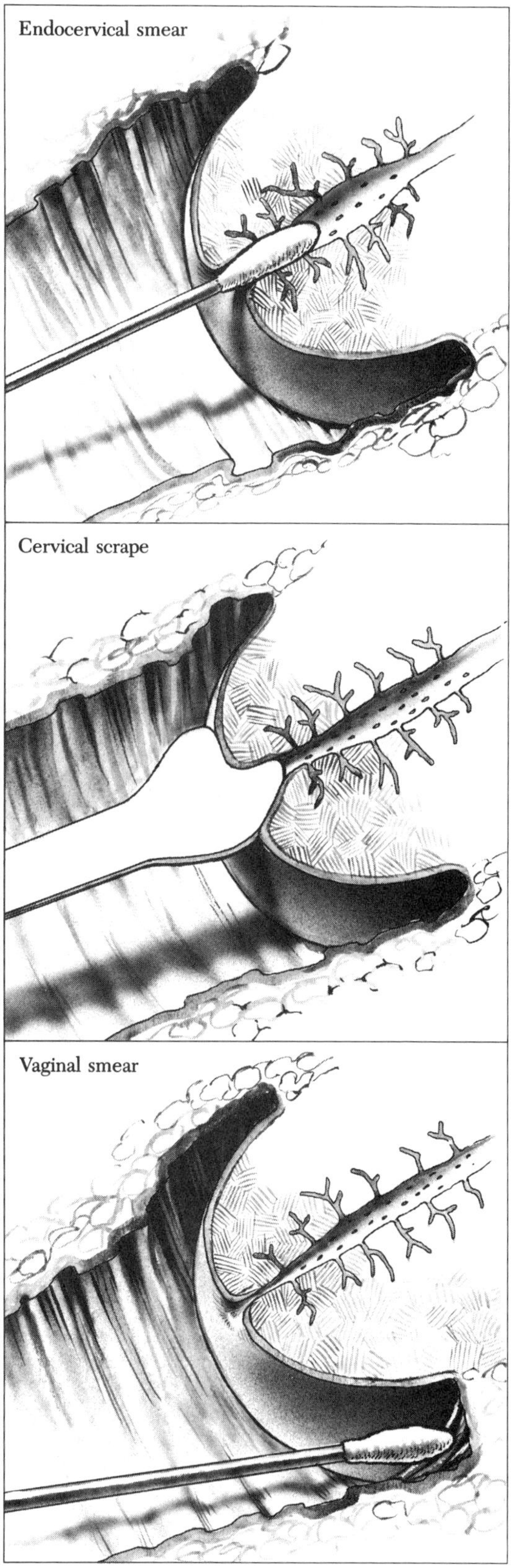

Figure 16-16 Sites and techniques for Pap test.

Technique for Bimanual Examination

1. Lubricate gloved examining finger.
2. Insert finger into vagina.
3. Characteristics of cervical palpation:
   Surface
   Consistency
   Movability
   Abnormalities
4. Place other hand on abdomen between umbilicus and pubic symphysis.
5. Place index finger on one side of the cervix and middle finger on the other side to steady cervix.
6. Press abdominal hand downward to palpate uterus.
7. Characteristics of uterine palpation:
   Size and contour
   Consistency
   Position
   Abnormalities
8. Place vaginal examining finger(s) in right lateral fornix.
9. Place abdominal hand in right lower quadrant.
10. Bring abdominal hand downward and vaginal fingers upward to attempt palpation of right adnexa.
11. Transfer abdominal hand to left lower quadrant and vaginal finger(s) into left fornix.
12. Press abdominal hand downward to meet vaginal finger(s) in attempt to palpate the left adnexa.
13. Withdraw finger(s) to vaginal opening.
14. Place tip of index finger slightly inside lateral aspect of vaginal introitus.
15. Place thumb in opposition on the outside.
16. Palpate Bartholin's gland area on either side of the vaginal opening.

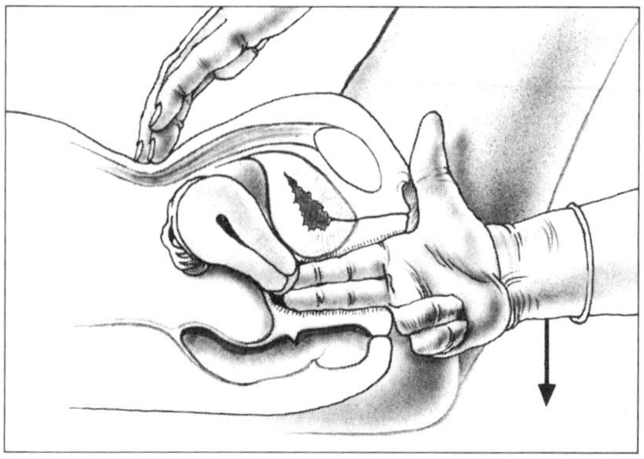

Figure 16-17 Bimanual palpation technique.

- Press the abdominal hand downward between the umbilicus and pubic symphysis to judge the size, consistency, position, and contour of the uterus.

Figure 16-18 illustrates retroversion, the backward tilting of the entire uterus (both body and cervix) in which the fundus of the uterus is palpable through the rectum, and retroflexion, the backward angling of the body of the uterus in relation to the cervix; the fundus of the retroflexed uterus may be palpable rectally.

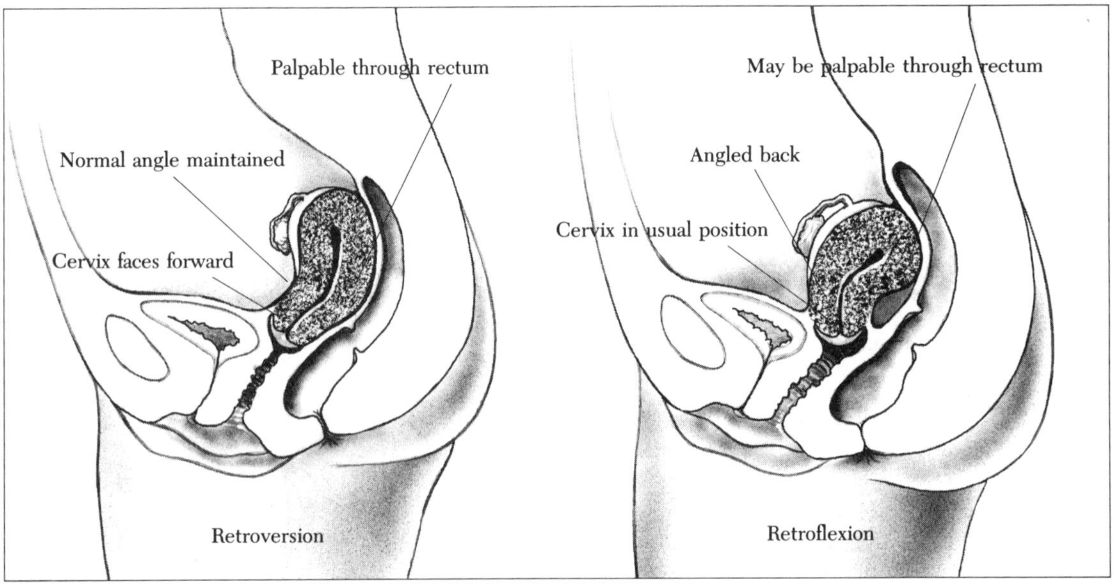

Figure 16-18 Retroversion and retroflexion of the uterus.

Palpation of the Adnexa Palpation of the adnexa (fallopian tubes and ovaries) (Fig. 16-19) is the most difficult maneuver of the pelvic examination, especially for the beginner. Even the expert is occasionally foiled if the client is obese, is tense, has a full bladder, or has abdominal-pelvic tenderness.

- To assess the right ovary, press the abdominal hand gently but deeply into the right lower quadrant while placing the vaginal finger firmly in the right lateral fornix.
- Try to palpate the adnexa between the finger inserted into the vagina and the hand, which is flat upon the abdomen.
- Reverse the positions of the vaginal finger and abdominal hand to assess the left ovary.

The normal fallopian tube and ovary are usually nonpalpable.

- As you withdraw the vaginal finger, at the completion of the adnexal assessment, palpate the area of the Bartholin's glands (Fig. 16-20).
- Firmly hold the area between your index finger, slightly inside the margin of the vaginal introitus, and your thumb, which on the outside perineal skin.

Normally, the Bartholin's glands are not palpable unless they are infected (Fig. 16-21).

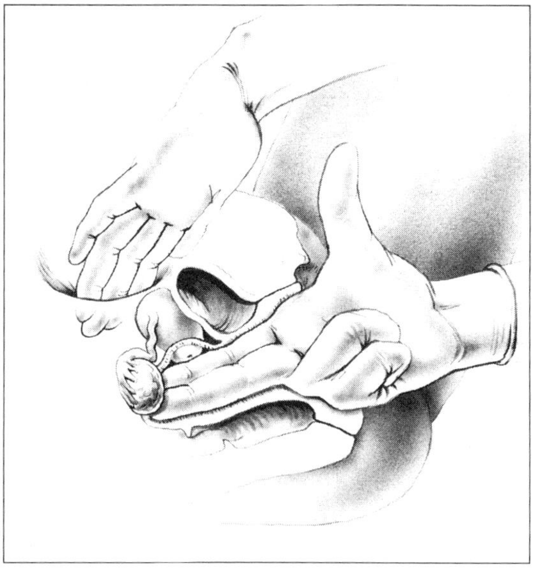

Figure 16-19 Bimanual palpation of the adnexa.

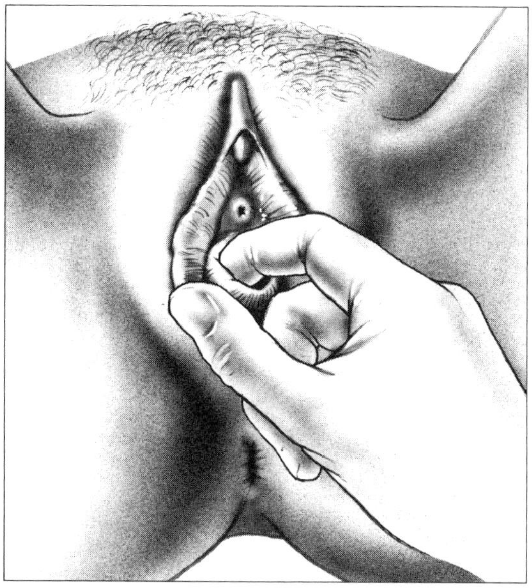

Figure 16-20 Palpation of the Bartholin's glands.

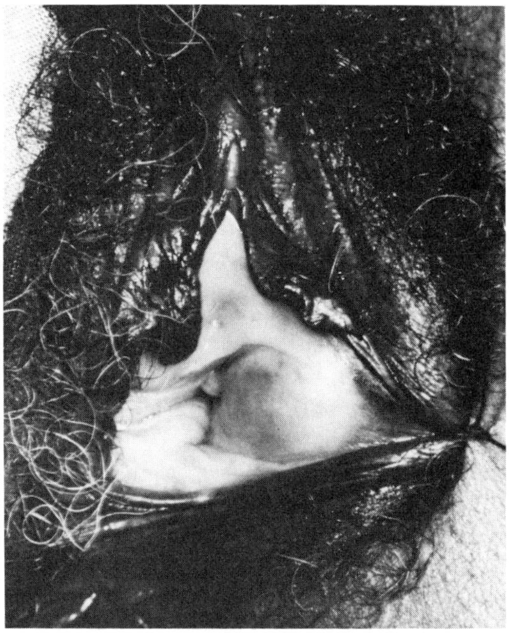

Figure 16-21 Bartholin abscess in an African-American woman. Note swelling of the left labia.

Technique for Rectovaginal-Abdominal Examination

1. If you have gloves on and have completed prior examination of the female genitals, put on new examining gloves.
2. Tell client that this may make her feel as if her bowels must move.
3. Insert lubricated index finger into the vagina.
4. Insert lubricated middle finger simultaneously into the rectum.
5. Assess strength of rectovaginal wall.
6. Next, place other hand on abdomen over uterus.
7. Push uterus backward, palpating posterior surface with rectal finger.

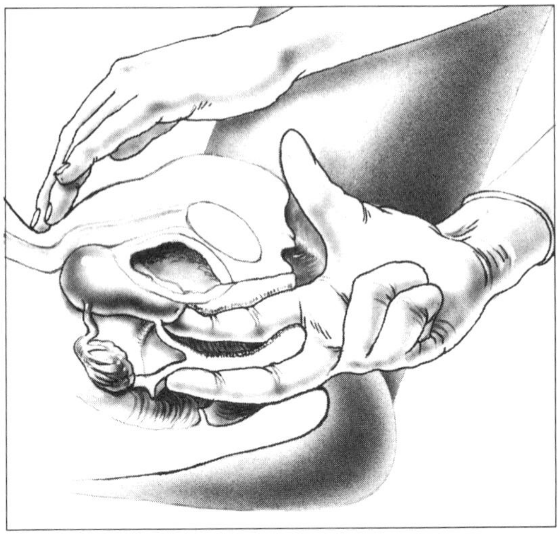

Figure 16-22 Rectovaginal-abdominal palpation technique.

Rectovaginal-Abdominal Examination

The last portion of the pelvic examination is rectovaginal-abdominal palpation (Fig. 16-22).

- Put on a new examining glove to prevent possible cross-contamination between the genitals and the rectum.
- Inform the client that this procedure may cause her to feel as if her bowels must move.
- Insert your index finger into the vagina and your middle finger into the rectum.
- Assess the strength of the rectovaginal wall. This technique makes it possible to detect herniation of the small bowel dissecting between the rectal and vaginal walls.
- Direct careful attention to the area beneath the cervix.
- Apply pressure with the abdominal hand to move the uterus backward so the posterior surface may be palpated with the rectal finger. Ordinarily, the pelvic tissues, particularly the broad ligaments, are inaccessible to manual assessment.

The rectovaginal-abdominal technique allows palpation of inflamed areas and indurated areas of malignant tumor invasion and can be done only via the rectum.

In conducting a pelvic assessment of virgins or elderly women in whom the introitus has become atrophied and small, use a single examining finger, a small vaginal speculum or a nasal speculum, or the bimanual examination with one finger in the rectum and a hand on the abdomen, whichever technique is most appropriate for comfort of examination. Figure 16-23 illustrates the different appearances of hymen in women.

STRUCTURE AND FUNCTION OF THE ANUS AND RECTUM

The anus is the most distal portion of the gastrointestinal tract. It is demarcated from the rectum by a line at which skin changes to the mucous membrane lining of the rectum. The anus has an abundance of somatic nerves, which renders

Technique for Inspection of the Anus

1. Position in Sim's or have client stand and lean over bed or examining table.
2. Spread buttocks gently with a hand positioned on each buttock.
3. Examine crevice of buttocks from sacrum to anterior genitals.
4. Characteristics of inspection:
   Anus
   Perineal skin surface
   Abnormalities
5. Instruct client to "bear down" while examining the anus.

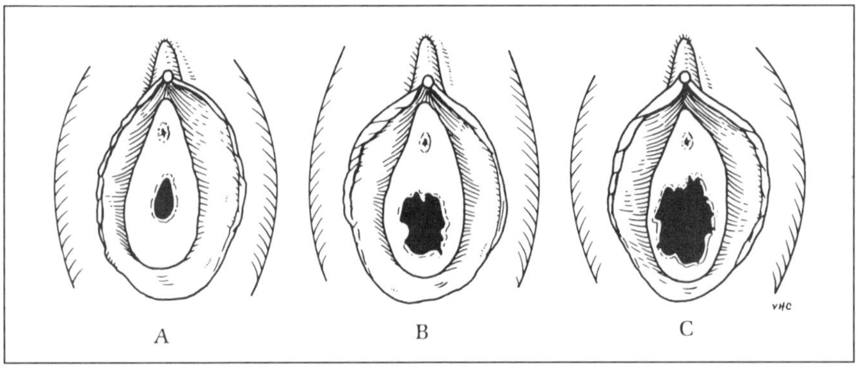

Figure 16-23 Different appearances of hymen in **(A)** a virgin, **(B)** a woman who has had sexual intercourse, and **(C)** a multiparous woman. (From Sana, J.M. and Judge, R.D. *Physical Assessment for Nursing Skills* (2nd ed.). Boston: Little, Brown, 1982, p. 325.)

it highly susceptible to discomfort caused by a rough examination technique.

The rectum, located between the anus and the sigmoid colon, is about 12 cm long. It is in the rectum that the urge to defecate is stimulated, a result of stretching of the nerve fibers by the bulk of descending feces.

CHARACTERISTICS AND TECHNIQUES OF EXAMINATION

The rectum is very accessible to physical examination, and the procedure takes but a few minutes. Rectal examination is an essential part of any routine assessment. It is a quick and easy means for early detection of carcinoma of the prostate gland in the male as well as of carcinoma of the rectum. Because early prostatic carcinoma produces no symptoms to prompt the client to seek medical attention, the rectal examination should be performed on an annual basis, especially for every man over the age of 40 because the risk of occurrence increases with age.

Out of fear that stimulating the vagus nerve will result in a decreased heart rate, physicians and nurses have been, and continue to be, reluctant to perform rectal exams on clients with acute myocardial infarction. The evidence, however, does not support this notion (see box).

The Earnest and Fletcher Study

A closely monitored study involving 86 clients admitted to a coronary care unit, none of whom displayed any symptoms of shock or life-threatening arrhythmias, was conducted, and no adverse effects from a gentle digital rectal examination were found (Earnest and Fletcher 1969). The clients were monitored before, during, and for 3 minutes following the examination. No negative effects were noted, either clinically or electrocardiographically, and there were no incidents of angina pectoris. The researchers concluded that there were no adverse effects and, furthermore, that immediate value may be forthcoming from a brief gentle rectal examination of clients diagnosed with acute myocardial infarction, assuming the absence of shock or life-threatening arrhythmia.

Information obtained from the rectal examinations of the study clients included 38 potential fecal impactions, 9 with 3+ to 4+ benzidine tests (occult-blood), 20 of 56 with prostatism, and 8 with symptomatic prostatism.

Inspection

- Inspect the superior cleft area of the buttocks for presence of a pilonidal cyst.
- Spread the buttocks in both male and female clients to best visualize the anus. This maybe very painful for the client with an anal fissure.
- Inspect the anus and perineum for any lesions, fistulas, fissures, or skin tabs. Skin tabs may be associated with a history of hemorrhoidal problems.
- Note the presence of hemorrhoids.
- Instruct the client to "bear down"; this normally causes the anal sphincter to contract and indicates intact innervation. However, prolapse of the rectum may be observed.

Technique for Palpation of the Anus

1. Have client remain in same position as for inspection of the anus.
2. If you have on examining gloves from prior examination of the genitals, put on a new pair.
3. Place your well-lubricated index finger gently against the anus.
4. As client relaxes, slowly insert index finger into rectum.
5. Note sphincter muscle action.
6. With the palmar aspect of your examining finger, palpate the posterior rectal wall.
7. Rotate your examining finger and palpate the left rectal wall.
8. Rotate finger to palpate the right rectal wall.
9. Rotate finger to palpate the anterior rectal wall.
10. Withdraw examining finger slowly.
11. Observe finger for presence of feces.
12. Note characteristics of feces.
13. If feces present, test for occult blood.
14. Wipe anus with tissue.

Palpation

If the genitals have been examined prior to the rectal examination, and particularly if gonorrhea is suspected, you should put on a new pair of examining gloves. Gonorrhea can infect the rectum as well as the genitals.

- Gently press against the anus with a well-lubricated finger; as relaxation occurs, slowly insert the finger into the rectum.
- Rotate your finger to palpate all sides of the rectal wall with the palmar aspect.
- Note any tenderness, nodules, or masses.
- Examine your finger after it is withdrawn; observe for the presence of feces.
- Feces should be tested for occult blood. Record the color of the feces as well as any presence of mucus or visible blood.

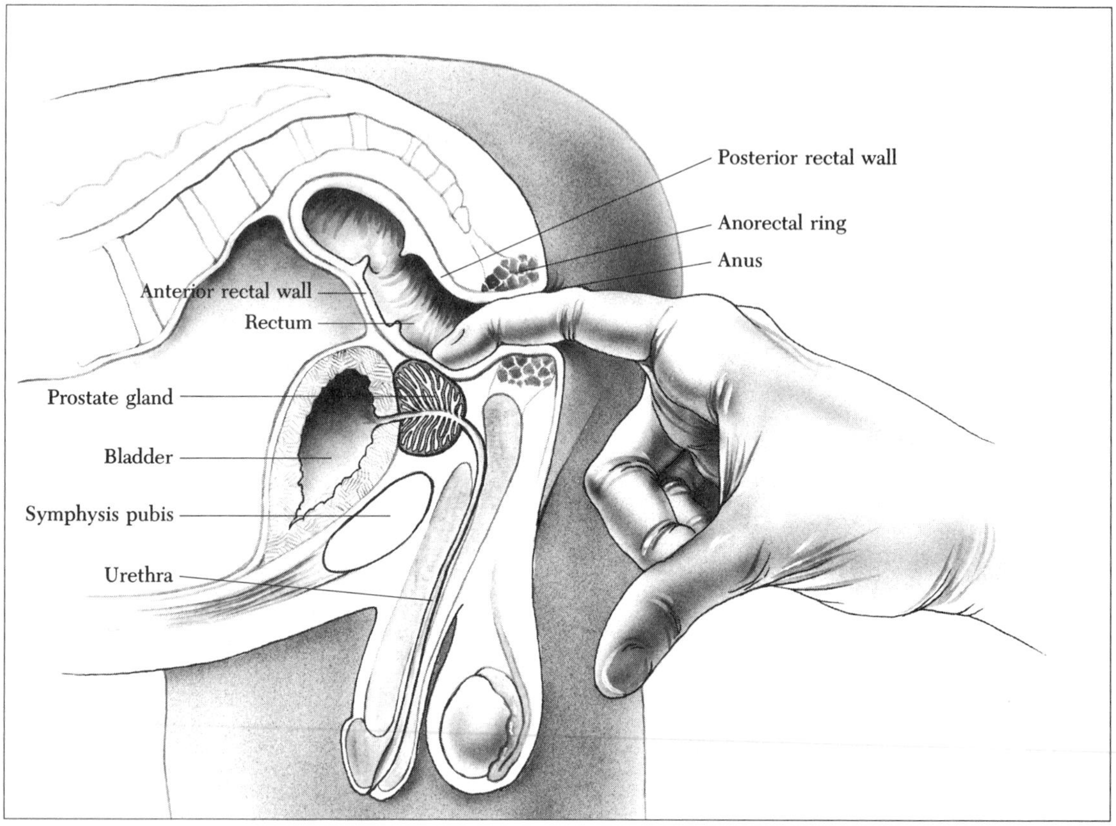

A

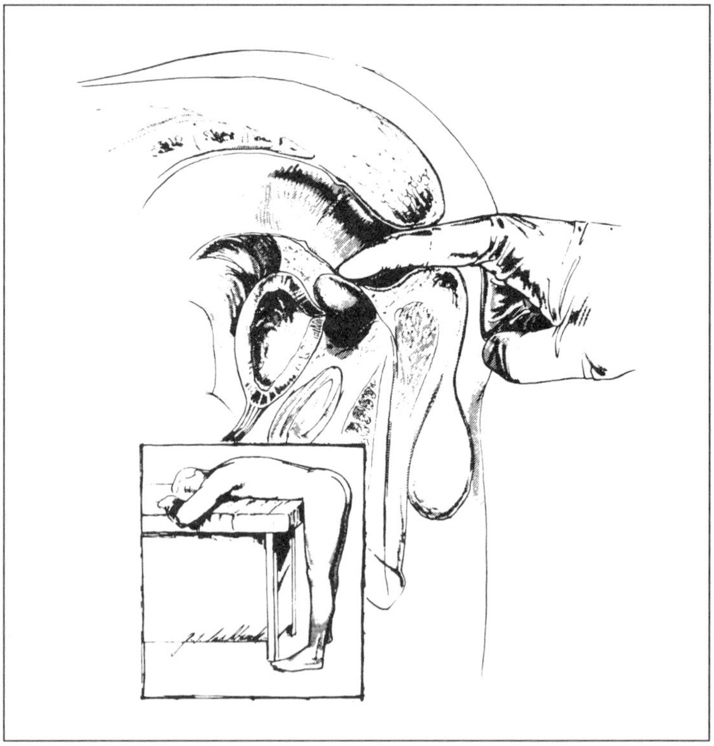

B

Figure 16-24 **(A)** Technique for palpation of the prostate gland. **(B)** Examination of the prostate gland. (From Sana, J.M. and Judge, R.D. *Physical Assessment for Nursing Skills* (2nd ed.). Boston: Little, Brown, 1982, p. 303.)

In the male, the prostate gland can be palpated through the anterior wall of the rectum. Figure 16-24A illustrates the technique for palpation of the prostate gland.

- The best position for palpation is to have the client stand and lean over the bed or table (Fig. 16-24B).
- Inform the client that he may experience the urge to urinate, but that there should be no tenderness.
- Identify the well-marked median sulcus, which divides the two lobes of the gland.
- The prostate is normally firm and rubbery, approximately 4 cm in diameter, and the borders are discrete.
- Normally, there is no fixation of the gland.

Tenderness of the prostate is commonly experienced during the examination of clients with benign prostatic hyperplasia and urinary abnormalities. The cause of prostatic hypertrophy is not known, although it is definitely linked with aging and is a common occurrence in men over 50 years of age.

See Table 16-1 for common abnormalities of the genitals.

Technique for Palpation of the Prostate Gland

1. Performed at completion of palpation of the rectum in men prior to withdrawing examining finger.
2. Tell the client to inform you if the area is tender.
3. Tell the client that he may experience the urge to urinate during the procedure and that this is common.
4. Through the anterior rectal wall, identify the median sulcus.
5. Palpate the surface of the left and right prostatic lobes.
6. Characteristics of palpation:
   Size
   Consistency
   Borders
   Movability
   Abnormalities
7. Wipe lubricant and feces from anus with tissue.

Table 16-1 **Common Abnormalities of the Genitals**

Condition	Characteristics	Comments
Phimosis	Narrow preputial orifice, resulting in inability to retract foreskin back over the glans penis	Health teaching regarding peri-care Acute stage treated with saline soaks Medical referral for evaluation of need for circumcision
Hypospadias	Congenital opening of urethra on underside of penis; congenital opening of urethra into vagina	Medical referral for evaluation regarding reconstructive surgery
Epispadias	Congenital opening of urethra on superior surface of the penis	Medical referral for evaluation regarding reconstructive surgery
Epididymitis	Swollen, tender epididymis; fever, chills, inguinal pain	Investigate medical history—may be complication of prostatic and urinary infections, mumps, TB, sexually transmitted disease, or prolonged use of Foley catheter. Medical referral; Rx consists of bedrest, scrotal support, antibiotics.
Prostatitis	Fever; chills; tender, swollen prostate, which frequently is slightly asymmetrical	Check for history of low back or perineal pains and urinary, erection, and ejaculation difficulties; urine culture; medical referral warranted. Prostatic massage may decrease congestion.
Hydrocele	Enlarged scrotal sac; transilluminates	Medical referral warranted
Varicocele	Varicose veins of the spermatic cord; occasionally purplish appearance, palpable full vessels on side(s) of scrotum	Investigate whether dull ache and/or dragging sensation in area of cord. Rx: suspensory; medical referral warranted with persistent symptoms
Syphilis	*Primary stage:* ulcerated papule or erosion (chancre); painless hard ulcer with shiny red, raw, scooped-out appearance; purulent secretion; generalized lymphadenopathy *Secondary stage:* skin rash, condylomata lata (syphilis warts) occurring 6–8 weeks after chancre *Latent stage:* usually asymptomatic	Primary syphilitic is highly contagious ulcer during chancre stage—wear gloves; examine rectum, mouth, genital area, woman's breast, and eyelids and conjunctiva; heals without leaving scar. Take culture and order serology. Medical referral warranted for antibiotic therapy.

Continued

Table 16-1 Continued

Condition	Characteristics	Comments
Gonorrhea	Men—thick opaque or purulent urethral discharge; red, swollen urethral meatus	Check for history of sore throat; urinary urgency; take throat (oral sex), urethral, and rectal culture.
	Women—may be asymptomatic carrier; purulent urethral discharge; cervical discharge; red, swollen Skene's or Bartholin's glands and/or edema of vulva is usual.	"Milk" urethra; check for history of sore throat, dysuria, and abnormal uterine bleeding; cervical, vaginal, rectal and throat secretions cultured. Increased incidence in 15- to 30-year-olds.
Genital herpes	Painful blisters or sores, which eventually form scabs and heal; occasionally headache, fatigue, fever, dysuria, and enlarged and tender inguinal lymph nodes	Most common STD in upper-income and college-educated people. Cervical Pap smear in women every 6 months (linked with cervical carcinoma). Check for history of headaches, anorexia, general malaise, premature deliveries, and spontaneous miscarriages. Medical referral warranted for pharmacologic control of disease.
Trichomoniasis	Women—vulvar irritation and pruritis, foul greenish-yellow foamy vaginal discharge; men—may be asymptomatic; urethritis; prostatitis	Obtain saline slides, Pap smear, and urinalysis.
Moniliasis *(Candida)*	Vulvar irritation and pruritis, thick cottage cheese-like vaginal discharge	Obtain culture of discharge, wet smear, Pap smear, and urine culture.
Crabs (pubic lice)	Pruritus—especially nocturnal; presence of parasite (gray colored but rusty red after feeding on human blood 4–5 times per day) in pubic hair, eyebrows, eyelashes, and/or beard; occasionally mild fever and cervical lymphadenopathy	Health teaching: spreads via close contact, clothing, bedding, toilet seats. Rx for patient and all sexual partners: Kwell cream or shampoo, and washing of clothing and bedding (Rand C Spray).
AIDS	General malaise, fever, 10–20-lb weight loss over few months; ecchymosis; painful and enlarged lymph nodes (over 10 days' duration); persistent herpes sores (over 5 weeks' duration); sensory or motor loss	Etiology unknown; higher incidence in homosexual men but rising in heterosexual women. Believed to be sexually transmitted and via contaminated blood or blood products. Check for respiratory signs and skin lesions. Check for history of syphilis, nitrate inhalants ("poppers"), and sexual practices—i.e., oral-anal, penile-anal, and manual-anal contacts.
Cystitis	Fever, pyuria	Check for history of burning on urination, urgency, low back or abdominal pain. Obtain clean-catch (midstream) urine for urinalysis. Health teaching: hot tub bath t.i.d., force fluids, avoid bladder irritants (alcohol, coffee, tea, and spices). Medical referral warranted.
Endocervicitis	White or yellow mucoid vaginal discharge, cervical erosion on inspection	Medical referral for electrocauterization of cervix
Ovarian carcinoma	Distended abdomen and/or ascites (shifting dullness), signs of hyperthyroidism, feminization or virilization; anemia and cachexia in advanced cases	Check for vague lower abdominal discomfort/pain and mild digestive complaints; medical referral warranted.
Cervical carcinoma	Friable cervical mass or ulcer on inspection	Obtain Pap smears; medical referral warranted.
Vaginal carcinoma	Tumor of vaginal wall on inspection (commonly posterior upper one third of vaginal wall), watery discharge, urinary frequency	Check for history of bleeding after coitus, dyspareunia; involvement of bladder or rectum may result in urgency and/or painful defecation. Obtain Pap smear, perform Schiller's test. Medical referral is warranted.
Uterine carcinoma	Recurrent metrorrhagia in menstruating woman, postmenopausal bleeding, mucosanguineous vaginal discharge with vaginal metastasis	Peak incidence 50–60 years of age. Check for stormy menstrual history, infertility, and suspicious predispositional factors (obesity, hypertension, diabetes mellitus, familial history). Obtain Pap smear and make medical referral.

Table 16-1 **Continued**

Condition	Characteristics	Comments
Prostatic carcinoma	Change in urinary stream, hematuria, pyuria, palpable stony hard induration and/or nodule(s)	Check for history of bone pain (pelvis and/or lumbar spine metastasis); medical referral warranted. Do annual rectal exam for all men 40 years of age and older.
Testicular carcinoma	Firm or cystic scrotal mass, occasionally painful	Health teaching: self-testicular exam, check for history of cryptorchid testis, trauma in young men 17–35 years old (increased incidence). Immediate medical referral when signs present.

RECORDING OF FINDINGS

Normal findings are presented in the first column. Abnormal findings are presented in the second column.

Male Genitals
Inspection: Diamond-shaped pubic hair distribution; urethral meatus at penile tip; uncircumcised; no lesions, scars, edema, discharge, or erythema.

Palpation: No nodules; foreskin freely movable; testicles descended; no tenderness.

Female External Genitals
Inspection: Inverted pyramid-shaped pubic hair pattern; labia majora/minora and perineum intact; no lesions, scars, fissures, excoriations, swelling, or erythema; normal clitoris; vestibule clear; meatus clear; fourchette intact.

Palpation: No urethral discharge with "milking"; Skene's and Bartholin's glands nontender and without inflammation.

Female Internal Genitals
Inspection: Vaginal walls intact—negative for cystocele and rectocele; mucosa pink; no discharge; cervix positioned posteriorly; cervix pink with no lacerations, erosions, or masses.

Palpation: Pap smears (3) done; bimanual examination: cervix firm, smooth, freely movable; uterus normal size and shape, smooth, firm, mobile, positioned anteriorly; adnexa nonpalpable; rectal wall normal consistency; cul-de-sac free of bulging and lesions; posterior uterine aspect smooth.

Anus and Rectum
Inspection: Anal sphincter intact; no lesions, fissures, skin tabs, or external hemorrhoids; stool brown with no visible blood or mucus; negative for occult blood.

Palpation: No tenderness, masses, or internal hemorrhoids; (male) prostate firm, discrete borders, mobile, normal size, no tenderness or nodules.

Male Genitals
Inspection: Severe bilateral scrotal edema; transillumination present.

Palpation: Unable to palpate epididymis or spermatic cord; nontender.

Female Internal Genitals
(Client has inflammation of a Bartholin's gland secondary to gonococcal infection)

Inspection: Left lower labial edema with tenderness; erythematous; copious purulent vaginal discharge; urethral orifice edematous and red.

Palpation: Tenderness and greenish yellow urethral discharge on "milking" urethra; dysuria; endocervical and urethral cultures done.

Anus and Rectum
(Client diagnosed as having prostatic carcinoma)

Inspection: Anal sphincter intact; no lesions, fissures, skin tabs, or external hemorrhoids; stool brown with no visible blood or mucus; negative for occult blood.

Palpation: No tenderness, masses, or internal hemorrhoids; enlarged prostate 6–7 cm with multiple stony-hard nodules, no tenderness, fixated.

CLINICAL CORRELATIONS

Phimosis is a condition in males in which the foreskin adheres to the glans, making it impossible to retract it back over the glans (Fig. 16-25). This condition promotes the build-up of smegma, which can serve as an irritant leading to inflammation of the glans penis, balanitis (Fig. 16-26). Paraphimosis is the condition in which the foreskin can be retracted but cannot be returned; it is tight, causing inflammation of the prepuce, swelling, and ischemic pain. Variations of the urethral meatus are hypospadias, in which the meatus is located on the underside of the penile shaft, and epispadias, in which it is on the top surface of the penis. Such abnormalities are generally corrected at a young age by plastic surgery.

Scrotal edema is usually associated with generalized edema, as in cardiac and renal disease (Fig. 16-27). A common abnormality that causes enlargement of the scrotum and is readily identified is a varicocele, a soft irregular mass within the scrotum resulting from varicosities. It has been appropriately termed a "bag of worms" because it feels like one. These varicose veins of the scrotum will collapse gradually as the scrotum is elevated while the client is lying down. Other causes of scrotal enlargement are hydroceles (clear fluid-filled cysts), spermatoceles (localized cysts containing spermatozoa of the epididymis or spermatic cord), testicular tumors, epididymitis (inflammation of the epididymis), orchitis (inflammation of the testis) that may accompany mumps, and indirect inguinal hernias (Fig. 16-28).

A deviated or poor urine stream suggests such conditions as urethral stricture, urethral polyp, or urethral obstruction from prostatic hyperplasia.

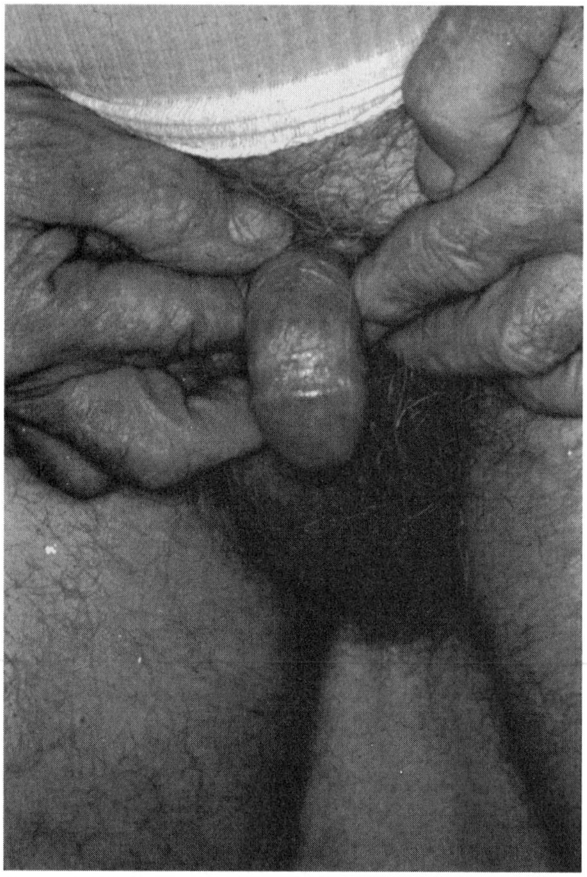

Figure 16-26 Balanitis.

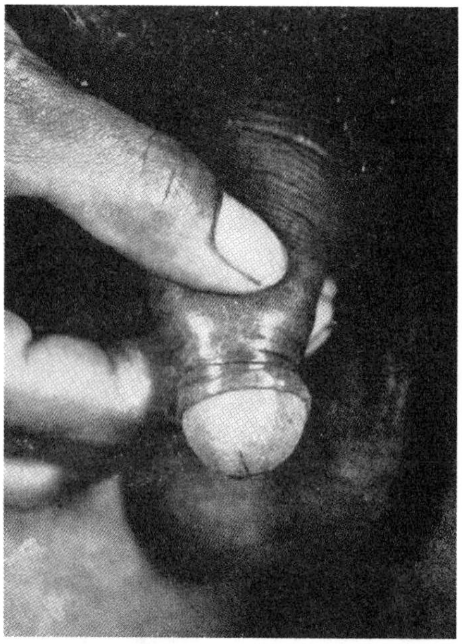

Figure 16-25 Phimosis of moderate degree. Note constriction of the glans as foreskin is retracted.

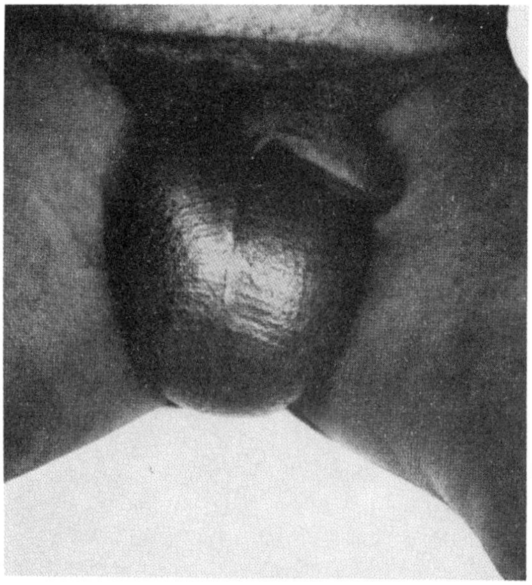

Figure 16-27 Edema of the scrotum and penis in congestive cardiac failure.

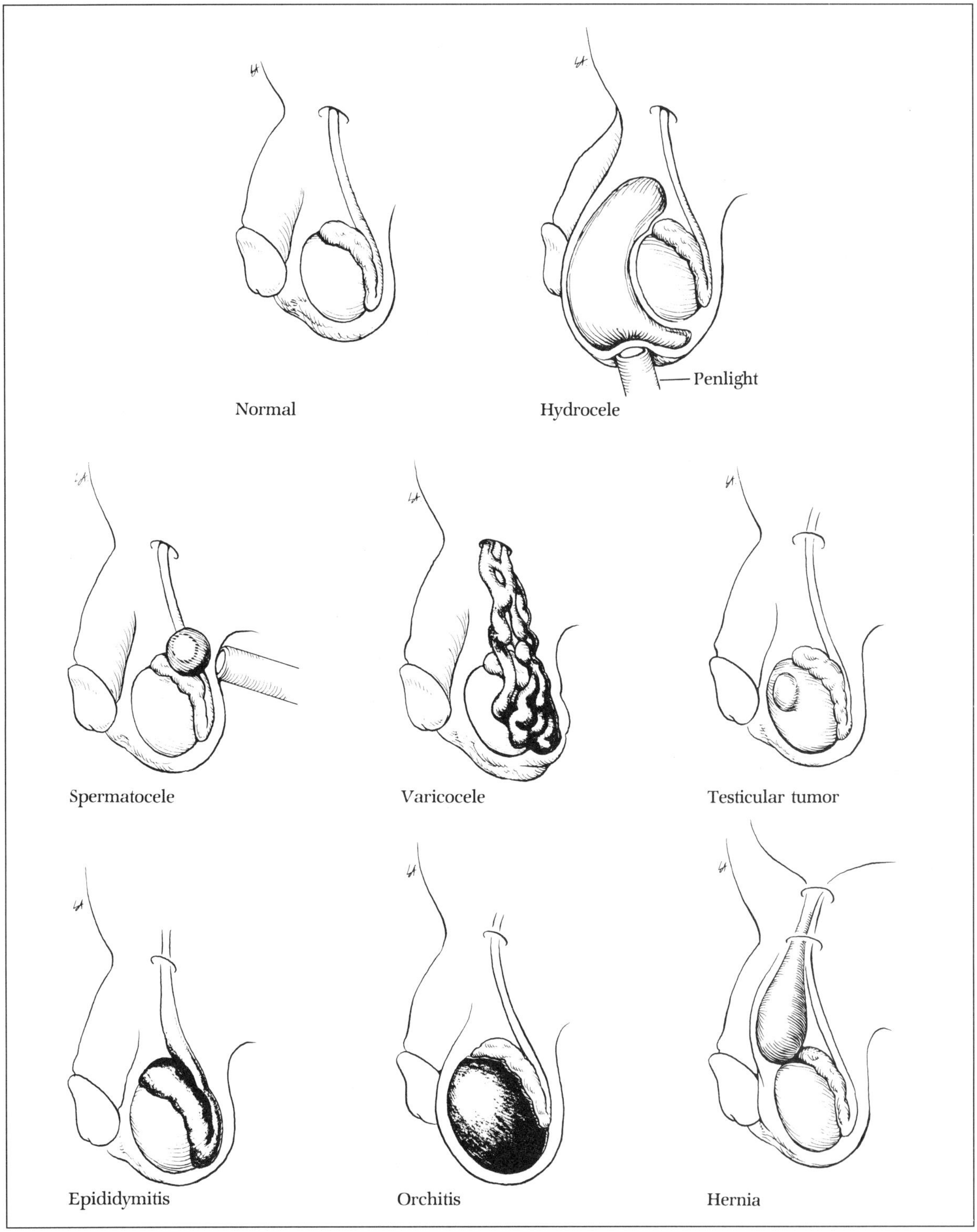

Figure 16-28 Some scrotal lesions. (From Sana, J.M. and Judge, R.D. *Physical Assessment for Nursing Skills* (2nd ed.). Boston: Little, Brown, 1982, p. 301.)

Herpes genitalis, herpes simplex virus type 2, is generally considered a sexually transmitted disease (STD). The viral infection presents with itching and soreness followed by a small patch of erythema and then painful vesicles that have about a 10-day duration. The virus can occur any place in the genitalia and anal region and mucosa. *Condylomata acuminata* also is caused by a virus that is transmitted sexually. It can be either a dry or moist single wart-like lesion or multiple groups on the skin of the external genitalia or near the anus. The chancre of syphilis evolves from a small red papule to a small ulcer to an indurated, hard oval lesion. Drawings of these conditions are provided in Fig. 16-29. Primary syphilitic chancres are shown in Fig. 16-30.

A thick, purulent discharge suggests gonorrhea. Gonorrhea may also manifest associated urinary symptoms. If un-

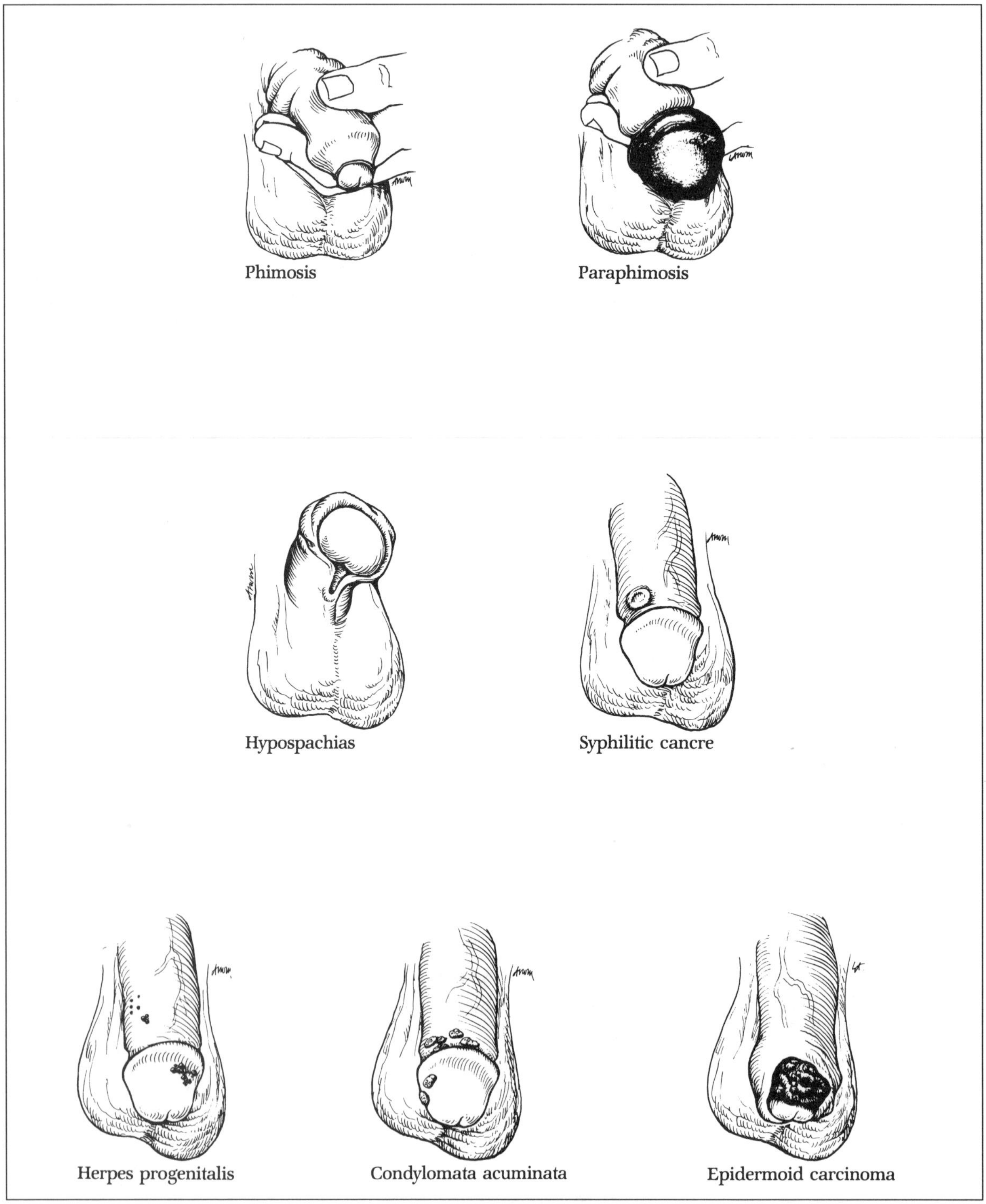

Figure 16-29 Some lesions of the penis. (From Sana, J.M. and Judge, R.D. *Physical Assessment for Nursing Skills* (2nd ed.). Boston: Little, Brown, 1982, p. 309.)

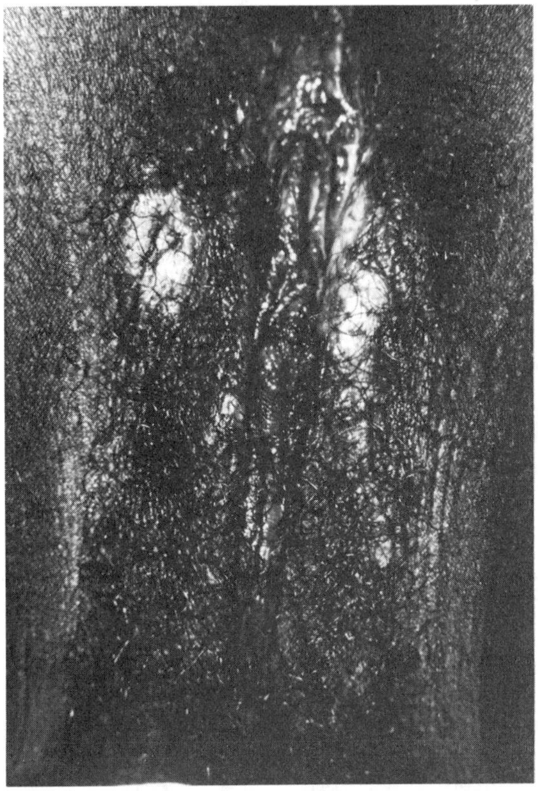

Figure 16-30 Syphilitic chancres of the left and right labia. Note scooped-out appearance and red-raw floor. This condition heals without leaving a scar.

treated, the disease process could lead to sterility, arthritis, and endocarditis. A thin, mucoid discharge may indicate urethritis.

In the female, on examination of the cervix, generally, a beefy red color will present with ulcerations and erosions. Early carcinomas can appear beefy red also, but with progression they may appear as a hard granulated or cauliflower-like growth. Both erosions and carcinomas bleed easily when daubed with an applicator or sponge stick.

If the cervix appears abnormal, a Schiller test is performed. In this test, normal areas of the cervix and upper vagina stain brown when painted with Lugol's solution (iodine in potassium iodide). Abnormal areas remain colorless due to the lack of glycogen; these areas warrant biopsy, which can be performed in the office with a biopsy punch. The bleeding that occurs with biopsy can be controlled easily by a tampon, silver nitrate stick, or electrocauterization. Biopsy specimens should be placed immediately in 10% formalin. Cervical cancer usually has its beginnings at or near the cervical os and may be present in a cervix that appears normal. Thus, it is important to have annual routine Pap smears (cytology studies) to increase early detection of cervical cancer. On bimanual examination of the pelvis, pain will occur with cervical inflammation, and the cervix may be immovable with PID or with malignant infiltration.

Other abnormalities that may be observed are cervical polyps, which are palpable as soft, spongy masses, and the "strawberry spots" associated with trichomonas vaginitis (Fig. 16-31). Translucent nabothian cysts (which accompany chronic cervicitis), eversion, and erosion are common abnormal phenomena (Fig. 16-32).

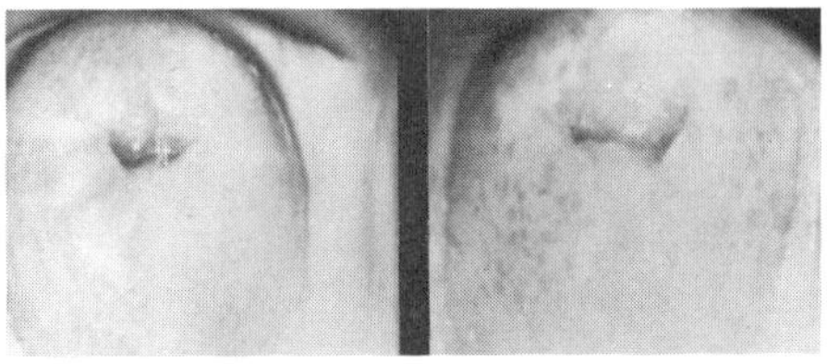

Figure 16-31 Trichomonas vaginitis.

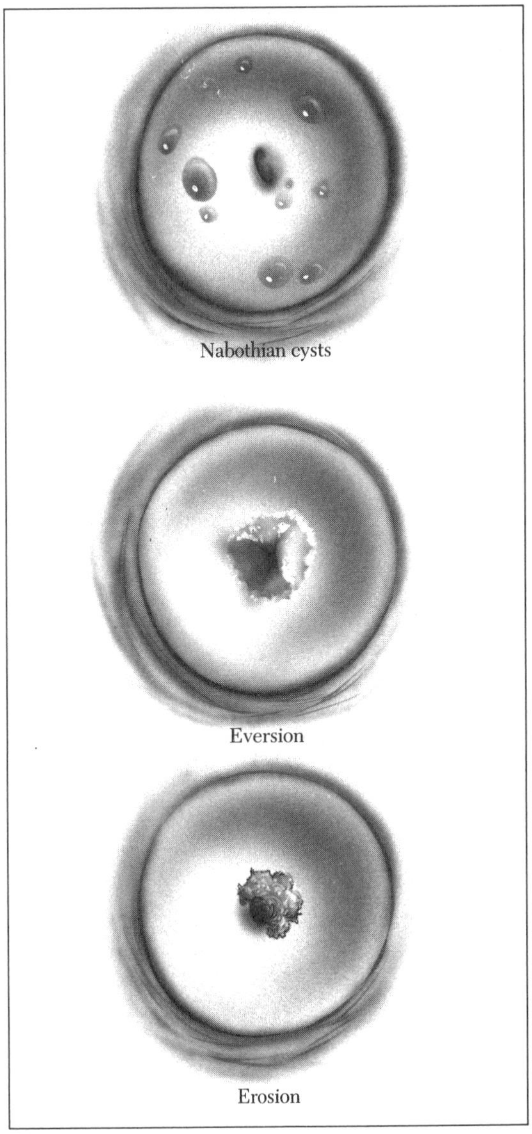

Figure 16-32 Surface irregularities of the cervix.

Table 17-5 **Continued**

Defect	Pathophysiology
Atrial septal defect (ASD) 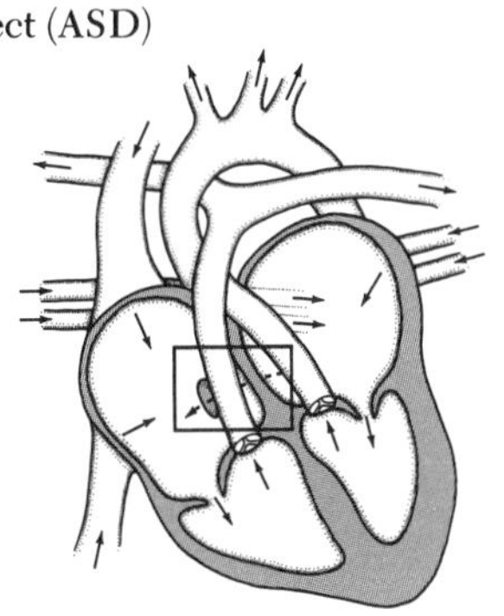	One or more openings located between the left and right atria, permitting left-to-right shunting of blood between the atria. Ostium secundum type located in an intermediate position of atrial wall. Ostium primum type is low in position and is a form of endocardial cushion defect. May be asymptomatic. If presenting behaviors occur, they usually do so by the third decade of life. Ostium secundum type most common, twice as common in females. Left atrial pressure is higher than right. Left-to-right shunt may cause pulmonary artery hypertension. If associated with cyanotic defects such as transposition, this defect may be life-saving.
Ventricular septal defect (VSD) 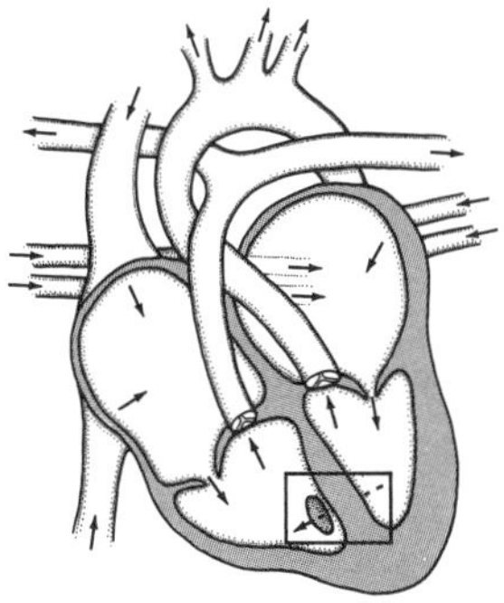	Abnormal opening in ventricular septum (usually membranous area), allowing shunting of blood between left and right ventricles. Blood usually shunts left to right due to less resistance in the pulmonary vascular bed than systemic arteries. The shunt causes an increased pulmonary blood flow. Simple ventricular septal defect most common More than 50% of small defects may close spontaneously. Closure usually occurs in the first 6 months of life. May be life-saving when associated with other defects. Mortality from a large VSD is highest during the first year of life due to cardiac failure.

Behavioral assessment	Diagnostic criteria	Medical therapy
Clinical findings and clinical course are dependent on degree of pulmonary hypertension and size of shunt. Characteristic machinery murmur maximal at second intercostal space and left sternal border and below left clavicle. Bounding pulses; pulse pressure is widened. Normal first heart sound; second sound is narrowly split.	X-ray findings negative with small shunts; left atrial and left ventricular enlargement with large shunts. ECG may be normal or may indicate left ventricular hypertrophy with large shunt. Evidence of increased oxygen saturation at the level of the pulmonary artery on cardiac catheterization.	Surgical correction is recommended, except in patients with pulmonary vascular obstruction. Patients with pulmonary hypertension and large left-to-right shunts should have surgery early (before 1 year of age). Simple patent ductus should be corrected after the child reaches 1 year of age. Indomethacin has proven successful in closing patent ductus in low-birth-weight infants.
If symptomatic, easy fatigability with severe murmurs Congestive heart failure uncommon. Pulmonary systemic ejection murmur heard best at the second left intercostal space, wide split second heart sound. Middiastolic murmur may be present. Arterial pulses are normal and equal. Atrial arrhythmias may result from right atrial overload.	Chest x-ray usually demonstrates slight cardiac enlargement. ECG may be normal or may indicate right ventricular hypertrophy. Echocardiography reveals two features: abnormal motion of right ventricular wall and ilation of the right ventricle. Cardiac catheterization reveals increased oxygen saturation at the atrial level.	Generally, defects do not require surgery early. Large defects are usually repaired before the child enters school. Surgical correction is direct closure of the defect with a dacron patch.

Continued

Table 17-5 Continued

Behavioral assessment	Diagnostic criteria	Medical therapy
Small left-to-right shunt usually asymptomatic. Child may have frequent respiratory infections in infancy and childhood. Large left-to-right shunts usually cause behaviors of dyspnea, poor weight gain, exercise intolerance, frequent respiratory infections. Congestive failure may develop in the first 6 months of life. Typical murmur is harsh and pansystolic, best heard at left sternal border in 3rd and 4th intercostal space.	X-ray and ECG findings normal with small defects X-ray findings with large defects demonstrate cardiac enlargement and increased pulmonary vasculature. ECG findings with large defects indicate combined ventricular hypertrophy.	Treatment by pulmonary artery banding may be performed to decrease pulmonary blood flow and relieve behaviors of congestive heart failure. Surgical repair is achieved through dacron-patch closure at defect. Age for elective surgery is becoming progressively earlier (usual range is 2 to 5 years) Pulmonary artery banding is generally being replaced by early total correction.

Defect	Pathophysiology
Pulmonary stenosis 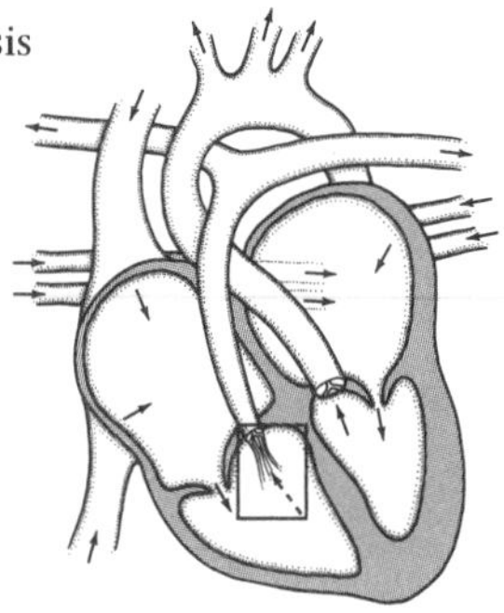	Cusps of pulmonary valve are fused to form a membrane with an opening in the center. Obstruction of blood flow across the pulmonary valve results in increased pressure developed by the right ventricle to maintain adequate output. Asymptomatic and acyanotic unless defect is severe Associated with maternal rubella Right ventricular pressure increases to overcome obstruction. Right atrial pressure increases, and finally systemic pressure rises. Right ventricular failure may result. In severe cases, a patent foramen ovale may persist.
Endocardial cushion defect	Results from incomplete fusion of membranous portion of ventricular septum, atrial septum, and leaflets of the tricuspid and mitral valves. Defect may be complete or incomplete. Complete form consists of a high ventricular defect and a low atrial defect continuous with the ventricular defect. A cleft is also present in both the septal leaflet of the tricuspid valve and the anterior leaflet of the mitral valve. The incomplete form involves as small atrial septal defect. Incomplete defect may present few problems. With severe defects, may develop congestive heart failure. Large defect allows blood flow between chambers of heart. First-degree heart blocks present in 50% of cases. High incidence of defect associated with Down's syndrome.
Aortic valvular stenosis 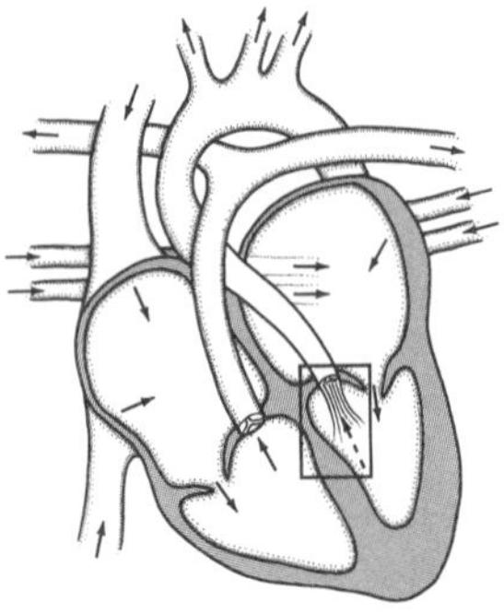	At valvular level may be caused by fusion of the valve cusps. The valve is frequently bicuspid rather than tricuspid and has thickened leaflets. Subaortic and supravalvular stenosis may also occur. Subvalvular obstruction may be due to fibrous ring or muscular obstruction below the aortic valve. Usually asymptomatic and acyanotic in infants and children. Severe obstruction causes increased left ventricular pressure to maintain aortic pressure. Left ventricular hypertrophy may result. Pulse pressure in the aorta is narrowed. More common in males

Table 17-5 **Continued**

Behavioral assessment	Diagnostic criteria	Medical therapy
Progressive cyanosis Easy fatigability Dyspnea on exertion Systolic ejection murmur associated with a thrill heard best at left sternal border.	X-ray findings in mild forms indicate normal heart. In moderate to severe cases, cardiac enlargement and decreased perfusion to the pulmonary vasculature may occur. ECG indicates varying degrees of right ventricular hypertrophy.	Surgical correction is recommended immediately for all children who have right ventricular pressure equal to or greater than systemic pressure or who have cyanosis. Valvotomy is performed for a valvular obstruction. Elective surgery is usually performed by 2 to 3 years of age.
In severe cases, chronic congestive heart failure, growth failure, and persistent respiratory infections may occur; a systolic thrill may be palpated. A loud, hard holosystolic murmur is heard best at the lower left sternal border. Diastolic flow murmur heard at the apex and lower left sternal border. Cyanosis may be present in severe cases and with predominant right-to-left shunts.	X-ray may reveal enlarged heart with increased pulmonary vascular markings. ECG shows left axis deviation and ventricular hypertrophy:	Corrective surgery involves patch closure of septal defect, and mitral and tricuspid valve repair. Surgery for incomplete forms has significantly higher mortality. Complete correction is advised in first year of life before irreversible behaviors occur. Primary repair is performed on children who have intractable heart failure or severe pulmonary hypertension.
If symptomatic, mild exercise intolerance Easy fatigability A prominent aortic ejection click Systolic ejection murmur with a thrill felt at the second right intercostal space.	Chest x-ray frequently shcws a normal heart. Dilation of ascending aorta may be seen with subvalvular aortic stenosis. ECG may be normal, even with severe obstruction. Left ventricular hypertrophy may be present. Cardiac catheterization demonstrates pressure differential between left ventricle and aorta.	Major criterion for considering surgery is a large resting pressure gradient of 60–80 mm Hg. Surgery frequently unsuccessful. Aortic insufficiency may result from repair. Surgical outcome is better for discrete subvalvular disease. Close follow-up and limitation of exertion are necessary for nonsurgical management.

Defect	Pathophysiology
Coarctation of the aorta 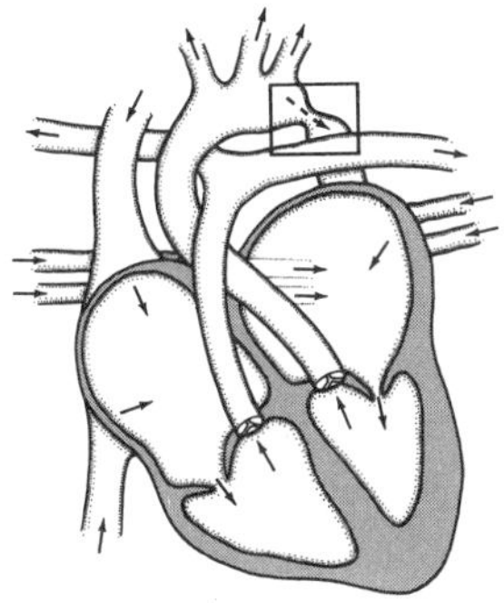	Constriction of aorta, occurring most frequently in thoracic portion of descending aorta Commonly classified as pre- or postductal; may, however, be juxtaductal. Usually associated with other anomalies, such as patent ductus arteriosus, ventricular septal defect, and bicuspid aortic valve

Behavioral assessment	Diagnostic criteria	Medical therapy
Hypertension Bounding pulses proximal to defect; weak or absent pulses distal to defect (femoral pulses) Stenotic murmur across the back	X-ray findings indicate left ventricular enlargement. Ascending aorta is usually normal in size. ECG may show evidence of slight left ventricular hypertrophy.	Infants with severe coarctation require measures to correct congestive heart failure. Surgical resection and end-to-end anastomosis of uncomplicated juxtaductal coarctation can be accomplished with excellent results.

Continued

Table 17-5 Continued

Behavioral assessment	Diagnostic criteria	Medical therapy
Systolic ejection murmur heard best at aortic area and lower left sternal border. Dizziness, fainting, headache, decreased exercise tolerance, easy fatigability Increased pallor and cool lower extremity on manual compression Behaviors of this defect usually occur in either early infancy or adulthood.	Infants with marked congestive failure indicate marked cardiac enlargement with right ventricular hypertrophy. Cardiac catheterization demonstrates severity, degree, and location of coarctation.	Asymptomatic children may have surgery delayed until 4 to 6 years of age.

Table 17-6 Findings and Medical Management of Cyanotic Congenital Heart Defects

Defect	Pathophysiology
Tetralogy of Fallot 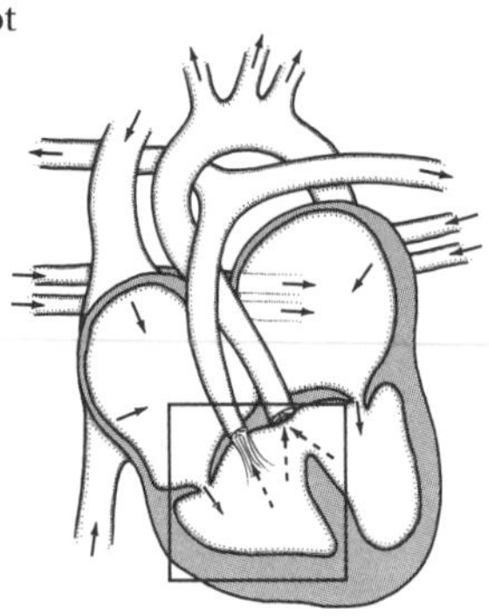	Consists of four anatomic abnormalities: ventricular septal defect, overriding aorta, pulmonary stenosis (right ventricular outflow obstruction), and right ventricular hypertrophy. Right-to-left shunting of blood results from severe right ventricle outflow obstruction and large ventricular septal defect. Unoxygenated blood shunted through ventricular septal defect. Partially oxygenated blood is pumped to systemic circulation. Most common cyanotic defect

Behavioral assessment	Diagnostic criteria	Medical therapy
Cyanosis (determined by size of defect and amount of outflow obstruction) Clubbing of nailbeds in older infants and children Dyspnea and easy fatigability Delayed growth and development Feeding problems Hypoxic spells Knee-chest position or squatting to relieve respiratory distress Rough, ejection type systolic murmur, best heard at left sternal border, 3rd intercostal space. Murmur radiates over anterior and posterior lung fields.	Chest x-ray usually reveals boot-shaped heart; aorta often on right; right ventricle may be hypertrophied. Pulmonary vascular markings are usually decreased. ECG indicates right ventricular hypertrophy. Cardiac catheterization demonstrates a right-to-left shunt at ventricular level.	Immediate palliative surgery is required for the cyanotic infant. Surgery may be postponed for infants who have minimal behaviors of distress. Most common palliative surgery is joining of right pulmonary artery to right subclavian artery (Blalock-Taussig). Waterston anastomosis is less frequently used. Procedure is an anastomosis between right pulmonary artery and ascending aorta. A third procedure involves an anastomosis between ascending aorta and main pulmonary artery. Palliative procedures are performed to reduce hypoxemia and reduced pulmonary blood flow. Total correction is recommended for nearly all patients. Total correction is achieved by relieving the pulmonary stenosis and patching the septal defect. Cardiopulmonary bypass under deep hypothermia is used for infants; heart/lung bypass in older children. Early repair, even in infancy, is advocated in most cardiovascular centers.

Table 17-6 **Continued**

Defect		Pathophysiology
Tricuspid atresia	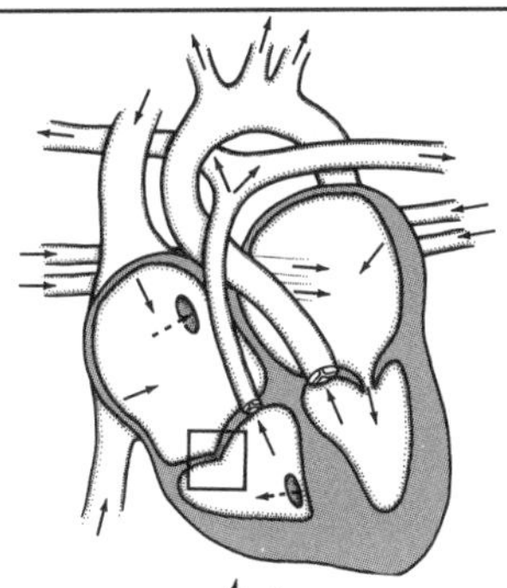	Tricuspid valve fails to form. No direct communication exists between right atrium and right ventricle. The two types are those with normally related great arteries and those with transposition of the great vessels. Right-to-left shunting occurs through a stretched foramen ovale into the left heart. Pulmonary blood flows through a left-to-right shunt at ventricular level. Relatively rare; often associated with other cardiovascular defects, such as ventricular septal defect
Transposition of the great vessels	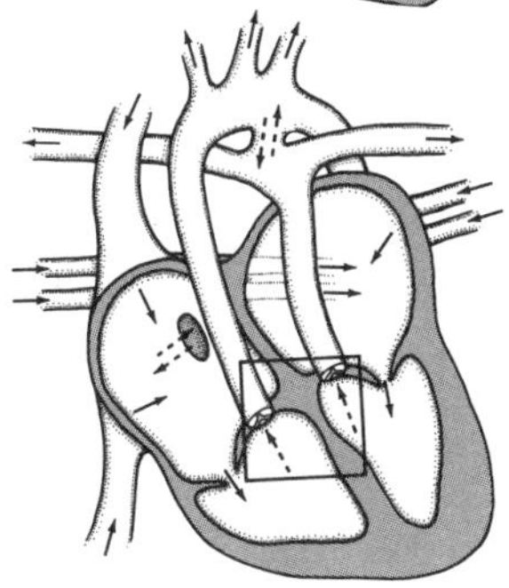	Pulmonary artery leaves the left ventricle, and aorta leaves the right ventricle. Oxygenated blood flows through left heart and is recirculated through lungs. Unoxygenated blood flows through right heart into aorta and through the systemic circulation. Second most common cyanotic defect Male-female ratio 3:1 May be associated with life-saving defects, ventricular septal defect, patent ductus, and artial septal defect. Newborns are often large for gestational age. May have family history of diabetes.
Truncus arteriosus	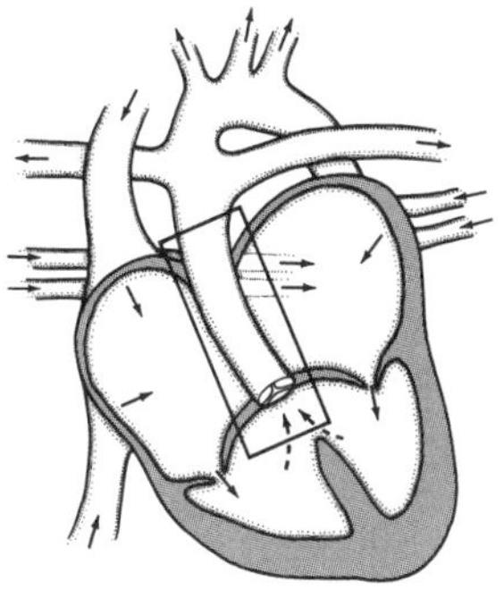	A great vessel arises from the heart supplying both pulmonary and systemic circulations. A high ventricular septal defect is always present. Valve leaflets usually number from 2 to 6. Clinical picture depends on the degree of pulmonary blood flow. Pulmonary vascular obstruction does not usually become restrictive until 1 to 2 years of age. Early development of pulmonary vascular obstructive disease is responsible for a poor prognosis in truncus arteriosus.

Behavioral assessment	Diagnostic criteria	Medical therapy
Severe cyanosis from diminished pulmonary flow Congestive heart failure may occur if ventricular septal defect is large. Delayed growth and development Easy fatigability on feeding Tachypnea, dyspnea, and hypoxic spells Clubbing may be present in older children. Harsh, blowing murmur best heard at left sternal border.	X-ray findings indicate diminished pulmonary vascular markings and a right atrium varying in size from huge to moderately enlarged. ECG findings of left axis deviation, right atrial enlargement, and left ventricular hypertrophy suggest tricuspid atresia in a cyanotic infant.	A palliative shunting procedure may be done in the neonatal period—Blalock-Hanlon septectomy or anastomosis of the superior vena cava to right pulmonary artery. Functional correction has been accomplished by insertion of a prosthetic conduit with a valve between right atrium and pulmonary artery. Closure of the interatrial communication (Fontan procedure) With appropriate palliative surgery in early life, approximately half of patients survive to first decade. Candidates for corrective surgery must have normal pulmonary vascular pressure and a mean pulmonary artery pressure less than 20 mm Hg, adequate left ventricular function, and pulmonary arteries of near-normal size.

Continued

Behavioral assessment	Diagnostic criteria	Medical therapy
Cyanosis (minimal with large PDA and VSD) Retarded growth and development after neonatal period Congestive heart failure, dyspnea, and hypoxia are the major complications. Murmur usually not a significant finding unless large ventricular defect is present.	Chest x-ray demonstrates cardiac enlargement with increased pulmonary vasculature. ECG findings include right atrial enlargement and right ventricular hypertrophy.	Palliative procedures are usually performed to create interatrial mixing of blood. Common procedures are Blalock-Hanlon (surgical creation of an atrial septal defect); balloon septostomy (passing a balloon catheter through the foramen ovale, inflating the balloon, and withdrawing it to rupture the atrial septum); pulmonary artery banding, and creation of a ductus arteriosus if pulmonic stenosis is present. Complete repair is done by performing a Mustard procedure. This physiologically corrects the defect by rerouting systemic and pulmonary venous return to heart with a pericardial intraatrial baffle.
Congestive heart failure and poor physical development occur early in infancy. Mild cyanosis becoming progressively more severe with age Harsh systolic murmur and low-pitched, rumbling middiastolic murmur and bounding pulses are usually present.	X-ray findings indicate gross cardiomegaly, with left or combined ventricular enlargement. Main pulmonary artery segment may be small or absent. Left ventricular hypertrophy, alone or in combination with right ventricular hypertrophy, is usually present on ECG.	A palliative procedure of surgical banding of one or both pulmonary arteries is usually performed to reduce blood flow to lungs. A corrective procedure is usually performed before 1 or 2 years of age. The procedure consists of closing the ventricular septal defect using a valve-containing prosthetic conduit to establish communication between right ventricle and pulmonary arteries.

Defect	Pathophysiology
Total anomalous pulmonary venous return 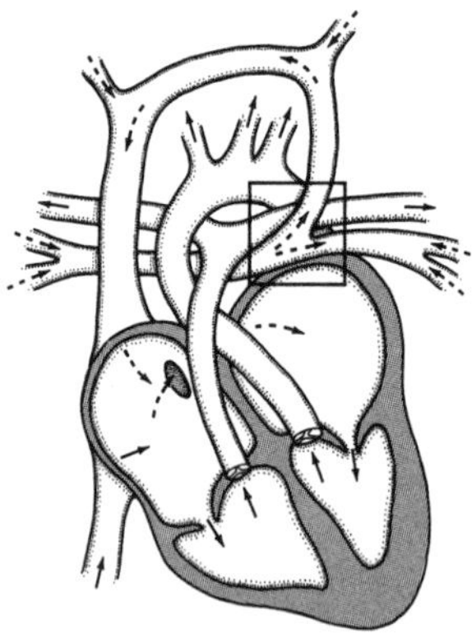	Total venous drainage empties into right atrium via a systemic venous connection. Malformation is classified by site of entry of pulmonary veins into right atrium: *Type 1* Left superior vena cava is point of entry (43%) or right superior vena cava is the point of entry (12%). *Type 2* Right atrium or coronary sinus is point of entry. *Type 3* Portal vein is usually point of entry. *Type 4* Multiple entry points Oxygen saturation is determined by ratio of systemic blood flow to pulmonary blood flow. If pulmonary vascular resistance is normal, pulmonary artery blood flow is greater than blood entering left side of the heart. Pulmonary return is increased with high O_2 saturation within the right atrium. If pulmonary vascular resistance is increased, ratio of pulmonary to systemic blood flow is lower. When equal amounts of blood flow in both directions, marked O_2 desaturation of blood occurs and child is extremely cyanotic. Defect is rare, accounting for 2% of all malformations. Right-to-left shunt is always present at the atrial level. Half of the infants with increased vascular resistance die by 6 months of age. High mortality due to congestive heart failure Children who survive beyond 2 years of age do not have pulmonary arterial hypertension.

Table 17-6 **Continued**

Defect	Pathophysiology
Hypoplastic left heart	Underdevelopment of the left heart Anomalies include underdeveloped left atrium and ventricle, stenosis or atresia of aortic or mitral orifices, and hypoplasia of ascending aorta. Following birth, there is marked impairment of circulation due to small left ventricle and obstructive lesions. Congestive heart failure usually occurs by first week of life.

Behavioral assessment	Diagnostic criteria	Medical therapy
Normal pulmonary vascular resistance: Majority of patients have an increased pulmonary blood flow. Mild cyanosis in early life Respiratory infections occur frequently. Growth failure may occur. Right ventricular heaving pulse may be present. Third and fourth heart sound may be heard. A systolic murmur is heard in the pulmonary area. A middiastolic flow murmur may be heard at the lower left sternal border. *Increased vascular resistance:* Cyanosis usually present at birth—pronounced by 1 week of age. Tachypneas is an early presenting behavior. Congestive heart failure may develop later in life. A very noticeable right ventricular point of maximum impulse is present. A systolic murmur grade I–IV/V is heard over the pulmonary area. Diastolic murmurs are uncommon.	*Normal vascular resistance:* Chest x-ray reveals cardiac enlargement. Pulmonary vascular markings are increased. ECG reveals right axis deviation with hypertrophy of right and left ventricle. *Increased vascular resistance:* Chest x-ray reveals marked pulmonary venous congestion with a small heart. ECG shows right atrial and right ventricle hypertrophy. Cardiac catheterization is diagnostic and confirms the presence of the defect along with associated features.	Atrial balloon septostomy should be performed at initial diagnostic cardiac catheterization, if immediate surgical correction is not contemplated. Surgical treatment during cardiopulmonary bypass involves anastomosing common pulmonary trunk to left atrium. The atrial septal defect is usually closed, and the systemic venous circuit eliminated. Surgical results have improved, even with symptomatic infants. The prognosis appears to be excellent if postoperative hemodynamics are normal.
Clinical picture depends on type of obstructive lesions. Dyspnea and hepatomegaly are usually present. Peripheral pulses are weak. A right ventricular lift is present due to cardiac enlargement. Murmurs, if present, are short and midsystolic. Cyanosis is usually present and visible early in life.	Chest x-ray may be normal at birth with rapid and progressive cardiac enlargement associated with pulmonary venous congestion. ECG frequently indicates right axis deviation and right ventricular hypertrophy with absence of left ventricular forces.	Therapy is symptomatic. Most patients die in first few weeks of life. Surgical procedures have been attempted to decompress left atrium by septectomy, creation of a systemic-pulmonary shunt, and banding of both pulmonary arteries. Heart transplant is becoming an increasingly viable option. The mortality associated with these procedures is high, and long-term prognosis is not known.

Source: From J. Servonsky and S. Opas. *Nursing Management of Children.* Boston: Little, Brown, 1987.

common finding, especially in African-American infants. These hernias vary in size from a few millimeters to 3 cm; however, any hernia that grows in size after 1 month should be referred and further evaluated.

The nurse should auscultate the abdomen with a stethoscope before palpating and percussing to prevent distorting the bowel sounds. During auscultation, the presence of bowel sounds should be verified. The nurse should also listen for vascular sounds in the abdomen. Venous hums may be found in cases of congenital problems in the portal system or in hemangiomas of the liver.

Palpation of the newborn's abdomen begins by assessing the skin for turgor. All four quadrants of the abdomen should be palpated lightly, then more deeply progressing to deep palpation for the purpose of specific organ identification. The liver edge is normally palpated 102 cm below the right costal margin; the border of the spleen is usually felt 1 to 2 cm below the right costal margin; the border of the spleen is usually felt 102 cm below the left costal marking. During deep palpation, the nurse should not feel any areas of weakness or muscle herniation; in addition, no tenderness should be apparent. The kidneys are able to be felt using deep palpation techniques. The lower pole of the right kidney can usually be felt. Because the left kidney is obliterated by the intestine and is also normally positioned higher in the abdomen, it is not as commonly palpable. Kidney size should be noted. The umbilical ring should be palpated. Generally, rings greater than 2 cm in diameter will not close spontaneously. Diastasis recti abdominis is palpated as a wide separation between the two rectus muscles and is a common finding in the African-American population.

Finally, the abdomen should be percussed to determine tympany and to confirm the presence and location of the liver, spleen, and the superior margin of the bladder.

ASSESSMENT OF THE GENITALS AND RECTUM

The newborn's genitals typically appear large in relationship to the rest of the body. Some edema of the genitals may be present in breech-birth infants. Genital development is a criterion used to determine gestational age (see Fig. 17-2).

Male Genitals

The size of the genitals varies in newborn male infants. Commonly, the penis is between 2 and 3 cm and the testes are between 1 and 2 cm. The foreskin should be retracted to visualize the urinary meatus and its placement on the glans. If the prepuce adheres to the glans, the end of the prepuce should be peeled back to ascertain the position of

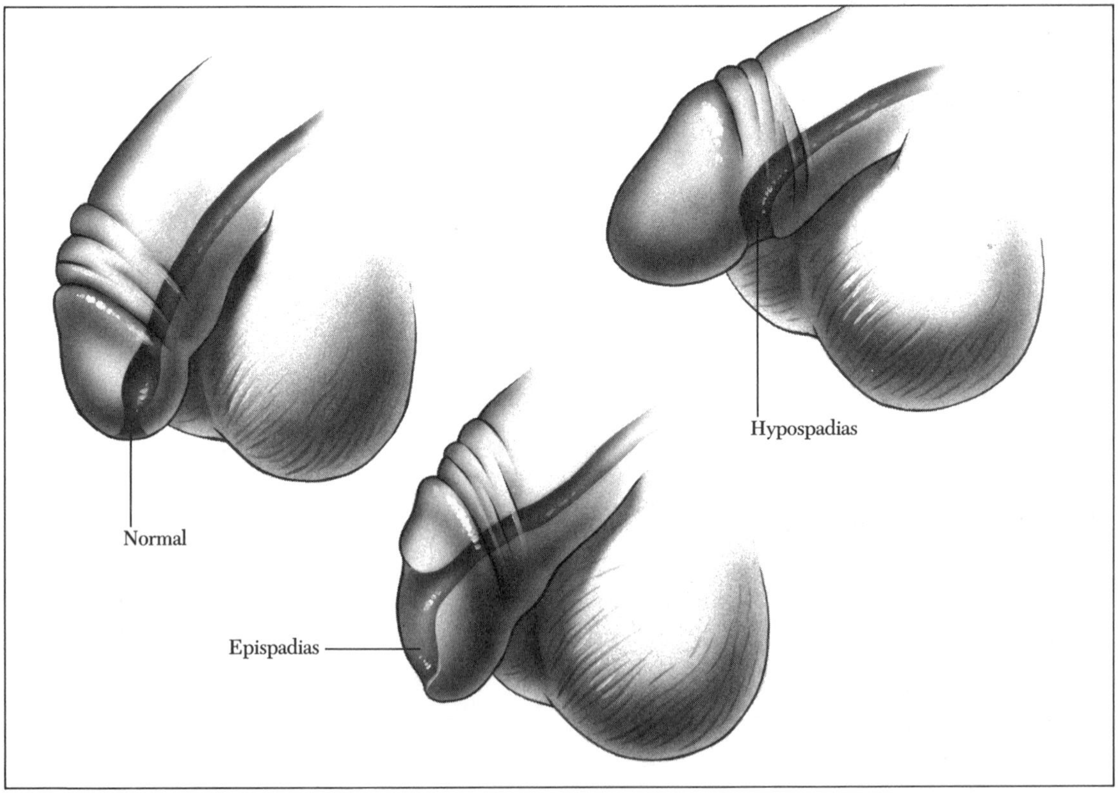

Figure 17-28 Three types of meatal openings: normal, hypospadias, and epispadias.

the urinary meatus. The meatus should appear as a slit centrally located on the glans. In epispadias, the urinary meatus is located on the dorsal side of the penis, and in hypospadias, the opening is found ventrally at the junction of the glans and the penile shaft (Fig. 17-28). Both conditions should be referred because surgical intervention is usually necessary. Phimosis, or a pinpoint opening of the urinary meatus, should also be referred. There should be no discharge from the urinary meatus.

Normally, the scrotum is slightly asymmetrical, with the left side appearing slightly larger than the right. The nurse should note the development of rugae on the scrotal sac and palpate both testes to confirm that they are descended. It is helpful to palpate using one hand to block the inguinal canal, which prevents the testes from slipping upward as the other hand palpates. *Cryptorchidism* is a term used to describe undescended testicles. The condition should be referred immediately. Hydrocele, whether unilateral or bilateral, usually disappears spontaneously and is insignificant.

Female Genitals

The nurse should inspect the female genitals for the presence of the gross structures. The labia majora and labia minora are often enlarged. In fact, the labia minora may be so prominent that they protrude over the labia majora. The urethral and vaginal openings are often obliterated by edema of the labia. Smegma and vaginal secretions are routinely present and are often blood-tinged in response to the withdrawals of maternal hormone. A mucoid vaginal discharge is often commonly present for about 7 to 10 days.

Anus

The nurse's finger-cotted little finger may be inserted into the anus to verify patency. Patency can also be determined by the presence of meconium or stool on a rectal thermometer. There should be no evidence of anal fissures, bleeding, or imperforate anus.

ASSESSMENT OF THE EXTREMITIES

The nurse should inspect the infant, confirming that no gross abnormalities exist and verifying that all body parts are present, intact, and symmetrically aligned. The infant generally assumes a flexed resting position, and the nurse can conduct full passive range of motion to determine the mobility of the extremities. Any paralysis of limitation of range of motion of an upper extremity may be due to a fractured clavicle, brachial or cervical plexus injury, or fracture of one of the long bones of the arm. Polydactyly is the presence of a supernumerary digit on the hand or foot. This is a common finding, and the digit is usually rudimentary. Syndactyly is an absence of a digit on the hand or foot.

Spine

The spinal curve is convex in the newborn, and as head control is gained, a cervical curve gradually develops.

Upper Extremities

The nurse may test muscle tone by unflexing the newborn's arm for about 5 seconds. When the arm is released, it should return to the flexed position immediately. This finding would suggest normal muscle tone. The length of the arms can be evaluated by holding the infant's arm down parallel with the thigh. If the arms appear to be unusually short, the existence of achondroplastic dwarfism may be indicated.

The hands should be inspected. Infants who have webbing between the fingers, an unusual curve and shortness of the little finger, and a simian crease may be suspected of having Down's syndrome. The range of motion of the wrist should be assessed. The radial pulses should be palpated and compared. The entire extremity should be palpated to rule out any fractures of the bones. The scarf sign may also be conducted as a test for gestational age (see Fig. 17-2). Shoulder muscle strength is assessed by lifting the infant under the arms. The infant should be able to maintain this position and not slip through the nurse's hands.

Lower Extremities

On inspection of the lower extremities, a mild degree of bowing or medial rotation is common. After a frank breech presentation, the lower extremities tend to be abducted and externally rotated; therefore, only gross abnormalities of the lower extremities are able to be confirmed immediately after birth.

The hip joint should be evaluated to determine whether it is intact. The nurse should inspect the anterior and posterior thighs for symmetry of medial skinfolds. The gluteal folds should also be even and bilaterally symmetrical. The nurse should perform the Ortolani maneuver by placing the index and middle fingers under the hip joints and laterally abducting and flexing the hips (Fig. 17-29). Normal range of motion is approximately 160 to 170 degrees in flexion and extension. When flexed at the hip, the thighs should abduct to an angle of 160 degrees between them. There should be no click or feeling of the hip joint slipping due to the head of the femur striking the acetabulum ridge. If such a click is noted, it should be referred and reported immediately, and the Ortolani maneuver should not be repeated, because subsequent motion will serve to further weaken and damage the hip joint.

The knee joint should be flexed and extended to verify range of motion. The legs should be aligned and inspected for an increased degree of bowing, which is termed *tibial torsion.*

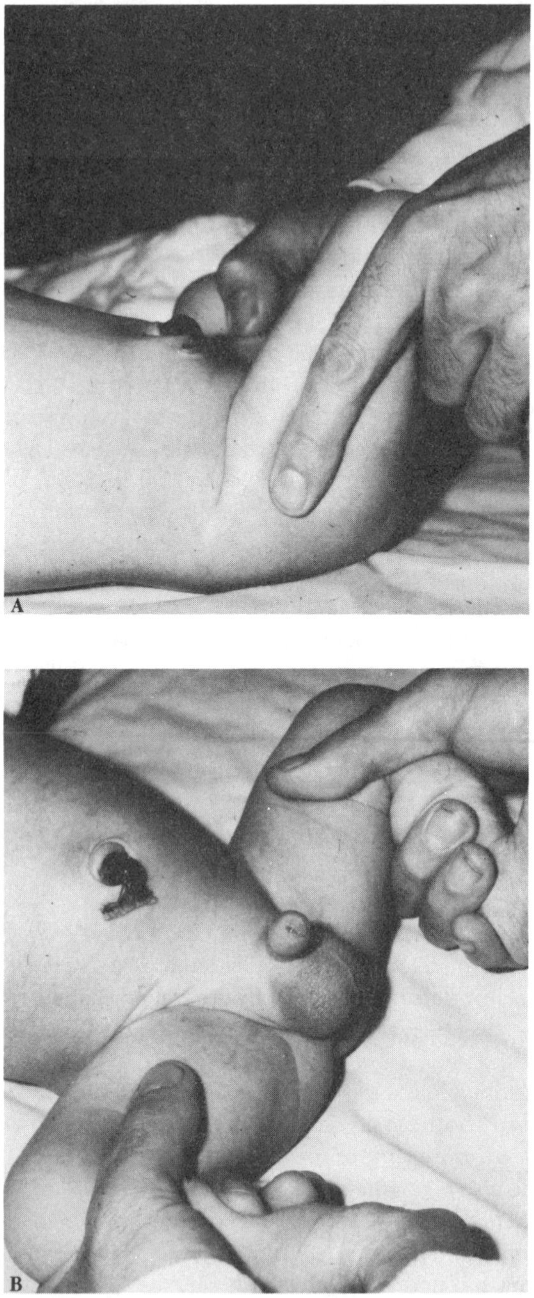

Figure 17-29 Method of inducing Ortolani's sign. **(A)** With the infant's knees bent, hips flexed to 90 degrees, the examiner's fingers are placed over the femoral head, exerting pressure downward. **(B)** The thighs are then fully abducted to induce the characteristic "click."

Foot position should be evaluated. The intrauterine position of the infant may have caused the feet to turn inward (varus). If the foot can be turned passively in the opposite direction without forceful manual stretching, this finding is usually transient and insignificant. Putting the ankle through range of motion determines the flexibility of the heel cords. Normally, 120 degrees of motion between flexion and extension is apparent. Any evidence of clubfoot (talipes equinovarus) should be referred promptly. Clubfoot is a relatively common deformity, which usually involves plantar flexion, inversion, and adduction. Angle clonus may be tested by sharply dorsiflexing the foot. One or two clonic beats are normal; however, any evidence of clonic movement should be referred.

ASSESSMENT OF THE NEUROLOGIC SYSTEM

Neurologic assessment of the newborn aims to determine the general integrity of the central nervous system (CNS). The CNS develops more rapidly than any other body system during the first year (Fig. 17-30). Many of the reflexive behaviors tested are present only during the first weeks of life. Persistence beyond the normal time may be a signal of CNS disease and should be referred, although many reflexes are variable and their significance is uncertain. The nurse should observe the infant's reflex pattern and development, motor skill development, and socialization development. Table 17-7 lists normal newborn reflexive patterns along with typical ages of onset and disappearance.

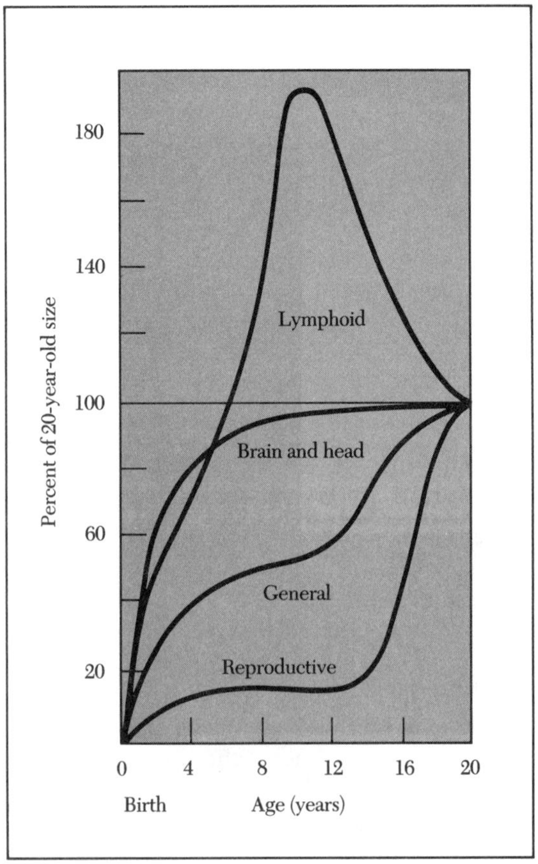

Figure 17-30 Growth patterns of various systems.

Table 17-7 Newborn Reflexes

Reflex	Stimulus	Normal response	Age of appearance/ disappearance	Comments
		Eyes		
Optical blink reflex	Shine penlight into infant's eyes.	Bilateral eyelid closure	Persists throughout life	Absence or unilateral blink may indicate cranial nerve III, IV, and/or VI damage.
Acoustic blink reflex	Clap hands next to infant's ear.	Bilateral eyelid closure	Persists throughout life	Absence may indicate acoustic nerve damage.
Pupillary reflex	Shine penlight into infant's eyes.	Pupillary constriction	Persists throughout life	Any asymmetrical response or evidence of fixed or dilated pupils may indicate cranial nerve II, III, IV, or VI damage.
Glabella reflex	Tap index finger on bridge of infant's nose.	Symmetrical eyelid closure	Persists throughout life	Absence may indicate cranial nerve III, IV, and/or VI damage.
		Mouth and throat		
Sucking reflex	Stroke infant's lips; place clean finger in infant's mouth.	Strong sucking movement; tongue pushes finger up and back.	Present at birth; diminishes by 3–4 months; disappears by 12 months	Absence is a strong indicator of possible brain damage.
Rooting reflex	Stroke infant's upper or lower lip or lateral aspect of lips.	Face turns toward the stimulus and mouth opens.	Present at birth; disappears by 3–4 months when awake; disappears by 7–8 months when asleep	Absence may be due to cranial nerve V damage.
Extrusion reflex	Touch infant's tongue.	Tongue thrusts outward.	Present at birth; disappears at 2–4 months	A continuous tongue protrusion may indicate Down's syndrome or macroglossia.
Gag reflex	Stimulate posterior pharynx with tongue blade.	Gag	Persists throughout life	Absence may indicate cranial nerve IX or X damage.
Swallowing reflex	Place an object on posterior tongue.	Swallow	Persists throughout life	Absence may indicate cranial nerve IX or X damage.
		Extremities		
Palmar grasp reflex	Place index finger in infant's palm from ulnar side.	Infant grasps finger and forcefully holds.	Present from birth until about 3–4 months; replaced by voluntary grasping	Any asymmetry of response may indicate a neurologic problem.
Plantar grasp reflex	Touch sole of infant's foot.	Plantar flexion of toes	Present from birth until 8–10 months	Absence may indicate defect of lower spinal column.
Babinski reflex	Stroke lateral surface of infant's sole beginning at heel and moving in a curve to great toe.	Fanning of toes; dorsiflexion of great toe	Present from birth until about 18 months	Absent response may indicate lower spinal cord defect; unilateral absence may be due to peripheral nerve damage on affected side.
Moro reflex (startle response)	May be elicited by jarring the infant's bed, using an auditory stimulus (loud hand clap, bell), or suddenly dropping infant's head (loss of equilibrium)	Extension of trunk and extension and abduction of limbs; also, extension of fingers followed by flexion and adduction of the limbs	Present from birth until about 1–4 months	Asymmetry of response may indicate fracture of clavicle or injury to brachial plexus. Consistent absence before 1–4 months may be due to brain damage.

Continued

Table 17-7 Continued

Reflex	Stimulus	Normal response	Age of appearance/ disappearance	Comments
		Extremities (continued)		
Parachute	Lower infant in prone position quickly downward.	Infant will extend arms, hands, and fingers out as if trying to break the fall.	Begins 7–9 months; persists	Absence is significant of CNS defect.
Tonic neck reflex	Rotate infant's head to one side in prone or supine position.	Arm and leg on same side as head is turned will extend; opposite arm and leg will flex; classic "fencer" position.	Appears at birth to 2 months and disappears at 4–6 months	Asymmetry may indicate cerebral lesion. Many normal infants never exhibit this response.
Trunk incurvation reflex (Galant's reflex)	Stroke dorsal skin along vertebral column from shoulders to buttocks using a sharp object (infant should be lying in a symmetrical, prone position).	Trunk curves toward side stimulated	Easily elicited at 3–6 days of age; disappears at 2 months	Absence may indicate spinal cord damage (T2 to S1).
Placing reflex	Hold infant upright with dorsum of one foot gently touching underside of a surface (table, shelf).	Knees and hips flex; stimulated foot should rise and be placed on surface.	Present from birth until about 6 weeks	May be difficult to elicit during first 4 days.
Step-in-place/ stepping reflex	Hold infant upright with feet flat on table.	Infant will demonstrate alternating stepping movements.	Easily elicited at 3–4 days; diminishes at 2–3 months; disappears at 7–8 months	Asymmetry may indicate neurologic abnormality. Some breech infants will not exhibit this reflex.
Landau	Hold infant in prone position and flex head downward.	Legs will flex.	Elicited at 3–12 months; disappears at 2 years	Absence is significant of CNS defect.

MENTAL ASSESSMENT

The newborn should appear quiet and content. A fretful or tense appearance is not typical.

Speech

The infant's basic verbal communication with the environment is the cry. The cry may normally be loud and even sound rather angry; however, a high-pitched, shrill cry should be noted and referred.

Cranial Nerves

Some cranial nerves can be tested indirectly by observation of the newborn's functioning. Cranial nerves III, IV, and VI can be assessed by observing the infant's ability to visually follow an object a short distance. Any total nonrecognition or absence of the blink reflex should be referred.

Cranial nerve V function can be demonstrated by observing the rooting reflex. This reflex is elicited by stroking the infant's upper or lower lips or the side of the cheek. The normal response is that the infant will turn his face toward the stimulus and open his mouth. This reflex is present at 32 gestational weeks and is fully developed by 34 gestational weeks. The rooting reflex tends to disappear by 3 to 4 months when the baby is awake, and by 7 to 8 months when the infant is asleep. It is important to note that this reflex may be depressed, especially after feeding. The rooting reflex also is somewhat less vigorous during the first 2 days of life.

The sucking reflex also indicates the integrity of cranial nerve V function. This reflex is vital to life, although it tends to be less intense during the first 3 to 4 days. The nurse can elicit the sucking reflex by stroking the lips. Complete evaluation of the suck can be made by placing the index finger in the infant's mouth and noting the action of the tongue, which should push the nurse's finger up and back. The rate, pressure, strength, and pattern of grouping of the suck should also be noted. The sucking reflex is normally strong at 32 weeks of gestation and is completely developed at 34 weeks. It tends to diminish by 3 to 4 months and gradually disappears by 12 months. It also is difficult to elicit in a recently fed baby. Absence of the sucking reflex is a strong indicator of possible brain damage.

Cranial nerve VIII function can be demonstrated by eliciting the startle, or Moro, reflex using an auditory stimulus. The nurse may ring a bell or clap her hands. A complete Moro reflex would include extension of the trunk and extension and abduction of the limbs. Extension of the fingers into a C formed by a thumb and index finger, followed by flexion and adduction of the limbs would also be present to constitute a complete reflex response (Fig. 17-31). The Moro reflex may also be elicited by any loss of equilibrium of the infant, as with sudden movement. However, when the establishment of disequilibrium is used as a stimulus, cranial nerve VIII function is not tested. The Moro reflex is typically present at 32 gestational weeks and tends to diminish and disappear between 1 and 4 months. A consistent absence before this time is a sign of possible brain damage. Unilateral absence of the Moro reflex may be due to brain damage, a fractured clavicle, or injury to the brachial plexus.

Cranial nerves IX and X can be tested by placing an object on the back of the tongue to assess the infant's swallowing reflex. This reflex is present at 34 to 36 gestational weeks and persists throughout life. The gag reflex is another indicator of cranial nerve IX and X function.

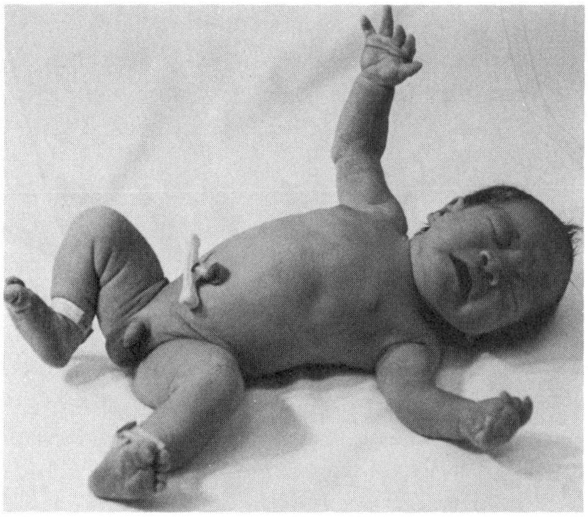

Figure 17-31 An infant demonstrating a Moro reflex.

Cerebellar Function

Cerebellar function, including proprioception, can be tested by observing the infant's spontaneous activity and noting symmetrical, smooth movements. The infant should also swallow easily. Sensory function is not normally tested in the newborn. Muscular tone and function can be assessed by inspecting the infant's resting position and using the pull-to-sit maneuver. Muscle tone should also be evaluated by holding the infant in a ventral position supporting the chest. A full-term infant should hold the head at 45-degree angle or less, exhibit a straight or slightly flexed back, flex the arms at the elbows, and partially extend at the shoulders and moderately flex the legs. Range of motion will also provide information as to motor function and muscle tone.

Other Reflexes

Deep tendon reflex testing is not usually done in the infant. Rather, a series of infant reflexes should be evaluated by the nurse. These include the optical and acoustic blink reflexes, which both result normally in eyelid closure but use different stimuli. In the optical blink reflex, a light source is used, but the acoustic blink reflex is elicited by using a loud clap or other sound stimulus. These reflexes might be difficult to elicit during the first days of life; however, if the infant is unable to demonstrate them after 203 days, the absence may indicate visual or auditory problems.

The glabella reflex is elicited by tapping on the bridge of the infant's nose. The normal response would be a symmetrical closing of the eyes.

The tonic neck reflex is an important one for the nurse to assess. The typical posture associated with this reflex consists of turning the face to one side with the jaw over one shoulder. The arm and leg on the jaw side will extend and the opposite arm and leg will flex, placing the infant in the classic "fencer" position (Fig. 17-32). The tonic neck, or fencing, reflex can be elicited by turning the infant's head. It usually appears from birth to 6 weeks and disappears at 4 to 6 months. Some normal infants never exhibit this response.

The palmar grasp reflex is tested by placing the nurse's finger in the palm of the infant's hand from the ulnar side. Typically, the infant will grasp the finger with her hand, and the grasp should be of sufficient strength that the nurse can lift the infant into a sitting position (Fig. 17-33). This reflex is present from birth until about 3 to 4 months of age and is then replaced by voluntary grasping.

The plantar grasp is elicited by touching an object to the sole of the infant's foot, resulting in flexion of the toes

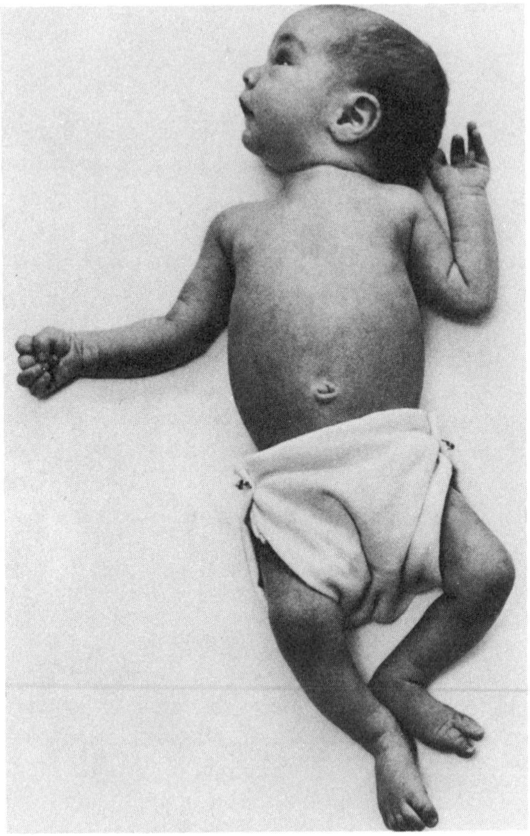

Figure 17-32 An infant displaying the tonic neck reflex.

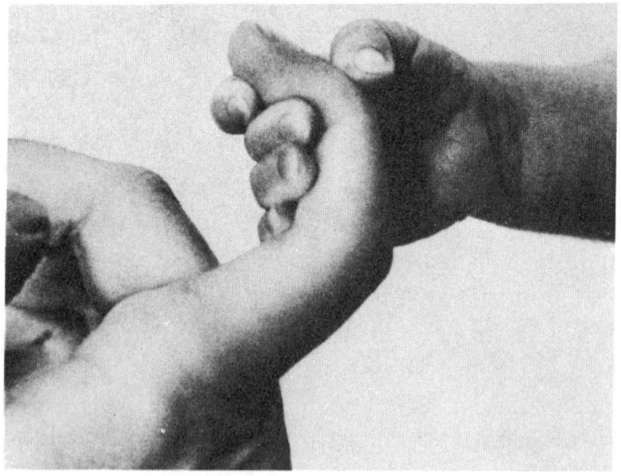

Figure 17-33 Palmar grasp reflex.

downward (Fig. 17-34). This reflex is normally present from birth to about 8 to 10 months.

The Babinski reflex is stimulated by stroking the lateral surface of the infant's sole, beginning at the heel and moving in a curve to the great toe. The normal infant response of fanning of the toes and dorsiflexion of the great toe is present

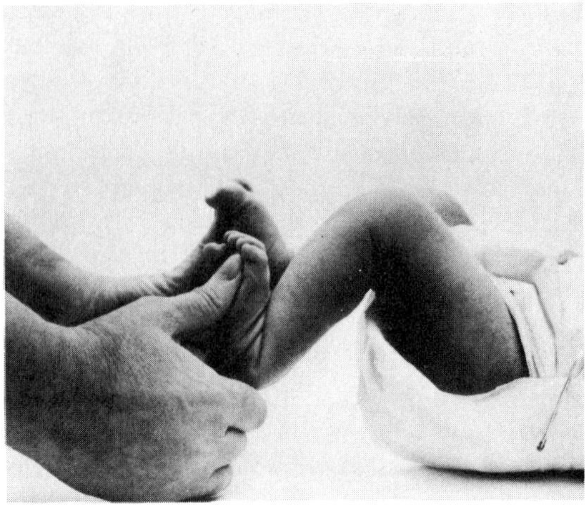

Figure 17-34

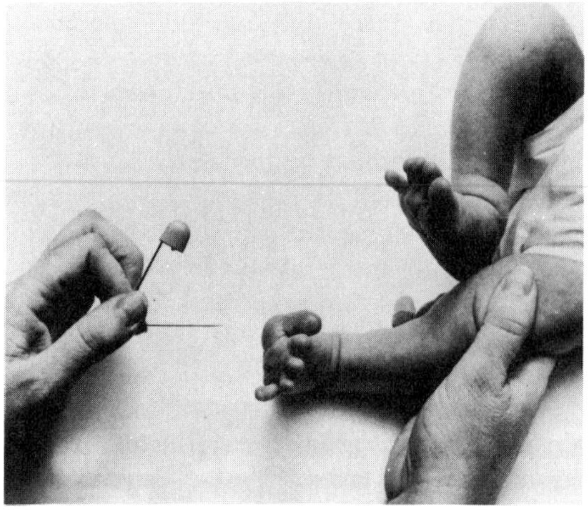

Figure 17-35 The Babinski reflex.

from birth to 18 months (Fig. 17-35). This is described as a positive response.

Galant's reflex, or the trunk incurvation reflex, is demonstrated by lightly scratching a pin or other sharp object from the shoulders to the buttocks parallel to the spinal cord at about 3 cm from midline. The trunk should curve toward the side stimulated. This reflex is easily elicited at about 5 to 6 days of age.

The placing reflex is elicited by holding the infant upright with the dorsum of one foot gently touching the table edge. The infant's knees and hips should flex, and the stimulated foot should rise and then come to rest on the table. This reflex may be difficult to elicit during the first 4 days. The step-in-place reflex is similar, but the baby is placed with feet flat on the table (Fig. 17-36). Normally, the infant will respond by demonstrating alternating stepping movements. This reflex is more difficult to elicit in the first 2 to 3 days and tends to fade at about 2 to 3 months. Some breech infants will not exhibit the stepping reflex.

Example of a Newborn History and Physical Examination

HEALTH HISTORY
Name: Megan M.
Address: 16 Clark Road, Amherst, New York
Sex: Female
Age: 2 days
Birthdate: 1/10/86
Race: Caucasian
Ethnic origin: Irish
Informant: Mother; reliable historian
History of present illness: Normal newborn assessment

Past History
Prenatal—Megan is the first child of Mr. and Mrs. M. Mother was in good general health throughout the pregnancy. Prenatal care was provided beginning in the first month through the ninth month by a private physician. Prenatal vitamin and iron supplement was taken as prescribed by the physician. No illnesses, infections, accidents, x-rays, or medications reported. Mother's blood type O+; father's blood type O+. A sonogram was done at 16 weeks to determine the EDC more exactly. Mother consumed a balanced diet; weight gain of 30 pounds. No alcohol, cigarette, or drug use. No previous abortions or miscarriages. Both parents were excited about this planned pregnancy.
Natal—Spontaneous rupture of amniotic membranes followed by a labor of 6½ hours. No anesthesia or medication. Father was present and coached throughout. Baby born at Sister's Hospital, Buffalo, New York. Gestational age 40 weeks. Vertex delivery. Length: 21″; weight: 7 lb 5 oz. Infant cried spontaneously. Apgar 8 and 10. No jaundice, cyanosis, or respiratory problems.
Postnatal—Infant placed in regular nursery. Breast-feeding successfully. Both parents very happy about and comfortable with baby.

Family History
Family members: Mother—29 years, good health; father—29 years, with seasonal allergies.
Family diseases—Denies history of diabetes, arthritis, TB, alcoholism, bleeding disorders, mental illness, stomach problems, liver disorders, hypertension, heart disease, kidney disease, birth defects, and infant deaths.
Family history significant for cancer and allergies.
Geographic exposure: not significant.

Review of Systems
Eyes, ears, nose, throat: No discharge, swelling, swallowing difficulties
Cardiorespiratory: No labored breathing, cyanosis
Gastrointestinal: No vomiting, diarrhea, constipation
Genitourinary: No irritation, rashes, discharge
Neurologic: No convulsions
Musculoskeletal: No dislocations, congenital malformations

Physical Assessment
General impression: Megan M. is a 2-day-old female, well developed, well nourished, and in no acute distress. No gross abnormalities.
Length—21″
Weight—7 lb 2 oz.
TPR—98.4F/136/38.
Integument: Color pink to reddish, somewhat mottled. No excoriations, fissures or lesions. No birthmarks evident. Numerous white papules over chin, nose, and forehead. Pale pink area over medial aspect of left eyelid that blanches with pressure. Finger and toe nails intact, pink in color. Fine, downy hair over the shoulders and back. Scalp hair fine, soft, and dark. Normal skin turgor.
Head, face and neck: Normocephalic, head circumference 35 cm. No molding apparent. Anterior fontanelle 2 cm × 2 cm. Unable to palpate posterior fontanelle. No bulging of fontanelles noted. Normal facial symmetry with full range of motion. Eyes, ears, and nose, symmetrically placed. Neck is symmetrical; no webbing. Full range of motion present. No apparent neck pulsations. Trachea at midline, thyroid not palpable.
Eyes: Normal alignment and position of eyes and eyebrows. Noted edema of eyelids. Palpebral fissures normal, no slanting noted. Sclerae white; corneas clear, shiny smooth, transparent. Lacrimal apparatus patent bilaterally. Corneal reflex intact. PERRL. Iris color slate gray. Blink response present. Hirschberg's test normal. No nystagmus. Bilateral red reflex present.
Ears: Symmetrically placed. Normal placement in relation to eyes. External ear canals pink. Startle reflex intact in response to sound stimulus.
Nose: Smooth, centrally placed. Nares patent bilaterally. No nasal flaring.
Mouth and throat: Lips are deep pink, symmetrically positioned. Inner lips and buccal mucosa pink. Tongue

pink and centrally located within the mouth. Hard and soft palates intact on palpation. Palatal arch normal. Sucking, rooting, gag, and extrusion reflexes intact.
Chest: Skin color pink. AP diameter = lateral diameter. Chest circumference 33 cm. No bulging or depression. Sternum straight, smooth. Clavicles smooth and straight, no fracture or dislocation. Nipples positioned symmetrically. No retractions. Vesicular breath sounds auscultated throughout. PMI palpated, normal heart sounds auscultated.
Abdomen: Cylindrical contour, no visible peristaltic waves. Umbilicus centrally located. Cord stump dry. No odor, discharge, or redness at stump site. Normal bowel sounds present. Liver edge palpable. Spleen not palpable. Lower pole of right kidney felt on deep palpation. General abdominal tympany.
Genitals and rectum: Labia majora and labia minora present, slightly enlarged. Urinary meatus patent. Vaginal meatus present.
Anus: Patent. No anal fissures or bleeding.
Extremities: Infant resting in a flexed position. All extremities present, intact, in appropriate alignment. No polydactyly or syndactyly. Complete range of motion of all extremities. Convex spinal configuration. Normal muscle tone in upper extremities. Lower extremities slightly bowed. Hip joints intact bilaterally. Foot position slightly inverted; able to passively straighten without force. No ankle clonus present.
Neurologic:
Speech—Cry loud and strong. No high-pitched or shrill sound.
Cranial nerves—III, IV, V, VIII, IX, and X intact. Rooting, sucking, startle, swallowing, and gag reflexes intact.
Cerebellar function—Movement is generally symmetrical and smooth. Normal muscle tone.
Other reflexive behaviors—Optical and acoustic blink, glabella, tonic neck, palmar and plantar grasp, Babinski, and placing reflexes present.

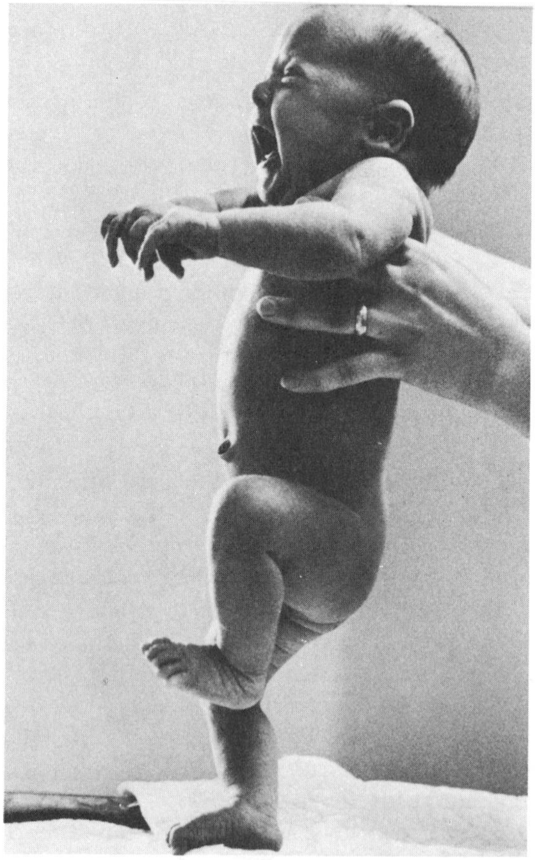

Figure 17-36 The step-in-place, or stepping, reflex.

SUMMARY

This chapter discussed the health assessment of the newborn infant, including the history. A complete newborn assessment comprises all aspects of physical assessment and provides the nurse with important baseline data about the infant's status. Many typical variations and conditions of the newborn were presented. The newborn assessment is a prime opportunity for the nurse to initiate rapport with the parents as well as to reassure and counsel the parents regarding any obvious deviations. The general techniques of physical assessment must be modified in many areas to apply to the newborn.

DISCUSSION QUESTIONS/ ACTIVITIES

1. Discuss the value of the newborn assessment in establishing rapport with the family.
2. Give the rationale behind having a flexible sequence of examination when doing a newborn assessment.
3. Collect a complete history on a newborn. What specific questions need to be answered?
4. What methods are utilized to assess gestational age?
5. What is the role of the nurse in counseling parents regarding birthmarks?
6. Name three types of birthmarks, and describe their characteristics and resolution.
7. Describe the resting position of a normal, full-term infant.

8. List three common birth-trauma–related head-shape deviations.
9. Describe the importance of infantile reflex testing as related to central nervous system function.
10. What symptomatology would lead the nurse to suspect Down's syndrome?
11. Describe the normal newborn's umbilicus at about 4 hours after birth.
12. Conduct an examination and evaluation of the health status of a newborn.

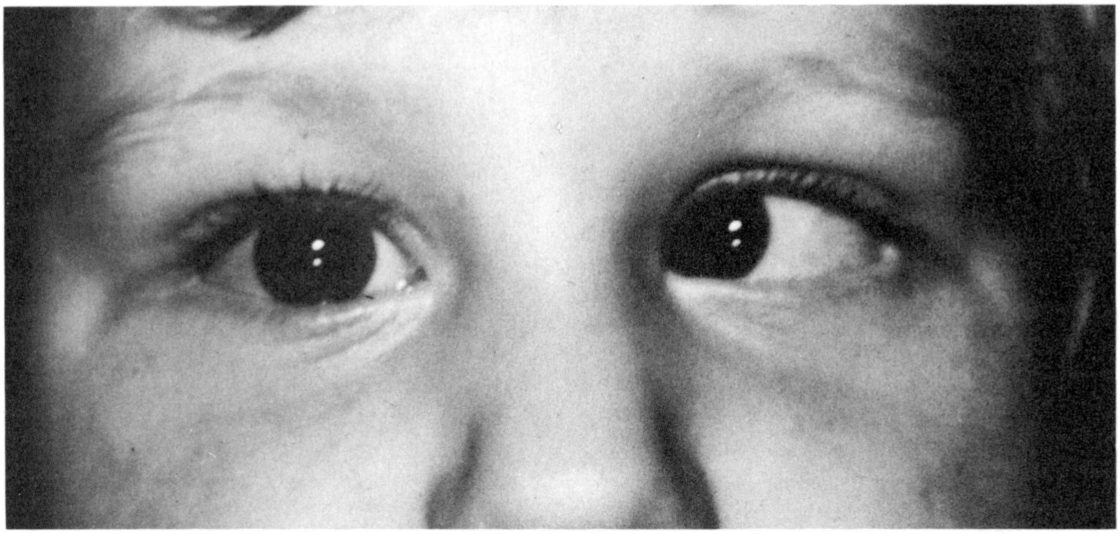

Figure 18-13 Convergent squint of left eye. Note asymmetry of light reflection.

kit. First, ascertain that the child knows the name of each picture. Then give the child one end of a 15-foot string, and while you hold on to the other end, ask him to walk that distance away from you. Test one eye at a time. Tell the child to place the plastic eye cover over one eye. Then present five pictures; the child normally should be able to identify at least three with each eye.

For children under 7 years old and for illiterate persons who are unable to read letters, as on the Snellen letter eye chart, you can use a Snellen *symbol* eye chart for distant vision screening. Es of various sizes and positions are on the chart. Ask the client to point in the same direction the "fingers" or the "legs" of the Es (or "tables") are pointing. Test each eye separately. A child stands 15 feet from the chart, while an adult would stand 20 feet away. The scoring is the same as for the conventional Snellen chart (Fig. 18-14).

A 20/30 vision is normal for children between the ages of 4 and 8. Children age 9 and older test out normally at approximately 20/20. If visual acuity is questionable, referral for further evaluation and ophthalmoscopic examination of the eyegrounds by an expert is warranted.

Visual fields of the preschool child and older are tested in the same manner as for the adult (see "Visual Fields" in Chapter 8). The same indices of fundoscopic examination are assessed in the child as in the adult (see "Ophthalmoscopic Examination" in Chapter 8), except that the retinal background of the child will present highlights (shiny light reflections) as the light of the ophthalmoscope falls on it.

Nose

The patency of the nares is assessed in the child by occluding one naris at a time and instructing the child to blow through her nose. A partially occluded naris will produce a higher pitch with forced nasal expiration compared with a nonoccluded naris; you may encounter this finding frequently, as toddlers and preschool children have a tendency to stick small objects in their body orifices.

Testing of the olfactory nerve (cranial nerve I) in the preschooler and younger aged child will not provide reliable findings.

Nose shape and symmetry should be noted. Palpation is performed to detect any deviation and tenderness. The nasal mucosa is normally free of lesions and red in color.

Sinuses

The sinuses are not usually assessed until the child is of school age. The frontal and maxillary sinuses are assessed by inspection, palpation or direct percussion, and transillumination in the same manner as for an adult (see Chapter 9). The difference, however, is in their changing anatomic locations throughout the growth stages from infancy to adulthood. In the infant, the sinuses are small and cylindrically shaped and lie near the bridge of the nose; in the child, the maxillary sinuses enlarge somewhat in a horizontal fashion toward the cheekbones. Prepubescence brings a widening and elongation of both frontal and maxillary sinuses; in the adolescent, the sinuses assume more of a block-like pattern, with the frontal sinuses positioned above the level of the brows. In the adult, the sinuses are larger, and the maxillary sinuses are distributed over a wider area of the cheeks.

Mouth

At about 6 months of age, the deciduous teeth begin to erupt and the complete set of 20 teeth is present by the age

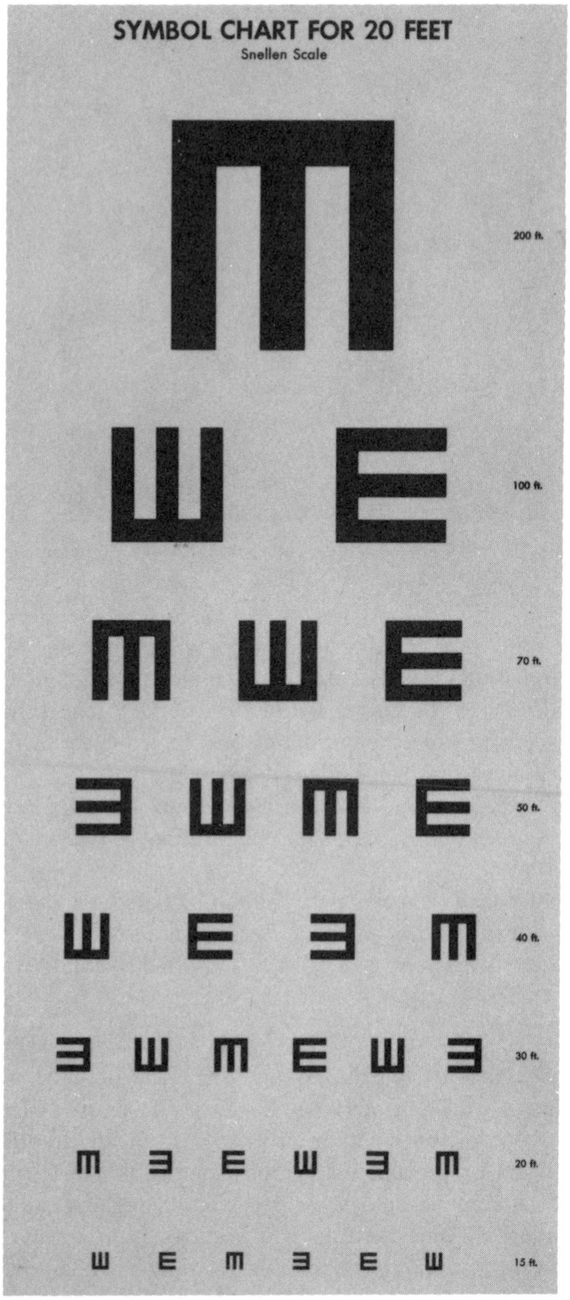

Figure 18-14 Snellen symbol chart.

of 3. There are 4 incisors, 2 canines, and 4 bicuspids on both the upper and lower jaws. The child begins losing these teeth by about the age of 6 or 7, and they become replaced by 32 permanent teeth (Fig. 18-15).

The uvular reflex can be assessed as the child cries or phonates, and the gag reflex is tested as it is in the adult (cranial nerves IX and X; see "Oropharynx" in Chapter 9). You will need to use a special approach with the infant to test whether the hypoglossal nerve is intact (cranial nerve XII; see "Tongue" in Chapter 9). The infant is unable to

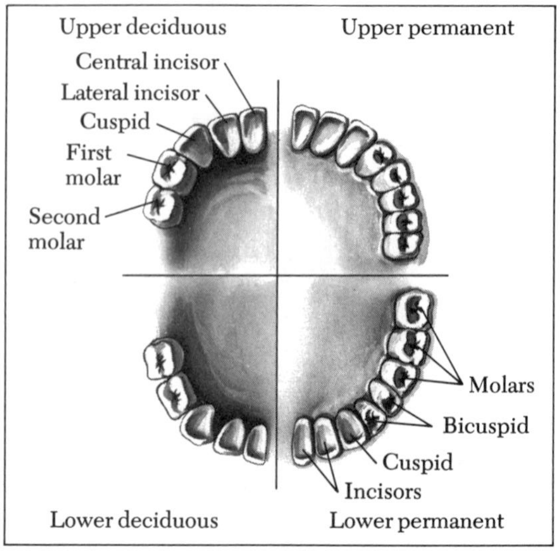

Figure 18-15 Maxillary and mandibular positions of both deciduous and permanent teeth at full eruption.

follow your instructions to "stick out your tongue and say 'aah.' " Instead, gently pinch the infant's nares closed. In response, he will open his mouth to breathe; with this, the tongue will normally extend out in the midline and up. Lateral deviation of the tongue would suggest pathology, just as in the adult.

Lymph nodes may be found in asymptomatic children under 12 years of age. Normally, the are nontender. If they are tender, you need to assess whether there are additional signs of infection, such as fever and erythema. Likewise, the tonsils are proportionately larger in the child than in the adult because they are a part of the lymphatic system. Further enlargement of the tonsils may interfere with eating and swallowing. Hypertrophied adenoids frequently accompany serous otitis media. Excessive mouth breathing and a voice of nasal quality may indicate enlarged adenoids. Mumps, a childhood disease affecting one or both of the parotid glands, manifests as swelling anterior to the lower part of the ear, which may extend behind the ear above the angle of the jaw to the mastoid process. This area is generally tender to palpation.

Respiratory System

Respiratory rate varies according to age (Table 18-12). You will note that the child up to approximately age 7 breathes abdominally rather that costally. Also, about age 7, the thorax of the child assumes a more elliptical shape, like that of the adult rather than the round, barrel-shaped characteristic of the newborn or preschooler. A round thorax in the school-age child would cause you to suspect respiratory dysfunction, such as asthma.

The intercostal spaces are carefully observed in the infant-child for retraction or bulging, which would indicate respiratory dysfunction. Inspection reveals as much as palpation in the infant because of the smallness of the chest.

Generally, the suprasternal notch is palpated to detect any abnormal cardiac pulsations in this area and to determine whether the trachea is midline. Increased fremitus may be indicative of consolidation in the lung tissue; however, in the infant and child, fremitus is normally of great intensity on palpation due to the thinness of the chest wall and paucity of adipose and muscle tissue in the area. For this reason, it is not usually necessary to palpate for fremitus in the child under 7 years of age.

In the infant and small child, the percussion note will be much more resonant than in the adult. It is best, therefore, to use a light, direct percussion technique. Direct percussion of the small chest is performed lightly by using the pad of the index finger and striking the chest directly, but gently, over the lung fields. Any area of decreased resonance is significant, as it would be in an adult, and warrants medical validation. The auscultory sites in the young child are fewer and somewhat different than those of the adult. It is best to use the bell of your stethoscope so that you will be better able to localize the source of sounds. It is preferable to use a bell that has soft rubber margins, because it makes more complete contact on the small, curved thorax of the infant and the small child.

The normal breath sounds that you will hear in the child are harsher than those heard in the adult. Even at the periphery of the child's lung fields, the breath sounds are bronchovesicular because of the thinness of the chest wall, which allows for greater transmission of sounds to the outside. Therefore, auscultation is of little diagnostic benefit in the young child. A technique to detect rhonchi in the infant is to hold our stethoscope in front of the mouth. This technique, however, does not reveal the presence of rales. Adventitious sounds within the lungs are able to be detected in the older child; thus, auscultation of the lungs is of greater diagnostic benefit in the school-age child. In prepubescence, the normal auscultated lung sounds become similar to those of the adult.

Cardiovascular System

Epigastric pulsations may be normally detected on inspection of the anterior thorax of the young child; they may also be detected in very thin adults. These pulsations are normal if they correspond to the timing of the arterial pulse. Abnormal epigastric pulsations in the infant may indicate an enlarged heart.

The point of maximal impulse (PMI), in contrast to being in the left 5th to 6th intercostal space to the left of the midclavicular line until the age of 7.

Auscultation of the heart reveals sinus arrhythmia. More than 50% of children have innocent systolic heart murmurs of grade III or less. Generally, they are heard loudest along the left sternal border at the level of the 2nd or 3rd intercostal space. There are no other associated cardiovascular symptoms. Murmurs heard in the child may or may not be pathologic, but they warrant medical referral for evaluation and follow-up.

Breast

Breast tissue growth begins in the preadolescent period. In the girl, the growth may begin in only one breast, and the breast may be tender. It is not uncommon during adolescence for boys to have some breast engorgement and tenderness. This may persist for several years. In this situation, there are no local or systemic signs of infection. Injury to the area must be ruled out at the onset. Stages of breast development have been identified by Tanner (Fig. 18-16).

Abdomen

Infants and toddlers have a round, slightly protruding abdomen, and it is not uncommon to see slight umbilical protru-

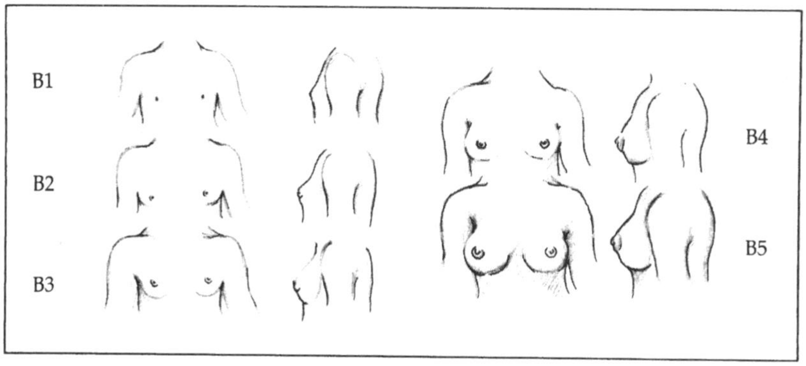

Figure 18-16 The Tanner stages of human breast development. (Adapted from G. Ross and R. Vande Wiele. The Ovaries. In R. Williams [ed.], *Textbook of Endocrinology* [5th ed.]. Philadelphia: Saunders, 1974; and from W.A. Marshall and J.M. Tanner. Variations in pattern of pubertal changes in girls. *Arch Dis Child* 44:291, 1969.)

sions in the toddler. Referral for further evaluation is needed if a child in this age range presents with a scaphoid abdomen. On inspection of the child's abdomen, the supervisional veins are readily observed, but they should not be prominent.

In the toddler and the preschool child, bowel sounds are normally heard every 10 to 30 seconds and are of greater frequency shortly after eating or when the stomach has been empty for several hours. The bowel sounds of the school-age child, as well as those of the adult, occur 5 to 6 times per minute. They will also increase in frequency with an empty stomach and after a recent meal.

Palpation of the liver in the infant is performed lightly, using only the fingertips to a depth of 1 to 2 cm. The liver edge may be felt 2 cm below the right costal margin in contrast to that of the adult, which is palpated immediately above or at the costal margin.

Percussion for liver size in the young child reveals a normal-sized liver of 4 to 6 cm approximately in the right midclavicular line. Normal liver size in the older child and adolescent ranges from 6 to 10 cm.

The kidneys are usually palpable in the infant and the thin child; the procedure is performed in the same manner as for the adult (see Chapter 12).

Palpation of a distended bladder above the pubic symphysis in the infant requires the retention of 90 mL of urine, whereas 180 mL is required to extend the adult bladder above the pubic symphysis.

Genitals

Developmental changes in pubic hair pattern and the genitals in the boy are heralded between the ages of 12 and 16. Before this age, there is no pubic hair. At development, sparse, soft, straight hairs begin to grow at the base of the penis, and the scrotal skin reddens and becomes thicker. Gradually, the pubic hair gets darker, coarser, and curlier and eventually covers the total pubic region. At the completion of puberty, the pubic hair distribution is diamond-shaped with the far ends at the level of the umbilicus and anus, and the genitals are of adult size and shape (Fig. 18-

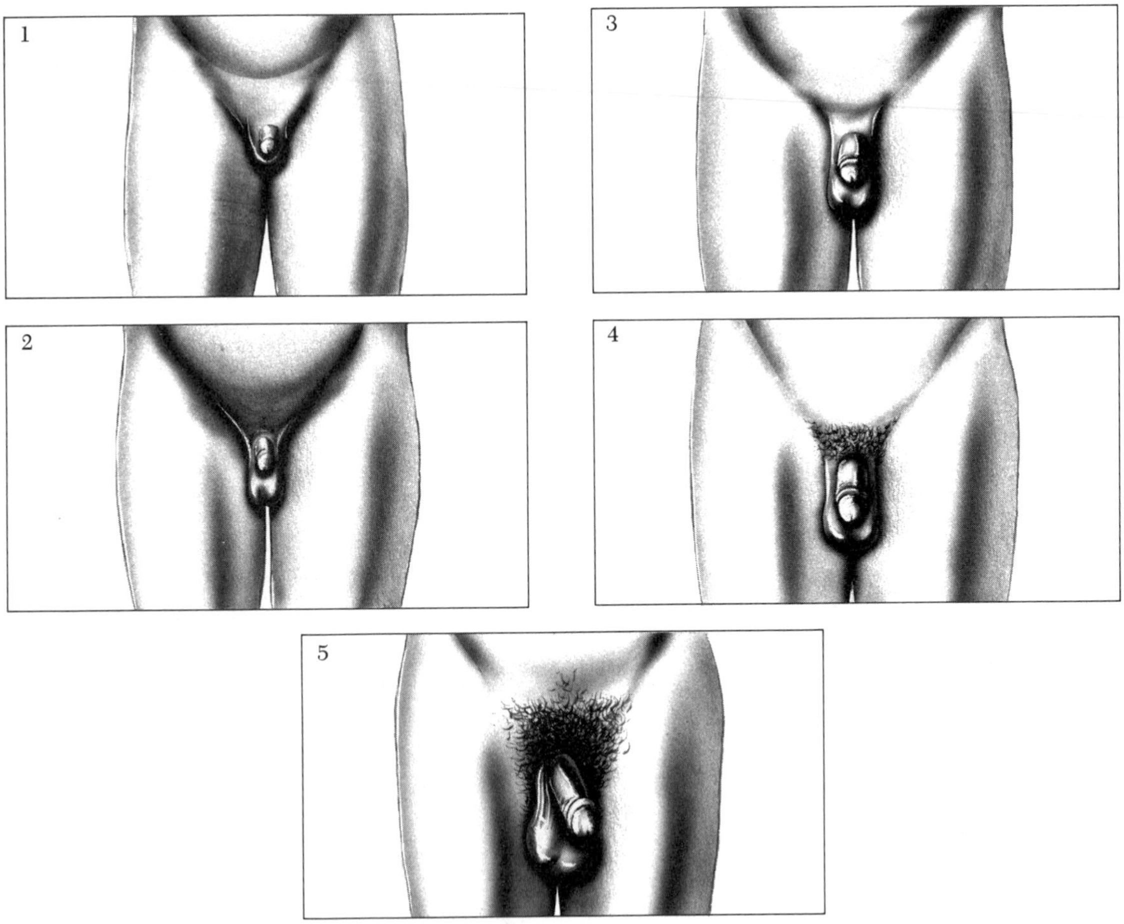

Figure 18-17 Stages of male genital development. **(1)** Prepubertal in which the size of the testes and penis is similar to that in early childhood. **(2)** Testes become larger and scrotal skin reddens and coarsens. **(3)** Continuation of stage 2, with lengthening of penis. **(4)** Penis enlarges in general size, and scrotal skin becomes pigmented. **(5)** Adult genitals.

17). Pubic hair growth and enlarged genitals in the boy prior to age 10 may indicate endocrine pathology. The penis is inspected and palpated with care to note any abnormalities (see Chapter 16). The prepuce may remain adherent to the glans until an infant is 6 months of age. After this age, however, it should retract easily.

The scrotum and its contents, testes and epididymides, are palpated in the same manner as that of the adult (see Chapter 16). The epididymis may be difficult to distinguish before school age. However, the epididymis and the inguinal ring on both sides of the scrotum are assessed in the school-age child. The little finger, rather than the index finger, is used to palpate the inguinal ring.

The best position in which to place the child for assessment of the anus and rectum is the supine position, with the legs flexed at the knees and laterally rotated at the hips (frog-legged). The prostate gland is not assessed until a boy is in adolescence.

Generally the pubic hair pattern of the girl is established between the ages of 11 and 13 (Fig. 18-18). It is shaped like an inverted triangle. Assessment of the genitals in girls employs only the techniques of inspection and external palpation. Internal vaginal inspection and palpation of the Bartholin's gland, vaginal walls, uterus, and adnexa are not performed. The position assumed by the female child for inspection of the genitals is the same as that for assessment of the anus and rectum (supine and frog-legged).

Adhesion of the labia minora may be present in infants and toddlers; these children will be more prone to urinary infections due to urine collected in a sac formed by the labial adhesion.

When performing a pelvic examination of the adolescent girl, use a small or medium vaginal speculum. A summary of pubertal development is provided in Table 18-13.

Musculoskeletal System

The center of gravity in the child before the age of 4 is higher than that in the adult, which is at about the level of the iliac crest. As a result, the child has a wide gait and stance. In addition, until the age of 4, the child normally has an increase in the lumbar curvature, giving a slightly swayback appearance. All children are examined for the presence of scoliosis, a lateral spinal curvature deviation. To inhibit further deviation of structure, the nurse must refer any sign of scoliosis, no matter how mild. The best method for inspection is to view the child from the back as she bends over at the waist and leans forward, dangling her hands toward her toes. With scoliosis, the scapulae are no longer on a horizontal plane; instead, the scapula on the deviated side is displaced laterally and superiorly (Fig. 18-19). In the young child, the Denver Developmental Screening Test is used to assess muscle strength. The school-age and the older child's muscle strength is assessed in the same way as in the adult. As muscle strength and intellect develop, so do the child's abilities.

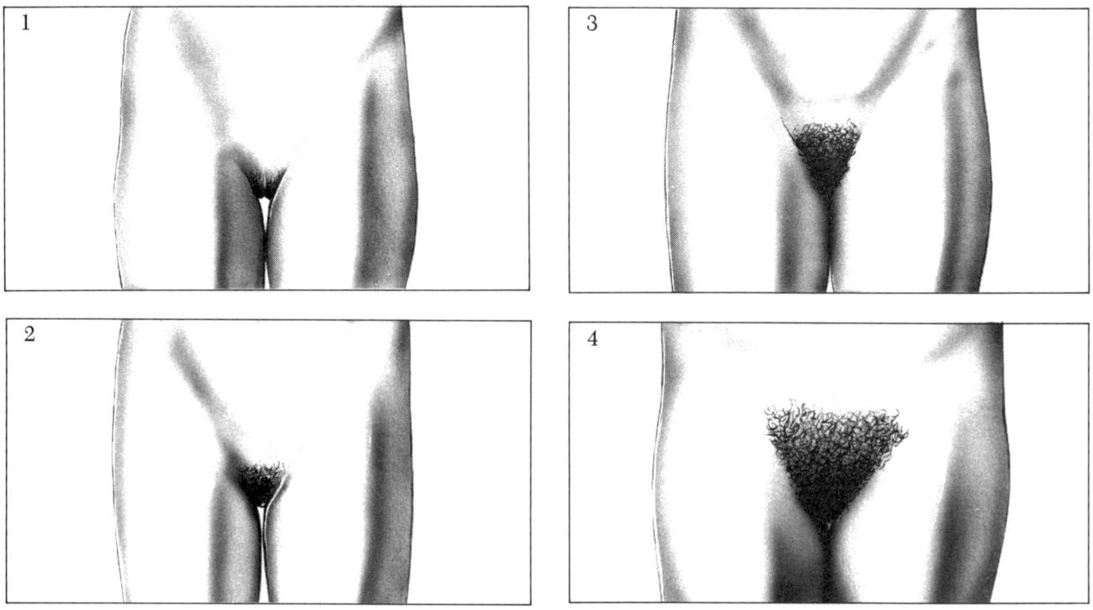

Figure 18-18 Stages of pubic hair development in adolescent girls. **(1)** Sparse growth of downy hair mainly at sides of labia. **(2)** Pigmentation, coarsening, and curling, with an increase in the amount of hair. **(3)** Adult hair, but limited in area. **(4)** Adult hair with horizontal upper border.

Table 18-13 Sequence of Pubertal Development

Male		
Average age onset	Physiologic changes	Average age completion
11.5 years	*Genital development* (see Fig. 18-17) —Testicular volume increases —Penile enlargement and lengthening	2–5 years after onset
12.5	*Adrenarche* (growth of body hair) —Pubic hair development (see Fig. 18-19) —Axillary and facial hair development	Late teens
About 2 years after onset of pubic hair growth 13.5	*Growth spurt* —Pattern: hands and feet, calves and forearms, hips, chest, shoulders, trunk —Height: increases about 7–12 cm/year at peak —Weight: almost doubles between 12 and 16 years —Larynx growth and voice deepening occur at end of penile growth	18–20
About 3 years after onset of genital development	*Ejaculation* via masturbation or nocturnal emissions —Mature sperm are produced between 14.5 and 17.5 years of age *Breast development* —Areola darkens and enlarges —Transient gynecomastia may occur between 10 and 16 years of age	14.5 to 17.5 years

Female		
Average age onset	Physiologic changes	Average age completion
9.0 to 11.0 years	*Breast development* (see Fig. 18-16) —Breast bud appears followed by general enlargement and raising of the breast and areola —Areola and nipple are raised from breast —Adult breast contour	14.0 to 17.0 years
About 1 year after breast buds appear About 1 year after onset of pubic hair growth	*Adrenarche* —Pubic hair development (see Fig. 18-18) —Axillary hair development	Late teens
10.5 years	*Growth spurt*—same sequence as male —Height: increases 6–11 cm/year at peak	16 years
12.5 to 13.5 years	*Menarche* (onset of menstruation) —Initial cycles are usually anovulatory and irregular —Ovulatory cycles usually occur within two years of menarche —Dysmenorrhea more often associated with ovulatory cycles	

Source: From J. Bellack and P. Bamford: *Nursing Assessment: A Multidimensional Approach.* Boston: Little, Brown, 1987, p. 192.

Neurologic System

The Denver Developmental Screening Test is used initially at the age of 3 months and is repeated about every 6 months up to around age 6. Children 5 to 6 years old can be tested like an adult for balance, using the Romberg test, and for coordination ability of upper and lower extremities (Figs. 18-20 and 18-21).

Children 6 years of age and older can be tested for sensory function as would an adult. Infants will respond to a pinprick (pain sensation) by crying and/or withdrawal. Hot and cold sensations and sharp and dull sensations can be tested in the 3-year-old. Vibration and position sense are not tested in the infant or toddler because of the difficulty in gaining cooperation. These sensations, as well as stereognosis and graphesthesia, can be readily assessed in children who are 6 years old and older (see Chapter 15).

At approximately 6 months of age, the superficial reflexes are present. When testing for the plantar reflex, you may normally observe a Babinski response up until the age of 2. The appearance of any pathologic reflexes after the age of 2 is abnormal and warrants referral. Any child, regardless of age, who displays a high-pitched cry, irritability, and extended posturing, or who is unresponsive, must be seen by a physician.

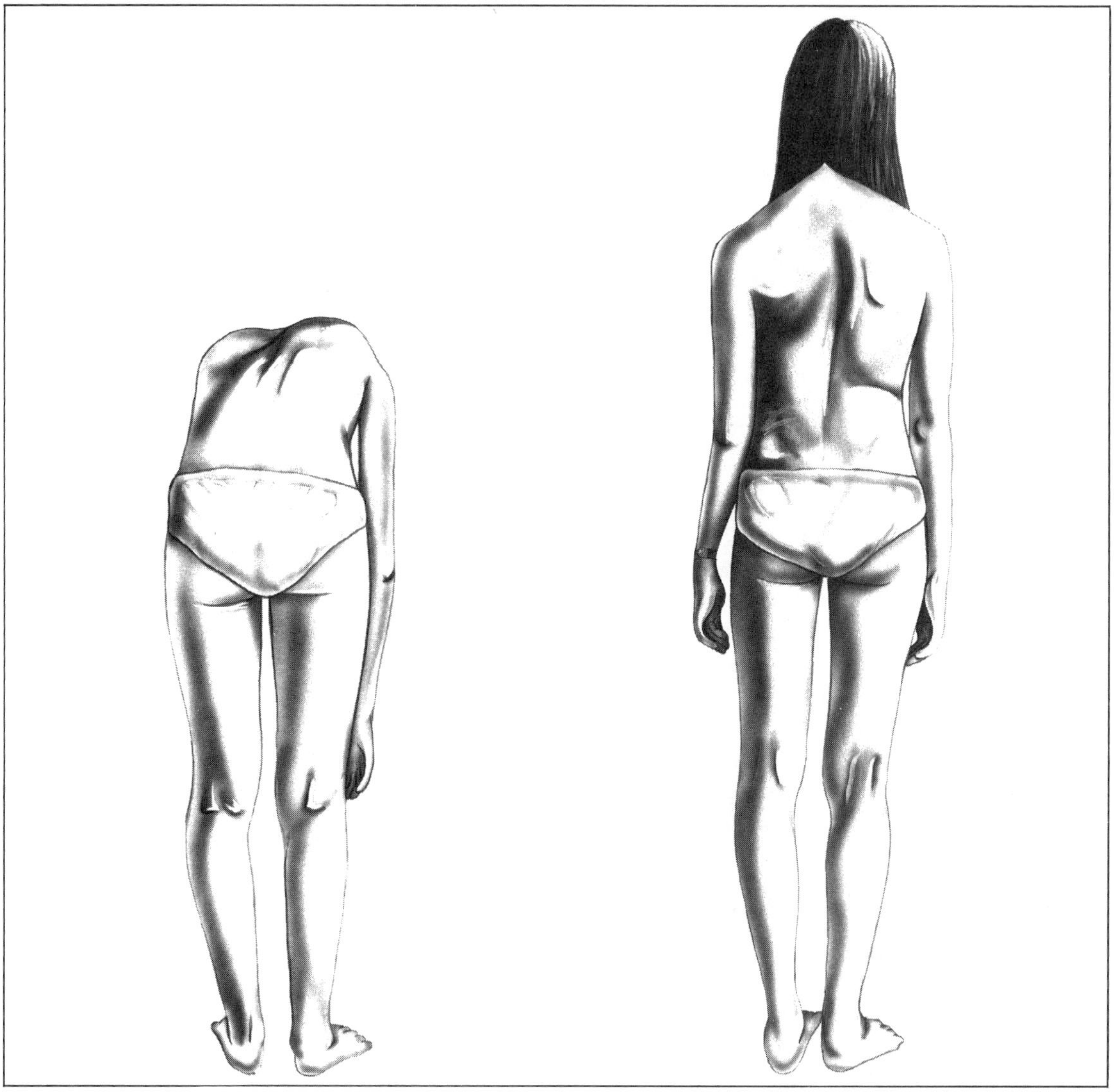

Figure 18-19 Screening procedure for scoliosis.

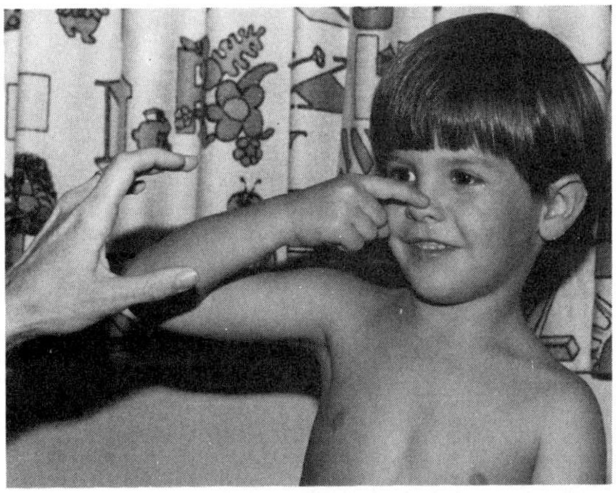

Figure 18-20 Finger-to-nose test for cerebellar functioning.

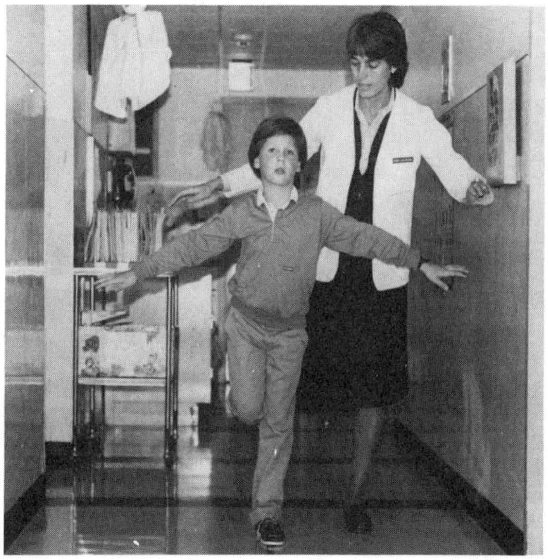

Figure 18-21 Assessing balance for cerebellar functioning.

Example of a Health Assessment of a Child

HEALTH HISTORY

Name: Kevin Cain Jones, Jr.
Address: 82 Brushlee St., Carlsburg, N.M.
Sex: Male
Age: 5 years
Birthdate: 5/9/82
Mother: Ann Marie *Age:* 30 *Address:* Same as client *Education:* High school graduate
Religion: Catholic *Race:* Caucasian *Ethnic origin:* Italian
Father: Kevin Cain Jones *Age:* 28 *Address:* same as client *Education:* B.S. in business
Religion: Protestant *Race:* Caucasian *Ethnic Origin:* English
Informant: Parents; reliable source
Chief Concern/Complaint: "Sore throat"

History of Present Illness (HPI)

Client has been "cranky" for past 3 days. Nonproductive cough and runny nose. Asking for more fluids. Appetite poor. Temperature 102°F since midnight. History of 1–2 strep throat infections/yr for past 2 yrs. No earaches, stomachaches, diarrhea, or changes in bowel habits.

Personal History and Patterns of Living

Prenatal—Healthy pregnancy. Kevin was 1st child. No x-rays, special diet, or hospitalization during pregnancy. Followed from 4th–9th month at Saver's Prenatal Clinic. On vitamins and iron for duration of pregnancy. No abortions or miscarriages. Mother, father, and client have RH + blood types.

Natal—Uneventful 10-hr labor. Father present most of labor and present at delivery. Vaginal delivery. Vertex presentation, caudal anesthesia at Carlsburg General Hospital. Apgar 9; birth weight: 7 lb 2 oz; length: 20 inches. Color was good—spontaneous cry; no O_2 needed.

Postnatal—Uneventful, mother and Kevin discharged on 2nd day postdelivery. Client had slight bilateral breast hypertrophy that lasted about 2 wks without tenderness or erythema. No jaundice or cyanosis. Cord and circumcision healed without complications. Breast-fed. Lost 5 oz 1st wk at home.

Present—Kevin attends kindergarten, which he enjoys; has formed friendships with peers. He gets along with most people. Protective and sharing with 3½ yr old sister, Cindy. Talks constantly; appropriate interaction content; asks relevant questions; egocentrism, normal for his age, displayed; talks about grandparents, aunts and uncles; knows his name, age, address, telephone number, and where his daddy works and mommy goes to school; knows basic colors, days of week; able to print name and few other short words and write numbers 1–20. Cindy spends time on weekdays at Happy Child Day Care Center. Mother attends Catholic church school most Sundays with both children. Father attends infrequently. No outstanding financial debts. Maternal grandparents are helping with cost for mother to attend baccalaureate nursing program at Carlsburg University. She is ending her 4th semester.

Family Health History

Denies family history of TB, alcoholism, mental illness, bleeding disorders, stomach problems, liver and kidney disorders, cancer, heart disease. Family history significant for hypertension, arthritis, and diabetes.

Geographic Exposure: Disneyland at age 4. Family has traveled and vacationed mainly in state and Texas.

Lifestyle

Sexuality—Mimics father. Plays with building blocks, tricycle. Has favorite teddy bear for naps and bedtime. Girls are mommies, boys are daddys.

Personal habits: Brushes teeth after breakfast and before bedtime. Likes soda and popsicles—allowed 2–3 times/wk. Has been on penicillin when strep throat past couple years. Tylenol liquid for fever.

Diet: Generally has good appetite. Meat, vegetables, fruit, cereal, and milk daily. Pasta 2–3 times/wk. Loves fruit. Weekdays has brown bag lunch—sandwich, cookies, raw carrots or celery, apple, carton of milk. No eating difficulties except when past strep throat and present "sore throat." Does not like raw tomatoes or cooked peas. Takes Flintstone daily vitamin.

Sleep and rest patterns: 8 P.M. bedtime. Wakes 7–8 A.M. Short nap in afternoons (½ hr). No bedwetting. "Bad" dreams—ghosts, witches 4–5 times/month. Sleepwalks 2–3 times/month.

Activities of daily living: Feeds, washes, and dresses self. Needs help with tying shoelaces and combing hair. Brushes teeth. Toilet trained at 3½ yrs. Picks up toys—usually after reminded to do so.

Home and neighborhood: Family rents small bungalow in young family residential area. No basement, small backyard. 3 BR (each child has own bedroom).

Interpersonal relationships: Contact with grandparents, aunts, and uncles. Closest to maternal grandparents. Father and mother share chores, child care, and responsibilities. Stressful at times—father works in bank; mother is college student. Discipline seems consistent, with father and mother consciously working at it. Removal of privileges seems most effective discipline with client—occasional spanking 2–3 times/yr.

Recreation: Likes to go for walks, to the local playground. Watches Saturday A.M. cartoons. Enjoys building with blocks, Leggos, Tinkertoys.

Previous experiences with illnesses

Mumps at 3 yrs of age. No history of measles, chickenpox, scarlet fever, or rheumatic fever.

Immunizations: DPT and TOPV 2 mos old, 4 mos old, 6 mos old, 18 mos old. Tine Test 1 yr old. Measles, rubella, mumps vaccine 1½ yrs old. DPT and TOPV booster 4½ yrs old.

Allergies: Animal fur—breaks out in rash.

Past illness, injuries, surgery: Strep throat past 2 years. Rx with penicillin by Dr. Rouse. Mumps at 3 yrs of age. Fell 2 mos ago at kindergarten and lacerated base of left palm—needed 3 sutures. No surgeries or hospitalizations.

Review of Systems

General health: Very strong and active except for strep throat. No history of polydipsia, ecchymosis, bleeding tendencies, easily fatigued.

Integument: Papular rash when around furry pets. No jaundice, diaphoresis, hives, pruritus, skin lesions. 3 cm diameter port wine birthmark on lower, lateral quadrant of left buttock. Lately, past couple of months, has begun biting nails. No changes in daily routine.

Head: Never complained of headache or held head when crying. No head injuries known.

Eyes: No history of infections or pain. No excessive lacrimation, crossed-eyes, or photophobia. No history of walking into walls or doors. Can see blackboard from seat.

Ears: Earache last winter with last episode of strep throat. No vertigo noted.

Nose, nasopharynx, and paranasal sinuses: No epistaxis, strep throat 1–2 times/yr for past 2 yrs with tenacious white-yellow nasal drainage.

Mouth and throat: No toothaches, sores of mouth or tongue. Dysphagia when strep throat episodes. Annual dental visits.

Neck: Complains of pain (see HPI).

Breasts: No scaling, edema, or discharge.

Cardiorespiratory system: Nonproductive cough past couple days (see HPI). No history of pneumonia or asthma. No dyspnea or wheezing. Dr. Rouse, pediatrician, told family that client had slight murmur but that it appeared to be "innocent." Annual pediatrician exam done.

Gastrointestinal system: Client goes to toilet by self; no known recent diarrhea or constipation. No bloody stools, pain, or vomiting. No food intolerances.

Genitourinary system: Straight, strong urinary stream. No dribbling, nocturia, hematuria, or polyuria noted.

Musculoskeletal system: No broken bones, sprains, pain, or swelling in joints, lameness, weakness, dislocations, or congenital defects.

Neurologic system: No history of convulsions, twitching, tremors, vertigo, "blackouts," fainting, or difficulty with motor activities. No stuttering or other speech difficulties.

PHYSICAL ASSESSMENT

General impression: Kevin Cain Jones, 5-year-old white male presents with "sore throat" and dysphagia. Appears within cognitive and physical developmental norms. Raspy cough and visible swollen glands in neck; nasal congestion. No gross deformities.

Ht.—45".

Wt.—43 lbs.

TPR—102.6°F./88/26.

BP—98/66 left arm lying.

Chest circumference—54.5 cm.

Integument: Moist, flushed, and warm to touch; skin turgor—fair; port wine birthmark noted lower, lateral quadrant of left buttock; curly, short blond hair; moderate degree of nail-biting observed; no clubbing of digits; no nailbed cyanosis; good capillary refill.

Head and neck: Normocephalic; atraumatic; clean clear scalp; tonsillar and anterior cervical lymph nodes enlarged and tender to touch bilaterally; trachea midline.

Respiratory: Rate 26; abdominal respirations; no ICS or sternal retractions noted; round thoracic cage; symmetrical breathing; no cyanosis; resonance; bronchovesicular breath sounds; no crackles, wheezes, or rubs.

Cardiovascular: Slight epigastric pulsations concomitant with arterial pulse; no heaves or thrills; PMI at left 4ICS slightly left of MCL; rate 88; sinus arrhythmia; summation gallop; physiological splitting of S_2; $A_2 = P_2$. Grade I systolic murmur at left 2ICS; no radiation into neck or axilla.

Abdomen: Flat, B.S. every 10–30 seconds; tympany; liver dullness = 5 cm; splenic dullness = 4 cm; no pain or masses with light and deep palpation.

Musculoskeletal: Full ROM; no joint tenderness or edema noted; good bilateral, proximal, and distal strength; normal gait; tires easily from present fever; no spinal deviations noted.

Neurologic: Scapulae on horizontal plane. Slow mental processes 2° to pyrexia. Sensitive to hot and cold, light touch, and vibration. Able to button and unbutton shirt. Can tap toes. Romberg sign absent. Able to touch nose with finger. Babinski sign absent. Abdominal, anal, and cremasteric reflexes present.

Eyes: No edema; sclerae white; corneas clear; no lid lag; EOMs intact; PERRLA/consensual reaction; convergence; Hirschberg test—symmetrical reflection; cover test—no jerking movements, no deviation. Snellen chart results—O.U. 20/30 does not wear glasses; field vision WNL by gross confrontation.

Example of a Health Assessment of a Child, continued

Ears: Appropriate placement; no lesions or drainage noted. No mastoid tenderness. TMs—pearly gray, landmarks visible, membranes movable; Weber without lateralization; Rinne—AC > BC. Watch ticking 12″ bilaterally.
Nose: Congested; thick, whitish yellow exudate; no deviation; pale bluish mucosa.
Mouth/pharynx: Free of lesions; all deciduous teeth (#20); tongue midline; uvular reflex; pink, firm gums; posterior pharynx erythemic; purulent, exudative, enlarged tonsils bilaterally; culture taken (to be referred to pediatrician, Dr. Rouse for medical Rx).
Genitourinary: No pubic hair; descended testicles; urethral opening and penile size appropriate; prepuce retracts easily; circumcised; no drainage, masses, or hernias noted.

		T	B	BR	P	A	PR
DTRs	L	2+	2+	2+	2+	2+	↓
	R	2+	2+	2+	2+	2+	↓

SUMMARY

The health assessment of the child and the adolescent uses developmental parameters for each age level as a base for evaluation. These activities and functions were incorporated throughout the chapter. How cultural history is pertinent to the health assessment of the child was discussed. Also presented were specific communication and interview principles that need to be used with the child and the adolescent. The components of the health history were reviewed in light of the areas of inquiry, and sample questions were given relevant to the child and the adolescent. The specific techniques of measurement (head, chest, and abdomen circumferences) for the very young child were included in the general appearance section. Rationales and examples for approaching the physical assessment of the child and of the adolescent in a particular way were given. Specific techniques used with the child for each body system, as well as the normal findings, were included. If an assessment technique is used for the child and the adolescent in the same manner as used for the adult, the reader was referred to the chapter or section in the text where it was originally described.

DISCUSSION QUESTIONS/ ACTIVITIES

1. Role-play a history-taking session with an adolescent and parents who do not allow the client to answer questions or talk very much to you.
2. Perform a health assessment on a toddler, preschool child, school-age child, prepubescent child, and a mid- to late-adolescent child.
3. Describe some ways that you might approach children and adolescents that would decrease anxiety and facilitate communication and examination.
4. List areas of history-taking that would likely be sensitive for the adolescent and how you would plan to approach these areas.
5. Discuss how cultural history is pertinent to the health assessment of the child.
6. Describe how aspects of your cultural history influence your health status and behavior.
7. Develop projects that will enhance wellness and health maintenance in children and adolescents.

REFERENCES

Hales, D. 1981. *The complete book of sleep.* Reading, Mass.: Addison-Wesley.

Oswald, I. 1972. *Sleep.* Baltimore: Penguin Books.

CHAPTER

19 Assessment of Wellness

Learning Objectives

1. Describe the techniques of anthropometric measurement.
2. Cite specific examples of undernutrition.
3. Explain what is meant by subclinical malnutrition.
4. Describe body density, lean body weight, and body fat.
5. Describe methods for determining body density and body fat.
6. Review tests used to measure cardiovascular function, strength, and flexibility.

Aesculapius, the Greek God of Healing, had two daughters, Panacea and Hygeia. Panacea believed that the best way to help people was to treat all illness. Hygeia believed the best way was to teach people how to live so that they did not become ill. The approach of Hygeia is related to the focus on wellness in our society. Wellness can be viewed as a process through which individuals become aware of and make choices toward a more satisfying and healthful existence. Wellness assessment includes mental and physical assessment; in addition, it is a review of lifestyle and the identification of health-related beliefs. The culmination of the wellness assessment is reached by helping clients gain increased control over their health. They do this by improving their personal health habits, lifestyle, and environment. Mental assessment was discussed in Chapter 3. This chapter focuses on nutritional and physical fitness assessments.

NUTRITIONAL ASSESSMENT

Good nutrition is a major prerequisite to health. An adequate and carefully planned diet can alleviate and modify disease states and current disease. Many scientists believe that reducing calories, fat, cholesterol, sugar, and salt and eating more whole grains, fruits, and vegetables will reduce heart disease, cancer, and strokes. There is evidence that the public is becoming more interested in human nutrition, as demonstrated by the number of new books dealing with eating better and staying healthy and slim. Increasing media attention has been devoted to food safety, exercise and diet, world hunger, drug and diet interaction, and the mental and physical effects of long-term nutritional excess or deprivation. Because it is believed that an improper diet and

Table 19-1 Ideal Body Weights Using the Height-Frame Rule

Frame size	Height data	Weight (lb) Men	Women
Medium	First 5 feet	106	100
	Each inch above 5 feet	6	5
Large	Each inch above 5 feet	110/100 × weight calculated for medium-frame person	
Small	Each inch above 5 feet	90/100 × weight calculated for medium-frame person	

Source: From H. Y. Hui: *Human Nutrition and Diet Therapy.* © 1983 Boston: Jones and Bartlett Publishers, p. 294. Reprinted with permission.

sedentary lifestyle are the major risk factors leading to disease and early death, it is only sensible that attention to these factors be an important part of wellness assessment and of the subsequent planning with the client for proper and healthful nutrition. Four major areas must be included in nutritional assessment:

1. anthropometric measurement
2. clinical examination
3. dietary evaluation
4. biochemical data evaluation

Anthropometric Measurement

This assessment involves measurement of height, weight, midarm and chest circumference, skinfold thickness, and—in infants and young children—head circumference. Height and weight tables can be used to determine normal values for specific sex, age, and body frame (see Appendix A). Care should be taken in determining whether a client is overweight or underweight based on these tables alone because they do not take into consideration the quality of body weight. For example, an athlete with well-developed muscles might be overweight according to the tables, yet he may not have excessive adipose tissue. Another individual, on the other hand, may be considered only slightly underweight according to the tables, but he may actually have lost significant body protein, which could be life threatening (Lewis 1984, p. 125). A method of determining ideal body weight is shown in Table 19-1.

Skinfold measurement is a method for determining body density, body fat, and lean body weight (Fig. 19-1). Body density describes the compactness of the body. Body fat refers to fat that is subcutaneous and stored in adipose tissue. Lean body weight is the body weight minus the fat stored in the adipose tissue. There are two ways to take skinfold measurements. The first is termed the *scientific pinch.* Because most body fat is subcutaneous, the thickness of a pinch of skin and fat can be a good indicator of total body fatness. Pinch the skin and fat on the back of the arm over the triceps muscle, at the lower tip of the shoulder blade, and at the abdomen. The thickness of these folds should average not more than three fourths of an inch. As the saying goes, if you can pinch an inch, you are too fat. A more accurate method is to measure the skinfolds with calipers and then use formulas to calculate body density and fat (Table 19-2).

Technique for Skinfold Measurement

- Grasp the skinfold between the thumb and forefinger. The skinfold should include two thicknesses of skin and subcutaneous fat, but not muscle.
- Apply the calipers approximately 1 cm below the fingers and at a depth equal to the thickness of the fold.
- Each fold is taken in the vertical plane while the client is standing except for the subscapular, which is picked up on a slight slant running laterally in the natural fold of the skin.
- Release the finger slightly so that most of the pressure is on the calipers, not the fingers.
- Read the dial to the nearest millimeter. Measurement should be made three times, and the average value of the two closest readings should be used as the actual measure (Getchell 1979, pp. 78–79).

The anatomic sites for measuring with the calipers are

- triceps—the back of the upper arm midway between the shoulder and elbow joints

Table 19-2 Triceps Skinfold Thickness Indicating Obesity (mm)

Age (yr)	Males	Females
5	≥12	≥14
10	≥16	≥20
15	≥16	≥24
20	≥16	≥28
25	≥20	≥29
30 and above	≥23	≥30

From C. C. Seltzer and J. A. Mayer. "Simple Criterion of Obesity." *Post Graduate Medicine,* August 1965. Copyright © 1965, McGraw-Hill, Inc.

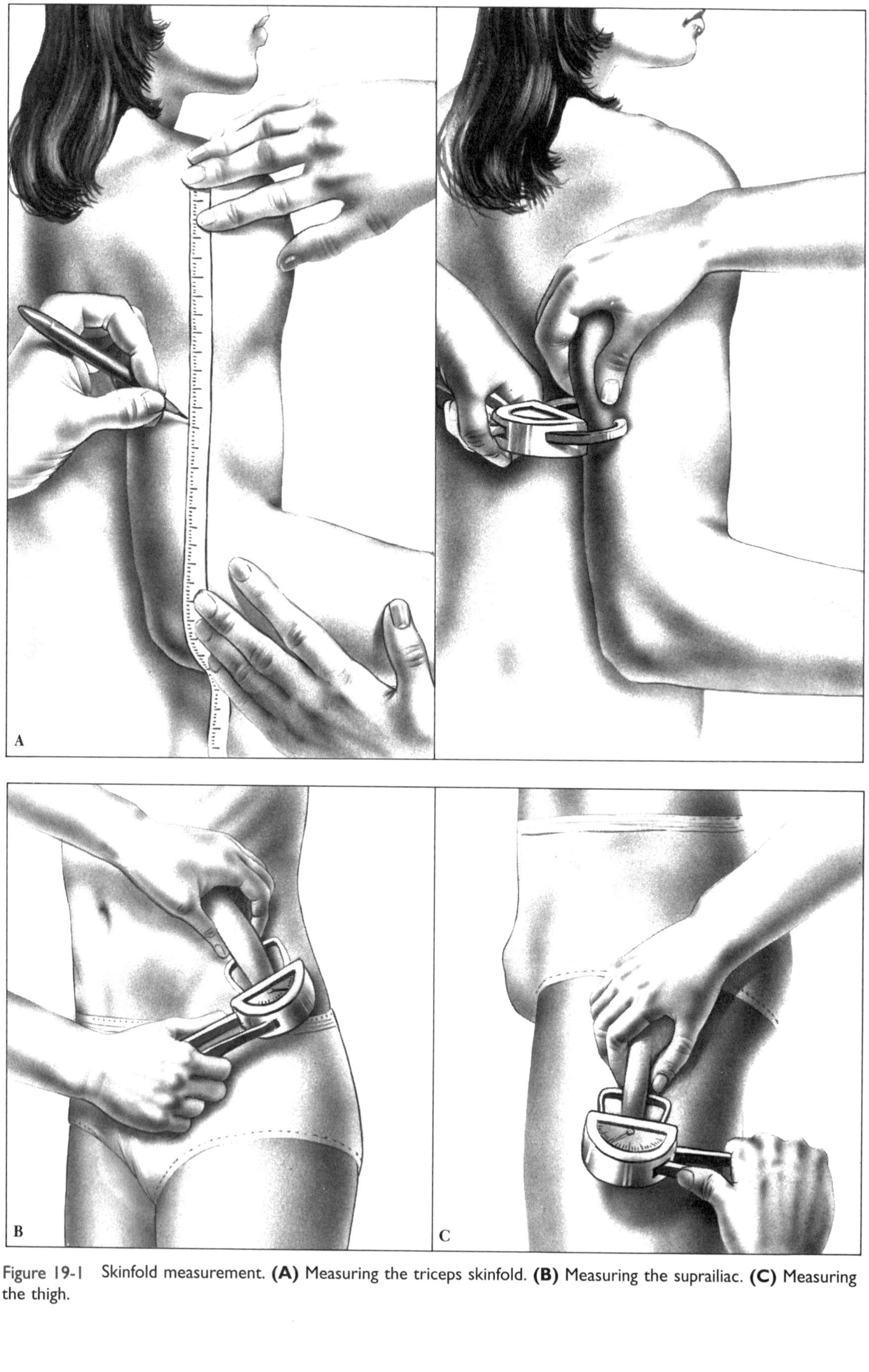

Figure 19-1 Skinfold measurement. **(A)** Measuring the triceps skinfold. **(B)** Measuring the suprailiac. **(C)** Measuring the thigh.

- subscapula—the bottom point of the shoulder blade
- thigh—the front side of the thigh midway between the hip and knee joints
- suprailiac—just above the top of the hip bone (crest of the ilium) at the middle of the side of the body

To take the measurement, you will need a skinfold caliper. Then you must decide on the measurement sites. All measurements are made on the right side of the body. Because of differences in males and females, measurements are taken at different sites.

Females are measured at suprailiac and triceps areas; males are measured at the thigh and subscapular areas (see Fig. 19-1).

The following formulas allow the nurse to calculate body density and then body fat.

Women

- Skinfold assessment of triceps: Calculate the mean of the three readings.
- Skinfold assessment of suprailiac: Calculate the mean of the three readings.
- Computation for body density (gm/cc):

Body density = 1.0764 − (0.00088 × tricep) − (0.00081 × suprailiac)

Men

- Skinfold assessment of subscapula: Calculate the mean of the three readings.
- Skinfold assessment of the thigh: Calculate the mean of the three readings.
- Computation for body density (gm/cc):

Body density = 1.1043 − (0.00131 × subscapula) − (0.001327 × thigh)

A good amount of body fat is between 10% and 12% of total body weight for men and between 18% and 20% for women. Body fat greater than 25% in men and 30% in women is too much and indicates obesity. The computation for percentage of body fat (male and female) is as follows (Fig. 19-2):

Percentage of body fat = (4.570/body density − 4.142) × 100

Another method of calculating body fat, without the use of calipers, is based on muscularity and height. Tables, such as Tables 19-3 and 19-4, have been developed at Ball State University to estimate ideal weight and body fat.

Women

Skinfold assessment (millimeters)

	Trial 1	Trial 2	Trial 3	Mean
1. Tricip	13.0	16.0	15.0	14.7
2. Suprailiac	7.5	8.0	7.5	7.7

Computation for body density (gm/cc)

Body density

= 1.0764 − (0.00088 × tricep) − (0.00081 × suprailiac)

= 1.0764 − (0.00088 × 14.7) − (0.00081 × 7.7)

= 1.0764 − (.01294) − (.00624)

= 1.057 gm/cc

Computation for percentage of body-fat:

Percentage body fat = (4.570/body density − 4.142)100

= (4.570/ 1.057 − 4.142)100

= .169 × 100

Percentage body fat = 16.9 %

Men

Skinfold assessment (millimeters)

	Trial 1	Trial 2	Trial 3	Mean
1. Subscapula	11.5	11.0	11.0	11.0
2. Thigh	15.0	15.0	—	15.0

Computation for body density (gm/cc):

Body density

= 1.1043 − (0.00131 × subscapula) − (0.001327 × thigh)

= 1.1043 − (0.00131 × 11.0) − (0.001327 × 15.0)

= 1.1043 − (.01441) − (.01991)

= 1.070 gm/cc

Computation for percentage of body fat:

Percentage body fat = (4.570/body density − 4.142)100

= (4.570/ 1.070 − 4.142)100

= (.1290)100

Percentage body fat = 12.9 %

Figure 19-2 **Male and female calculations of body density and body fat.**

Clinical Examination

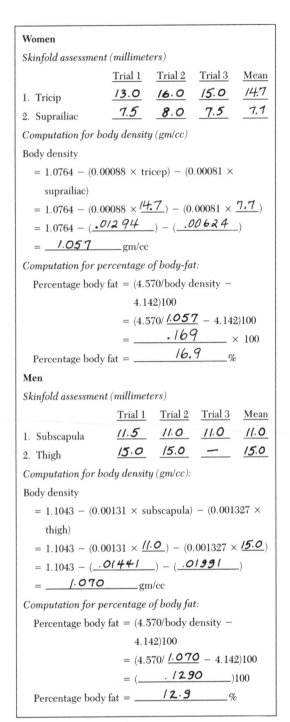

Nutritional status is observed during all phases of physical assessment. Indications of nutritional health may be noted in all body systems, but of particular note are the hair, face, eyes, lips, gums, skin, nails, glands, muscular and skeletal systems, and gastrointestinal and nervous systems. The signs of malnutrition, until the late stages, are often nonspecific and must be considered in connection with the total information obtained from the physical assessment and the client history. The overt signs of malnutrition are dry brittle hair, changes in skin pig-

Table 19-3 Ideal Weights for Women*

Height (inches)	Degree of muscularity Low	Medium	High
56	78	84	90
57	82	88	94
58	86	92	98
59	90	96	102
60	94	100	106
61	98	104	110
62	102	108	114
63	106	112	118
64	110	116	122
65	114	120	126
66	118	124	130
67	122	128	134
68	126	132	138
69	130	136	142
70	134	140	146
71	138	144	150
72	142	148	154
73	146	152	158
74	150	156	162
75	154	160	166
76	158	164	170

*Based on 18% body fat and degree of muscularity.

Source: From B. Getchell with W. Anderson. *Being Fit: A Personal Guide*, pp. 88–89. Copyright © 1982 John Wiley & Sons. Reprinted by permission of John Wiley & Sons, Inc.

Table 19-4 Ideal Weights for Men*

Height (inches)	Degree of muscularity Low	Medium	High
60	129	135	143
61	132	138	146
62	135	141	149
63	138	144	152
64	141	147	155
65	144	150	158
66	147	153	161
67	150	156	164
68	153	159	167
69	156	162	170
70	159	165	173
71	161	168	176
72	164	171	179
73	167	174	182
74	170	177	185
75	173	180	188
76	176	183	191
77	179	186	194
78	182	189	197
79	185	191	200
80	188	193	203

*Based on 12% body fat and degree of muscularity.

Source: From B. Getchell with W. Anderson. *Being Fit: A Personal Guide*, pp. 88–89. Copyright © 1982 John Wiley & Sons. Reprinted by permission of John Wiley & Sons, Inc.

ment over different parts of the body surface (loss of elasticity), loss of 20% to 25% of body weight, edema, decreased cardiac output and blood pressure, decreased respirations and slow-down of the basal metabolic rate, hormonal modifications, malabsorption, diarrhea, and nervous system effects such as apathy or irritability (Table 19-7).

Extreme cases of malnutrition in Africa have been shown by the media. Degrees of malnutrition can be observed in groups of underserved people in the United States. These people are poorly nourished due to lack of food, unsanitary conditions, inadequate water, lack of education, and other social, geographic, and cultural factors. In the past few years, there has been increasing concern for what is termed *subclinical* malnutrition. This affects everyone in the United States and is a result of extreme processing of food and the addition of chemicals to enhance appearance and increase shelf life.

Dietary Evaluation

With all of the published data related to diet, it is relatively easy to calculate the approximate amounts and proportions of fats, carbohydrates, proteins, vitamins, and minerals that should constitute a healthy diet. Most people, however, do not read nutritional charts, nor do they know how to define nutritional requirements in terms of actual food consumption. They tend to eat what and when they like or can afford, regardless of whether the meal has the right nutrients. In the United States, for instance, many students dash off to classes, having had no breakfast at all or else a quick meal of coffee and toast. A lunch consists of a hamburger and fries, supplemented with candy or soft drinks. This kind of diet can provide an adequate number of calories to get through the day but inadequate nutrients to nourish all of the body systems. A common form of malnutrition in the United States is overconsumption of food, which can create serious health problems such as obesity and heart disease and contribute to certain forms of diabetes.

Humans differ widely in their caloric requirements, depending on their size, age, sex, occupation, and so on. The average middle-aged man needs about 2600 calories a day, a woman about 1900, and a 12- to 15-year-old girl or boy from 2500 to 3000. Methods for calculating caloric need are

Technique for Calculating Body Fat

1. Determine muscularity: Measure girth of calf at widest circumference, or measure wrist at smallest circumference.
2. Check Tables 19-5 and 19-6 to see if you have low, medium, or high muscularity.
3. Refer to the ideal weights in Table 19-3 or 19-4. Find your height in inches, and then move across the table to find your degree of muscularity. At that point you will find your ideal weight. Note that these weights are based on optimum percentage of body fat.
4. Calculate your percentage of body fat by using the following formula (Getchell 1982, pp. 86–87):

Women:

$$\frac{\text{existing weight} - (.82 \times \text{ideal weight})}{\text{existing weight}} \times 100 = \%\ \text{fat}$$

Men:

$$\frac{\text{existing weight} - (.88 \times \text{ideal weight})}{\text{existing weight}} \times 100 = \%\ \text{fat}$$

Example:

$$\frac{185 - (.88 \times 165)}{185} = \frac{185 - (145.2)}{185}$$

$$= \frac{39.8}{185}$$

$$= .215$$

$$.215 \times 100 = 21.5\%\ \text{fat}$$

Table 19-5 **Calf Girth Measurements**

Degree of muscularity (estimate)	Women (inches)	Men (inches)
Low	12½ and below	14 and below
Medium	12½–13½	14–15½
High	13½ and up	15½ and up

Source: From B. Getchell with W. Anderson. *Being Fit: A Personal Guide*, pp. 88–89. Copyright © 1982 John Wiley & Sons. Reprinted by permission of John Wiley & Sons, Inc.

Table 19-6 **Wrist Girth Measurements**

Bone structure (estimate)	Women (inches)	Men (inches)
Low	5¼ and below	6¼ and below
Medium	15½–6	6¼–7
High	6 and up	7 and up

Source: From B. Getchell and W. Anderson. *Being Fit: A Personal Guide*, pp. 88–89. Copyright © 1982 John Wiley & Sons. Reprinted by permission of John Wiley & Sons, Inc.

Table 19-7 **Physical Signs and Symptoms of Undernutrition**

Organ/tissue	Undernutrition	Good nutrition
Hair	Dry, wirelike	Shiny, lustrous
	Stiff often brittle	Healthy scalp
	May exhibit some bleaching of normal color	
	Easily pluckable (pediatric form)	
Eyes	Thickened, opaque bulbar conjunctivae with angular lesions	Bright, clear, moist
	Increase in vascularity, conjunctival injection	
	Xerosis conjunctivae (the conjunctivae, on exposure by holding the lids open and having the subject rotate the eyes, appear dull and lusterless and exhibit a striated or roughened surface	
	Bitot's spots—small circumscribed grayish or yellowish dull, dry, foamy superficial lesions of the conjunctiva; seen most often on lateral aspect of conjunctiva and in children; not to be confused with pterygium	

Table 19-7 Continued

Organ/tissue	Undernutrition	Good nutrition
	Xerophthalmia—recorded when bulbar conjunctiva and cornea are dry and lusterless with a decrease in lacrimation; often associated with evidence of infection or, in extreme cases, keratomalacia	
	Keratomalacia (pediatric form shows corneal softening with deformity, either localized, usually central part of lower half of cornea, or total)	
Mouth and tongue	Lips—angular lesions and scars, indicating cheilosis	Reddish-pink color to lips, tongue, and mucous membrane
Mucous membranes	Tongue—Filiform papillary atrophy (smooth slick), hypertrophy/hyperemia, geographic tongue, fissure/serrations or swelling, red, scarlet, beefy (glossitis), magenta colored (color of alkaline phenolphthalein)	Absence of lesions Adequately moist
Teeth and gums	Teeth—visible caries	Surface papillae present on tongue
	Gums—atrophy, recession, inflammation; marginal redness or swelling (marginal redness is a definite red border along dental margin of gum, marginal swelling in a swollen border of gum, which may be spongy or firm); swollen red papillae; bleeding gums, which either bleed spontaneously or bleed on slight pressure with a swab stick	Teeth straight, bright without crowding, no evidence of caries Gums firm, reddish pink with no evidence of swelling or bleeding
Skin	Follicular hyperkeratosis—rough, dry	Smooth, slightly moist, good color
	Xerosis—dry or scaling	
	Hyperpigmentation—seen most frequently on dorsa of hands and lower forearms, particularly where skin hygiene is poor; skin is rough and dry, and often has a grayish cyanotic base	
	Thickened pressure points (other than elbows and knees); look especially at belt area, ischial tuberositis, sacrum, over greater trochanters	
Abdomen and lower extremities	Potbelly (pediatric form only), hepatomegaly	Abdomen flat
	Pretibial edema (bilateral)	No tenderness, weakness, or swelling of feet and legs
	Calf tenderness (adult form only)	
	Absent knee/ankle jerk (adult form)	
	Absent vibratory sense (adult form): test with tuning fork over lateral malleoli; record as positive only if absent bilaterally	
Skeletal (pediatric form only)	Beading of ribs	Good posture
	Bossing of skull	No malformations
Face and neck	Malar pigmentation (adult form)—areas of dark brown pigmentation over malar eminences	Skin of face and neck clear, smooth
	Nasolabial seborrhea—a definitive greasy, yellowish scaling or filiform excrescences on nasolabial area, which become more pronounced on slight scratching with a fingernail or tongue blade	No thyroid enlargement
	Parotid glands visibly enlarged	
	Thyroid enlarged	
Muscles	Flaccid underdeveloped, or wasted in appearance, tender	Well developed, firm

presented in Tables 19-8 and 19-9. These approximations assume a moderate amount of physical activity. If an individual consumes more calories than are burned, the extra calories are converted to fat and the person gains weight. If one does not consume enough calories, the body begins to convert its own tissue into the calories it needs, and weight is lost. Reducing diets based on this principle are often extreme and do not provide the necessary vitamins and minerals.

For individuals to meet all their nutritional requirements, they must eat a variety of foods, which nutritionalists have grouped into four broad categories. Nurses need to have

Table 19-8 One Method of Calculating Daily Caloric Needs According to Basal Metabolism and Activity Level

Physical activity	Total calories needed daily
Sedentary to light	$\frac{130}{100} \times$ basal caloric need
Moderate	$\frac{150}{100} \times$ basal caloric need
Strenuous	$\frac{(175 - 200)}{100} \times$ basal caloric need

Source: From H. Y. Hui: *Human Nutrition and Diet Therapy.* © 1983 Boston: Jones and Bartlett Publishers, p. 295. Reprinted with permission.

Table 19-9 USDA Rule of Thumb for Calculating Daily Caloric Needs

Physical activity	Total calories needed daily*	
	Women	Men
Sedentary	Ideal body weight × 14	Ideal body weight × 16
Moderate	Ideal body weight × 18	Ideal body weight × 21
Strenuous	Ideal body weight × 22	Ideal body weight × 26

*All ideal body weights expressed in pounds.

Source: From H. Y. Hui. *Human Nutrition and Diet Therapy.* © 1983 Boston: Jones and Bartlett Publishers, p. 296. Reprinted with permission.

Table 19-10 Milk Products That Contribute As Much Protein and Calcium As 1 Cup of Fluid Whole Milk

Milk product	Amount of product containing given amount of nutrient	
	9 g Protein	280 g Calcium
Nonfat milk	1 c	1 c
Cheddar cheese	1⅓ oz	1⅓ oz
Cottage cheese	1⅓ c	⅓ c
Ice cream	1½ c	1½ c
Cream cheese	30 T	9 T

Source: From H. Y. Hui. *Human Nutrition and Diet Therapy.* © 1983 Boston: Jones and Bartlett Publishers, p. 253. Reprinted with permission.

Table 19-11 Foods in the Fruit and Vegetable Group

Varieties rich in vitamin A and carotene
- Dark green leafy vegetables: beet greens, broccoli, chard, collards, watercress, kale, mustard greens, spinach, turnip tops, wild greens (dandelion and others)
- Orange-colored vegetables: carrots, pumpkins, sweet potatoes, winter squash, yams
- Orange-fleshed fruits: apricots, muskmelon, mangoes

Varieties rich in vitamin C
- Citrus fruits: grapefruit, oranges, lemons, tangerines; juices of these fruits
- Other good and excellent sources: muskmelon, strawberries, broccoli, several tropical fruits (including guavas), raw sweet green and red peppers
- Significant sources: tomatoes, tomato juice, white potatoes, dark green leafy vegetables, other raw vegetables and fruits

Other fruits and vegetables
- Vegetables: asparagus, lima beans, green beans, beets, cabbage, cauliflower, celery, corn, cucumber, eggplant, kohlrabi, lettuce, okra, onions, green peas, plantain, rutabagas, sauerkraut, summer squash, and turnips
- Fruits: apples, avocados, bananas, berries, cherries, dates, figs, grapes, nectarines, peaches, pears, pineapple, plums, prunes, raisins, rhubarb, watermelon; juices and nectars of many fruits

Source: From H. Y. Hui. *Human Nutrition and Diet Therapy.* © 1983 Boston: Jones and Bartlett Publishers, p. 255. Reprinted with permission.

knowledge of recommended dietary allowance if they are to adequately assess a client's dietary history. Several excellent books on nutrition are available in bookstores and libraries, and, whenever possible, nurses should consult with nutritionists for help with assessment and planning. The following information about the four food groups is brief, but will be of assistance in the assessment process.

Food Groups

There are four groups: milk and milk products, meats and meat equivalents, fruits and vegetables, and breads and cereals. Each group contributes a substantial amount of the major nutrients necessary for good health.

1. Milk and milk products (Table 19-10)
   - Fluid milk: whole, low-fat, skim, fat-free
   - Dry milk: whole, low-fat, skim, fat-free
   - Other milk: evaporated, condensed
   - Milk products: yogurt, cheese, cottage cheese
   - Milk alternates: soy milk, powdered soy milk, soy cheese
2. Meat and meat equivalents
   - Lean meat: beef, veal, lamb, pork, liver
   - Variety meat: heart, brain, tongue, kidney
   - Fish: shellfish, fresh- and saltwater varieties
   - Poultry: all fowl (chicken, turkey, guinea hen, duck, goose) and their giblets
   - Miscellaneous meats: "turkey ham," hot dogs
   - Dry legumes: navy beans, lima beans, lentils, and peanuts
   - Peas: All split, dried peas, pinto beans, chick peas, and pigeon peas
   - Eggs, cheese
3. Fruits and vegetables: The daily food guides recommend four or more servings of fruits and vegetables each day (Table 19-11).

4. Breads and cereals
   - Breads: yeast breads, rolls, quickbreads, biscuits, buns, muffins, pancakes, waffles, crackers
   - Breakfast cereals: ready-to-eat types, including flaked, rolled, and puffed forms; cooked types, including whole grain and rolled forms
   - Other grain foods: macaroni, spaghetti, noodles, flour, rice, cornmeal
   - Whole grain products: wholewheat flour and its products, bulgur, dark rye flour, brown rice, whole ground cornmeal

Table 19-12 lists the recommended number of servings from the four food groups. Table 19-13 outlines the nutrient contributions of foods in each of the groups. Tables 19-14 and 19-15 offer suggested meal plans.

Dietary History

A component of the nutritional assessment that is very useful in determining the client's nutritional status is the dietary history. The nurse asks the client to keep a record, usually for 24 hours, of all food eaten and at what times of the day. This is probably the most common way to make this assessment. One example of a dietary history format is shown in Table 19-16. Because there are many variations, the nurse should use the one that is most helpful in obtaining the needed information. Information obtained in this assessment can be used by the nurse to develop a teaching plan to meet the client's specific needs. It is helpful to use the guidelines provided in Table 19-17, or similar ones, when helping clients plan an adequate diet.

Biochemical Data Evaluation

The final component of nutritional assessment is the biochemical analysis of blood, urine, feces, saliva, and mucus. This analysis is a valuable adjunct to clinical and dietary data. Actual or subclinical deficiencies can be determined. Substances analyzed are in three categories: (1) blood

Table 19-12 **Recommended Numbers of Servings from the Four Food Groups**

Food group	Serving size	No. of daily servings
Milk and milk products		
Fluid milk	1 c, 8 oz, ½ pt, ¼ qt	Children under 9: 2–3 Children 9–12: ≥3 Teenagers: ≥4 Adults: ≥2 Pregnant women: ≥3 Nursing mothers: ≥4
Calcium equivalent	1 c milk 2 c cottage cheese 1 c pudding 1¾ c ice cream 1½ oz cheddar cheese	
Meat and meat equivalents	2–3 cooked lean meat without bone 3–4 oz raw meat without bone 2 oz luncheon meat (e.g., bologna) ¾ c canned baked beans 1 c cooked dry beans, peas, lentils 2 eggs 2 oz cheddar cheese ½ c cottage cheese 4 T peanut butter	≥2
Fruits and vegetables	Varies by item: ½ c cooked spinach 1 potato 1 orange ½ grapefruit	≥4, including 1 of citrus fruit and another fruit or vegetable that is a good source of vitamin C and 2 of a fair source 1, at least every other day, of a dark green or deep yellow vegetable for vitamin C ≥2 or more of other vegetables and fruits, including potatoes
Bread and cereals	1 slice of bread, 1 oz ready-to-eat cereal ½ to ¾ c cooked cereal, cornmeal, grits, macaroni, noodles, rice, or spaghetti	≥4

Source: From H. Y. Hui. *Human Nutrition and Diet Therapy.* © 1983 Boston: Jones and Bartlett Publishers, p. 251. Reprinted with permission.

Table 19-13 Approximate Nutrient Contributions of the Different Food Groups

Food group	Major nutrient contributed	Proportional contribution to the American diet
Milk	Protein	⅓
	Calcium	⅔
	Riboflavin	½
Meat	Protein	½
	Thiamin	¼
	Iron	>⅓
	Niacin	>⅓
Fruits and vegetables	Vitamin C	practically all
	Vitamin A and carotene	¾
	Iron	¼
Bread and cereals	Iron, thiamin, niacin, other B vitamins, fiber	>¼
Supplementary foods		
Fats, oils	Calories, fat-soluble vitamins	varies
Sweet products	Fluids, calories, small amount of nutrients	varies
Spices and seasonings	Iodine	varies
Alcohol	Calories	insignificant to ⅓

Source: From H. Y. Hui. *Human Nutrition and Diet Therapy.* © 1983 Boston: Jones and Bartlett Publishers, p. 258. Reprinted with permission.

Table 19-14 Suggested Meal Plan

Breakfast	Lunch	Dinner
Fruit juice, ½ c/1 serving	Soup, ½ c	Soup, ½c
Cereal: hot/6 oz; dry/1 oz	Meat (regular/substitute), 2–3 oz	Meat (regular/substitute), 3–4 oz
Egg (regular or substitute), 1 serving	Vegetable (cooked/salad), ½ c	Fruit/juice, ½ c/1 serving
Meat: 2 strips bacon; 2 sausages; 1 oz regular meat	Potato (regular/substitute), ½ c	Vegetable (cooked/salad), ½ c
Bread, 1–2 slices	Salad dressing, 1 T	Potato (regular/substitute), ½ c
Butter/margarine, 1–3 t	Bread/roll, 1–2 servings	Salad dressing, 1–2 t
Jelly/jam/preserves, 1–3 t	Butter/margarine, 1–3 t	Bread/roll, 1–2 servings
Milk, 1 c	Dessert, 1 serving	Butter/margarine, 1–3 t
Hot beverage (coffee/tea), 1–2 c	Milk, 1 c	Dessert, 1 serving
Cream (regular/substitute), 1–3 t	Hot beverage (coffee/tea), 1–2 c	Milk, 1 c
Sugar, 1–3 t	Cream (regular/substitute), 1–3 t	Hot beverage (coffee/tea), 1–2 c
Salt, pepper	Sugar, 1–3 t	Cream (regular/substitute), 1–3 t
	Salt, pepper	Sugar, 1–3 t
		Salt, pepper

Source: From H. Y. Hui. *Human Nutrition and Diet Therapy.* © 1983 Boston: Jones and Bartlett Publishers, p. 259. Reprinted with permission.

components such as proteins, albumin, hemoglobin, and fibrinogen; (2) minerals and specific substances such as cations, hydrogen-ions, adenosine triphosphate, and glutathione; and (3) nutrients and their metabolites, such as amino and fatty acids, glycerol, phospholipid, cholesterol, triglycerides, carbohydrates, vitamins, minerals, and hormones. Body wastes to be analyzed include carbon dioxide, water, bilirubin, urea, and creatinine.

Table 19-15 Menu Plan Providing 2,400 kcal and 95 g of Protein

Breakfast	Lunch	Dinner
Orange, ½ c	Pea soup, ½ c	Chicken broth, ½ c
Oatmeal, 6 oz	Crackers, 2	Fried chicken, 3 oz
Egg, 1	Ham, 2 oz	Spinach, ½ c
Bread, 2 slices	Lettuce/tomato salad, ½ c	Rice, ½ c
Margarine, 2 t	Noodles, ½ c	Bread, 1 slice
Jelly, 1 t	Toast, 1 slice	Margarine, 1 t
Milk, 1 c	Margarine, 1 t	Milk, 1 c
Coffee, 1 c	Milk, 1 c	Coffee, 1 c
Cream, 1 t	Ice cream, 1 c	Cream substitute, 1 t
Sugar, 2 t	Coffee, 1 c	Sugar, 1 t
Salt, pepper	Sugar, 1 t	Salt, pepper
	Salt, pepper	

Source: From H. Y. Hui. *Human Nutrition and Diet Therapy.* © 1983 Boston: Jones and Bartlett Publishers, p. 259. Reprinted with permission.

Table 19-16 Dietary History Format

Record of foods eaten and drinks	Amount (cups, tbsps)	Record of foods eaten and drinks	Amount (cups, tbsps)
Morning		Afternoon	
Food		Food	
Drinks		Drinks	
Midmorning		Evening	
Food		Food	
Drinks		Drinks	
Noon		Before bed	
Food		Food	
Drinks		Drinks	
Vitamins or mineral supplement (list kind and number taken)			

Table 19-17 Guidelines for Assisting the Client in Dietary Planning

Current dietary patterns		Recommended dietary goals	
42% fat	16% saturated	10% saturated	30% fat
	19% monounsaturated	10% monounsaturated	
	7% polyunsaturated	10% polyunsaturated	12% protein
12% protein			
46% carbohydrates	28% complex carbohydrates and naturally occurring sugars	48% complex carbohydrates and naturally occurring sugars	58% carbohydrates
	18% refined and processed sugars	10% refines and processed sugars	

Source: From *Dietary Goals for the United States.* U.S. Senate Select Committee on Nutrition and Human Needs. Washington, D.C.: Government Printing Office, December 1977.

PHYSICAL FITNESS ASSESSMENT

Physical fitness has taken the United States by storm. Health clubs are bustling, aerobic classes are full, and the streets are noticeably busy with walkers, bikers, and joggers. They are on a quest for wellness, fitness, and an improved lifestyle.

Fitness is important at all ages. For children, optimum fitness assists their normal development and helps them to be strong enough to meet life's challenges. For young adult and middle-aged clients, a fit body helps to prevent degenerative conditions such as coronary heart disease, obesity, and musculoskeletal disorders. For older clients, maintaining fitness improves quality of life by helping to maintain or improve physical capabilities and, often, social interactions. Research has demonstrated a link between physical fitness and an improvement in self-esteem (Ben Leslies & Short 1983, pp. 11–28).

Complete physical fitness assessment can be complex and may require specialized equipment and space. The nurse can do an initial assessment, which is helpful in making overall plans for client care. The basic components of health and fitness are cardiovascular function, body composition, strength, and flexibility.

Cardiovascular Function

Cardiovascular function is the most important component in health-related fitness. Cardiovascular disease is the leading cause of death among adult populations of most industrialized societies. An alarming aspect of this is the prevalence of heart disease among younger adults. This problem, however, is not confined to adults. In two recent studies of boys and girls ages 7 to 12, it was noted that 60% exhibited at least one of the risk factors associated with increased coronary heart disease in the adult population (obesity, high serum cholesterol and/or triglycerides, elevated blood pressure, or low work capacity) (Baylor & Dishman 1980, p. 40).

Various laboratory tests, stress tests, and ECG examinations are the most definitive in making an assessment of cardiovascular fitness. Some tests can be performed easily by the nurse when conducting a cardiovascular assessment. The first is the step test. This test is an easy-to-use field test, which can give preliminary information on the cardiovascular fitness of the client. It is not stressful for most clients, but caution should be used in testing clients over age 40, those who are obese, and those who have a history of cardiovascular problems.

A step 17 to 18 inches high is needed. The client should be instructed to step up and down on the step, 30 steps per minute for men and 24 steps per minute for women. The following sequence should be used: right foot up, left foot up; right foot down, left foot down. After the client has continued stepping for 3 minutes (4-count sequence), the pulse is measured. Apical, carotid, or radial pulses may be used. Pulse rates are counted for 30 seconds at the following intervals:

- 1 to 1½ minutes following exercise
- 2 to 2½ minutes following exercise
- 3 to 3½ minutes following exercise

The 30-second pulses are added and the sum is called the recovery index (Getchell 1979, pp. 70–73) (Fig. 19-3).

Body Composition

Body composition is the relative percentage of fat and fat-free body mass. Body composition is an important correlate to cardiovascular function, as far as health-related fitness is concerned. Excess fat is excess baggage and causes the body to have to increase energy expenditure, which in turn causes the circulation to work harder. In addition to increased coronary heart disease among obese persons, there is also greater risk of developing hypertension, diabetes mellitus, gallbladder disease, arthritis, and kidney disease. In addition to assessing body density, fat, and weight (methods described earlier), body proportions should be considered. If the body is well proportioned, the individual generally feels better about self-image. Norms for determining girth measurements (Pender 1982, p. 87) are as follows.

Women

- Bust and hips: same
- Abdomen at waist: 25 to 26 cm less than bust and hips
- Thigh: 15 cm less than waist
- Calf: 18 to 20 cm less than thigh
- Ankle: 13 to 15 cm less than calf
- Biceps (upper arm) relaxed, 2 times the size of wrist

Men

- Chest and hips: same
- Abdomen (at waist): 13 to 18 cm less than chest and hips
- Thigh: 20 to 25 cm less than abdomen
- Calf: 18 to 20 cm less than thigh
- Ankle: 15 to 18 cm less than calf
- Biceps (upper arm) relaxed: 2 times the size of wrist

Strength

Strength, defined as the capacity of a muscle to exert or resist force, is the third component of fitness. Strength is important to the athlete and to the average individual. Strong muscles protect joints, which in turn protect against strain, sprains, and pulls. Toned muscles help to prevent sagging abdomens, round shoulders, and back pain. Lack of strength can impair the client's ability to perform even the simplest of activities of daily living.

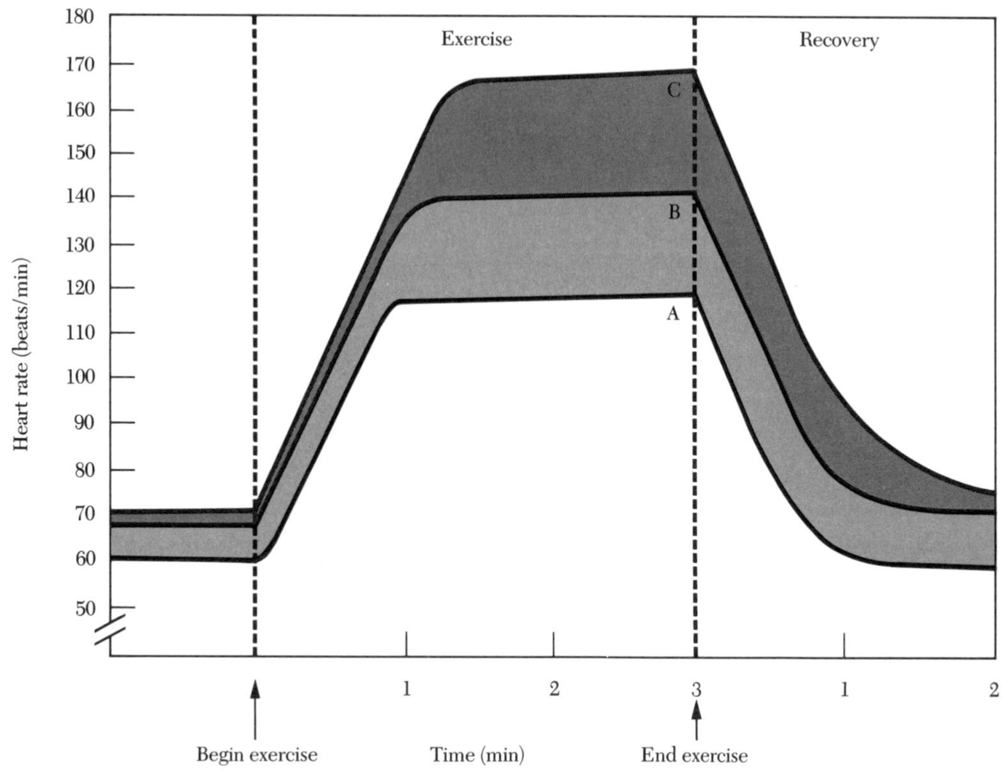

Figure 19-3 Heart rate response to step test. Examples are given for three people **(A, B, C)**.

Bent-knee sit-ups can be used as a test of muscular strength. Clients who have not maintained their fitness level will often find them difficult to do. For women, the number of sit-ups is calculated for 1 minute; for men, the number in 2 minutes. Clients with cardiovascular disorders or other chronic illnesses and the elderly must be observed carefully. The nurse may make the judgment that performing bent-knee sit-ups would be too distressing for a client, assuming that muscle strength is poor. A client's needs and capabilities can guide development of a plan that would help to build reasonable muscle strength.

The procedure for assisting the client with bent-knee sit-ups is as follows:

- Have the client lie on her back on a mat or firm support and bend the knees approximately 90 degrees with feet flat on the floor.
- Hands should be interlocked behind the neck, with elbows pointed toward the knees.
- The nurse can hold the feet while instructing the client to curl the back and raise the trunk until it is perpendicular to the floor.
- It is important to keep the knees bent during the entire exercise.

For further information, refer to Fig. 19-4 and Table 19-18.

Table 19-18 Evaluation of Bent-Knee Sit-Ups

Rating	Women (no. of sit-ups per 1 min.)	Men (no. of sit-ups per 2 min.)
Excellent	33 or up	69 or up
Good	27–32	60–68
Average	20–26	52–59
Low	16–21	42–51
Poor	16 or under	41 or under

Source: Adapted from B. Getchell. *Physical Fitness: A Way of Life*, 2nd ed. (New York: Wiley, 1979), pp. 56–57.

Flexibility

Flexibility refers to the degree to which a joint may move throughout its maximal possible range of motion. Maintenance of the ability to move, bend, and stretch provides good protection to muscles during activity. Flexibility decreases with age and with a sedentary lifestyle. Poor flexibility may result in misalignment of body structures, crowding of internal organs, and low back pain. Lack of flexibility also makes it difficult for clients to maintain activities of daily

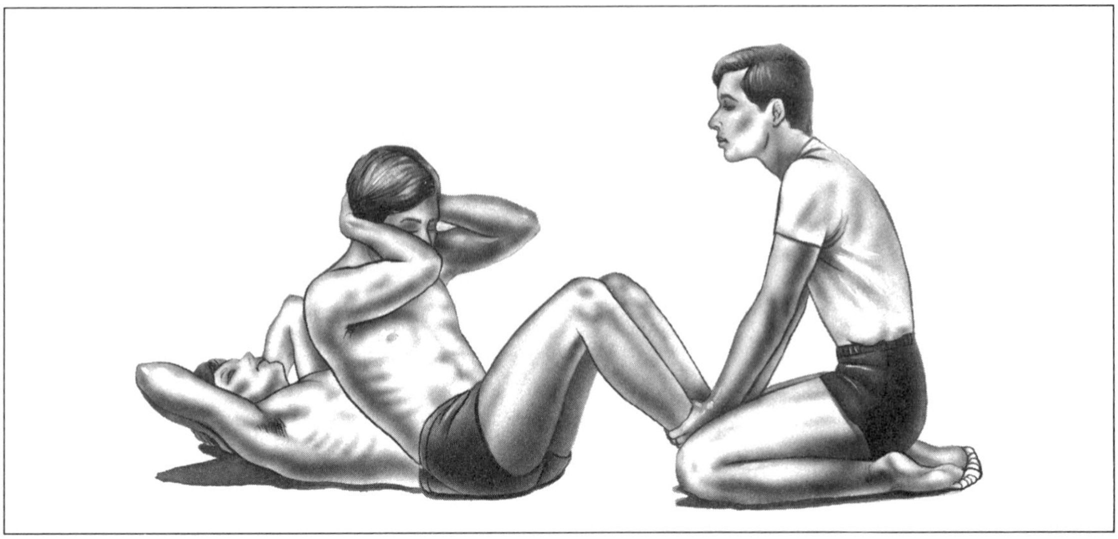

Figure 19-4 Bent-knee sit-ups.

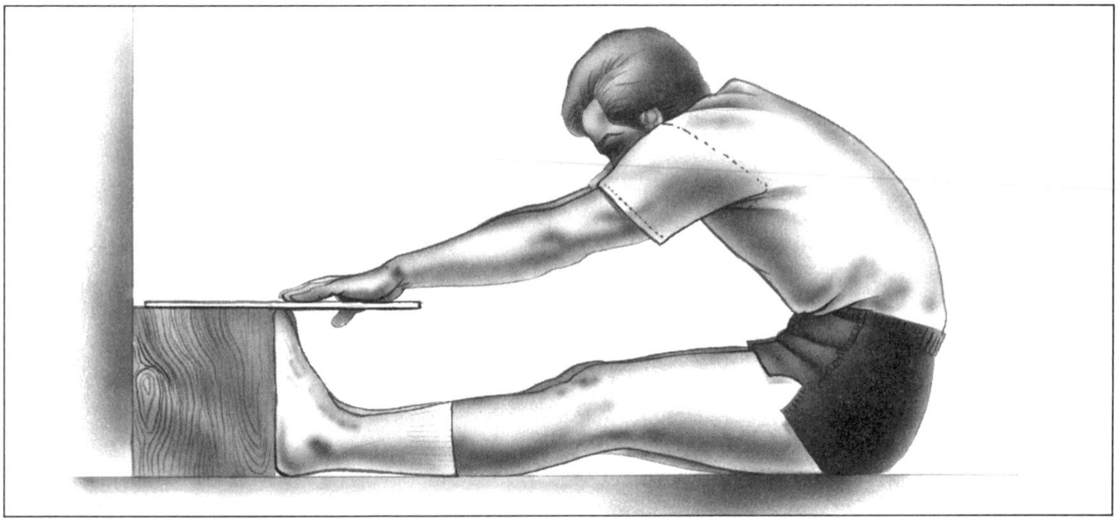

Figure 19-5 Measuring trunk flexion.

living. A quick test of flexibility is to have the client bend forward and, keeping his knees straight, touch his toes. Poor flexibility is indicated by an inability to reach the toes.

Another test of flexibility measures the client's ability to stretch back and thigh muscles (Fig. 19-5). The procedure for measuring this is as follows:

- Have the client sit on the floor with legs fully extended and feet flat against a box, which has been stabilized against the wall.
- Instruct the client to extend arms as far forward as possible, stretching from the waist.
- With a ruler, measure the distance the client can reach beyond the proximal edge of the box.
- If the client cannot reach the edge, report the distance of the fingertips from the edge as a negative number.

SUMMARY

There is little doubt that what we eat has a tremendous impact on our health. It is essential that the nurse gather information from each client about eating habits. This assessment initially occurs when the client's history is being gathered. Information obtained at this time will help the nurse to determine if a more in-depth nutritional assessment is needed.

Cardiovascular fitness, body composition, muscular strength, and flexibility are critical components in the overall evaluation of client fitness. The nurse can assess these as separate components in the health evaluation or include them when evaluating various body systems. For example, cardiovascular fitness can be determined while assessing the cardiovascular system. Body composition can be determined while assessing the musculoskeletal system. It is up to the nurse to determine the appropriate time to assess each component.

DISCUSSION QUESTIONS/ ACTIVITIES

1. Choose a classmate or family member and have that person keep a food diary for 24 hours. Review the diary with the individual. Help the individual plan a more healthy diet, if necessary.
2. Discuss your personal diet and exercise program with the class.
3. Using the techniques described, assess a client's cardiovascular status, strength, and flexibility.

REFERENCES

Ben Leslies, S., and Short, M. 1983. The effects of physical exercise on self-attitudes. *Occupational Therapy in Mental Health* 3:11–28.

Getchell, B. 1979. *Physical fitness: a way of life.* 2nd ed. New York: Wiley.

Getchell, B., and Anderson, W. 1982. *Being fit: a personal guide.* New York: Wiley.

Lewis, C. M. 1984. *Basic and family nutrition: a self-instructional approach.* Philadelphia: F. A. Davis.

Pender, N. J. 1982. *Health promotion in nursing practice.* Norwalk, Conn.: Appleton-Century-Crofts.

CHAPTER

20 Assessment of the Older Adult

Learning Objectives

1. Appreciate the ways in which culture dictates the behavior of the older adult.
2. Recognize that chronologic age is a poor index of mental functioning and physiologic performance.
3. Acquire a general understanding of the older adult.
4. Identify changes in lifestyle patterns of the older adult.
5. Analyze physical assessment findings in light of criteria that includes physiologic changes of aging.

The United States grows grayer every year, despite the obsession with youth. In the past decade, according to the U.S. Census Bureau, the number of people over age 65 has increased 37%, which is more than double the growth of the general population. According to the Bureau's projections, this country will continue to age, and by 2010 people 55 and older will number about 74 million, or one quarter of the total population. This fact alone warrants that this group of people needs to be understood in regard to the influence of the aging process on health status. The "elderly image" has been one of frailness, confusion, and doddering; however, research is shattering the myths of aging. The elderly are not a homogeneous group with identical developmental changes and behaviors that can be categorized. Indeed, they are unique individuals with the commonality merely of having lived a longer time than other people. The perceptions of old age are based on obsolete information and have been associated with the term *elderly;* therefore, in an attempt to move away from such an undeserved image, we have chosen to discuss health assessment of the *older adult.*

The quality of health assessment is dependent on not stereotyping or making assumptions. Moreover, it is dependent on the awareness, understanding, and attitudes of each nurse regarding each age group, including the older adult.

It has been said that aging is a process to become old. But what does this mean? Does this mean that the individual is decrepit and cannot or should not be salvaged? Chronologic age is a poor index of mental functioning and physiologic performance. Aging is highly individualized. Therefore, a careful health assessment must be performed. More research is needed in the area of health and health status regarding the older adult to better meet the needs of this large population group. Contained in this chapter is a discussion of specifics regarding the health assessment of the older adult with indices inherent in cultural, mental health, and physical assessment aspects—the knowledge divisions of health assessment used throughout this text.

CULTURAL ASSESSMENT

Investigation of a client's cultural background brings out the beauty and uniqueness of the individual. For the most part, the older adults within our society are the ones who uphold and transmit culture and ultimately are the preservers of culture. The many life experiences—some difficult learning experiences and others emotionally, intellectually, and physically pleasurable—have profited the value system formation of the older adult. If the adage "practice makes perfect" is true, the older adult has much to teach each of us if we will only listen. Moreover, by being aware of the values, beliefs, attitudes, and practices of older individuals, which may differ greatly from our own, we can conscientiously afford them respect as individuals and come to understand the rationale behind some of their behavior.

Health Practices

The majority of older adults today continue to view the use of health care systems as a source of help only in times of severe illness or injury. They are often reluctant to leave their homes and forfeit their independence.

Religion

As one ages, the concern of mortality becomes more paramount, and the spiritual sphere enlarges. Faith is a tenet of everyday living, though it is not often verbalized. If the older adult had interrupted formal religious practices earlier in life, it is not uncommon for her to return to active participation in the later years of her life. Most likely the return is due to a combination of religious reawakening and a means for socializing.

Social Aspects

In the many years of lifework, the person has developed networks for socialization and support systems to help cope with stressful life events. Most central to an individual's social support network is the family. Research by Preston and Grimes (1987) found that married persons rely a good deal on their spouses as confidants for help. The married man relies significantly more on his spouse, whereas the married woman tends to rely on family and friends as well as her spouse. Therefore, if the wife should die first, the social support system of most widowers is devastated. The nurse can help the married man, preferably with the aid of his wife, to broaden his network. To identify the social support system with the older adult becomes a mutual task within the cultural assessment component of the total health assessment. A good social support system is highly correlated with well-being. Along with knowledge of support systems, the nurse needs to consider the available resources, the client's assets, and his effective coping skills.

The occupational history aids in the identification of predisposing factors to particular disease entities and infirmities and may be of significance in determining a diagnosis. When assessing the older adult, you would be greatly amiss if you ceased investigation of occupational experiences at the mention of "I am retired." A person may have worked as a clerk in a hardware store for a few years prior to retirement; however, as you continue investigation, you may find that he spent 10 years as a coal miner and another 30 years shoveling coal into blast furnaces in a steel mill. This would call your attention to the possibility of existing or potential respiratory problems. Inadvertently you may learn about interests and support networks as you have the client talk about his lifework. For instance, you may hear a client say, "I've worked with Joe for the past 30 years; he will always be my friend. We go fishing together almost every weekend, and we help each other in planting our gardens."

Lifestyle

The eating habits of the older adult sometimes fail to change, although exercise and other physical activities are generally modified. Given the sustained daily caloric intake, the client tends to put on weight. With a lowered basal metabolic rate (BMR), the need for high caloric intake no longer exists. Or the client may have lost weight and is thin or actually malnourished; this may have an etiology of just not cooking for oneself for a variety of reasons or of not having financial means, or it may be due to a disease state.

The sleep pattern changes with age. Around the age of 50, the fourth stage of sleep is decreased by 20% of what it was during the second decade of life. The void is replaced by an increase in stages two and three and is accompanied by an increase in the frequency and duration of spontaneous awakening.

Most nurses probably do not pursue an assessment of sexuality in the older adult. Once again, though, research has debunked the myth that sexuality and sexual activity are dead past age 50. However, the older woman may find that suitable partners are lacking. Because women tend to live longer than men, the ratio of women to men becomes greater with age. Many times, social customs must be breached for the older woman to satisfy this social-physical need. She may engage in an alternative lifestyle, find a younger partner, have a married partner, or cohabit with a widower. The practice of marriage may not be exercised by the older adult at times because of the attitudes of children or other relatives. Thus the older adult makes a sacrifice of moral values in the name of love for his family. Perhaps family members do not have difficulty accepting the sexuality of parents, but they are fearful of losing part or all of an inheritance if marriage occurs. Premarital contracts regarding already accrued property and assets may be a solution (Fig. 20-1).

Those older adults in nursing homes find themselves deprived of human intimacy. Nurses can be advocates by ensuring privacy and coupling activities that promote the expression of sexuality by the residents. Despite long-term institutionalization, illness, and disease, sexual needs continue. Because of cultural attitudes and myths, the older adult may experience feelings of guilt and embarrassment. Sexual activity may even be avoided in order to conform to these cultural "norms." However, some older adults may have never had much interest and enthusiasm in sexual matters. Some may have a decreased self-image and lack the self-esteem necessary for a healthy expression of sexuality. Ebersole and Hess (1981) point out that impaired physical health may interfere directly or indirectly with sexual activities. Effects of chronic illness, such as fatigue, shortness of breath, and alterations in blood or nerve supply, may impair sexual functioning. Also medications used by the older adult can alter sexual behavior. The phenothiazines increase libido in older women; L-dopa increases libido in older men. This effect may be very distressing for the client. Medications commonly used by older adults that depress sexual behavior are listed in Table 20-1.

If the older adult is aware of the effects of medications and is knowledgeable of the changes in sexual response that commonly occur as a normal part of the aging process, he will understand the effects rather than fear that sexual powers are being lost (Table 20-2).

The use of alcohol by the older adult should be investigated. Because of the diminished BMR in the older adult, alcohol tends to remain in the body longer. Thus, even though the older adult drinks less, he may not necessarily be less intoxicated. The same alcohol intake criteria for other ages cannot be used, because the older adult has changes in fat and water composition and in body weight. The older adult who lives alone is at greater risk; the identification of alcohol abuse is more difficult. Many times, well-caring families are not aware that such a problem exists. The family members may live far away; they may lack knowledge to identify the signs and symptoms; they literally may not care, or they may be preoccupied with their own lives. In addition, the older adult may tend to withdraw and isolate himself from the family so as not to be a burden or interfere. He may attempt "to drown in the bottle" feelings of unworthiness, guilt, loneliness, and the like. A stigma remains attached to seeking help, and fear of being institutionalized is common.

Signs of alcohol abuse in the older adult are similar to many other problems frequently observed in this age group. For example, memory loss can be due to decreased cardiac output; alcohol will exacerbate this memory loss problem. This could have a ripple effect, wherein the older adult

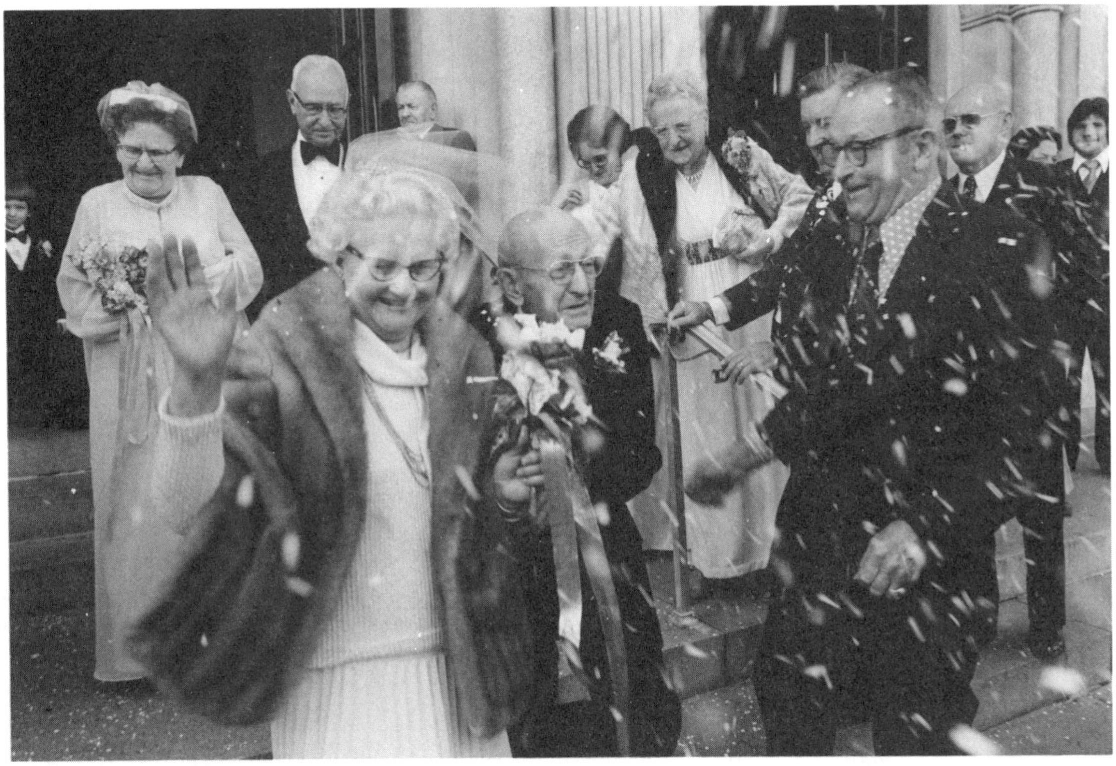

Figure 20-1 Marital bliss can be a reality for the older adult.

Table 20-1 Drugs That May Suppress the Libido in the Older Adult

Antianxiety agents (in large doses causing CNS depression)
Clorazepate dipotassium
Chlordiazepoxide
Diazepam
Meprobamate
Oxazepam
Antidepressants
Monoamine oxidase (MAO) inhibitors
Tricyclics
Antihypertensives
Chlorothiazide
Guanethidine
Hydralazine
Methyldopa
Pargyline
Rauwolfia alkaloids
Antispasmodics/Anticholinergics
Atropine
Diphenhydramine
Propantheline bromide
Trihexyphenidyl
Narcotics
Codeine
Heroin
Meperidine
Oxycodone
Sedatives
Alcohol
Antiasthmatics
Barbiturates
Flurazepam
Stimulants
Amphetamines
Anorexic agents
Caffeine (small amounts)
Ephedrine
Epinephrine
Methylphenidate
Tranquilizers
Butyrophenones
Dihydroindolones
Haloperidol
Phenothiazines
Thioxanthenes

Source: B. H. Glovers. Sex Counseling of the Elderly: *Hospital Practice* 12:101–113, June 1977.

becomes less and less capable of handling his household and everyday affairs. The effects of alcohol may become altered because of the pattern of polydrug use by this age group. Older adults constitute about 25% of the users of prescription tranquilizers such as Valium and Librium. They are generally heavy over-the-counter drug users. The use of a combination of drugs and alcohol is practiced by over half of the older adult population. This is a deadly combination; unintentional overdose can be a result. The interaction of drugs and nutrition needs to be analyzed (Table 20-3).

Table 20-2 Age-Related Changes in Sexual Response

Phase of response cycle	Age-related changes
Excitement phase	Female—may require from 1–5 minutes of sexual play for vaginal lubrication Male—less intense and slower erection
Plateau phase	Female—less change in labia color; clitoral hood and fatty tissue of mons decrease Male—decreased or absence of Cowper's lubrication.
Orgasmic phase	Female—fewer orgasmic contractions Male—fewer penile and rectal sphincter contractions; decreased force of ejaculation; decreased semen
Resolution phase	Female—vasoconstriction of clitoris and orgasmic platform quickly subsides Male—refractory period lengthens (time required for another erection ranges from several to 24 hours or longer)

The stereotypic image of exercise in the older adult is knitting in a rocking chair or playing checkers. This image is rapidly fading as we see our mothers, fathers, grandmothers, grandfathers, and even great-grandparents, aunts, and uncles running in marathons. The older adult can sometimes have more stamina than the most active of the young. Also, research is showing that walking, gardening, and similar activities contribute to health maintenance almost as much, if not as much, as aerobic dancing, jogging, and swimming. The older adult need not exercise to the point of severe sweating for 20-minute periods three times a week to maintain health as was previously thought. In fact, this type of regimen may be detrimental. Particularly when initiating an exercise regimen that is vigorous and a great change from normal exercise activity, the older adult needs to begin gradually and consult with his physician (Fig. 20-2).

The nurse can explore thoughts and plans about retirement with older adults. What changes do they anticipate? What are their goals in regard to retirement? Do they belong to groups and engage in activities with persons other than co-workers? Do they enjoy activities with their spouse? Do they foresee financial problems? If already retired, how are they enjoying it? How and why does it seem to be miserable for them? Are they setting goals and identifying realistic ways to meet them? What are the stumbling blocks and problems? Have their living arrangements changed?

Table 20-3 Nutrient/Drug Interactions to Be Aware of in Elderly Persons

Drug	Nutritional effects
Alcohol	Can lead to deficiencies in all nutrients, especially B vitamins Can replace eating
Aminopterin Methotrexate (used to treat leukemia)	Inhibits folate utilizations. However, if folate is supplemented, drug may not be as effective.
Antacids	Magnesium salts can cause diarrhea, limiting absorption of all nutrients. Protein absorption may be adversely affected when stomach acidity is reduced. Aluminum hydroxide binds phosphates.
Antibiotics	1. Tetracycline can bind iron, magnesium, and calcium salts. 2. Many antibiotics are antagonistic to folic acid and can result in deficiencies of other nutrients. 3. Can lead to malabsorption. 4. Neomycin binds bile acids and affects fat-soluble vitamin absorption 5. Neomycin causes intestinal structural changes that result in malabsorption of N, Na, K, Ca, lactose.
Anticoagulants	Can cause vitamin K deficiency
Anticonvulsants	Primadone, phenobarbitol induce folate deficiency and vitamin D deficiency.
Antidepressants	Some cause accelerated breakdown of vitamin D. If the monamine oxidase (MAO) inhibitor-type is used, patients become intolerant to foods containing tyramine, such as aged cheese, red wine, beer, dry salami, and chocolate. These foods can precipitate hypertensive crisis when MAO inhibitors are being used.
Aspirin and other antiinflammatory drugs	1. Many cause gastrointestinal bleeding; arthritic patients who ingest large quantities may develop iron-deficiency anemia secondary to blood loss. 2. Aspirin usage can affect folic-acid status. 3. Aspirin and indomethacin can increase need for vitamin C by impairing its effectiveness.
Barbiturates	1. Some cause breakdown of vitamin D 2. Excessive sedation of nursing home patients for behavior control can result in missed meals. 3. Folic acid is malabsorbed.
Cathartics	Reduce intestinal transit time necessary for proper absorption of some nutrients
Cholesterol-lowering drugs such as chlofibrate	Any drug altering blood lipids can affect absorption of fat-soluble vitamins. Vitamin K deficiencies can be produced.
Colchicine, used in gout	Causes malabsorption of fat, carotene, sodium, potassium, vitamin B12, folic acid, and lactose
Diuretics	Most diuretics cause potassium to be lost in urine. Blood levels of potassium must be monitored, because mental confusion can result from low levels of potassium. Dietary sources of potassium should be consumed. (Magnesium may be deficient in long-term diuretics.)
Glucocorticoids, used in allergy and collagen disease	Impair calcium transport across mucosa
Hormones	1. ACTH and cortisone therapy increases excretion of sodium, potassium, and calcium, and may contribute to the development of diabetes, hypertension, obesity, and water retention. Calcium and potassium supplements may be needed, as well as special diet prescriptions if hypertension and diabetes develop. 2. Calcitonin treatment: Decreases serum calcium levels as calcium is deposited into bone. Tetany may develop without oral calcium supplements. 3. Estrogen therapy: Over an extended period, may result in deficiencies of folic acid and vitamin B6. Patient should not receive folic acid supplements until vitamin B12 status is confirmed to be satisfactory. 4. Hormone therapy can cause peptic ulcers, which require dietary management. 5. Prednisone causes malabsorption of calcium.
Isoniazid (INH) (a drug used to treat tuberculosis)	Causes B6 deficiency in some persons because it is an antagonist to the vitamin
Laxatives	Harsh laxatives may cause diarrhealike effects: Food passes through the GI tract too fast to be absorbed. Mineral oil absorbs vitamins A and D, preventing them from being absorbed.

Continued

Table 20-3 Continued

Drug	Nutritional effects
Licorice candy	Limits potassium absorption
Metformin and Phenformin Hypoglycemic agents used in diabetics	Competitively inhibit vitamin B12 absorption
Para-amino salicylic acid, used to treat tuberculosis	Can cause malabsorption of fat and folic acid; blocks absorption of vitamin B12
Potassium chloride, used to replenish potassium lost due to diuretic use	Depresses absorption of vitamin B12

Source: From Kart/Metress/Metress: *Aging, Health and Society.* © 1988 Boston: Jones and Bartlett Publishers. Reprinted with permission.

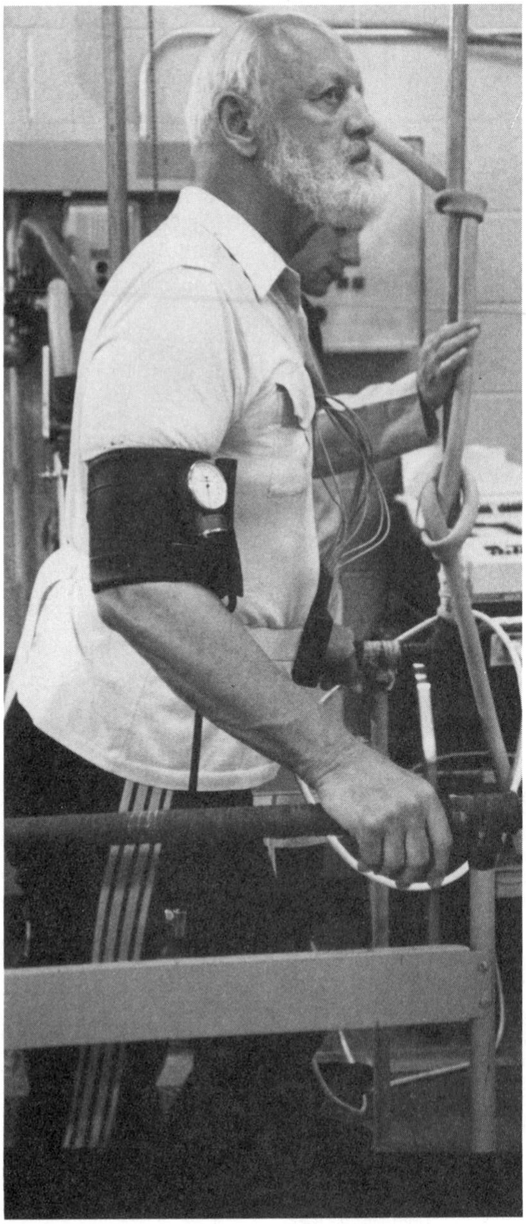

Figure 20-2 Older adults should not begin an exercise program without first getting a physical examination and physician input.

Economic Status

The stereotype is that the older adult is in the lower income bracket. About 15% to 20% of older persons fit this picture, and of this percentage, 40% are minority groups, with the African-American woman being at the lowest level. Conversely, the majority of older adults are in a higher income bracket; they usually own their homes and have relatively low expenses.

Stress

It has been said that aging is the ability to survive stress and, laughingly, that gray hair is hereditary—you get it from your kids! However, changes attributed to aging are most apparent when the individual is under stress. Such is the source for comments like "That took 10 years off my life!" and "He looks 40 years older!" The nurse must assess the degree of stressful life events that the older adult has experienced. The more common ones are dealing with death, disease, accidents, and retirement. The major health problems of older adults fall into the category of chronic disease. Commonly occurring conditions are accidental injuries, mental health problems, nutritional problems, colon/breast/cervical cancer, hearing and visual defects, anemia, diabetes, renal disease, poorly fitting dentures, dental caries, and periodontal disease. The leading causes of death in people over age 65 are congestive heart failure, stroke, cancer, and accidents.

MENTAL HEALTH STATUS ASSESSMENT

In the not too distant past it was thought that chronic and acute organic brain syndromes were consequences of aging. Any signs of disorientation, delirium, confusion, decreased cognitive ability, excitement, or poor judgment were attributed to the aging process. Yet young and middle-aged clients who are afflicted by such conditions as hypoglycemia, hypokalemia, anemia, dehydration, cardiac failure, and stroke will manifest many of these same mental changes. The old stereotype of intellectual decline in the older adult has become a self-fulfilling prophecy in many cases. Most people assume that intellectual decrement in the later years of life is a universal and unavoidable phenomenon. In a 7-year longitudinal study of older adults (Schaie 1985), it was found that on the average, intellectual functioning did decline in the sixth decade of life; however, even by age 81 about 50% of the subjects maintained their intellectual functioning level over the 7 years. Other than genetic factors, those individuals who maintained function were free of cardiovascular disease, were of at least middle-class socioeconomic status, and had a stimulating and engaged lifestyle. They also described themselves as having flexible attitudes and behaviors during the middle-aged years. In light of these findings, professionals and the media need to educate the public and focus attention on those 95% of the elderly who are not institutionalized, who are living in the community, and who possess full cognitive competence.

The older adult must be approached with respect and value of equal worth and importance. Nurses can play a significant role in teaching and encouraging the older adult to seek compensation for sensory changes and to remain active in lifestream activity. More effort needs to be placed on developing flexible retirement plans and on preretirement counseling. Chronologic age, in the form of mandatory retirement, has become nothing more than a constraining time frame.

The usual parameters of mental health and techniques used for assessing intellectual functioning are the same as described in Chapter 3. Depression and suicide have a high incidence in the older age group and are due to the same kind of problems experienced by persons of a younger age group who also manifest depression and attempt or commit suicide. A decrease in self-esteem may be a basis. Disengagement from society may contribute to a lowered self-image. Sensory deprivation brought about by living alone and ignored by society may give rise to depression. Sensory stimulation, or "future shock" due to increased technological changes, may also be the cause of mental stress and dysfunction. Research has shown that the degree of participation in family and community is positively correlated with an individual's mental state and functioning. Assessment therefore needs to include an investigation of family life and participation in such aspects of community life as volunteer work, senior citizen groups, and pastoral visits (Fig. 20-3).

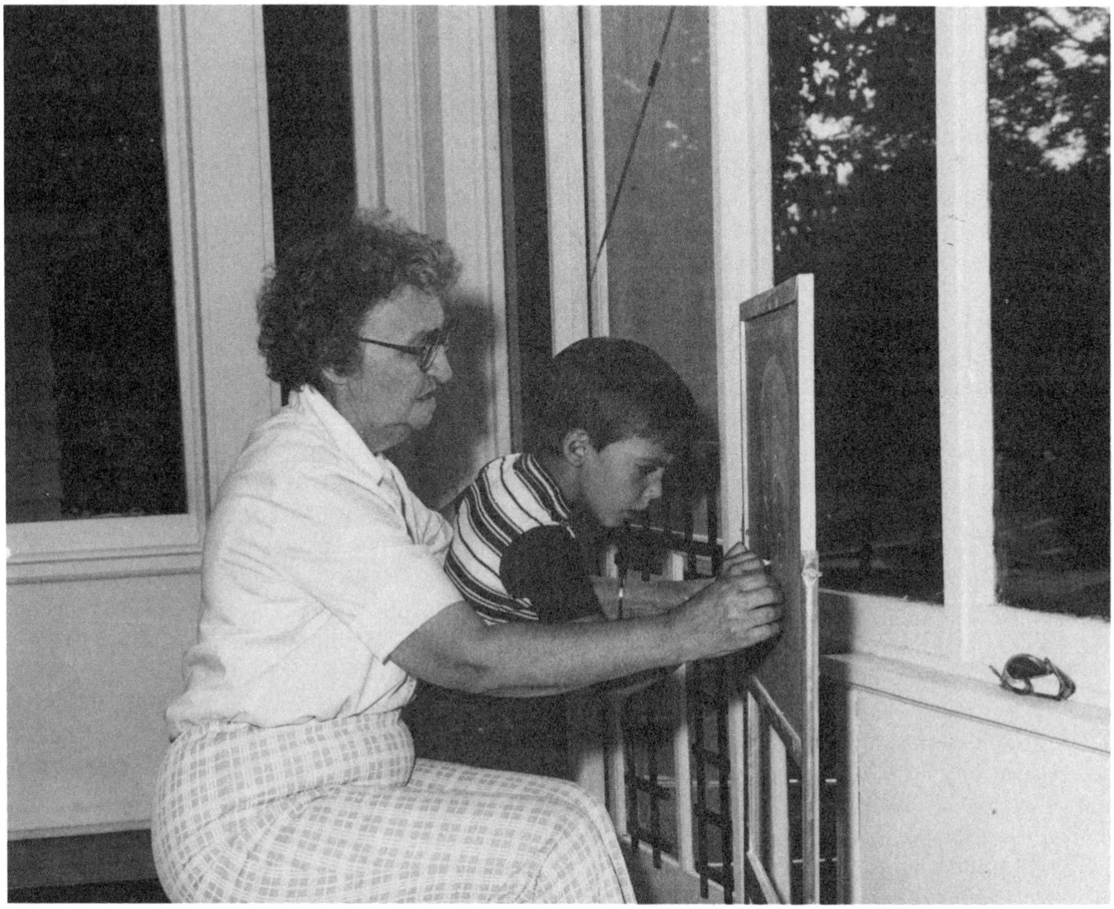

Figure 20-3 Involvement has been highly correlated with an individual's mental state and functioning.

PHYSICAL ASSESSMENT

The following information addresses the physical assessment of the older adult in ways that differ from the process of assessment found in the major portion of the textbook. For example, the normal physiologic changes attributed to the aging process will be reflected in criteria of norms for this age group. However, at the present, there is much doubt regarding whether the changes commonly observed in the older adult are due to aging, because wide variations are observed. In other words, in regard to physical changes that are thought to be due to aging, a 70-year-old may actually be in better physical shape than a 30-year-old. This is dependent on many things, such as lifestyle, genetics, life stresses, and environment. Logically, though, one would expect that such changes would be present after many years of wear and tear on all of the body parts and systems. Therefore, in assessment of the older adult, you must be careful not to stereotype; you must approach the process with an objective attitude.

Assessment of the Integument

Assessment techniques or procedures learned in earlier chapters will not be repeated.

Inspection

Over the years, the skin begins to lose its elasticity and becomes thinner, particularly over the dorsum of the hands. Skin turgor is poor to fair, and because of the thinning phenomenon, the superficial blood vessels are more visible. The skin appears wrinkled, and sagging is prominent. The skin color is generally paler than in the middle-aged adult, even in the absence of anemia. However, anemia is a common problem; it may be due in part to decreased iron absorption in the stomach. Hydrochloric acid is needed for this iron absorption, and the production of hydrochloric acid by the gastric mucosal cells diminishes with age. Because of the iron deficiency state, vascular skin lesions such as petechiae and ecchymosis may be frequently observed. Another reason for the presence of vascular lesions may be medications such as anticoagulants and aspirin. Types of nonpathologic lesions commonly seen are cherry angiomas (small ruby-red round papular lesions) and hyperkeratosis (raised flat brown-black lesions). Because of the increased incidence of diabetes in the older adult, xanthomas are common. In the presence of diabetes, the older adult, like the younger client with diabetes, will be prone to yeast, fungal, and bacterial infections.

The hair of the older adult may be thinner on all parts of the body as well as on the head. Older women may develop upper lip and chin whiskers. Older men do not usually need to shave as often because facial hair growth is retarded. The color of the hair may vary from the natural coloring of the middle years to a dull gray, silver, white, or yellow.

The nail growth slows and the thickness increases.

Palpation

The skin of the older adult is dry to the touch because of diminished functioning of the sebaceous and sweat glands. Additional factors promoting dryness are exposure to wind and sun, hot climates, increased use of soap with inadequate rinsing, frequent bathing, and central heating systems. Frequently, pruritus becomes a problem with dry skin.

Assessment of the Neck

Inspection

Difficulty in swallowing (dysphagia) may be noted due to diminished salivary gland function. Jugular venous distention may be noted with regard to the common incidence of impending or existing heart failure (see discussion in Chapter 11).

Palpation

Palpation of the carotid pulses must be performed with caution so as not to massage the carotid bodies, thereby causing bradycardia to occur. Moreover, both carotid arteries should not be palpated at the same time; this could result in vertigo (dizziness) or syncope (fainting) if the vertebral arteries, which extend up the posterior portion of the neck, have a high degree of atherosclerosis.

Auscultation

Because of the potential of a higher degree of atherosclerosis, which begins early in childhood (about age 9), the carotids should be auscultated for the detection of bruits (see Chapter 11).

Assessment of the Eye

Inspection

Loss of the lateral third of the eyebrows is a common sign accompanying hypothyroid state, especially in the older woman. There may be increased signs and symptoms of irritation and infection because of diminished tearing and the subsequent loss of protection afforded by this process. Increased vulnerability to irritation and infection can be caused by the commonly occurring condition of extropion (eyelids turn outward), in which the palpebral conjunctiva is readily observed, giving the eyes a sagging or "sad sack" appearance. With entropion (eyelids turn inward), the inward turning of the lashes onto the bulbar conjunctiva and cornea gives rise to mechanical irritation. These conditions may cause enough discomfort to require correction; this is a relatively simple surgical procedure. It is not unusual to see a thinning and yellowing of the conjunctiva. Arcus senilis, particularly in the older adult, is considered a normal variation and is of no significance (see Chapter 8). Because of changes in the neurologic system, some decrease in the range of upward gaze may be observed when checking the extraocular muscle movements (EOMs). In addition, the eyes may be unable to converge. Also, decrease in the peripheral fields of vision is commonly noted. The older adult requires corrective lenses because of the atrophied/fibrosed condition of the ciliary bodies and resultant loss of accommodation and loss of elasticity in the lens per se. Cataract phenomenon is common, and the nurse should carefully check for this via oblique lighting (see "Ophthalmoscopic Examination" in Chapter 8).

Ophthalmic examination of the eyegrounds typically reveals tortuosity and silver-wire retinal vessel changes despite the blood pressure of the older adult. Be aware, though, that the presence of A-V nicking signifies arteriosclerosis of the retinal arteries. The incidence of diabetes in the older adult is higher than in any other age group. It is therefore common to observe the fundoscopic changes characteristic of diabetics, such as hard exudates, cotton wool patches, flame-shaped hemorrhages, microaneurysm, and narrowed arteries (see "Ophthalmoscopic Examination" in Chapter 8).

Palpation

Palpation for extraocular pressure may reveal an increase. Because glaucoma commonly occurs in the older adult, a more accurate assessment of intraocular pressure should be performed every 2 years in persons over 40 years of age, using a tonometer (see "Intraocular Pressure" in Chapter 8).

Assessment of the Nose, Mouth, Pharynx, and Ear

Inspection

With aging, especially in older men, there is an increase in hair growth in the nares. Additionally, it is not unusual for the sense of smell to be diminished bilaterally and for taste acuity to be decreased due to the atrophy of the taste buds. The latter change may account for the practice, often observed with aging, of increasing the use of seasoning on food. Conditions attributing to inadequate intake of vitamins, whether decreased finances, loss of teeth, or inability to exercise social desire for eating due to being alone, may manifest as cheilosis, crusted or tender lips, and an edematous tongue. The mouth should also be carefully inspected for abrasions and sores caused by ill-fitting dentures. It is not unusual to find a decreased response to the gag reflex. The cilia in the ear become coarser and stiff with aging and present interference with the sound waves reaching the tympanic membrane. In addition, there appears to be an accumulation of cerumen, which is influential in the decreased hearing commonly observed in the older adult. Otosclerosis and neurosensory changes further compound the problem. The chief difficulty begins with the perception of high-frequency tones; communication may be impaired, resulting in inadequate history taking. This inability to communicate adequately due to hearing loss tends to give the older adult the appearance of being confused or unsociable. This problem could be an impetus for withdrawal from interacting with others because of embarrassment and frustration and for the state of depression frequently observed in the older adult. The older adult should be screened for hearing defects and should undergo dental examination every 2 years.

Assessment of the Lungs

Inspection

An increased anteroposterior diameter may be observed due to senile emphysema, secondary to loss of lung tissue elasticity and resulting from degenerative changes in the ribs and vertebrae and an increase in rigidity of the rib cage. The first sign of these changes is a shortness of breath. Adding to this is the atrophy and decreased strength of the respiratory muscles and the decreased efficiency of neurologic innervation of the respiratory muscles. There is debate as to whether a Tine test should be done once in this age group (60–80 years old). However, the older adult is at risk for tuberculosis, even though the incidence of tuberculosis is rare today. The theory underlying this belief is that the older adult lived through a time when tuberculosis had a high incidence and treatment was inadequate and that the disease can surface years after the primary infection dissipates.

Percussion

When percussing the lung fields, pay careful attention to the apices of the lungs, which extend above the level of the clavicles, because that is the most common site for tuberculosis. Also, the diaphragmatic excursion is generally decreased in the older adult due to the changes that occur in the respiratory system.

Auscultation

Auscultation is not as diagnostic in the older adult as in the younger client because there is less movement of air, particularly in the bases of the lungs, compared with the apices. This is because of the gradual decrease in lung tissue elasticity and limitation of chest movement and expansion due to calcification of the costal cartilages.

Assessment of the Cardiovascular System

Inspection

The face and extremities may be pale or mottled. At 80 years of age, the person has approximately one half the cardiac output (amount of blood forced out of the heart with ventricular contraction) of the younger years. With the decrease in stroke volume, there is a decrease in circulation to all of the organs, including the heart.

Palpation

The extremities, especially the feet, are generally cold to the touch. Wearing socks or "footies" to bed is recommended. Overall, the arteries are more easily palpated because of the loss of connective tissue and thinning of the overlying skin. However, due to generalized and localized arteriosclerosis, weak and absent pulses in the lower extremities may be found without additional local signs of decreased circulation.

Auscultation

Heart rate does not change with age at normal rest. Progressive arteriosclerosis, however, leads to peripheral resistance. A significant rise in the systolic blood pressure occurs, and there is a slight rise in the diastolic pressure. This results in an increase in pulse pressure (the difference between the systolic and the diastolic pressure; see sections on heart sounds in Chapter 11).

Systolic murmurs are present in 60% of the older population. Diastolic murmurs and ventricular gallops are significant of pathology and deserve referral to the physician and follow-up (see "Heart Murmurs" in Chapter 11). Any complaint of chest pain, even mild chest pain, should be thoroughly investigated because the older adult does not experience pain to the degree that the younger person does. A slight feeling of tightness in the chest may be a manifestation of cardiac angina. The typical pattern of precordial site and radiation down one or both arms will be seen. In the older adult, the primary symptom of myocardial infarction may be fatigue. Because the pain is of less intensity than in the younger person, it may be ignored in light of the more apparent signs of dyspnea and confusion. Thus, the clinical picture may not appear as serious as it realistically is. Attention must be given to chest pain, no matter how mild, in the older adult.

Assessment of the Breast

The procedure for examining the breasts of the older adult is the same as for any age group (see Chapter 12). However, the incidence of breast carcinoma increases with age. Therefore, breast examination screening should be done annually by a professional, and the examiner can review the procedure for self-breast examination with the client at that time. A regular time each month, perhaps the first day of each month, should be earmarked by the postmenopausal woman for performing the self breast examination.

Inspection

The breasts may have a sagging appearance, and the nipple line, which is usually at the level of the fourth rib, may fall lower. Gynecomastia may be seen in the older man. This may be due to the decrease in testosterone, leaving a greater effect on the body by adrenal-produced estrogen; it has also been seen in clients who are taking digoxin. In the woman, diminished breast tissue is noted.

Palpation

The consistency of the breast tissue in the older woman may be stringy and more nodular in character. You might detect small, nontender, firm, mobile axillary lymph nodes due to minor trauma and infection that occurred in the hands.

Assessment of the Abdomen

A large number of gastrointestinal problems are commonly found in the older adult. The etiology of most is secondary to decreased circulation. For example, the following sequence of events can follow decreased circulation to the stomach: (1) degeneration of the gastric mucosa results in decreased hydrochloric acid production; (2) achlorhydria or decreased gastric acidity leads to bone disease and iron deficiency anemia, because an acid medium is necessary for the absorption of calcium and iron. Also, periumbilical pain may be due to ischemia of the colon.

The weakening of musculature also results in gastrointestinal problems. Diverticulosis is common, as is the incidence of hiatal hernia. Approximately 80% to 90% of persons age 70 and older have a hiatal hernia. In the older adult who has an acute abdomen, the characteristic sign of abdominal muscle rigidity may be missing. Medications frequently taken by the older adult, such as aspirin and cortisone for arthritis and muscular aches and pains, may cause gastric ulcers. Antacids, such as calcium carbonate, have a constipating effect, and they slow gastrointestinal motility. However, constipation can also be caused by emotional stress via the stress response of sympathetic stimulation, which inhibits intestinal peristalsis. Sedatives, opiates, and tranquilizers all tend to diminish gastric motility. Prolonged use of laxatives tends to weaken the intestinal musculature and contributes to decreased motility and constipation. Laxatives also tend to deplete the body of potassium, further compounding the situation, because potassium is essential for neural transmission in muscular contraction.

Inspection

Lipid distribution tends to be concentrated in the trunk of the older adult, and the extremities tend to be thin with little fat deposit. Increased visualization of the vascularity of the abdomen may be noted due to thinning of the skin and abdominal distention secondary to muscular weakness of the abdominal rectus muscles and flatus accumulation secondary to decreased intestinal motility.

Palpation

The liver may be palpable below the right costal margin, but it will be smooth and nontender. Percussion for size will reveal a normal-size liver. The downward displacement of the liver in absence of disease is due to senile emphysema, wherein the overinflation of the lungs maintains the diaphragm at a lower position. Refer to Chapter 13 for the palpation and percussion techniques used in assessing the abdomen. Palpation of the lymph nodes in the groin may reveal nontender, small, mobile nodes secondary to multiple minor injuries and infections in the feet and legs.

Auscultation

Abdominal aortic aneurysms resulting from weakening of the vessel wall may give rise to a bruit heard mid-abdomen above the umbilicus. The bruits of stenotic renal arteries will be heard above the umbilicus on either side of the midline area (see Chapter 13). Decrease in the frequency of bowel sounds may be observed.

Assessment of the Musculoskeletal System

Osteoporosis is common in the older adult; postmenopausal Caucasian women are at highest risk. Other factors predisposing the client to osteoporosis are inadequate calcium intake and lack of vitamin D, although the latter does not occur as often if the person is exposed to sunshine. Good sources of vitamin D are milk, eggs, liver, and fish. Osteoporosis presents the hazard of fractures occurring. Osteoarthritis can be seen due to the wear and tear of joint motion over the years.

Inspection

Height may decrease 1 to 4 inches from lifetime maximum height. Changes in the joints and tendons influence the overall appearance of the older adult. The appearance may be one of some kyphosis and slight flexion of the elbows, knees, and hips. There is generally a decrease in muscle mass, and with this, the bony prominences are usually more visible. Because of fibrotic changes in the muscles, tendons, and joints, range of motion is limited and the arms swing less when the client is walking. The use of Brudzinski's sign to diagnose meningitis is futile when the older adult has difficulty bending his head forward because of cervical spondylosis.

Palpation

Atrophy of the musculature can most often be detected by palpation.

Assessment of the Neurologic System

Inspection

With diminished neurologic functioning, primarily affected by vascular changes and decreased oxygen, it is not uncommon to observe senile tremors in the older adult. These are benign involuntary movements involving the head, face, and hands. They appear slightly as a jerking vertical or horizontal movement of the head and continuous facial and tongue movements.

Percussion

The voluntary and automatic reflexes are more sluggish. This is seen in the pupillary response to light and also at times with the deep tendon reflexes. Although the deep tendon reflexes remain present in the healthy aged, the lack of elasticity of the tendons and arthritic involvement of the joints may result in a diminished or absent deep tendon reflex, particularly of the knees and the Achilles' tendon reflex. The sense of light touch, pain, and vibration is depressed in the feet, but if this occurs above mid-shin level, pathology such as peripheral neuropathies or spinal cord tumor may be present.

Assessment of the Genitals and Rectum

Inspection

Decreased cardiac output from reduced cardiac muscle efficiency and arteriosclerosis results in less blood flow to the kidneys and thus decreased filtration rate. The degenerative changes in the kidneys per se lead to a decrease in the number of nephrons. The tubular walls become less permeable, and toxic levels of drugs accumulate as a result of decreased tubular excretion. On the other hand, dehydration occurs because of diminished tubular reabsorption. You must therefore be attuned to observing for drug overdose signs and symptoms and hallmarks of dehydration. Decreased urine output could be a sign of dehydration, but it should be thoroughly investigated because there are many additional problems that would cause this sign as well. With polyuria, a urinalysis should be done, because there is an increased incidence of diabetes in this age group. Furthermore, a routine urinalysis should be done every 4 to 5 years for the purpose of screening for diabetes. An annual urinalysis is recommended for the older woman because urinary tract infections are common and many times asymptomatic.

A prolapsed uterus is a commonly observed problem in the older woman due to muscle weakness. When inspecting the perineum, pay special attention to the vestibule (the area beneath the clitoris and urethra), because this is a common site for carcinoma of the genitals in the woman. During a pelvic examination the nurse may find that the vaginal walls appear thinner and drier; it is not uncommon for vaginal pruritus to result. Additionally, narrowing and shortening of the vaginal canal may be noted. In the older man, the size of the testes is decreased.

Palpation

Rectal examination may reveal constipation or fecal impaction and commonly occurring problems like a cystocele in women and benign prostatic hyperplasia in men. The incidence of colonic cancer increases with age and should, therefore, be an object of screening in annual health history

Example of a Health Assessment of an Older Adult

HEALTH HISTORY

Name: James Guisweite
Address: RD#3, Easton, Maryland
Sex: Male
Age: 70
Birthdate: 12/3/18
Marital status: Widower since 10/86
Occupation: Retired dairy farmer since 2/84, worked 5 years in sawmill as a young man 21–26 yrs of age.
Religion: Methodist (attends church regularly)
Race: Caucasian
Ethnic origin: German
Education: High school graduate
Informant: Client, a reliable historian

History of Present Illness

Comes to clinic every third week for blood pressure check. Stiffness and discomfort in hands due to arthritis has increased over the past three months. Grief acceptance (see next topic).

Personal History and Patterns of Living

Was "always self-sufficient." Very close relationship with wife—"We worked, played, laughed and cried together." Acceptance of wife's death as "God's will." Was very depressed and antisocial first year following her death. Youngest daughter strongest support. Quite active recently in farmers market and livestock auction—selling vegetables and regular socializing. Sold all of farm buildings, equipment, and land at the time of his retirement. Retained home, 1 acre orchard and 1 acre garden area (total 3.5 acres). Traveled to Europe and across the United States with wife before her death. These trips and photos taken provide pleasant reminiscing. He states no financial difficulties. Has health insurance—Mutual Benefit Corporation, and Medicare.

Family Health History

Denies family history of cancer, diabetes, heart disease, alcoholism, bleeding disorders, mental illness, stomach problems, liver disorders, kidney diseases. Family history significant for arthritis, hypertension, and TB.

Geographic Exposure

Within-state travel until retirement, then trip to Europe and across U.S. and to sons in Vermont and Pennsylvania and eldest daughter in Delaware.

Lifestyle

Sexuality: Very polite and traditional gentleman behavior, i.e., opening doors, standing when woman enters room, jokes tastefully with both young and older women. Traditional values of monogamy. Discomfort/conflict with separation of eldest daughter from her husband. Recently spending time with a "lady friend." His children encourage and support the latter relationship. "Too soon to think about marriage—I'll cross that bridge when I come to it!"

Personal Habits: Drinks a beer or wine cooler 1–2/wk. No coffee or tobacco. Takes over-the-counter pain pills for arthritis (Advil, Excedrin extra-strength) 2–4 tabs/day in the past 3–4 months.

Diet: Cooks for self. Eats 3–4 evenings at youngest daughter's home. Has cut down on his salt intake. Reads labels and buys low-salt food products and no-caffeine products. Breakfast—fruit, cereal, milk, toast. Lunch—soup and sandwich. Dinner—meat or fish (trying to eat more chicken and turkey than red meats), baked or broiled potatoes, vegetable, milk. Snacks on saltless pretzels before dinner and/or before bedtime. Has taken daily multivitamin capsules for last 5–6 years. Appetite is "not as good as it used to be."

Sleep and rest patterns: Slept 10–12 hrs/24 hr day after wife died. Lately is sleeping 6–7 hrs—feels rested. Up usually one time during night to urinate around 3–4 A.M.

Activities of daily living: No difficulties caring for self. Daughter does laundry and "helps keep the house clean."

Home and neighborhood: Close neighbor across the road and several good friends within 2–3 miles. Sleeps and lives mostly on first floor of home.

Interpersonal relationships: Doesn't see sons and eldest daughter as much as he would like, but youngest daughter "has been a blessing—I don't know what I would have done without her and the grandchildren."

Recreation: Loves to walk in the woods. Works about his home, garden and orchard almost every day. Helps youngest daughter and her husband frequently with projects for home improvement. They live 8 miles from the client. Enjoys socializing every Tuesday and Thursday nights at the livestock auction barn. Going square and round dancing "some" on Saturday nights with lady friend. Doesn't watch much TV. Reads the local daily newspaper.

Previous Experience with Illness
Had measles and mumps as a young child. Smallpox vaccination when 6 years old and before traveling to Europe (3 years ago). Flu shot—5 years and 3 years ago. Denies any known allergies. Hospitalized for fractured left leg at 56 years of age (kicked by a bull). Appendectomy at age 23.

Review of Systems
General health: No significant loss or gain in weight; denies fatigue, weakness, night sweats, cold or heat intolerance, easily bruised, excessive thirst or perspiration.
Integument: No history of skin diseases; some brown "liver" spots on face and arms. Nails—"seem thicker than younger years." Denies jaundice, eczema, psoriasis, hives, rashes, boils, ecchymoses, nevi that have changed in color or size, open sores that are slow to heal. Hair—"is thinning." Some pruritus and dry skin experienced. Mild seborrhea of scalp.
Head: Denies unusually frequent or severe headaches.
Eyes: Wears bifocals. Last eye exam two years ago. No history of infections or pain. Denies blurring, diplopia, photophobia, excessive lacrimation. No spots or halo-rainbows experienced.
Ears: "Hearing is somewhat diminished." No history of infections. Denies pain, discharge, tinnitus, auditory hallucinations and vertigo.
Nose, nasopharynx, and paranasal sinuses: No discharge. Denies epistaxis, allergies, postnasal drip, pain, and tenderness. Very seldom had colds except the past two years had winter-spring seasonal change cold. Smell lost when colds present.
Mouth and throat: New dentures in May of this year (old dentures were loose and rubbed). Denies bleeding gums; soreness of mouth, tongue, and throat; dysphagia, hoarseness. Edentulous.
Neck: Denies pain, edema, swollen glands, limitation of movement. Some stiffness in early morning experienced past 6 months.
Breasts: Denies drainage, soreness, masses, hypertrophy, skin changes. Did not realize men should examine breasts monthly.
Cardiorespiratory system: Chest x-ray when had severe cold 2 years ago (Dr. Madison). Denies cough, sputum, dyspnea, orthopnea, and PND. No chest pain, history of anemia, heart disease, palpitations, and varicosities. Takes hydrodiuril tablet 2 times/day when edema occurs (Rx Dr. Madison).
Gastrointestinal system: Denies nausea, vomiting, anorexia, dyspepsia, pyrosis, bright blood in stools, tarry stools, flatulence, pain, rectal pain. Hemorrhoidal discomfort when straining with "hard" stool. Switches to Bran Buds and more fruit in diet when this occurs. Does not drink much water (1–2 glasses/day), likes milk 3–4 glasses/day.
Genitourinary system: Denies frequency, burning upon urination, dribbling, hematuria, difficulty in starting stream, pain, polyuria, and discharge. Has not been sexually active with a partner since death of wife.
Musculoskeletal system: (see neck) Stiffness and some "turning of my fingers and knuckle-swelling." Occasional ankle swelling every 3–4 months for past year (hydrodiuril). Denies muscular pain, weakness, leg cramps, sprains, deformities, limp. Fracture of left femur (see previous experience with illness). Some hip and knee pain when cold, damp weather. No joint swelling except "knuckles."
Neurologic system: No history of unconsciousness, seizures. Denies vertigo, syncope, difficulty walking, pain in arms or legs, decreased strength in arms and legs, weakness in one part of his body. Has not experienced tingling, numbness, burning, or crawling sensations anywhere in body. Was "very down in the dumps after my wife died." Has had more energy recently and enjoys friends, family, and activities more. His memory "isn't what it used to be."
Client profile
Mr. James Guisweite, 70-year-old white male, appeared jovial and cooperative. Essentially healthy appearance. Logical thought processes. Mild discomfort presently with arthritis of hands. Able to care for self.

PHYSICAL ASSESSMENT
General impression: Mr. James Guisweite, a 70-year-old white male in NAD. WD/WN. Ruddy complexion, stocky frame, "laughing eyes," friendly but quiet manner. No gross abnormalities noted. 5′10″, 180 lb (weight stable for past 10 years ± 5 lb).
TPR—98.2°F, 76, 22.
BP—148/86 left arm sitting; 140/86 right arm sitting; left leg BP 160/82 (see clinic BP flow sheet for record of BP readings).
Integument: Thinning of skin over hands; good skin turgor; ruddy complexion; small brown macular lesions (½–1½ cm) on face, forearms, and hands; hyperkeratosis—mild, generalized over body (papular, flat black lesions, approx. ¼–½ cm). Silver, thin hair slightly receding. Nails—no clubbing and good capillary refill. No cyanosis noted; no ecchymosis; a few cherry angiomas on shoulders and anterior chest; skin warm, rough-dry texture.
Head: Normocephalic; atraumatic; scalp clear; no tenderness. Face—symmetrical. No sinus tenderness.
Neck: Limited flexion, extension, and lateral flexion:

Example of a Health Assessment of an Older Adult, continued

10–15 degrees short of normal range of motion. No JVD noted. Carotids equal bilaterally. No bruits noted. No thyroid enlargement; no masses; trachea midline; no lymphadenopathy.

Eyes: Arcus senilis noted; eyebrows full; no edema. Sclera white; small opacities noted left cornea; EOMs intact; PERRLA. Consensual reaction; sluggish on accommodation; unable to converge smoothly or sustain convergence. Corneal reflex. Peripheral fields slightly decreased 10–20 degrees by gross confrontation technique. Fundoscopy—red reflex; well-demarcated disk; slight arterial narrowing; no A-V nicking, exudates, or hemorrhages noted. Referral for visual acuity and tonometry check. No increase in ocular tension noted on palpation.

Nose, mouth, pharynx: No nasal obstruction; nasal mucosa red; lips, tongue, buccal mucosa, pharynx free of lesions on inspection and palpation; sluggish gag reflex; uvular reflex symmetrical; tongue midline.

Ears: No lesions; no discharge; no mastoid tenderness; large amount cerumen bilaterally—Rx with cerumenex. T.M.'s pearly gray; landmarks present; Weber $\bar{s}$ lateralization; Rinne—AC > BC; can hear whispered voice; clock ticking 10″ from right ear and 8″ from left ear.

Respiratory: Mild increase in AP diameter; respirations 22–24; pink skin color; symmetrical respirations. No use of respiratory accessory muscles; fremitus present; resonant percussion notes; bilateral diaphragmatic excursion, 3–4 cm; vesicular breath sounds.

Cardiovascular: NSR; 76 apical; feet warm, good color. Peripheral pulses:

	T	C	B	R	F	P	PT	DP
L	1+	2+	2+	2+	2+	2+	2+	1+
R	2+	2+	2+	2+	2+	2+	0	1+

No abnormal pulsations; no thrills; PMI at left 5ICS/MCL; MSL → LCBD = 10 cm at 5ICS; Grade I systolic murmur at apex—does not radiate; heart sounds distant; normal S_1 and S_2; $A_2 = P_2$; no abnormal splitting, ventricular gallops, or rub noted.

Breast: No tissue enlargement; everted nipples; no dimpling or retraction; no discharge; slight sagging; no masses noted; no lymphadenopathy—axillary, supra, and infraclavicular.

Abdomen: Flat and symmetrical; no hernias noted; B.S. present. No renal/aortic/femoral bruits noted; tympany in all four quadrants; spleenic dullness—7 cm at left MAL; liver dullness at right MCL = 10 cm; palpable liver 2 cm below RCM—smooth and nontender. Kidneys nonpalpable; palpable lymph nodes in left inguinal area—small, nontender, mobile.

Musculoskeletal: Mild kyphosis; body and limb symmetry; tenderness in PIPS, MIPS, and DIPs of all fingers. Slight enlargement of MIPS: Full ROM except for neck, fingers, and hips—latter 10–20 degrees less than norm; no crepitation. Muscles—symmetrical and good strength; proximal—distal muscle strength equal; muscle atrophy noted in biceps and fine muscles of the hands; no muscle tenderness; no edema or masses noted.

Neurologic: Slight horizontal tremors of head; no difficulty with gait; Romberg sign absent; smooth coordination of upper and lower extremities; CN I—not tested; CN II—referred for eye exam and tonometry; CN III–XII grossly intact (taste not tested); sensitive to pain, light touch, and vibration; position sense intact. DTRs:

	B	T	BR	P	A	PR
L	2+	2+	2+	1+	1+	↓
R	2+	2+	2+	2+	1+	↓

Abdominal reflex intact; no clonus, Babinski absent.

Mental status—Logical thought processes; alert; no speech difficulties; has calendar for notes to remind him of events; recent and remote memory intact; affect and mood congruent; "Christian—law abiding man"; intellectual functioning intact; cultivating new affectional and satisfying roles with family, friends, and initiating social activities appropriate to health, energy, and interests.

Genitals/rectum: Urinalysis WNL; circumcised; normal male pubic hair distribution; body and pubic hair thinning; no lesions or discharge noted; urethral meatus at end of penis; foreskin easily retracted; no abnormalities noted; no testicular masses; no indirect inguinal or femoral hernia noted; no rectal masses; several small anal tabs noted; sphincter and cremasteric reflex intact; stool negative for occult blood; prostate slightly enlarged, nontender and firm consistency.

taking. Also, the occurrence of prostatic carcinoma rises for older men. Men over 40 years old should have an annual rectal examination.

SUMMARY

The older population is steadily growing faster than any other age group; therefore, it is important that the older adult be understood in order to promote well-being and meet health needs. Stereotyping has placed limitations on how the older adult is viewed by the general society and on how older adults live in order that their behavior conforms with society's expectations. Sexual behaviors, living arrangements, need for privacy, capability to make decisions, and control of personal finances are a few of the areas in which U.S. society questions and restricts this group by stereotyping. Fears of institutionalization and an invasion of privacy deter the older adult from seeking health care. Fear of losing independence and self-sufficiency keep them from enlarging their social support networks. Fear of the stigma of being considered a "charity" case results in avoiding welfare and free services. Older adults have, to a great extent, become the victims of society. Ironically, they are the primary transmitters of culture.

The many signs and symptoms attributed to the aging process must be regarded cautiously. Myths surrounding mental abilities have been shattered with research revealing that intellectual functioning, learning, and decision making continue to grow. Also, physiologically, some older adults are in "better shape" than persons of much younger years.

The older adult is fitting into a self-fulfilled prophecy of what society dictates. However, the myths and stereotypes are gradually dissipating as older adults are becoming more assertive and active in such spheres as academia, politics, and sports. The lifestyles of older adults are changing accordingly. In this chapter, each phase of physical assessment was discussed in light of norms of the older adult and health risks of the older adult age group.

DISCUSSION QUESTIONS/ ACTIVITIES

1. Give some examples to illustrate how culture dictates the behavior of an older adult.
2. Choose a seemingly healthy older adult and take his health history.
3. Compare the similarities between the health histories of several older adults.
4. Compare the health history and physical and mental status of two older adults—one with a broad social support system and one without such a support system.
5. Analyze physical findings from several physical assessments of older adults and identify physiologic changes that are attributed to the aging process.
6. Role-play the part of an older adult with normal mental functioning who is institutionalized and is being cared for by a nurse's aide who holds stereotypic beliefs regarding the older adult.

REFERENCES

Ebersole, P., and Hess, P. 1981. *Toward healthy aging.* St. Louis: C. V. Mosby.

Preston, D., and Grimes, J. 1987. Study in differences in social support. *Journal of Gerontological Nursing* 13(2):36–40.

Schaie, K. W. 1985. *Adult intellectual development in a life-span context.* 2nd Annual Research Lecture. College of Human Development. The Pennsylvania State University.

CHAPTER

21 Assessment of Women's Health

Learning Objectives

1. Discuss the morbidity and mortality rate for women, and describe the differences in these rates between men and women.
2. Review and describe the physiology of menstruation.
3. Describe the components of a health history pertinent to distinguishing between primary and secondary dysmenorrhea and amenorrhea.
4. Describe the characteristics and symptoms of metrorrhagia and dysfunctional uterine bleeding.
5. Describe premenstrual syndrome.
6. Identify common physical changes of menopause.
7. Discuss anorexia nervosa and bulimia, and describe specific changes noted during assessment.
8. Describe those components of the health history specifically related to pregnancy.
9. Identify physiologic changes occurring throughout pregnancy.

Female mortality has always been less than that for males; however, the morbidity rate for women is higher than that of men. Women of all ages make more visits to the physician than men. Several theories have been advanced to explain this phenomenon. For example, women report more illness than men, presumably because it is more culturally acceptable for them to do so. Women's social role carries with it more stresses and anxiety, especially in confronting the more nurturant and circumscribed roles defined by society. Also, women are urged to seek more help in relation to contraception, prepartum and postpartum care, and relief of menopausal symptoms.

In the 1960s the women's movement drew attention to the special health needs of women resulting from their anatomy and physiology and the demands placed on them as they gave birth, raised families, and entered the workforce in increasing numbers. Greater numbers of women expressed dissatisfaction with the health care options available to them. Parameters of health or the absence of health were described by men who appeared to know little about normal functioning of women because most of the parameters of pathology had been gathered using male subjects as guides. Women became aware that functions such as menstruation, menopause, childbearing, and lactation are normal, healthy functions and in fact do not mean that women are less than or weaker than men. Women became critical of treatment that directly impinges on their lives as women, such as gynecologic examinations, birth control, sexuality, childbirth, and psychotherapy.

This chapter provides guidelines for assessing specific events that affect women's lives and health. Assessment data are presented for normal events and for several deviations from normal.

MENSTRUATION

One of the most constant reminders women have of their uniqueness is the occurrence of menstruation every month. This important event prepares women for other unique functions, such as pregnancy, lactation, and menopause. Menstruation has been misunderstood by many, and in fact many women have been socialized to feel that it is shameful, dirty, and to be considered an illness. Increased understanding of the event and education are helping women to view menstruation as a healthy and essential biologic and emotional experience.

Problems that occur with menstruation should never be dismissed lightly. The menstrual history must include information regarding onset of menarche, pattern of menstruation, method of contraception, reproductive history, sexual activity, feelings about menstruation, understanding of the event, and the effect of menstruation on lifestyle.

Abnormal vaginal bleeding or lack of bleeding can cause great anxiety for clients. Both are common symptoms, and emotional support must be provided while the cause is determined and treatment prescribed. Women may seek care for absence of bleeding (amenorrhea), painful menstruation (dysmenorrhea), or changes in the menstrual cycle.

Menstruation starts generally at age 11 or 12, although some girls have begun menstruation as early as 9 or as late as 18. Very few have an absolutely regular cycle. The length of the cycle ranges from 20 to 36 days, with the average cycle at 28 days. The menstrual flow lasts 2 to 8 days, with the average flow from 4 to 6 days.

It is important that adolescents and adult women understand menstruation and be aware that it is normal. Old wives' tales warning against activity, bathing, and sexual activity should be ignored. These fears have been passed from one generation to the next, creating fear, anxiety, and embarrassment that continues through life.

The menstrual fluid contains cervical and vaginal mucus as well as degenerated endometrial particles and blood. Sometimes clots appear in the fluid. About 2 to 3 ounces of fluid are lost with the menses, but the amount of flow is highly individual. The fluid does not smell until it makes contact with bacteria in the air and begins to decompose. Sanitary napkins and tampons are common methods of absorbing the flow. Caution is advised when using tampons, however, because toxic shock syndrome appears to be linked to the heavy use of them.

The nurse should also be aware of several other methods to absorb the flow. For instance, some women use a natural sponge. Before insertion, a piece of dental floss is tied around the sponge and the sponge is dampened. When the sponge is full, it is removed, washed in cool water and soap, and squeezed to remove excess water before being reinserted. A diaphragm with a little K-Y jelly or contraceptive cream on the edge to hold it in place can be used to collect the flow. In another method, called menstrual extraction, a small tube attached to a suction device is inserted in the uterus when the flow starts and the menstrual fluid is sucked out in 5 minutes. Advocates of this method note that there is no research to indicate the long-range effects of regular menstrual fluid extraction.

Problems Related to Menstruation

Dysmenorrhea

Dysmenorrhea, painful menstruation, is one of the most common gynecologic problems of women. More than half the women in the United States experience some discomfort; about 10% are so incapacitated they miss work or school. One study found that 35% of older adolescent girls, 25% of college students, and 60% to 70% of single women in their 30s and 40s experience discomfort severe enough to interfere with normal activities for 1 or 2 days (Green 1977). The degree of pain or discomfort varies with the individual and may be manifested as lower abdominal cramping pain, backache, or aching thighs. Two types of dysmenorrhea are *primary dysmenorrhea,* in which pelvic organs are normal, and *secondary dysmenorrhea,* in which a diagnosed pelvic disease or condition is present.

Primary dysmenorrhea usually develops 1 to 2 years after the onset of menstruation. It appears to be self-limiting and primarily a problem of teenagers and young adults. It disappears or is markedly better by age 25 or following pregnancy. The pain is either sharp or a steady dull ache accompanied by bearing down sensations with referred pain to the legs and suprapubic area. Many women also experience abdominal distention, breast tenderness, nausea and vomiting, dizziness, headache, palpitations, and flushing.

Secondary dysmenorrhea may occur due to such conditions as large uterine or cervical polyps, submucous fibroids, endometriosis, pelvic infection, a fixed malpositioned uterus, the presence of an intrauterine device, or cervical stenosis following recent gynecologic surgery or procedures. Secondary dysmenorrhea generally occurs after a pattern of problem-free periods had been present for some time. The pain is generally more constant in nature and continues throughout the period. A careful history must be obtained to distinguish between primary and secondary dysmenorrhea.

Information must be elicited as to when the client's periods began, because this is an important factor in determining whether primary dysmenorrhea is occurring. Although this problem is now thought to be related to the presence of prostaglandins, some experts still feel the problem is partly or wholly due to psychogenic factors. For this reason, the nurse should explore with the client the type of preparation she received prior to onset of menarche and attitude of the client and siblings or female relatives to menstruation.

Information on frequency and duration of menstruation is important so that the nurse can note where the client falls within the range of normal responses. Changes in the character and amount of flow should be noted. The nurse must also determine the time when cramps begin, their duration, and their severity. The relationship between pain and bleeding is significant. Any clotting should also be noted.

The client should be asked about the use of contraceptives because they may affect cramping. The IUD is often associated with more severe cramping, while oral contraceptives suppress ovulation and thereby alleviate dysmenorrhea associated with ovulation. Reproductive history is important because traumatic labor and delivery, cervical lacerations, infections, and gynecologic procedures predispose to secondary dysmenorrhea.

The client's pain threshold and response to pain should be determined. As mentioned previously, the nurse should explore the client's and family's attitudes toward menstruation to help determine whether there is a psychological component to the problem.

Amenorrhea

Amenorrhea, the absence of menstruation, is classified as primary or secondary. It is termed *primary* if the client has never menstruated and *secondary* if she has had normal periods. Primary amenorrhea exists if the client has had no menstrual period by age 14 and there is absence of growth and development of secondary sexual characteristics or if there is no menstrual period by age 16 regardless of the presence of secondary sexual characteristics. It may be caused by a variety of factors, including hormonal imbalance, chromosomal disorders, infection, congenital absence of the uterus (müllerian abnormalities), disorders of the anterior pituitary, and disorders in the central nervous system or hypothalamus.

Secondary amenorrhea exists when a client has been menstruating and stops for a period of at least 3 months. The existence of pregnancy should be determined; however, pregnancy is just one of many causes of secondary amenorrhea.

A careful history to determine whether the mother and grandmother had a late menarche can be significant to the diagnosis of primary amenorrhea, because girls tend to menstruate at the same time as their mothers and grandmothers. A history of systemic disease such as diabetes mellitus, tuberculosis, hyperthyroidism, or mitral stenosis may give a clue to the cause of secondary amenorrhea. It is also significant if the client is taking oral contraceptives or tranquilizers, especially chlorpromazine or phenothiazine. Some women experience "post-Pill" amenorrhea in which menstruation is not reestablished up to 12 months following discontinuation of the Pill. A history of stress, anxiety, and fatigue may also be significant. Women athletes frequently stop menstruating when they train very hard. This probably occurs because they have a low ratio of body fat to body muscle, resulting in an excessive secretion of prolactin, which in turn decreases release of gonadotropin releasing factor, causing a decrease in FSH, follicular development, and estrogen levels. Anorexia nervosa may cause stress-related anovulation due to the same increase in prolactin seen in athletes. In the obese client, it may be the result of increased conversion of androstenedione to estrone by adipose tissue.

Menorrhagia and Metrorrhagia

Menorrhagia is an abnormally excessive menstrual flow. It can occur as the result of anovulatory cycles just prior to puberty and in women nearing menopause. As you assess the client, you must determine what the client considers a heavy flow. For example, women who have discontinued the Pill often describe heavy flow when it may be normal. A woman who saturates a pad every hour for more than 2 hours has an excessive flow, as does a woman who saturates a tampon or pad every 2 hours for 7 to 9 days. Women using IUDs often experience a very heavy flow. Heavy flow may be indicative of anemia, endometriosis, a blood dyscrasia, or the presence of a tumor. A single episode of excessive bleeding may be due to a spontaneous abortion or an ectopic pregnancy. Women at menopause are at great risk for uterine cancer, which often has as a symptom increased bleeding.

Metrorrhagia describes bleeding between periods. Vaginal bleeding is a symptom of ovarian cysts and uterine cancer. When such bleeding occurs for more than 1 month and the client is not taking oral contraceptives, there is cause for concern. There are instances when this is normal. For example, some women have spotting at the time they ovulate. Women who take oral contraceptives may have "breakthrough" bleeding for the first 3 to 4 months. Vaginal infection may also be responsible. Any bleeding in the postmenopausal woman is considered to be abnormal. Bleeding that is continuously occurring in women around the time of menopause is referred to as dysfunctional uterine bleeding. This specific type of metrorrhagia is usually caused by prolonged estrogen stimulation of the endometrium after long periods of no ovulation secondary to faulty neuroendocrine or ovarian function. These factors cause the continuous proliferation of the endometrium.

A list of causes of menstrual alterations is provided in Table 21-1.

Premenstrual Syndrome

In recent years, a cluster of symptoms appearing just before menstruation and disappearing with the menstrual flow has been referred to as *premenstrual syndrome* (PMS). The awareness that the menstrual period is about to start is experienced by almost all women. For some, the symptoms are more dramatic and incapacitating. Examples of symptoms range from mild abdominal fullness, breast tenderness, and mild irritability to severe nervousness, fatigue, crying spells, decreased concentration, and depression.

Katharina Dalton, a pioneer in work on PMS, defines the syndrome as recurrent premenstrual difficulties followed by at least 1 week entirely free of symptoms. If a woman is

Table 21-1 Causes of Menstrual Alterations

Alteration	Causes	Alteration	Causes
Amenorrhea		Amenorrhea	
Primary	Anatomical alterations Imperforate hymen Blind end to vagina Cervical stenosis Agenesis of cervix Agenesis of uterus Gonadal alterations Turner's syndrome Androgen-secreting ovarian tumor Pituitary alterations Hypopituitarism Hypothalamic tumors Adrenal alterations Adrenogenital syndrome Androgen-secreting tumor Chronic disease Renal failure Inflammatory bowel disease Collagen-vascular disease Hypothyroidism Cushing's syndrome Addison's disease Cardiopulmonary disease	Secondary	Pregnancy Psychological alterations Crash dieting (anorexia nervosa) Drugs: cytotoxic agents phenothiazines, contraceptives, narcotics Pituitary or ovarian tumors Chronic disease (as per primary amenorrhea)
		Dysmenorrhea	Anatomical alteration Intrauterine device Prostaglandin overproduction Infection Endometriosis
		Menometorrhagia	Idiopathic Anovulatory cycles (dysfunctional uterine bleeding) Hematological disorders Hemophilia von Willebrand's disease Thrombocytopenia Spontaneous abortion Ectopic pregnancy Birth control pills Trauma Tumor

Source: J. Servonsky and S. Opas. *Nursing Management of Children.* Boston: Little, Brown, 1987.

experiencing difficulties in her life, these difficulties may not go away completely during the week that is free of premenstrual symptoms but will certainly become more severe premenstrually. For example, a woman whose symptom premenstrually is depression will have at least 1 week free of depression; on the other hand, a woman who is generally depressed will not have a week during which she is not depressed, but her depression will be more severe premenstrually.

Many theories have been offered to explain PMS symptoms. Explanations have included progesterone deficiency, estrogen excess, or a relatively high estrogen-progesterone ratio, vitamin deficiency, hypoglycemia, hormone allergy, fluid retention, prolactin excess, stress, endorphins, and psychosomatic causes. Several studies have been carried out in an attempt to correlate a wide variety of symptoms and behaviors with the premenstrual phase of the menstrual cycle. Most of these have been inconclusive and in fact have been criticized for their methodology. Much research needs to be done, not only related to the premenstrual phase but about all the phases of the cycle.

As nurses, we must be aware of the problems experienced by women related to menstruation and assess the health and symptoms that are occurring, with a goal of helping them take steps to alleviate those symptoms. When taking the history of the client, keep in mind several characteristics that are suggestive of premenstrual syndrome:

1. Painless periods are more common than painful ones.
2. The onset is often seen at puberty, after stopping birth control pills, after pregnancy, or after a period of amenorrhea.
3. The severity also seems to increase after stopping birth control pills, pregnancy, amenorrhea, tubal ligation, or hysterectomy.
4. Pregnancies may be complicated by miscarriage, toxemia, or postpartum depression.
5. There may be an onset of acute symptoms, such as

migraine headaches, panic attacks, epilepsy, or severe depression after long food gaps (5 hours in the day or 13 hours overnight).

6. The woman may experience food cravings, binges, or increased sensitivity to alcohol premenstrually.
7. The client may notice significant weight gain, water and salt retention, abdominal bloating, and mastalgia.

Women who have symptoms should be encouraged to use a calendar to chart which symptoms are occurring and when they occur. Those who are ovulating can correlate their temperature change with symptoms. At ovulation, the body temperature rises 0.5° to 1.0° and stays elevated until the next menstrual period.

Many women can be helped to alleviate or minimize their symptoms by changing their lifestyle (improved diet and exercise). Some may have to be medicated with progesterone. All women with symptoms need to have support and encouragement to manage their lives and avoid the stereotype of women as unreliable or out of control once a month because of menstruation.

MENOPAUSE

Menopause is the end of a cycle that began at puberty with the menarche. The most common age for the onset of the menarche is 12, while menstruation stops from 45 to 53. Unfortunately, menopause has been felt by many, including health professionals, to be a negative experience and is often described by the symptoms of dysfunction, rather than as a healthy and normal part of life's experience. *The Merck Manual* lists menopause, not under "Gynecology" as a natural physiologic function, but under "Ovarian Dysfunction." In her informative book about menopause, Rosetta Reitz objected to this approach because the attitude promotes the idea that a woman's life is normal for the 30 years she ovulates and abnormal before and after (Reitz 1977). The nurse can help to convey the normality of the period of menopause. Changes take place in the woman's body during menopause, and some of these can cause discomfort, just as with the menarche. Discomfort can be minimized through education of the client about the changes, a healthy mental and physical lifestyle, and, occasionally, the use of hormone therapy.

When taking the health history of the premenopausal client, ask the age at which menopause occurred for the client's mother. As with menarche, mothers and daughters appear to begin and end their menstrual periods about the same time. Menopause that occurs through the normal process of age tends to happen gradually. Many authorities feel it takes about 5 years to complete the cycle. The events of the climacteric can be divided into three phases:

1. *Premenopausal*—a time in which menstruation is still occurring but may become irregular. At this stage, estrogen decline begins and the fertility index declines.
2. *Menopausal*—at this stage, the ovaries are unable to respond to gonadotropins, resulting in the cessation of the menses and infertility.
3. *Postmenopausal*—all traces of ovarian activity are gone and signs of estrogen decline may occur.

During the history taking, the nurse must determine how the client views this experience. Often there is a fear of aging, and some women will still anticipate this time in their lives as one in which they will not feel well. Some women may view the menses as having been bothersome and are happy that it is ending. However, as many or more women equate the menses with femininity and may react with depression at the loss of this function. Some women find the period of menopause to be one of renewed interest and satisfaction in themselves. With a sense of how the client views this time, the nurse can help the client achieve a positive state of wellness.

Several physical changes occur with menopause. Vasomotor instability, referred to as "hot flashes," is the sensation of overwhelming heat spreading from the chest upward over the neck, face, and arms. The skin on the affected areas may become flushed, and excessive perspiration may occur. The episodes last from several seconds to a minute and occur most frequently at night, disturbing sleep. The precise mechanism for the vasomotor instability is unknown. One factor relates to the increased production of follicle-stimulating hormone (FSH) in response to the decreased production of estrogen and progesterone. The large amount of FSH upsets the delicate balance in the relationship between the ovaries, hypothalamus, and pituitary gland. The overactive pituitary is responsible for the increased production of FSH. Another cause given is the decreasing production of estrogen. Hot flashes are harmless, but they can cause great distress for some women. For those experiencing great discomfort, estrogen replacement may be prescribed. Other suggested means of controlling the symptoms of this instability are the use of the herb ginseng, vitamin B complex, and vitamin E.

Changes due to estrogen decrease can occur in the vulva, vagina, and uterus. The epidermis of the *vulva* thins, causing the labia and introitus to shrink. The vagina loses elasticity and becomes shorter and narrower. There is increased susceptibility to irritation and vaginal infection. This may result in atrophic vaginitis. Regular sexual activity makes these changes hardly noticeable and helps to prevent this condition. The use of vaginal creams has also helped some women. Dyspareunia occurs as a result of thinning of the vulva, but it can be helped by using K-Y jelly.

The *uterus* decreases in size and weight after menopause, and the cervix shrinks and becomes pale. The usual position of the uterus is anteroflexed. During menopause, the uterosacral ligaments may relax, and the position of the uterus will change.

Changes in the structure and function of the *ovaries* relate to the decrease in fertility and the decrease in size of the organs. Normally, they are nonpalpable.

Estrogen decline at menopause causes a negative nitrogen balance and subsequently causes the *skin* to thin and the subcutaneous fat to atrophy and lose elasticity. Clients should be advised that these changes can be minimized by a good skin care regimen, including the use of skin oils, avoidance of drying soaps and detergents, and adherence to a healthy diet. About this time, some women also develop freckles and brown spots, particularly on the face and hands. These skin changes appear to be due to the build-up of melanin that occurs as a process of aging. Occasionally, these spots will develop into wartlike growths referred to as seborrheic keratoses. None of these changes is harmful unless the warts change in size or shape or begin to bleed. Many clients are upset about these brown spots, especially if they are on the face. Some women have suggested that the spots can be lightened by using diluted lemon or cranberry juice on them before going to bed or dabbing yogurt or buttermilk on them during the day.

On assessment, no changes can usually be detected in the cardiovascular system. Women appear to be more susceptible to coronary artery disease after menopause, but it should be noted that the death rate for both sexes increases with age. Smoking, hypertension, and obesity are all risk factors that women should be counseled to control.

Musculoskeletal disorders, osteoporosis, and joint and muscle pain occur often in postmenopausal women. Both men and women lose bone after about age 35. The rate of bone loss appears to be greater in women. The many theoretical explanations given for the development of osteoporosis include inadequate intake of dietary calcium, fluoride, and vitamin D; alteration in the calcium-phosphorus ratio, probably precipitated by the lowered levels of estrogen and the subsequent increased removal of bone by parathyroid hormone; and lack of physical activity. An individual's lifestyle, diet, and cultural group may determine the increased likelihood of developing the condition. For example, people who are from vegetarian societies seem to have lower incidence than those from meat-eating societies like our own (Seaman & Seaman 1977). African-American women are less likely to suffer from the muscular and joint complaints and fractures (Seaman & Seaman 1977). At greatest risk seem to be Caucasian women who smoke and have a family history of osteoporosis. Estrogen therapy seems to have some positive effects on preventing or retarding this condition but only for the short term. Long-term therapy may contribute to decrease in bone formation.

To reduce the process of osteoporosis, women should be encouraged to select a diet with foods high in calcium and low in phosphorus, and some authorities recommend calcium supplements. Regular exercise should also become a part of the woman's lifestyle, because exercise not only helps to retard osteoporosis but also helps to control weight and improve circulation.

EATING DISORDERS

Our society's emphasis on slimness has contributed to an increase in the incidence of serious eating disorders, such as anorexia nervosa and bulimia. Anorexia nervosa, or self-induced starvation, affects about 1 of every 200 American girls between the ages of 12 and 18. Bulimia, a cycle of food binges followed by purging (induced by vomiting or by laxative or diuretic abuse), appears to be more prevalent, affecting an estimated 5% of adolescent and young adult females. Although both disorders occur less often among males, they are also victims of these ailments. A common feature of both disorders is the overwhelming desire to become and remain thin. Although a specific cause is unknown, a combination of interacting factors including psychological, familial, sociocultural, and biologic determinants contributes to these complex disorders.

Psychoanalytic theory suggests that anorexia nervosa is an attempt to delay or prevent puberty. Psychodynamic theory attributes the problem to the individual's problems with self-image and adequacy, social interactions, and overcompliance. The pursuit of thinness is viewed as the struggle to exert control and self-direction. Family dynamics, including disturbed patterns of interactions, have also been thought to contribute.

Our society's emphasis on extreme thinness remains pervasive. Two cultural factors, idealization of the thin female form and pressures on women to be independent and successful, are believed to have contributed to the recent increase in the numbers of women with eating disorders.

Anorexia Nervosa

The typical client with anorexia nervosa is a white adolescent girl from a middle- to upper-middle-class family. She is often described by her parents as the "perfect child." The anorectic tends to be a perfectionist, obedient, overcompliant, highly motivated, successful academically, well liked by peers, and a good athlete. Frequently, the anorectic's family is one that emphasizes high achievement, perfection, and physical appearance. Such families have been described as being overinvolved with one another, having a low tolerance for conflict, and being highly controlling.

Reason for Seeking Health Evaluation

Parents, alarmed by the girl's obvious weight loss, bizarre eating habits, purging, and often a loss of interest in school, may force their daughter to seek help. Other notable behavioral characteristics are extreme irritability, excessively overcontrolled behavior, an obsession with exercise, and changes in sleep patterns. In some cases, amenorrhea initially brings the client into contact with the health care system.

Current Health Status or History of Present Illness

In appearance, these girls are emaciated, resembling walking skeletons. They do not see themselves as particularly thin, and often they underestimate their own body size and the size of others. Hunger is usually denied, and in fact, appetite is described as too good.

Physical Assessment

On physical assessment, the nurse will usually find weight loss of 20% to 25% or more of total body weight or a reduced weight 20% to 25% below average for the age-appropriate height. Reduced body fat and wasting of muscle can be noted along with other symptoms of decreased metabolic rate, such as bradycardia, hypotension, and hypothermia. The anorectic client may also have abdominal tenderness, decreased motility, constipation, increased sensitivity to cold, dry inelastic skin with a yellowish caritonemic hue, brittle hair and nails, lanugo, and peripheral edema. Either during the history taking or during the physical assessment the nurse should determine whether the client vomits to control her weight and uses laxatives. Typical laboratory values show leukopenia, anemia, hypoglycemia, hypercholesterolemia, and reduced gonadotropins.

Mental Status Assessment

Impaired mental performance may be found. In addition, anorectics have a disturbed body image, insisting that their body size is normal. Awareness of the usual senses of hunger and appetite is missing. Another misinterpretation of stimuli is their inability to acknowledge fatigue associated with their constant hyperactivity. They also display a tremendous sense of ineffectiveness, a feeling that they are helpless to change their lives. This is usually expressed as extreme negativism and stubborn defiance.

Most anorectic girls have difficulty accepting their sexual identity and fear pregnancy, which is described as getting fat. Anorectics are often very hostile. The hostility is usually toward their mothers, who are frequently overprotective and overcontrolling. These clients try to solve their problems by changing their body through starvation and hyperactivity.

Bulimia

Bulimia is defined as recurrent episodes of rapid uncontrollable ingestion of large amounts of food in a short period, usually followed by purging, either by forced vomiting or by abuse of laxatives or diuretics. The purging techniques are used to prevent weight gain, relieve fullness, and restore the individual's sense of control. Like anorectics, bulimics have an exaggerated fear of fatness and are intent on pursuing slimness as a means of bringing control and a sense of effectiveness into their lives.

The typical bulimic is a white, single, college-educated woman of normal weight-for-height in her early to middle twenties who has been involved in bulimic behavior for 4 to 6 years before seeking treatment. Bulimics tend to be slightly older and of more varied socioeconomic status than anorectics. While most are women, about 10% to 13% are men.

Reasons for Seeking Health Evaluation

The reasons for seeking help vary. Using open-ended questions, which allow the client to express feelings, is the best approach and will probably elicit several reasons for finally entering the health care system.

Mental Status Assessment

Studies reveal that normal-weight bulimics have problems with impulse control (evidenced by stealing, abuse of alcohol or drugs), are chronically depressed or even suicidal, are intolerant of frustration, and have an exaggerated sense of guilt and recurrent anxiety. They feel alienated and self-conscious, are overly dependent on approval by others, and have low self-esteem and difficulties expressing feelings, especially anger.

Physical Assessment

Chronic self-induced vomiting can lead to enlarged parotid glands, esophageal inflammation, and many dental problems, such as caries and erosion of the enamel. Vomiting can also result in fluid and electrolyte disturbances, the most serious being hypokalemia. The client may also have urinary infections, renal failure, and cardiac arrhythmias. Laxative abuse may result in colon damage, disturbances of intestinal motility, and metabolic acidosis. Abuse of diuretics can lead to dehydration and hypokalemia and metabolic alkalosis. Bulimics complain of chronic indigestion, sore throats, facial puffiness, menstrual disturbances, muscle weakness, constipation, and lethargy.

ASSESSMENT OF PREGNANCY

Pregnancy is a normal physiologic process that affects every organ system. The genital tract reflects the earliest changes; the others are more subtle and frequently develop later. During the prenatal period, complex emotional adjustments affect the women and also her family and significant others. Health care must include the assessment of the client's physiologic and emotional status as well as provide health education during pregnancy and assistance in preparing for labor, delivery, and the postpartum period.

Health History

Although the components of the history are similar to those described in Chapter 4, some areas should be given special emphasis. The information obtained in the initial interview assists the nurse in identifying the many factors that will affect the client during pregnancy. These factors include information about the client's past physical history as well as her emotional response to the pregnancy. Each woman is different, and the nurse must allow her to express her feelings and concerns about the pregnancy in an open, nonjudgmental fashion.

Age

Extremes of age put the woman in a high-risk category. Adolescents are considered at risk because they are still developing physically and psychologically. In addition, the very young mother might find the routine and responsibility of child care time consuming and an interference to a developing social life. Women who are older may resent additional responsibility and fear that they do not have the physical strength to raise a child. Genetic defects in the fetus are more often seen in older women. Other more common complications in this age group include hydatidiform mole, placenta previa, twinning, and low birth weight. Early identification and referral of high-risk clients enables the nurse to achieve maximal benefit for both client and fetus.

Marital Status

Obtain information about the length of the marriage and about the husband's name, age, and occupation. The father's effect on the pregnancy relates to his ability to give emotional and financial support. Some evidence suggests that the father's occupation as reflected in the family's socioeconomic status is related to the incidence of prematurity and infant mortality. Unmarried women face additional stress in U.S. society. Mortality and morbidity rates are higher; prenatal care and advice are often not sought. When care is sought, the professional's advice is less likely to be followed. It may be that this is a denial of the pregnancy or that there is no significant other to give emotional support.

Current Occupation

The client's job is important in relation to the occupation's stress level and the degree to which heavy physical labor is required. Although women are encouraged to maintain an active lifestyle during pregnancy, certain physical activities may have to be altered as the pregnancy progresses. Of increasing importance is the exposure to possible toxic contamination at the place of employment. For example, women exposed to radiation are at definite risk. There is some question as to the health risks to the fetus for the mother who works daily with computers. Some are being advised to wear aprons with a lead shield during pregnancy. There is hard evidence that smoking causes low birth weights and a direct increase in infant mortality. A relationship between passive inhalation of environmental smoke and low birth weight has also been found in preliminary studies.

Ethnic Background and Religion

Ethnic origin may affect pregnancy outcome, as some diseases are more prevalent in certain races—for example, Tay-Sachs disease in Jews, thalassemia in Mediterranean and Asian populations, and sickle-cell anemia in those of African heritage. Beliefs and practices specific to pregnancy, childbirth, and child rearing are common to every cultural group. Cultural beliefs about diet, role of the father, activity, labor, and delivery should be incorporated into prenatal care. Examples of cultural variables affecting health care can be seen in many groups. Spanish-speaking women view pregnancy as natural and are often reluctant to seek health care (Gibbs, Martin, & Gutierrez 1974). Some Chinese women are afraid that iron will harden their bones and make delivery difficult; as a result they don't want to take iron supplements (Mead 1956). Also, some Asian and Mexican-American women, because of lactose intolerance, may not follow the nurse's advice to use dairy products (Rosenberg 1977). Food restrictions are noted almost universally. For example, Polynesian, Vietnamese, and Filipino pregnant women are forbidden to eat fruits that do not grow singly. They believe that fruits like bananas may cause twins (Brown 1976).

In many cultural groups, excessive modesty and submissiveness to men are cultural patterns that may influence a woman's use of the health care system. To ensure the pregnancy's successful outcome, the nurse must understand and accept certain rituals prescribed by the woman's cultural group and use this awareness in carrying out the health assessment.

Because of religious beliefs, some women might object to using any contraceptive method. More research must be done on religion's influence on pregnant women's beliefs about contraception. The accuracy of information in this area is questionable because of the hesitancy of members of some cultural groups to share their beliefs on this sensitive subject (Orque 1981).

Reason for Seeking Health Evaluation or Chief Complaint

Generally, the client has experienced one or more of the signs and symptoms of pregnancy, which include amenorrhea, breast changes, nausea, and perhaps a positive pregnancy test. Because self-administered pregnancy tests are now available, the client may have confirmed her belief with one of these. The client may indicate at this time that this is an unwanted pregnancy, which is an extremely stressful experience for the woman. The nurse must have the skill to assist the woman in arriving at a decision and counsel her about preventing future unwanted pregnancies.

Current Health Status

The client's physiologic and emotional health has a bearing on whether she will experience a normal or high-risk pregnancy. Health habits such as cigarette smoking and alcohol or drug use can affect the growth of the fetus. The client's age may have a bearing on the pregnancy's progression. Clients who are suffering from diseases such as hypertension, diabetes, heart disease, or endocrine disorders certainly are at greater risk (Table 21-2). Acute factors, such as viral or bacterial infections, can adversely affect the developing fetus.

Menstrual history should include such data as date of menarche and characteristics of the menstrual cycle, including length and amount of flow and date of last menstruation. This date is helpful in estimating the expected date of delivery. Frequently, clients will have difficulty remembering the date of the last menstrual period, particularly if the pregnancy was not planned. The skilled interviewer can use events that occur seasonally, such as Christmas or Valentine's Day, or special events in the client's life to help her remember.

The estimated delivery calculation (EDC) can be computed using Nagele's rule. Three months are subtracted and 7 days added to the first day of the last menstrual period. In simple terms, add 7 days to the last menstrual period (LMP) and count forward 9 months. The majority of women will deliver during the period extending 7 days before and 7 days after the EDC. This is only one determination of delivery date. If a woman does not know the date of her LMP or is very irregular, other methods are used to determine due date. In fact, ultrasonic measurement is being used more frequently to assess progress and determine the EDC.

At this time, ask the client to indicate whether fetal movement has been felt and, if so, when it was first felt. This is also a good time to gather information about obstetric history. Previous childbearing experiences can influence the course of the present pregnancy and can also be helpful to the nurse in predicting possible complications. The following are areas to explore:

1. *Number and dates of previous pregnancies*
2. *Duration of pregnancies:* If full-term deliveries, note date of delivery and birth weight of infant. If not full-term deliveries, note cause (if known) and gestational age of infant. *Gravida* and *para* are terms frequently used to describe pregnancy and the outcomes of pregnancy. A pregnant woman is described as gravida, and para is the number of pregnancies ending in the delivery of a baby or in the delivery of one weighing 500 g or of more than 20 weeks' gestation, either alive or stillborn. For example, a woman who has had three pregnancies, delivered two at term, and has had one miscarriage at 12 weeks would be described as gravida 3, para 2, or 3/2. A system referred to as G/TPAL is a five-digit means of expressing the woman's obstetric history more accurately:

Table 21-2 **Pregnancy Risk Factors**

Physical	Psychologic	Environmental and social
Age: younger than 18 or older than 35	Family disorganization	Poverty
Height: less than 5 feet	Conflict about pregnancy	Poor nutrition
Obesity	Drug abuse	Poor access to health care
Poor weight gain	Reluctance to accept pregnancy	Contaminants in home
Pelvic inadequacy	Low self-esteem	Lack of education
Uterine incompetency	History of mental illness	Poor housing
Nutritional deficiency	Mental retardation	Highly mobile lifestyle
Bleeding after 20 weeks' gestation		Occupation involving dangerous or contaminated substances
Exposure to carcinogens		Lack of significant support person
Postmaturity		
Multiple gestation		
Presence of major illness (diabetes, hypertension, renal disease, heart disease, pulmonary disease, endocrine disorder, sickle-cell disease, anemia, pelvic inflammatory disease)		
Poor gynecologic or obstetric history		
History of child with congenital abnormalities		

G = *gravida*

T = number of babies born at *term* alive or stillborn

P = number of babies born *prior* to term, alive or stillborn

A = number of pregnancies ending in *abortion*

L = number of children currently *living*

In this example the recording would be 3/2102.

3. *Labor and delivery experience:* Onset—specifically, was labor spontaneous or induced? If induced, what was the reason for induction and the method? Also, what was the length of labor, complications, anesthesia, type of delivery (vaginal or Cesarean), and presentation of infant (vertex or breech).

4. *Abortions:* Spontaneous or induced

5. *Problems experienced:* Types of complications and treatment

6. *Postpartum experience:* Infections, hemorrhage, emotional difficulties, and course of recovery

7. *Problems of the infant:* Jaundice, respiratory distress, infection, or stillbirth

8. *Living children:* Course of growth and development and current health

Personal History and Patterns of Living

Of particular concern is a family history of multiple pregnancy, cardiovascular disease, diabetes, renal disease, congenital abnormalities, genetic disorders, blood dyscrasias, and emotional problems. There is a familial and hereditary nature for many health problems. For example, if the client's mother suffered from hypertension, she is more likely to develop hypertension with pregnancy.

Because diet and lifestyle are implicated in maintaining wellness in the general population, they are certainly important in the pregnant woman. Increasing evidence links the mother's diet and habits to the infant's welfare. Note the wide dissemination of material related to smoking and drinking and infant wellness. Typically at risk are unmarried women, poorly nourished, often with a history of alcohol, drug, or tobacco abuse, chronic physical illness, or previous obstetric complications. Poor support systems and emotional disturbances may further complicate the problem. Poverty underlies many of these problems (Fogel & Woods 1981).

Previous Experience with Illness

Knowledge of past illness, including hospitalizations and surgery, helps the nurse determine whether any past problems may cause difficulties during the current pregnancy. Of particular importance are any past surgeries or injuries to the pelvis, urinary tract, bowel, or abdomen. Weakness or abnormalities in these areas could impede the progress of the pregnancy. Some previous conditions, such as hypertension, rheumatic fever, asthma, venereal disease, and allergies, may be exacerbated by the pregnancy.

Physical Assessment

A complete assessment should be performed when the client is first seen. She is then examined once a month until 32 weeks' gestation, every 2 weeks from 32 to 36 weeks, and weekly from that time until delivery. During these examinations, special attention is paid to the breasts, abdomen, and pelvis. Changes can be noted in practically every body system during pregnancy. Most become more pronounced as the pregnancy progresses.

Developing a General Impression

During the general inspection, you must focus on the client's state of consciousness, age, race, and development. As previously mentioned, age and concomitant physical and emotional development are important considerations. Nutrition may be one of the most important factors affecting the outcome of the pregnancy. Nutritional deficiency can have many consequences, such as retardation of fetal growth, increased incidence of spontaneous abortion, increased incidence of congenital malformation, and retarded motor and intellectual development. Observation of nutritional state should be made during the first visit, and the nurse might also carry out a complete nutritional assessment, as described in Chapter 5. In addition, a note should be made about the client's general state of health at the time of initial assessment.

Height and Weight

The client's weight is often an indicator of nutritional status. Optimal weight gain is approximately 24 to 27 pounds during pregnancy (Figs. 21-1 and 21-2). The pattern should be no less than 3 pounds during the first trimester and 0.8 pounds each week after that unless the client is overweight at the beginning of pregnancy. There should be no more than 0.5 pound each week during the first 20 weeks of pregnancy and 1 pound each week after that period unless the client is underweight at the beginning of pregnancy. An overweight status is much more common, even among the poor in the United States. Clients with high weights prior to pregnancy face an increased risk of developing preeclampsia, and those who are underweight have low-birth-weight babies more frequently.

Blood Pressure

The client's blood pressure (BP) in the first trimester should remain unchanged if she is healthy. A slight drop may be noted in the healthy client during the second trimester. This is the result of a decrease in peripheral resistance. Blood pressure should be measured in both arms on initial visit. If the pressure is elevated, measure again after a rest period

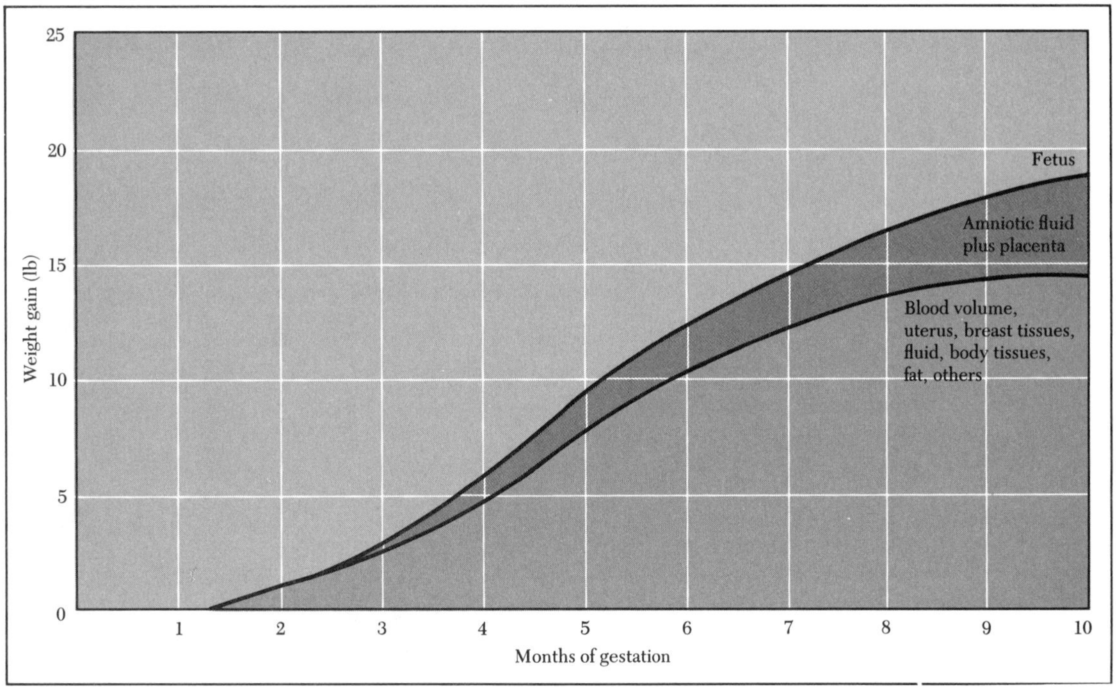

Figure 21-1 Components of weight gain in pregnancy.

with the client in the left lateral position, because the pressure is lowest in this position in the pregnant woman. The rollover test should be carried out on all nulliparous women between 28 and 32 weeks' gestation. If positive, this screening test indicates the woman is more likely to develop preeclampsia. To conduct the test, take one BP reading with the client in the left lateral position. Then have her roll on her back, let her rest for 5 minutes, and retake the pressure in the supine position. If the diastolic pressure is 20 mm Hg greater in the supine position than in the lateral position, the test is positive.

Assessment of the Integument

The hormonal changes that occur in pregnancy can be observed in some clients beginning about the 16th week. Pigmentation of the nipple and areola may be seen, particularly in dark-haired women. This increased deposition of melanin may also occur in the eyelids, vulva, and perianal area. Hyperpigmentation down the middle of the abdomen is called linea nigra. Mottling of the cheeks and forehead is called chloasma, or the "mask of pregnancy" (Fig. 21-3). Clients may express concern about these changes, especially those on the face. Dark pigmentation fades but does not completely go away after delivery. Other changes to note in the integument are localized areas of erythema over the fingers, fingertips, and palms. Striae may develop on the abdomen, breast, or buttocks. Fiery-red spider angiomas and bluish venous stars, the latter usually near varicose veins, may be observed.

Assessment of the Head, Face, and Neck

An increase in facial and body hair may occur during pregnancy. It usually begins about the third month and appears as fine lanugo on the face and chest. This disappears 2 to 3 months after delivery. Hair on the head tends to straighten and hair loss occurs, usually beginning about 2 to 4 months after delivery. Regrowth occurs without treatment.

On palpation, the thyroid is often found to be enlarged. This is due to hyperplasia of the glandular tissue and increased vascularity. Pregnant women have a marked increase in their metabolic rates, most pronounced close to the delivery. This occurs because more oxygen is needed to maintain the metabolic activity of the mother and fetus.

Assessment of the Ear, Nose, Mouth, and Pharynx

No changes are usually noted in the ear, although some women complain of mild hearing loss due to Eustachian tube blockage. Nosebleeds are not uncommon during pregnancy and are the result of hormonal changes. Tissues of the mouth and gums may become hyperemic and swollen. Even brushing the teeth may cause bleeding. Hypertrophy of the gums causing epulides, which are small benign vascular lesions, may develop. These disappear after pregnancy.

Assessment of the Breasts

The breasts become progressively larger, and areolar hypertrophy causes them to have a nodular consistency. Areolar pigmentation deepens and widens; the veins in the breast

Table of standard weight for height*
(height without shoes, plus 1 inch)

4′10″	= 104
4′11″	= 107
5′ 0″	= 110
5′ 1″	= 113
5′ 2″	= 116
5′ 3″	= 118
5′ 4″	= 123
5′ 5″	= 128
5′ 6″	= 132
5′ 7″	= 136
5′ 8″	= 140
5′ 9″	= 144
5′10″	= 148
5′11″	= 152
6′ 0″	= 156

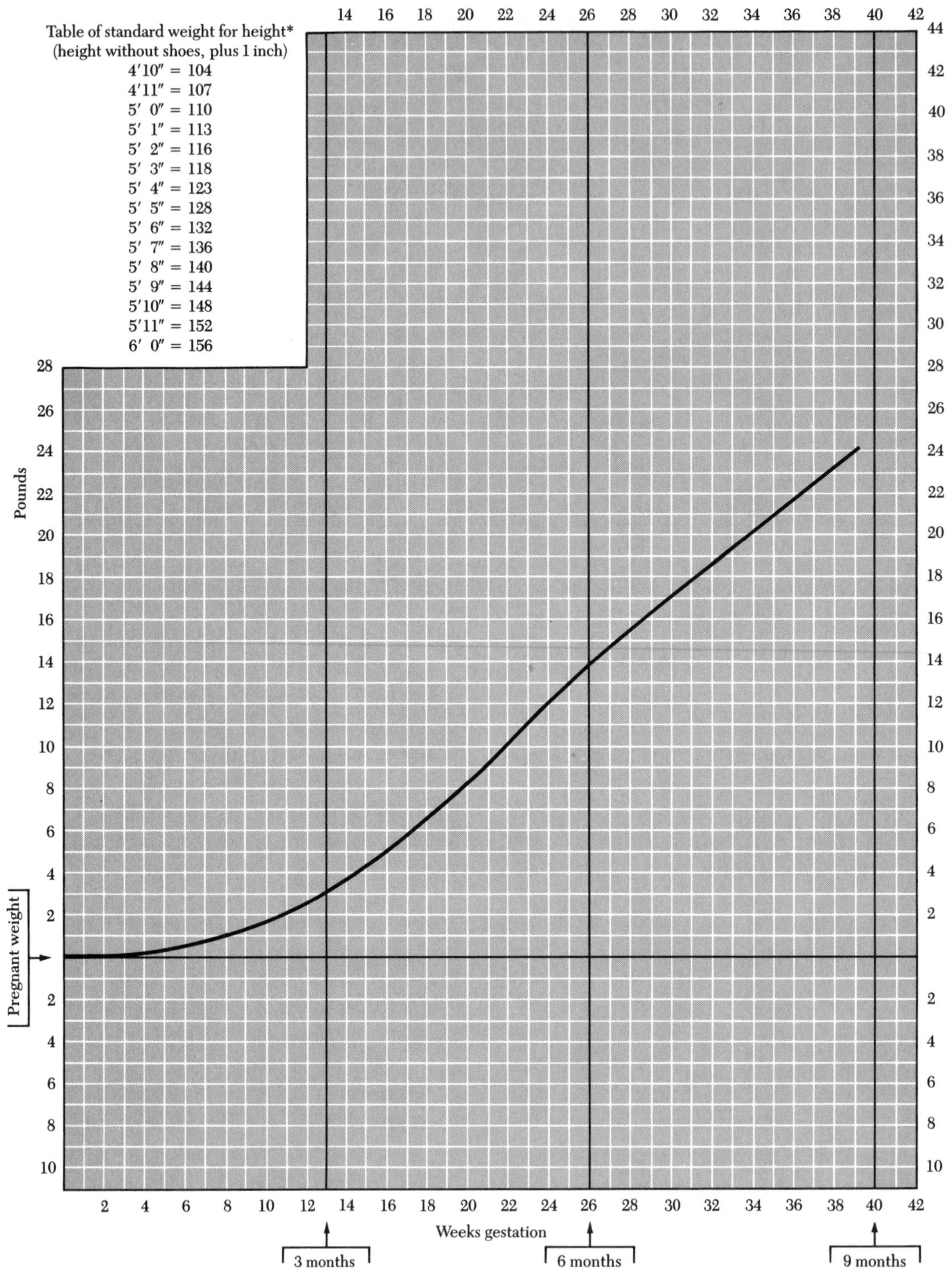

*The above weights were taken from Metropolitan Life Insurance Company Actuarial Tables, 1959 and adjusted to comply with instructions appearing on the Prenatal Weight Gain Grid, namely height in inches without shoes plus 1 inch to establish a standard for heels. Patients should be weighed with shoes as normally worn. The table above is for medium body build and, except for extreme body build deviations, these figures should be used. For example, a patient whose height, measured without shoes, is 5 feet 4 inches would have one inch added, therefore, her standard weight for height would be 128 pounds. Ranges are not acceptable in estimating standard weight since this is an objective observation and represents the mid-point. This mid-point must be used for recording purposes. For patients under age 25 one pound should be deducted for each year.

Figure 21-2 Prenatal weight gain grid.

become increasingly prominent (Fig. 21-4). About the 10th week, a secretion called colostrum may be expressed with gentle massage. The nurse should provide information regarding preparation for breastfeeding and should advise the client to wear a good, well-fitting bra for support.

Assessment of the Thorax and Lungs

There is an increase in respiratory rate as oxygen consumption increases. Breathing changes from abdominal to thoracic about the 24th week, and shortness of breath may occur late in pregnancy. Shortening and widening occurs at the base of the thoracic cage, and there is upward displacement of the diaphragm to allow for the expansion of the uterus.

Assessment of the Heart

As the uterus enlarges, it causes the diaphragm to elevate, which displaces the heart slightly upward and to the left, while at the same time causing a counterclockwise rotation (Fig. 21-5). The transverse diameter of the heart increases. The PMI is displaced laterally about 1 to 1.5 cm. Percussion and palpation of the heart will detect these changes. On auscultation, systolic murmurs may be heard. They are generally soft and blowing and are usually heard best in the pulmonic area and at the apex.

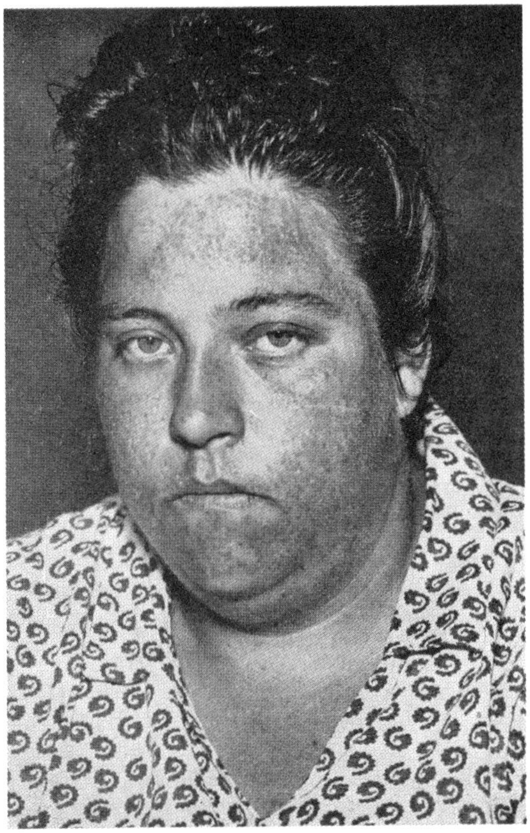

Figure 21-3 Mottling of cheeks and forehead, called chloasma of pregnancy.

The resting pulse is about 10 to 15 beats/min faster during pregnancy. There is a slight fall in the BP in the second trimester and then a rise as the pregnancy progresses. Any dramatic changes in the BP are suspect and should be noted. A sustained systolic increase of 30 mm Hg or diastolic increase of 15 mm Hg after 20 weeks' gestation may be indicative of pathology.

There is an increase in plasma volume, which may cause a pseudoanemia. Hematocrits should be done periodically, and an iron supplement is usually necessary to keep the hemoglobin levels normal.

Assessment of the Abdomen

A complete abdominal examination, including palpation of the kidneys, liver, and spleen, should be done at the first prenatal visit because as the uterus enlarges it becomes more difficult to palpate these organs. In subsequent visits, the abdominal examination is an objective measurement of fetal growth, as the fundal height changes at various gestational ages (Fig. 21-6).

Ask the client to empty her bladder before beginning the examination. Have her positioned with head slightly elevated and knees gently flexed. This position will relax the abdominal muscles. The liver and spleen should be palpated, although functions of both are normally unchanged during pregnancy. The kidneys should be palpated. Remember that renal blood flow increases by 25% during the first and second trimester. Percuss the abdomen, noting tympany. The bladder is more sensitive at this time and the enlarging uterus puts more pressure on it, resulting in frequency of urination during the first and third trimesters.

Inspection

The nurse should note the presence or absence of scars and striations. These will vary for each client, depending on past physical occurrences. Contour should be observed. Skin changes such as the linea nigra are not usually seen until the 16th week.

Palpation

From the 12th week of pregnancy on, the abdomen should be palpated to note fundal height and fetal presentation and position. In Fig. 21-6 you can see that at the 12th week the fundus is just above the symphysis pubis and at the 36th week it almost reaches the xiphoid.

To palpate the uterus, stand at the right side of the client, who is in the supine position. Select a point about 3 to 4 cm above where the fundus is expected to be at that point of gestation. Using the ulnar surface of the hand or the fingertips, palpate downward until the soft abdomen becomes the firm, round, fundal edge. When you have located the fundus, measure its distance from the symphysis. There are several methods of doing this and the method used should be documented each time. It is also recommended that the same person measure the fundus throughout the

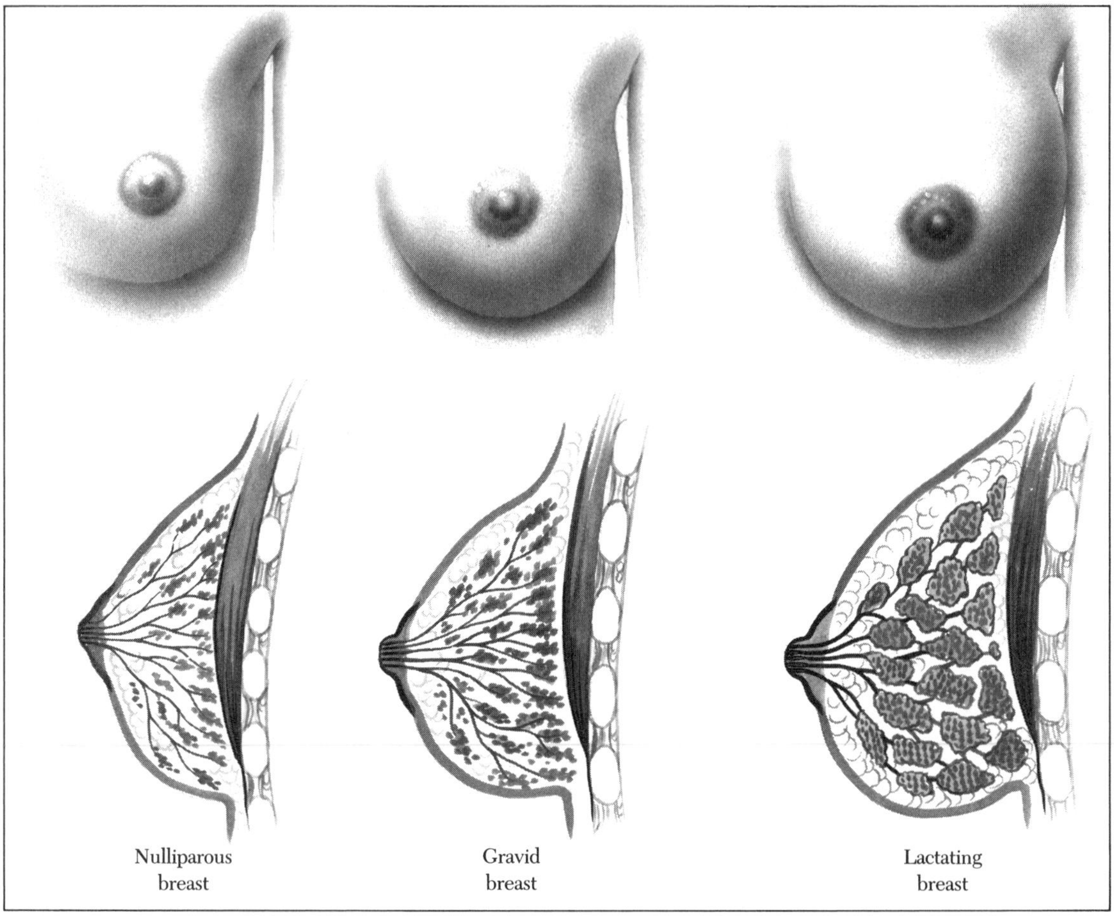

Figure 21-4 Changes in the breast during pregnancy and lactation.

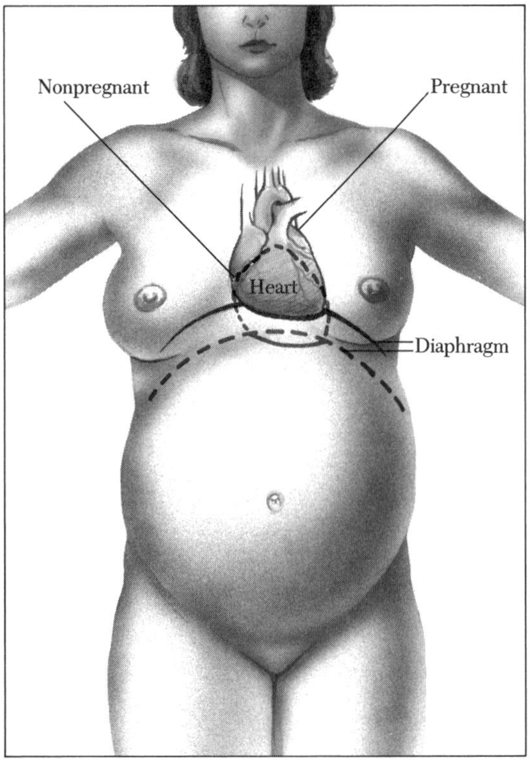

Figure 21-5 Changes in the heart and diaphragm during pregnancy.

pregnancy. The first method, using fingerbreadth measurements, is the most inaccurate. For example, you would record the fundus as being a certain number of fingerbreadths from the symphysis, umbilicus, or xiphoid (Fig. 21-7). The use of a measuring tape is more accurate. Place the tape at the superior border of the symphysis pubis and draw it up to the midline of the abdomen to the top edge of the fundus. After 22 to 24 weeks, the number in centimeters should equal gestation (Fig. 21-8).

Following the measurement of fundal height, the nurse should palpate the abdomen for lie, presentation, and position of the fetus. The relationship of the long axis of the mother to the long axis of the fetus is the lie. The lie can be longitudinal, oblique, or transverse (Fig. 21-9). Presentation denotes the part of the fetus that overlies the maternal pelvic inlet. The presentation can be vertex, brow, face, shoulder, or breech (Fig. 21-10). Position is the relationship of a designated point of the fetus (denominator) to a designated point in the maternal pelvis. For example, the occiput is the denominator in a vertex presentation. If the fetus has its occiput in the left inguinal area of the mother, the position would be described as left occipital anterior (LOA). The denominator in a breech presentation is the sacrum, and in a face presentation it is the chin.

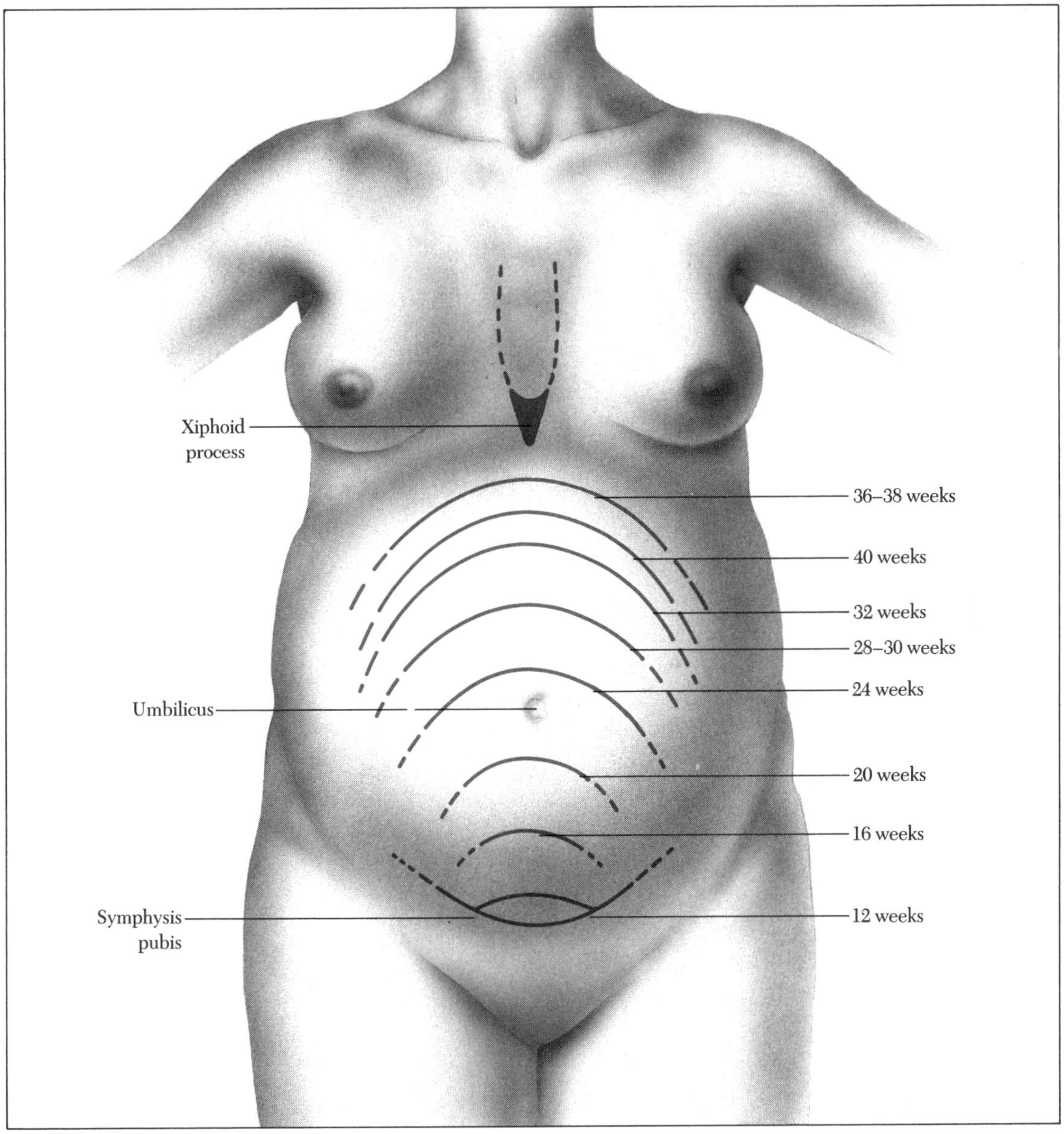

Figure 21-6 Fundal heights at various stages of pregnancy.

One method of determining lie, presentation, and position is called Leopold's maneuvers (Fig. 21-11). For these to be most effective, the fetus should be large enough so that different parts can be felt through the uterine and abdominal walls, about 26 to 28 weeks' gestation. For step 1 of these maneuvers, stand facing the client and place both hands on the abdomen. With fingertips nearly touching, cup your hands around the part of the fetus in the fundus. Usually the buttocks is in the fundus and it is rounded and somewhat soft. When moved, it causes the whole fetus to move. If the head is in the fundus, it is round and hard and moves independently of the rest of the fetus.

In step 2, continue to face the client and place your hands on either side of her abdomen. Hold one hand steady and apply pressure to the fetus with your other hand. If the hand you are applying pressure with feels a long, smooth part, you are probably feeling the fetus's back. If the part is bumpy and has indentations and angles, you are probably feeling the arms, legs, and knees. You will most likely feel movement on this side as the fetus gets older. On each side, palpate the flank to the midline, taking special note of the fetal back as a landmark in determining fetal position. If you feel the back more easily on the anterior abdomen, and the legs, knees, and so on, more on the flank, the fetus is in an anterior position. If you feel the back more on the flank and the arms, legs, and so on, more on the anterior abdomen, the fetus is probably in the posterior position.

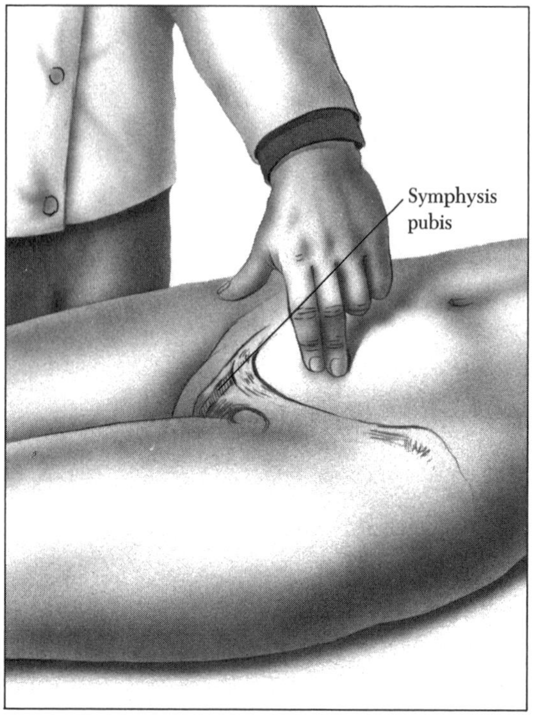

Figure 21-7 Measuring fundus using fingerbreadths.

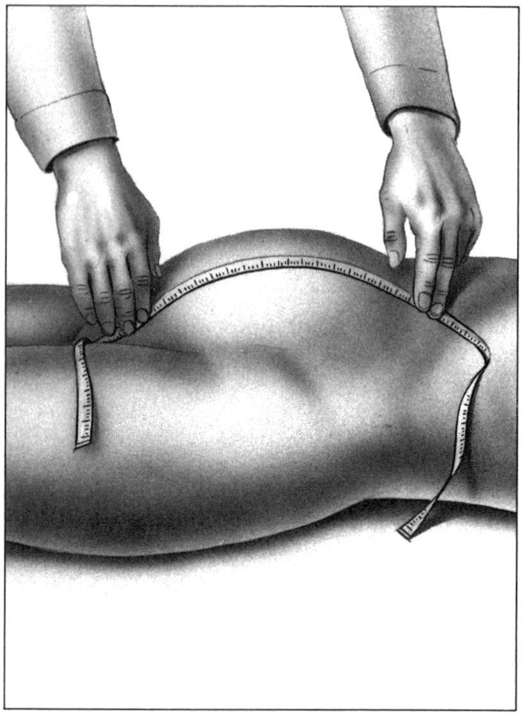

Figure 21-8 Measuring fundus with tape measure.

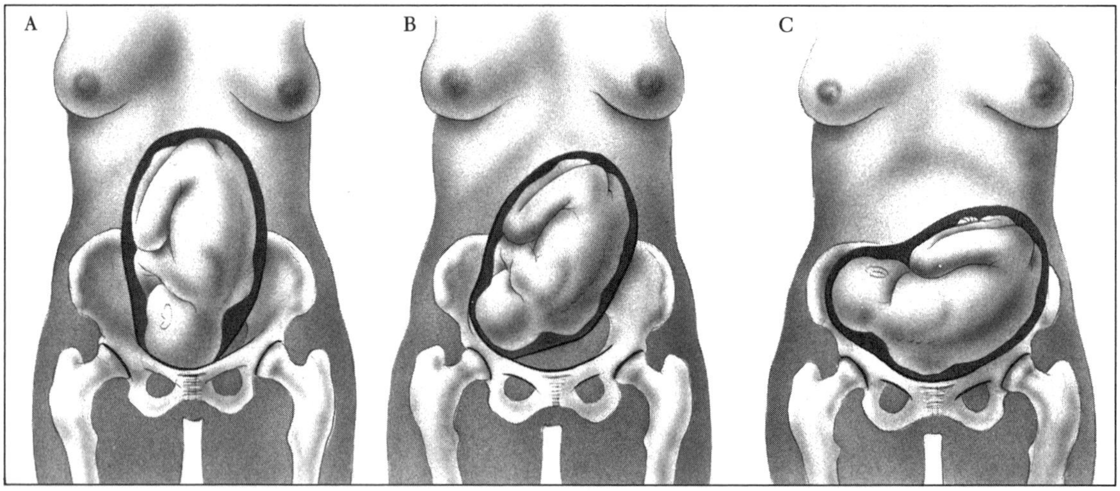

Figure 21-9 Examples of fetal lie. **(A)** Longitudinal lie. **(B)** Oblique lie. **(C)** Transverse lie.

To perform step 3, face the client and take the thumb and middle finger of your right hand and place them at the symphysis pubis with your fingers on the left side and thumb on the right side. Grasp the presenting fetal part. If the presenting part is hard and rounded and can be moved independently of the part in the fundus, it is the head. If it is soft and rounded and causes the whole fetus to move when grasped, it is the bottom, or breech.

Step 4 will help you to determine how far into the pelvis the presenting part has descended. Remain on the right side but face the patient's feet. Place both hands on either side of her lower abdomen just above the symphysis pubis. Ask the client to take a deep breath and then dip your fingers deep into the pelvis to determine which side the cephalic prominence is on. The brow should be felt on the same side as the arms, legs, and elbows. If the bony prominence is felt on the same side as the back, it indicates that the head is extended, which may result in problems during labor.

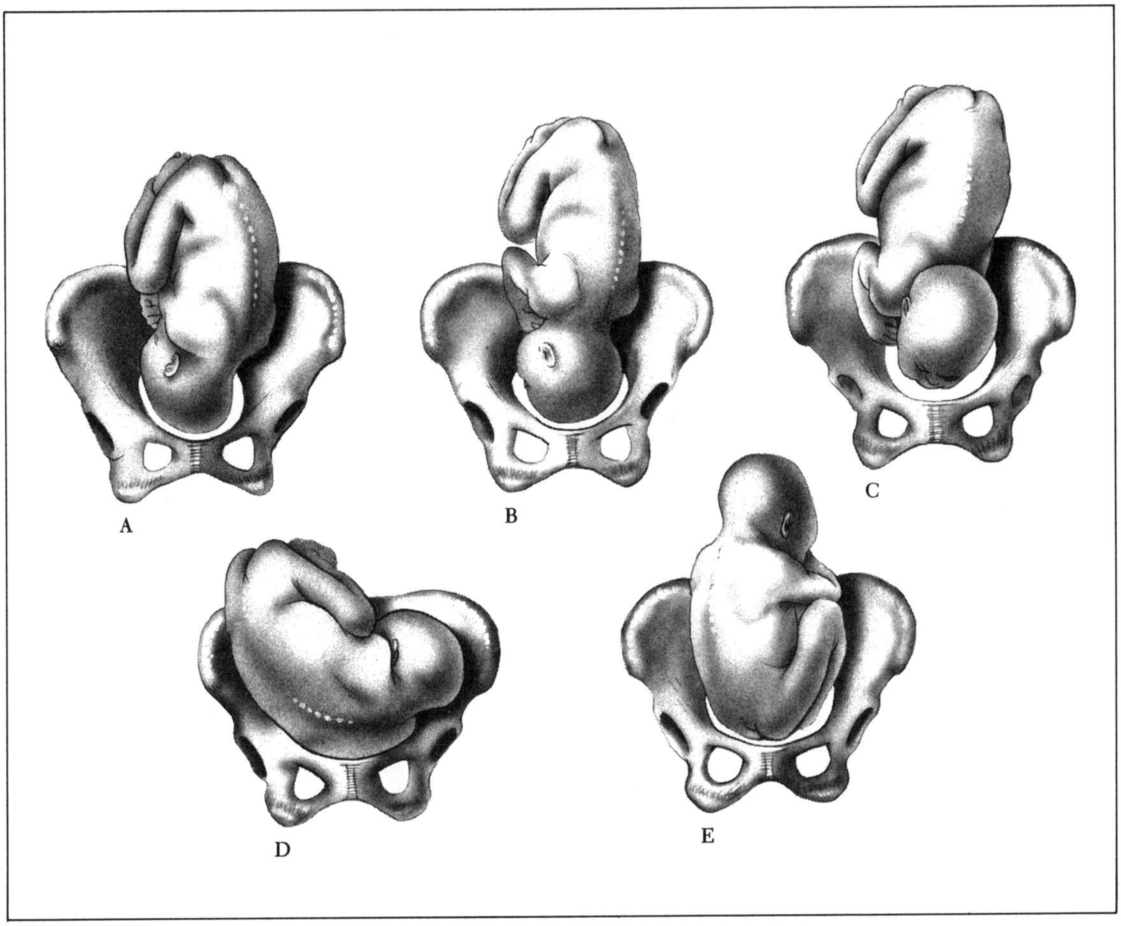

Figure 21-10 Examples of fetal presentation. **(A)** Vertex. **(B)** Brow. **(C)** Face. **(D)** Shoulder. **(E)** Breech.

Auscultation

Monitoring the fetal heartbeat is an important part of each prenatal visit. Electronic equipment can be used to hear the heartbeat at about 10 weeks' gestation. The standard fetoscope is used from 20 weeks (Fig. 21-12). The normal heart rate is 120 to 160, but it varies according to length of gestation. Usually, the heartbeat slows as the fetus grows and is closer to term. You can make some determinations about fetal presentation and position by locating the point of greatest intensity of fetal heart tones. Fetal heart sounds are heard best over a bony prominence. Therefore, if the fetal attitude is flexion, sounds will be best heard through the fetal scapula and shoulder. If the fetal attitude is extension, sounds will be best heard through the fetal anterior chest. When the fetus is in the anterior cephalic position LOA or ROA, you should place the stethoscope below the umbilicus to the right or left, depending on which side the back was felt. If the position is posterior, cephalic sounds are best heard by placing the stethoscope at the mother's flanks, again on whichever side the fetal back was felt. If the sounds are heard best above the mother's umbilicus, the fetus is probably in the breech position.

The fetal heart is rapid and sound. It is not synchronous with the mother's rate, so you can differentiate it by palpating the mother's pulse while auscultating the abdomen. Another sound that can be heard is called the uterine souffle, a blowing noise synchronous with the mother's pulse and heard best in the lower portion of the uterus. This sound, which is normal in the pregnant woman, is the result of the increased blood supply to the uterus.

Assessment of the Pelvis

The technique for pelvic examination is described in Chapter 16. Some changes in pregnancy can be noted early in pregnancy. The first of these is *Goodell's sign,* in which softening of the cervix can be detected at about 5 to 6 weeks. *Hegar's sign* is noted at about 6 to 7 weeks. Place two fingers of one hand behind the cervix in the posterior vaginal fornix. Then compress the lower part of the corpus anteriorly by retropubic pressure with the other hand (Fig. 21-13). On palpation, the dramatically enlarged globular uterus feels almost detached from the still not completely softened cervix. This occurs because the isthmus of the uterus is the first part to soften. At about the same time, the examiner can easily flex

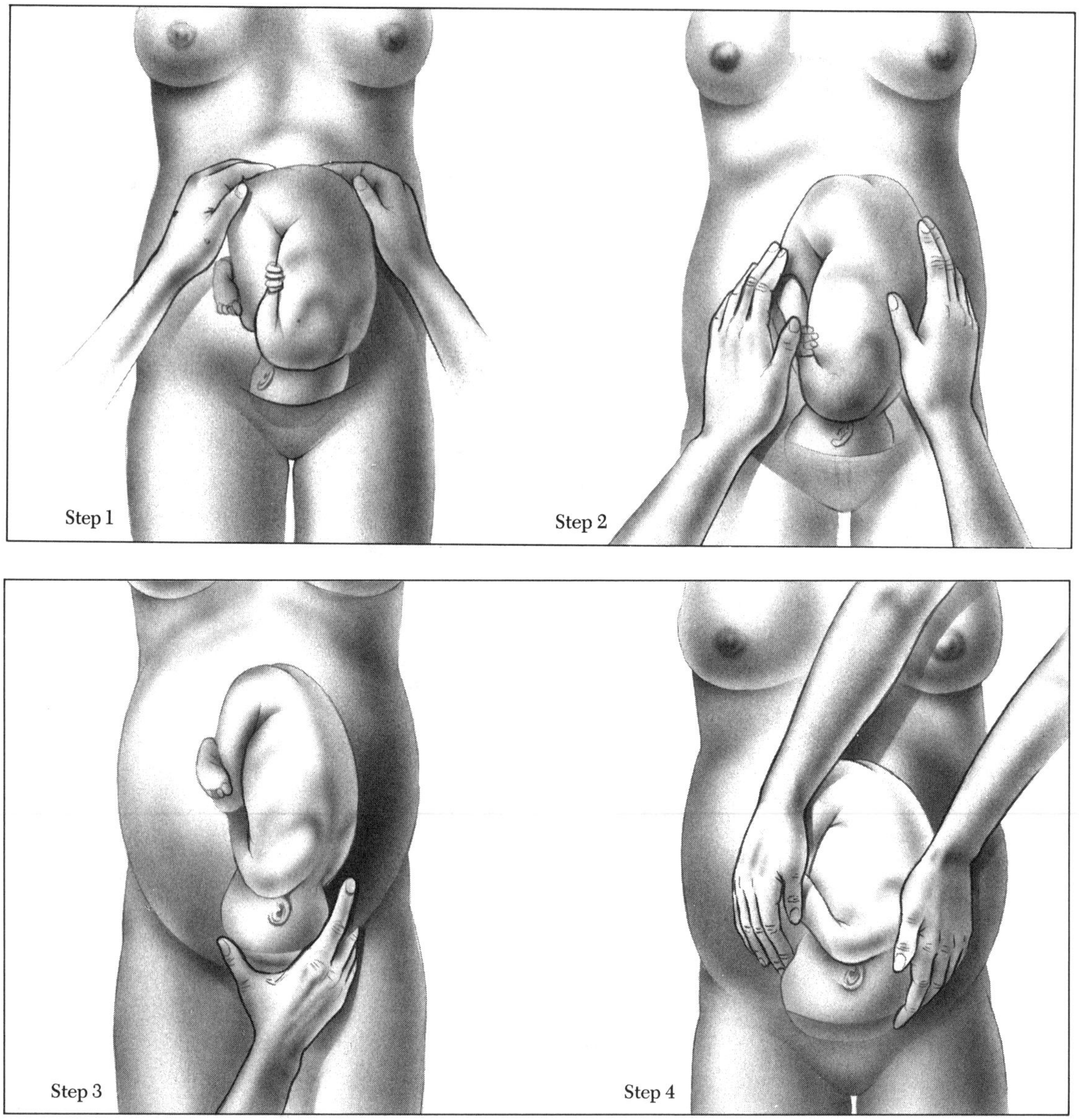

Figure 21-11 Leopold's maneuvers.

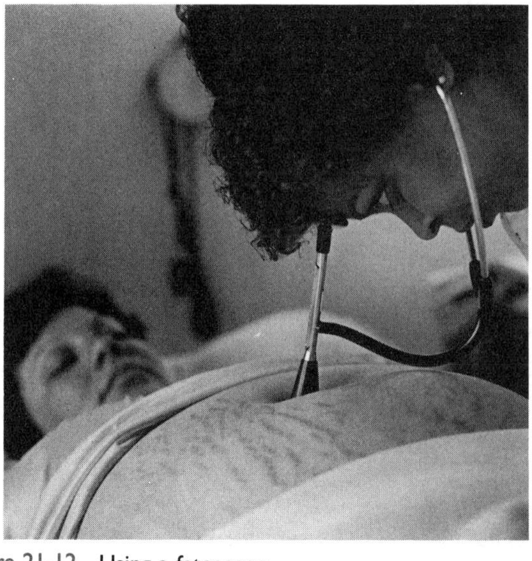

Figure 21-12 Using a fetoscope.

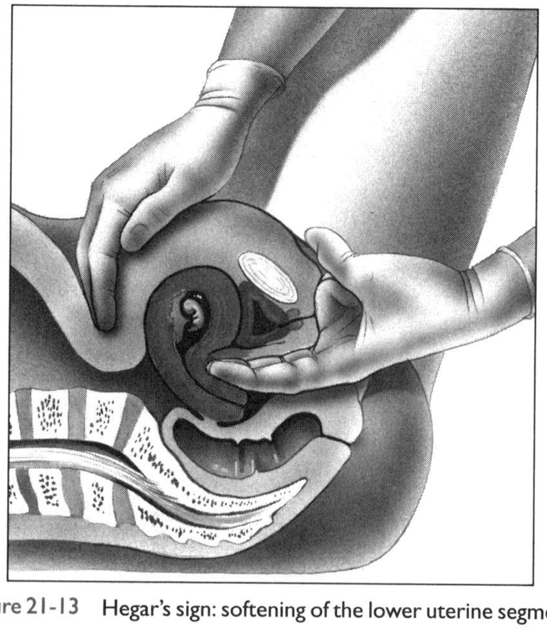

Figure 21-13 Hegar's sign: softening of the lower uterine segment.

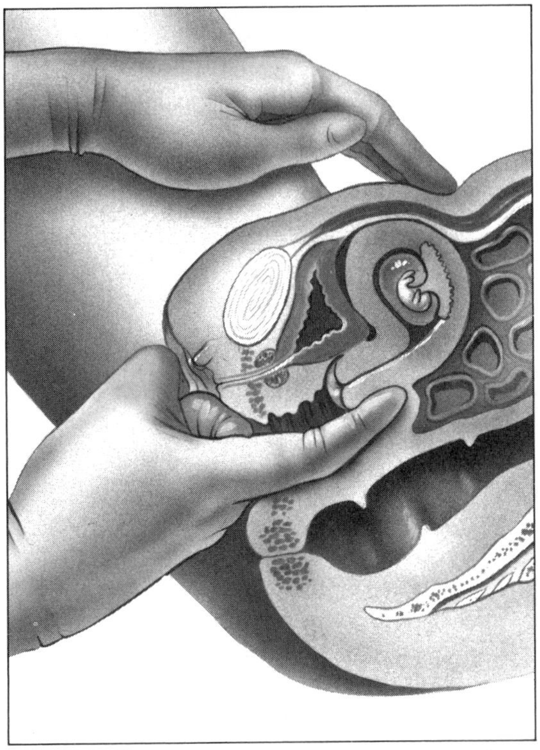

Figure 21-14 McDonald's sign: uterine body and cervix can be flexed against one another.

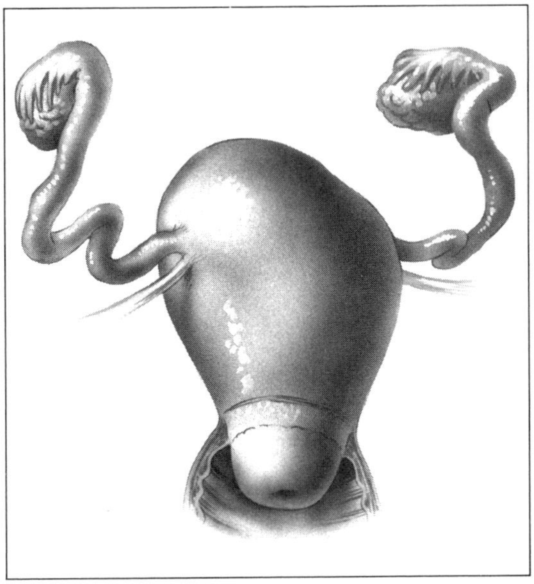

Figure 21-15 Piskacek's sign: asymmetrical enlargement of the uterine fundus.

the uterine body and the cervix against one another on bimanual examination. This is called *McDonald's sign* (Fig. 21-14). Frequently, the uterus can be palpated asymmetrically, softening at the cornua when the ovum has implanted

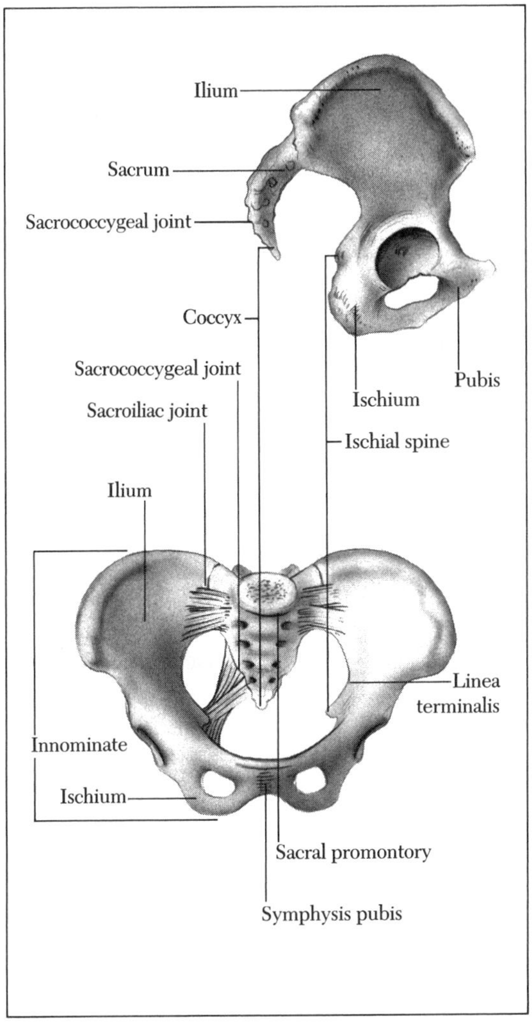

Figure 21-16 Bones and joints of pelvis.

there. This is referred to as *Piskacek's sign* (Fig. 21-15). *Chadwick's sign* results from increased vascularity and is evidenced by the bluish violet of the vulva, vagina, and cervix.

Pelvic measurements should be obtained to evaluate whether the pelvic cavity is big enough to accommodate the fetus at delivery. The pelvis is composed of four bones: the two innominate bones, the sacrum, and the coccyx (Fig. 21-16). The innominates join in front at the symphysis and at the sacrum by sacroiliac synchodroses. That portion above the linea terminalis is referred to as the false pelvis, which supports the enlarged uterus (Fig. 21-17). The true pelvis, below the linea terminalis, is the bony birth canal through which the baby must pass at delivery. If any of the planes or conjugates of this area are shortened or distorted, vaginal delivery may be difficult or impossible. The joints of the pelvis soften slightly during pregnancy in preparation for labor; the sacrococcygeal joint actually allows the coccyx to bend backward as the head is delivered.

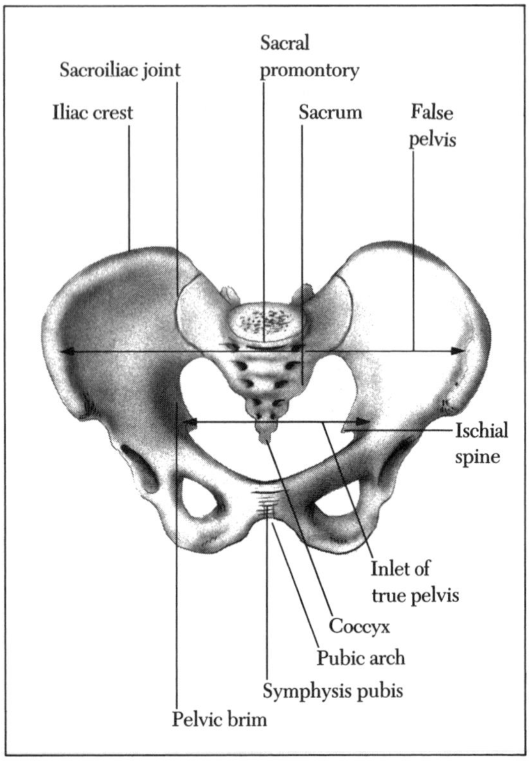

Figure 21-17 The pelvic cavity.

Race, sex, and age are responsible for the greatest variation in pelvic shape and size. Four types of pelvises have been identified (Fig. 21-18). Most often, the pelvis is a mixture of types.

1. *Gynecoid*—the classic female type. The inlet is wide and the pubic arch is wide. This pelvis is found in about 40% of women and is fairly easy for the fetus to move through.

2. *Anthropoid*—resembling the pelvis of anthropoid apes. This is a long, narrow pelvis. The inlet is oval-shaped, ischial spines are prominent, and the pubic arch is narrow. This shape is found in approximately 25% to 35% of women.

3. *Android*—resembling the male pelvis. This pelvis is long and narrow. The pubic arch is narrow and the ischial spines are sharp and prominent. This pelvis is found in 15% to 20% of women and is a difficult passage for the fetus.

4. *Platypelloid*—the flat pelvis. The inlet is wide with a narrow anterior-posterior diameter. The ischial spines are wide apart, the sacrum is short, and the pubic arch is wide, creating a shallow pelvis. This type is found in 3% to 5% of women.

The pelvis can be measured on the initial prenatal visit and repeated at 32 to 36 weeks if there is an indication of a problem or if the client's tenseness and resulting muscular contraction make the examination too difficult. Because the joints and ligaments relax more in the third trimester, the examination may be more accurate at that time. Another assessment can be made at the time of labor to compare pelvic measurements with data obtained on the presentation, position, and size of the fetus.

The first area to be assessed is the subpubic arch. To do this, press your right hand against the client's left ischiopubic ramus and the left hand against the right ischiopubic ramus so that the thumbs meet in the midline of the symphysis pubis (Fig. 21-19). Palpate the subpubic arch downward under the pubic bone until your right thumb rests on the left ischial tuberosity and the left thumb on the right ischial tuberosity. Mark each tuberosity with a small dot or *x* and then measure. Normally the line from the midline of the symphysis to the ischial tuberosity should form an angle measuring slightly more than 90 degrees, which is a right angle.

To assess the thickness and inclination of the symphysis pubis, palpate the internal surface with the middle finger of your left hand and the external surface with the index and middle fingers of your right hand. The inclination can be estimated by sweeping the examining fingers under the symphysis. Judgments to be made at this time are related to screening for an unusually long or steeply inclined symphysis and for an angular rather than a rounded forepelvis (Fig. 21-20).

Next, assess the curvature of the right and left anterior segments of the pelvic inlet and the ischial side walls to gain an idea of overall pelvic symmetry. With your right hand, follow the client's right pubic bone from the symphysis to the right side of the pelvic inlet. Then sweep downward over the right ischial side wall to the right ischial tuberosity.

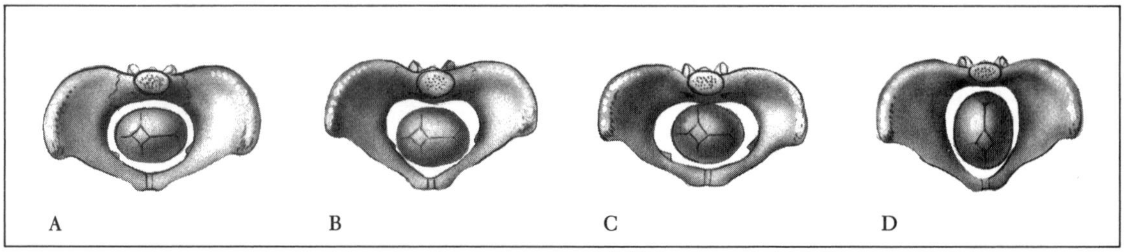

Figure 21-18 Four major pelvic types: **(A)** gynecoid, **(B)** android, **(C)** platypelloid (flat), and **(D)** anthropoid.

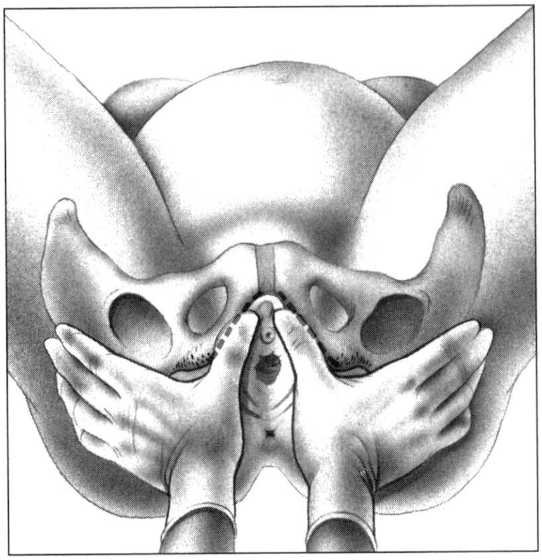

Figure 21-19 Method of estimating the angle of the subpubic arch.

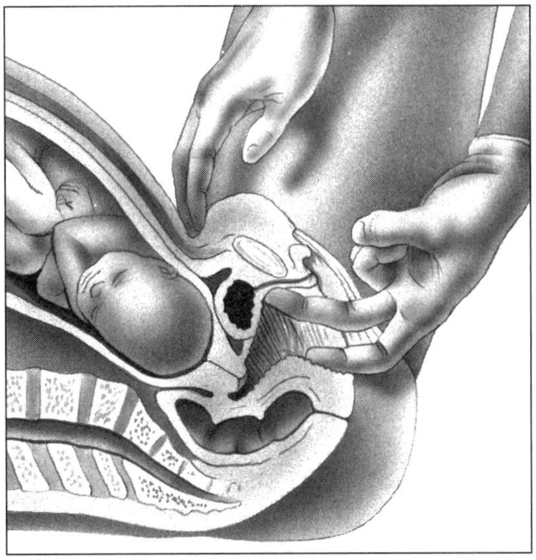

Figure 21-20 Estimation of the length and inclination of the symphysis pubis.

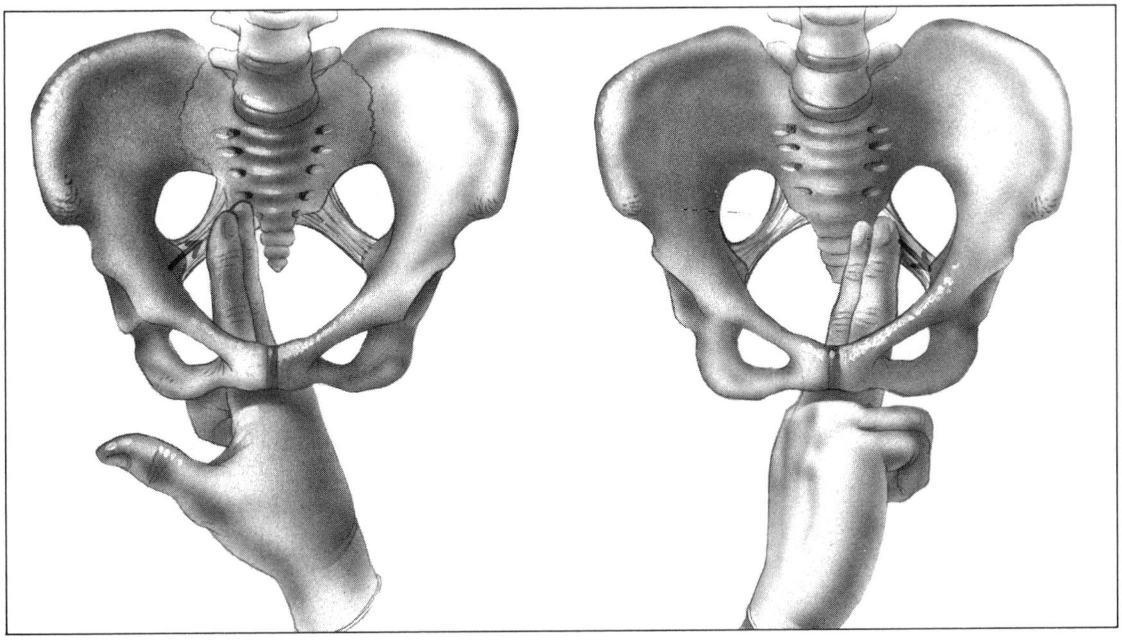

Figure 21-21 Measurement of the width of the sacrosciatic notch.

Repeat the procedure on the left anterior segment, using your left hand.

Examine the ischial spine and the sacrospinous ligament. Assess the spine as being blunt, prominent, or encroaching. If possible, the sacrosciatic notch is outlined with palpating fingers and the width determined in fingerbreadths or centimeters (Fig. 21-21). To do this, place the index and middle fingers of your right hand in the client's vagina. Palpate the right spine and then pass fingers across to the left ischial spine by pronating the right examining hand and following the conformation of the pelvic soft parts. This maneuver can be repeated several times. Ischial spines may be difficult to identify if they are not prominent. If that is the case, follow the sacrosciatic ligaments to their origins and reassess the spines during the rectal examination.

Measuring the transverse diameter of the midpelvis, also called the interspinous or bispinous diameter, can be accomplished by using an examining finger or a pelvimeter. Insert

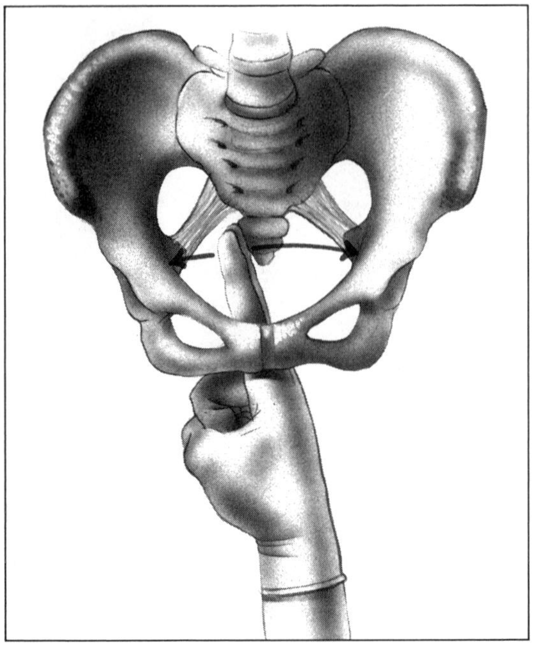

Figure 21-22 Measurement of the transverse, or interspinous, diameter.

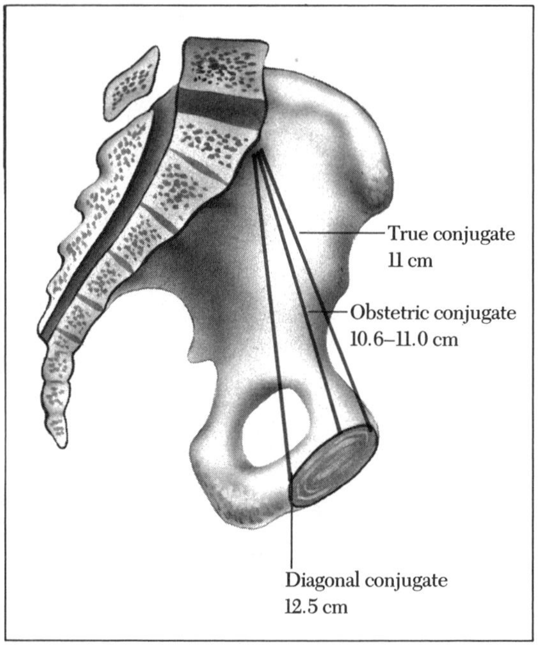

Figure 21-23 Assessing the anterior-posterior diameter of the pelvic inlet.

the examining fingers into the vagina and move them in a straight line from one spine to the other. You may have to pronate your hand to do this estimation. The estimate is measured in centimeters, and the average measure is 11 cm (Fig. 21-22).

The next important assessment is of the anterior-posterior diameter of the pelvic inlet (Fig. 21-23). There are three measurements of this diameter:

1. *True conjugate*—distance from the top of the symphysis pubis to the middle promontory of the sacrum
2. *Obstetric conjugate*—distance between the posterior surface of the symphysis and sacral promontory
3. *Diagonal conjugate*—distance from the inferior border of the symphysis to the sacral promontory

The diagonal conjugate is the only diameter that can be measured without the use of x-ray. This examination may produce discomfort, so you should instruct the client to relax and focus her attention on breathing slowly. A moderate amount of pressure is needed to depress the perineum. Position your own right foot on a small stool so that your right knee is bent and your right thigh elevated. For this examination, your fingers and wrist should be in a straight line with the forearm. Locate the sacrum with your examining fingers, and with the middle finger, walk up the sacrum until the promontory is reached or until your finger can no longer reach the sacrum. Keeping your middle finger in place, raise your right wrist until your hand touches the inferior border of the symphysis pubis. Withdraw your hand and measure from the tip of the middle finger to the point on the examining hand that has touched the symphysis (Fig. 21-24). Normally, the diagonal conjugate is greater than 12.5 cm. Estimation of the true conjugate can be made by subtracting 1.5 cm from the diagonal conjugate. An estimate of the obstetric conjugate can be determined by subtracting 2 cm from the diagonal conjugate.

The transverse diameter of the pelvic outlet is measured by the distance between the ischial tuberosities. The measurement can be made with a Thom's pelvimeter or can be estimated by placing a closed fist between the protrusions of the ischial tuberosities (Fig. 21-25). The usual distance is 10.5 cm.

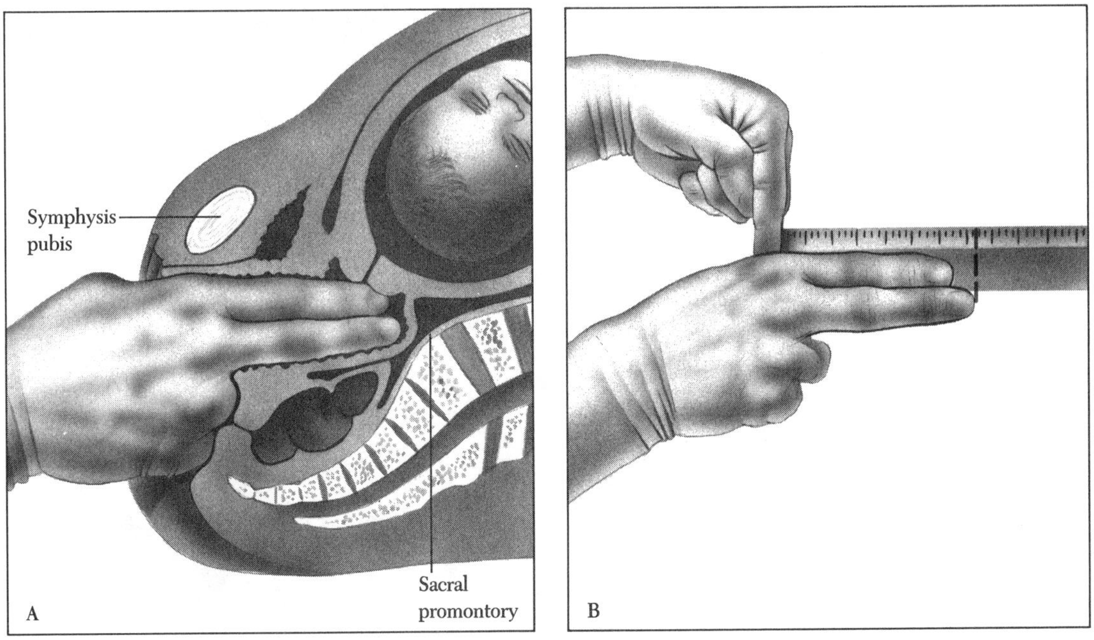

Figure 21-24 Measurement of the diagonal conjugate.

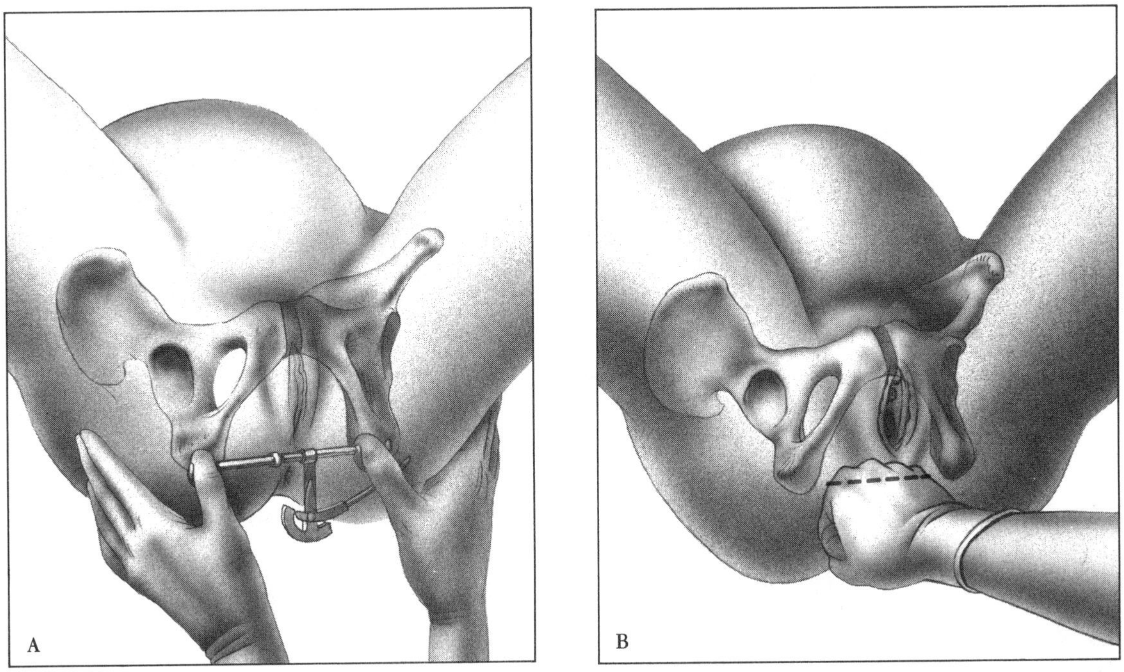

Figure 21-25 **(A)** Use of the Thom's pelvimeter to measure the intertuberous diameter. **(B)** Use of a fist to estimate the intertuberous diameter.

Example of a Health Assessment of a Pregnant Woman

HEALTH HISTORY
Name: Marianne Phillips
Address: 27 Lincoln Place
Sex: Female
Age: 34
Birthdate: 7/17/52
Marital status: Married since 1976
Occupation: Teacher
Religion: Protestant (attends church infrequently)
Race: Caucasian
Ethnic origin: English and Scotch
Education: College and graduate school
Informant: Client, a reliable historian

Reason for Seeking Health Care
Client has missed two menstrual periods and has been slightly nauseated on arising for the past 10 days. Has also noted more frequent urination for several weeks. Client feels she is probably pregnant. She expresses hope that she is and states that she and her husband have been hoping to have a third child.

Personal History and Patterns of Living
Client states she is happily married, has been teaching in a local college for two months, and in addition cares for two young children (both boys). She is able to handle all of these because her husband is very supportive, and she describes herself as being very ambitious. Her salary is $24,000 per year and her husband's is $50,000 per year. She describes financial status as very adequate for family needs; family has Blue Cross and Blue Shield health care coverage.

Family Health History
States family has a history of diabetes. Denies history of arthritis, alcoholism, bleeding disorders, kidney disease, hypertension, heart disease, endocrine disease, or mental illness.

Lifestyle
Client is currently attending diet classes but describes the plan as well balanced and one that with modifications for age and sex she can use for planning meals for her family. Wants to lose about 10 lb and, most important, to change the eating habits of herself and family to ensure good health. Client does not smoke and drinks only socially and then just wine. Describes family as very close and also close to grandparents, cousins, etc. Family is very active, swimming 3 times per week, cross-country skiing, and hiking.

Previous Experience with Illness/Hospitalization
Childhood illness: Mumps, age 8, chickenpox same year; measles (not sure of year); immunizations DPT.
Allergies: Allergic to grass and roses. Had series of allergy shots in early 1970s, which she describes as only moderately helpful. Uses over-the-counter medication (antihistamines) during June and August. She is aware that pregnancy will require change in that.
Past illness, injuries, surgery: Appendectomy age 11, hospitalized 6 days. Hospitalized for C-section in 1979 and 1981. Length of stay 2 weeks. Says she had to have sections due to high blood pressure and swelling.

Review of Systems
General health: In good health but has felt more fatigued in last few weeks with feeling of nausea and occasional vomiting in the morning. States she had same experience with previous pregnancies. Problem disappeared in several months. Never took medication to control symptoms in the past.
Integument: No history of skin disease but developed hyperpigmented areas on forehead and cheeks during last pregnancy. No itchy skin or scalp, denies rashes, hives, nevi, open sores, hair loss, or problems with nails. Has acne, which has become worse in last month.
Head: Denies frequent or severe headaches, dizziness.
Eyes: Denies infection or pain; does not wear glasses; last eye exam in 1983; denies diplopia, excessive lacrimation, blurring of vision, photophobia, or halo-rainbows around lights.
Ears: Has slight hearing loss in left ear since frequent infections as a child. Denies pain, discharge, tinnitus, auditory hallucinations, and vertigo.
Nose, nasopharynx, and paranasal sinuses: No discharge at present, infrequent colds, has allergies to roses and grass with seasonal copious discharge, itching, and sneezing. Notices decrease in sense of smell during middle and last part of pregnancy.
Mouth and throat: Denies bleeding gums at present but during last pregnancy noticed that gums were sensitive and bled easily when teeth brushed. Visits dentist yearly and was informed that gums often bleed more easily during pregnancy. Was advised by dentist to use softer

bristles when brushing and to call if there was any increase in bleeding or increased soreness of gums. This did not occur.

Neck: Denies pain, edema, limitation of movement, swollen glands.

Cardiorespiratory system: Reports significant elevation in BP during both pregnancies especially during last trimester. States that following delivery BP returned to normal. Denies cough, sputum, othopnea, dyspnea, and PND. No history of pneumonia, TB, pain, wheezing, hemoptysis, anemia. Has some leg varicosities. Wears support hose.

Gastrointestinal system: Has had nausea and vomiting for last 10 days; denies blood in stools, melena, flatulence, pain. Has hemorrhoids since last pregnancy, occasional pain associated with constipation (infrequent). Usually has soft, formed stool daily after breakfast.

Genitourinary system: Has had frequency in last few weeks; denies pain, itching, blood. Describes sex life as very satisfying.

Gynecologic and obstetric: Menarche age 13, LMP 1/2/86. Has irregular cycle 28–35 days, flow moderate, uses tampons and pad interchangeably due to fear of toxic shock. Denies metrorrhagia, menorrhagia, dyspareunia. Has noted slight spotty bleeding following intercourse recently. Para 2 gravida 2—Had 2 C-sections following rapid increase in BP and significant swelling of feet and hands. No abortions. When practicing birth control, uses diaphragm.

Musculoskeletal system: Denies muscular pain, edema (currently). Had significant hand and pedal edema during last trimester of previous pregnancy.

Reproductive: Normal pubic hair pattern; external genitals normal in appearance; labia and vaginal walls show increased vascularity (positive Chadwick's sign); Skene's and Bartholin's glands not inflamed; normal vaginal discharge, no odor or itching. Cervix oval, external os appears as transverse slit. Cervix soft (Goodell's sign) at 12 weeks' gestation. Adnexa—nothing significant.

Uterus: Bimanual exam reveals uterus slightly antiflexed, larger and soft (Hegar's sign present). Pap smear to lab. Fundal height: 1.2 cm above symphysis pubis. Client notes periodic tightening across abdomen (Braxton-Hicks contractions). No cyctocele, rectocele, or prolapse.

Rectum: One small internal hemorrhoid; sphincter tone good; test for occult blood.

Bony Pelvis Examination

Subpubic arch—above 90 degrees
Side walls—parallel
Ischial spines—average
Sacrospinous notch—8.5 cm
Sacrospinous ligament—4 cm
Interspinous diameter—10.5 cm
Sacrum—straight
Coccyx—projects posteriorly
Diagonal conjugate—12.5 cm
Intertuberous diameter using Thom's pelvimeter—10.5 cm

Based on Mrs. Phillips's last menstrual period the expected date of delivery is: October 9, 1986.

SUMMARY

This chapter has presented assessment in selected areas of women's health. The areas do not constitute a complete picture of women's health needs, however. Menstruation and menopause were presented because they are events all women experience. Specific health problems related to these events, such as amenorrhea, dysmenorrhea, and PMS, are frequent occurrences. Eating disorders were discussed, and there is evidence of increased incidence occurring particularly among younger women.

The women's movement has had a profound influence on the care of women during pregnancy. The need to understand both physiologic and psychological aspects of pregnancy is essential to the practice of nursing. Throughout the chapter, normal findings, as well as selected deviations from normal, were described.

DISCUSSION QUESTIONS/ ACTIVITIES

1. Describe the social factors that affect the health status of adolescent girls. Plan a health education program to counteract the negative responses that occur.
2. Research and discuss the historical development of women's health care as a specialty.
3. Plan a health education program related to menstruation and menopause.
4. Describe the assessment of the pregnant client on her initial health visit, at 16 weeks, and just prior to delivery.

REFERENCES

Brown, M. S. 1976. A cross-cultural look at pregnancy, labor, and delivery. *J.O.G.N. Nursing* 5:35–38.

Fogel, C. I., and Woods, N. F. 1981. *Health care of women.* St. Louis: C. V. Mosby.

Gibbs, C. E.; Martin, H. W.; and Gutierrez, M. J. 1974. Patterns of reproductive health care among the poor of San Antonio, Texas. *Am. J. Pub. Health* 64:37–40.

Green, T. H. 1977. *Gynecology: essentials of clinical practice.* 3rd ed. Boston: Little, Brown.

Mead, M. 1956. Understanding cultural patterns. *Nursing Outlook* 4(5):260–262.

Orque, M. 1981. Cultural components. In *Maternity care: the nurse and the family,* eds. M. Jensen, S. R. Bensom, and I. Bobak. St. Louis: C. V. Mosby.

Reitz, R. 1977. *Menopause: a positive approach.* New York: Penguin Books.

Rosenberg, F. 1977. Lactose intolerance. *Am. J. Nurs.* 77:823–824.

Seaman, B., and Seaman, G. 1977. *Women and the crisis in sex hormones.* New York: Rawson Associates.

CHAPTER

22 Assessment of Men's Health

Learning Objectives

1. Identify the impact of culture on men's health.
2. Analyze the value-belief pattern relative to male identity and its effect on client-health professional interactions.
3. Discuss the implications of male identity and health practices and status.
4. Identify the risk factors for cardiovascular disease.
5. List mental status alterations that may suggest cardiovascular difficulties.
6. Identify the physical findings that are reflective of cardiovascular disease.
7. State risk factors for lung cancer.
8. List signs and symptoms of lung cancer and potential metastatic sites and related symptomatology.
9. Discuss the ethnic epidemiologic findings associated with prostatic cancer.
10. Identify signs and symptoms of benign prostatic hyperplasia and prostatic cancer.
11. Discuss nursing implications relative to the incidence of testicular cancer.
12. State the signs and symptoms of testicular cancer.
13. Identify the primary causes of sexual dysfunctions.
14. Discuss the approach and components of history taking with the client experiencing sexual dysfunction.
15. Cite diseases, surgeries, and drugs that are commonly associated with male sexual dysfunctions.

> Gender is perhaps the single characteristic which most fundamentally determines perceptions, behaviour and position in most societies. No other characteristic of individuals may be subject to the same degree of cultural and social learning (Dean 1989, p. 138).

The medico-nursing system readily attends to the pathophysiology, diagnosis, and treatment of injuries and illnesses of prevalence in men (e.g., suicide, fractures, head and spinal injuries, cancers, hernias, peptic ulcers, cardiorespiratory diseases, and sex-related illnesses such as benign prostatic hyperplasia). Basic assessment skills and techniques of psychological and physical examination relative to these health problems that plague men are included in earlier chapters and will not be repeated here. This chapter initially focus on the value-belief pattern pertinent to gender identity that is learned within the sociocultural context of men's lives. This will assist the nurse in generating a more holistic view of the male client when assessing his health. Then data associated with selected health problems encountered by men will be addressed.

MALE IDENTITY

Most cultures have child-rearing practices that instill a gender identity for the male as one who is in control of his emotionality; therefore, a boy is taught to be inexpressive—to hide his emotions. Feelings of hurt, pain, anxiety, and depression are not to be freely shared or overtly manifested. To do so would constitute a sign of weakness and inferiority. Whether each of us is male or female, we generally have a similar cultural view of how men and women are to behave. Our society teaches us that a man is competitive; he is a warrior. To live up to society's expectations, compensatory masculine role behaviors may take the form of risk-taking, aggression, and violence. Traditionally, the male is thought of as being self-sufficient and strong. It follows then that these stereotypic characteristics of male identity will impact on health behaviors and health practices of clients and on practices and care rendered by health professionals.

Commonly, men feign good health to keep within society's expectations of the male identity as healthy and strong in spite of the fact that they might be ill. If not overtly, subconsciously the view that only the weak, dependent, and inferior become ill prevails in our society. It is not surprising that this ingrained belief leads men to psychologically deny health needs and find it difficult to seek preventive as well as curative care, and to accept assistance from others. This is a sad state in light of present health knowledge, and it likely contributes to the health statistics for men.

Chronic illnesses related to the leading causes of death, such as chronic ischemic heart disease and chronic obstructive pulmonary disease, are of a higher prevalence in men than in women. Men also have a higher risk of all the leading causes of death in the United States and a higher rate of injury at all ages compared with women. The higher rate of injuries may be related to occupational hazards in jobs done primarily by men and could be attributable somewhat to the more risk-taking behavior of men (Dean 1989). Issues of masculinity surround the high morbidity and mortality rates of motor vehicle accidents, homicides, and suicides involving men. Men tend to use seat belts less than women. Men have a greater use of alcohol and street drugs than women (Waldron 1982). The greater use of alcohol also is a contributing factor to men's higher morbidity and mortality from cirrhosis, laryngeal and bladder cancer, as well as from heart disease. Men are more likely to use alcohol and tobacco as coping behaviors. Alcohol and cigarette smoking act synergistically, increasing the risk of development of cancer of the lungs and of the esophagus (Doll and Peto 1981).

Traditionally, more men have smoked than women, and men have a greater mortality rate from lung cancer. Men ingest smokeless tobacco far more than do women and suffer a higher incidence of oral cancer as a result. The sex difference in cigarette smoking has lessened. In light of evidence and media focus on the dangers of tobacco, and legislation for "smoke-free areas" and individuals trying to "break the habit," it will be interesting to follow the morbidity and mortality rates for ischemic heart disease, lung cancer, emphysema, bronchitis, and other smoking-related diseases. Another interesting data find is that men have longer hospital stays than women (Dean 1989). Yet, in view of these statistics, men do not seek medical and nursing attention as frequently as do women (Forrester 1986).

Women are more active in preventive spheres and adhere to regular check-ups that include cancer screening (pap smears, stool examinations for occult blood, breast examinations, pelvic examinations, mammograms) and routine monitoring of blood pressure, weight, and blood chemistry. At present, the majority of men are not attentive to preventive screening and to practices that safeguard their health, social beliefs being one influential factor; and neither men nor women health professionals are attentive to men's preventive health needs. This lack of preventive health measures by and for men was a major tenet of men's health that prompted Bozett and Forrester (1989) to propose the educational preparation of a nurse practitioner in men's health.

A male movement is growing out of the recognition of high morbidity and mortality rates for men and because of social emphasis on preventive practices and the reach for greater longevity in general. This holds implications for nursing practice and research. "One positive potential for the men's health movement would be to identify linkages between the way men die and the way they live as *men*" (Allen & Whatley 1986, p. 8).

MEN AND HEALTH PROFESSIONALS

Sex stereotyping occurs in health professionals as well as in other individuals. Most professionals hold traditional values and beliefs about masculinity and find it difficult to address and accept emotionality in men. Most male professionals find it difficult to deal with feelings and emotionality in either men or women clients. Men as professionals and as clients generally do not share health concerns on an emotional level but interact in a more factual, business-like exchange. Even more difficult is sharing health problems associated with sexuality. It is generally believed that "men do not discuss such things with each other" and that women "cannot possibly understand the unique male experience" (Forrester 1986, p. 17). The stereotypic beliefs that men must "bite the bullet," that men are strong and self-sufficient, that men don't cry, and that men are stoic and do not show their feelings shape the male client's responses not only to health practices but also to illness and health personnel. So too, the practices of health professionals are influenced.

Quite some time ago, Jourard (1971) challenged health professionals to become aware of their cultural beliefs about men and to begin to help change the stereotypic image of men held by society in an effort to improve men's health and longevity. He emphatically addressed the need to encourage men to express their feelings of sorrow, pain, fear, tenderness, and love. He pointed out that, in turn, health professionals must be accepting of overtly manifested emotionality that does not fit the social stereotype. This is difficult for most individuals to do because of our deeply ingrained cultural values.

Some changes in values and attitudes surrounding masculinity are slowly evolving in parallel with the women's movement. Men are no longer viewed as the sole family breadwinner. When we find ourselves thinking this way, further investigation brings home to us the reality that today the breadwinner role is shared or reversed in some cases from the traditional role responsibility. Conversely, it is more acceptable for the man to engage in housekeeping chores and caring physically for the children without the shame that accompanied such behaviors in the past. It would seem that adaptation of a more androgynous model for social behaviors by health professionals, authors, media producers, teachers, parents, and society as a whole would decrease health risk behaviors in men. Health educators, nurses, and physicians need to convey the health hazards inherent in the traditional concept of masculinity. Health care professionals and those in the media and media production can incorporate guidance and reinforcement of positive health practices in their work so that more positive health behaviors may be fostered in men. All persons need to be conscientious role models. Storylines of books, films, and television programs could greatly help in this cause by incorporating positive health practices in the lifestyles of major male characters. In addition to the family, the public entertainment sphere is strongly influential in helping to form social values and beliefs.

SELECTED HEALTH PROBLEMS

Cardiovascular Disease

Health problems related to the heart and the cardiovascular system are heavily focused on in nursing and medical education and are commented on in most discussions of men's health. This is because heart disease is the major cause of death for men and the major cause of differences in mortality rates between the sexes. Incident rates for coronary occlusions and myocardial infarctions are substantially higher for men than for women. Being male is in and of itself a documented risk factor for heart disease. Credence has been given to the presence of estrogen for the lower risk of heart disease in women. With menopause and the decrease of estrogen, the risk for heart disease in women increases. The woman's risk for heart disease also increases with high blood pressure, diabetes mellitus, hyperlipidemia, and when menopause is premature. White men between the ages of 35 and 55 are 5 times likelier to die of ischemic heart disease than white women in the United States. A bald man, reflective of higher testosterone levels, has an even greater risk than other men for cardiovascular disease. Such research findings have lead to the androgen hypothesis. However, not all research findings support this hypothesis.

Foreman (1986) pointed out the logic that if this androgen hypothesis were valid, then men of all cultures and races would demonstrate similar rates of incidence of cardiovascular diseases. The incidence of cardiovascular heart disease is greatest in white American males and lowest in African-African males. Furthermore, Foreman cited literature that attributed atherosclerosis to emotional inexpressiveness (a stereotypic characteristic of male identity). In addition, he stated that a relationship was found between socially held beliefs of competitive and aggressive men and the characteristics of the type A personality. Type A personality with underlying anger has been associated with an increased risk for heart disease. Another risk for cardiovascular heart disease is age—as one grows older, the risk of heart disease increases.

Reason for Seeking Health Evaluation

Signs of cardiovascular disease in men may be detected in a routine employment history and physical. Clinical symptoms may include weakness; extreme fatigue; palpitations; peripheral edema; extremity pain, tingling, and/or numbness in the arms or legs; dyspnea on exercise; hypotension; syncope; cyanosis; and chest discomfort. Severe chest pain that persists is a symptom that most likely motivates the male client to voluntarily seek medical attention with expediency.

Sociocultural Aspects, Lifestyle and Habits

Stress is a relevant factor in the development and progression of cardiovascular heart disease. Lifestyle, including leisure activities, habits of sleep-rest, recreation, exercise, drug use, eating patterns, and diet, as well as values, beliefs, job satisfaction, family relationships, stressful life events, health practices, coping behaviors, and support systems require investigation and evaluation. Specifically, we will comment on smoking, drug use (alcohol consumption, caffeine intake), diet, and exercise habits.

A history of smoking is important to ascertain because of a strong association between tobacco and cardiovascular disease. The responses of the cardiovascular system to the nicotine component of tobacco include a rise in both systolic and diastolic blood pressure, heart rate, myocardial oxygen uptake, force of cardiac contraction, myocardial excitability, and peripheral vasoconstriction. Free fatty acids, cortisol (an antidiuretic hormone), glucose, and platelet aggregation also have been found to increase with nicotine use. Epidemiologic studies of industry reveal that more disability due to chronic illness and more workdays lost are found among cigarette smokers than nonsmokers. Male smokers have a 60% to 70% greater risk for cardiovascular heart disease than nonsmokers. Respiratory problems that may cause cor pulmonale (enlargement of the right ventricle secondary to respiratory diseases) include the following disorders: pulmonary vascular disease, airway obstruction from tracheal stenosis, obstructive sleep apnea syndromes (which occur more in men than women), respiratory symptomatology of medullary dysfunction (hypoventilation and central sleep apnea syndromes), physical limitation of lung expansion and function by spinal-thoracic deformities (kyphoscoliosis, funnel breast, and pigeon breast), and obesity. Chronic obstructive lung disease, which is of higher prevalence in men, is viewed as an occupational hazard secondary to greater air pollutant exposure, including cigarette smoke. Cessation of smoking is associated with a dramatic decline in risk for both respiratory and cardiovascular heart disease.

Smokers drink more alcohol, coffee, and tea (Braunwald et al 1987). If caffeinated coffee and tea are used, the amount consumed on a daily basis should be assessed. The use of street drugs or recreational drugs needs investigation. Cocaine use is especially a risk for cardiovascular heart disease. Endocarditis frequently occurs from "mainlining" habits (intravascular use of drugs). The use of tobacco, alcohol, and other psychoactive drugs by men is more culturally acceptable or tolerated. The use of such substances by women, particularly by pregnant women, is frowned on because of the known influences on the fetus.

Alcohol can induce tachyarrhythmias (holiday heart syndrome); they frequently occur after a drinking binge. Alcoholic cardiomyopathy manifests a low cardiac output and peripheral and cardiac vasoconstriction. Progression of this cardiomyopathy may be halted by alcohol abstinence. If alcohol consumption continues, severe heart failure and death ensues generally within 1 to 3 years. The caffeine content in coffee and tea stimulates the heart and also may be a cause of arrhythmias. Chocolate may produce a similar effect; therefore diet investigation should question whether foods such as chocolate candybars, cocoa, and brownies are frequently eaten.

Other aspects of diet need assessment in relation to cardiovascular disease risks. It is believed that a diet consisting of fried foods, high salt, and high animal fats promotes the progression of atherosclerosis. Diet habits such as times for eating, amount of calories eaten, and types of foods consumed may be a cause of obesity, which is considered to be another risk factor for cardiovascular disease. Obese men, especially over the age of 50, are more prone to cardiovascular heart disease. Lack of exercise may also be a proponent of obesity.

Exercise is viewed within the lifestyle; assess whether a regular exercise regimen is followed, and the amount of activity inherent in the type of occupation held, that is, the sedentary state versus degrees of physical activity. Exercise is postulated to clear the blood vessels of cholesterol and to raise the concentration of the high density lipoproteins.

Last, the family health history and the client's personal health history are scrutinized for any incidences of such diseases as hypertension, hypo-or hyperthyroidism, obesity, diabetes mellitus, peripheral vascular disease, thrombophlebitis, pulmonary embolism, pulmonary infection, anemia, rheumatic heart fever, heart attack, and congestive heart disease.

Mental Health Assessment

Because type A personality with underlying anger is strongly associated with the development of cardiovascular problems, it is important to assess if the characteristics representative of type A personality, as well as undertones of anger, are manifested (see Chapter 3). Memory and other cognitive functions require evaluation, as alterations characterized by forgetfulness, difficulty in concentration, headaches, anxiety, insomnia, and confusion are reflective of cerebral arteriosclerosis, diminished cerebral blood flow, and arterial hypoxemia as observed in severe congestive heart failure. Depression is a common finding in chronic, long-standing heart failure.

Physical Assessment

Abnormal blood pressure, and pulse and respiratory changes, may be found when checking the vital signs. The client may appear underweight and even cachectic as a result of congestion of the intestinal veins causing poor GI absorption of nutrients. The increased oxygen needs of an enlarged heart, and extra work demands met by the respiratory muscles, further deplete calories. Also, the decreased intake of food may occur in conjunction with congestive hepatomegaly with associated anorexia and nausea. Weight loss, anorexia, and nausea also may be signs of digoxin toxicity.

For integumentary assessment, check for pallor of poor cardiac output and slow capillary refill of the nails. Note for the presence of intense rubor of the feet observed in Buerger's disease (thromboangiitis obliterans). Buerger's disease typically occurs in young men in the age range of 20 to 40. Observe for signs of cyanosis, particularly in the lips and nailbeds, and on the earlobes, tip of the nose, and under the tongue. Look for jaundice that appears late in congestive heart failure. The skin needs to be inspected for lesions such as skin ulcers, stasis dermatitis, petechae, and venous stars. Check for clubbing of the nails and increased thickness in the nails, especially the nails of the toes. Examine the fingertips for signs of nicotine stains from cigarette smoking. Look at the palms of the hands and the soles of the feet for Osler's nodes. The nodes are purple in appearance and are painful and tender; they are seen in infectious endocarditis. Observe the skin for diaphoresis and palpate for the presence of generalized or localized coldness. Increased tactile warmness and flushing may indicate fever that accompanies cardiovascular inflammation in such conditions as rheumatic heart fever and thrombophlebitis. Check for edema, especially in the pretibial area, about the ankles, and the flank and sacral region of clients who are bedfast. With cardiovascular disease, the hair may be sparse and brittle and may lack luster.

In assessment of the eyes, the appearance of the eyes may be dull in severe congestive heart failure. Check the lids and perinasal areas for any sign of xanthelasma. Note any pallor of the palpebral conjunctiva. Examine the eyegrounds for retinal changes such as papilledema, A-V nicking, hemorrhages, and exudates.

When assessing the throat and neck, check for sore throat, as it may be a sign of rheumatic heart fever. Observe for the presence of jugular venous distention that is found in heart failure. Also look for abnormal pulsations in the neck region. Hemoptysis may signal pulmonary venous hypertension. Weak or absent carotid pulse(s) may be detected in heart failure and advanced arteriosclerosis. A carotid bruit may be auscultated in conjunction with a stenosed carotid artery or disorder accompanied by a dynamic blood flow.

For thorax and breast assessment, observe for thoracic deformities that may hamper adequate heart and lung function. Observe for the presence of gynecomastia that may be a sign of digoxin intoxication.

Within the cardiovascular assessment, check for paroxysmal nocturnal dyspnea, orthopnea, and dyspnea on exertion. Note whether there are any abnormal thoracic and epigastric pulsations or the presence of a cardiac heave (lift, thrust). Note the presence of the point of maximal pulse at a location other than the apex of the heart. Palpate the thorax and the epigastric area for sign of a cardiac thrill. A thrill is associated with a grade IV, V, or VI heart murmur. Check the chest x-ray for mention of cardiomegaly and/or percuss the left cardiac border (LCBD) to grossly assess heart size. Auscultate the cardiac region for abnormal heart sounds (e.g., murmur, gallop rhythm, wide-, fixed-, or paradoxical splitting, $A_2 < P_2$ ratio in the adult, opening snap, ejection click, and pericardial friction rub). Observe for varicose veins. Check for Homan's sign with any presence of vascular inflammation. Palpate the peripheral arteries for detecting weak, thready, and absent pulses. Review the ECG for any abnormalities.

During respiratory assessment, observe for abnormal breathing patterns and use of respiratory accessory muscles and sternal retraction. Note any retraction or bulging of intercostal spaces. Percuss for the dullness of pleural effusion or atelectasis. Auscultate for rales that accompany congestive heart failure.

When assessing the abdomen, note abnormal contour and abdominal asymmetry that may accompany congestive hepatomegaly. Check if the liver is palpable. Also, percuss to assess whether the liver dullness span in the adult is greater than 12 cm. Abdominal pain and fullness generally is associated with hepatic congestion. Serum SGOT and SGPT enzymes are frequently elevated. Tricuspid valvular disease and constrictive pericarditis manifest marked ascites. Ascites is typically observed in clients with congestive heart disease. Percuss to detect the dullness of ascites and check for a fluid shift and fluid wave. Auscultate for bruits over the abdominal aorta, renal arteries, and femoral arteries that may denote such disorders as stenotic arteries and vascular aneurysms.

Renal changes within cardiovascular disease may include oliguria that results from a decrease in blood flow to the kidneys. Check urine for proteinuria and a high specific gravity. Investigate any signs of impotence that could result from diminished penile blood circulation.

Lung Cancer

Carcinoma of the lung is increasing throughout the world and is the leading cause of death in the United States. The great majority of incidence is linked with cigarette smoking. The younger the age when one starts to smoke, the more years one smokes, and heavy daily smoking (one pack per day) all increase the risk for lung cancer. The high-risk profile is the man over 45 years of age who smokes two or more packs of cigarettes a day.

Reason for Seeking Health Evaluation

Lung cancer and other pulmonary conditions may manifest similar symptoms, and therefore the client may seek care for what may seem to him to be insignificant or nonserious respiratory symptoms. Such symptoms may be chronic cough, fatigue, wheezing, and a feeling of chest tightness. Some clients may put off seeking assessment until the symptoms become more frightening and include such events as hemoptysis, extreme weight loss, and the type of problems that arise with metastasis. Regional metastasis can cause tracheal obstruction and dyspnea, esophageal compression and dysphagia, and hoarseness. Neurologic defects would suggest brain metastasis. Bone pain, pathologic fractures, spinal cord compression syndromes, and cytopenias may herald skeletal and bone marrow involvement. Liver metastasis could result in anorexia, jaundice, and abdominal pain. Vascular occlusion can occur from metastasis and result in signs of cardiac failure and arrhythmias.

Sociocultural Aspects, Lifestyle and Habits

The incidence of lung cancer is highest in men, more in African-Americans than whites, and is steadily increasing in women. Variables that need investigation in association with lung cancer are the exposure to carcinogens in the workplace and home. Foremost is to assess smoking habits and exposure to the cigarette smoke of others. Were there smokers in the home when the client was growing up? Do other family members smoke in the home? Are there nonsmoking areas at work and in places that are frequented by the client? It is important to question exposure to asbestos. Asbestos has been used in insulation, pipes, filters, floor tiles, and highways. It has been detected in drinking water and acid rain. Nonsmokers with asbestos exposure have a 5 times greater risk of developing cancer of the lung than nonsmokers who have not experienced exposure to asbestos. Another toxic substance is nickel; it is found in asbestos as well as in coal and crude oil. Nickel is used in the stainless steel industry and as a fuel additive. Possible exposure to carcinogens is scrutinized through a careful occupational history. Increased risk also has been linked with exposure to uranium, chloromethyl ethers, synthetic rubber, pitchblends, radioactive ores, soaps, detergents, paints, industrial gas, and pharmaceutical preparations. Occupations that have an element of chronic irritation to lung tissue increase the risk (e.g., farmers, bakers, hairdressers, painters, gas station attendants, coal miners, truckers, auto body repairmen, stockcar and horse racers, cattlemen, and sawmill and grain mill workers, to name only a few). The home location may contribute to risk as well, depending on the degree of air pollution. The risk for lung cancer is twice as great in urban dwellers than in those living in rural areas. Lastly, the existence of a family history of cancer is important. The type of cancer that has occurred in a relative, and at what age, in addition to the age of death, if applicable, is helpful assessment information.

Mental Health Assessment

A diagnosis of cancer may result in feelings of anxiety, fear, and depression. Maladaptive coping may be present. Brain metastasis could display a difficulty with cognitive functioning and other neurologic dysfunctions, depending on the areas involved.

Physical Assessment

An overall appearance may or may not be cachexia. Integumentary assessment may reveal cyanosis, jaundice, and clubbing of the fingers. In assessing the respiratory system, observe particularly for an increased AP diameter, the use of respiratory accessory muscles, abnormal fremitus findings, dullness in percussion (detected over tumor and areas of pleural effusion), unequal diaphragmatic excursions with elevation of hemidiaphragm secondary to phrenic nerve involvement, and any adventitious lung sounds such as crackles, wheezes, and pleural friction rubs. Signs and symptoms of heart failure and arrhythmias should be noted when assessing the cardiovascular system. Abdominal assessment may reveal a liver mass or tenderness, and musculoskeletal examination may reveal localized bony pain and aching joints (hypertrophic pulmonary osteoarthropathy). With brain and nervous system metastasis, neurologic signs within a broad range could emerge, depending on the specific site(s) of metastasis (e.g., cerebellum [ataxia, tremors] and cerebrum [personality changes, cognitive functioning difficulties]). Tumors of the lung apicies that involve the bracheal plexus will produce symptoms of paresthesias and shoulder and arm pain, especially shoulder pain that tends to radiate down the ulnar distribution area of the arm.

Benign Prostatic Hyperplasia and Prostatic Carcinoma

Benign prostatic hyperplasia (BPH) is a common condition that occurs in 80% of men in the fifth to seventh decades of life and increases to over 95% thereafter. With the increase in longevity of men, there is an associated increase in the incidence of BPH. An increase in the number of prostatic cells thought to be caused by hormonal changes increases the overall size of the gland. Because of the location of the prostate gland, surrounding the prostatic urethra, the signs of BPH are urinary problems. Symptoms may include frequency, decreased size and force of the urinary stream, dribbling, hematuria, and urinary retention.

Similar symptomatology may occur in carcinoma of the prostate. However, metastasis may result in additional symptoms of back pain, hip pain, pathologic fractures, or pain from bony metastasis to the skull, ribs, thoracic vertebrae, and the long bones. Lymphedema can be secondary to cancer invasion of the pelvic lymph nodes, and ejaculation may be painful. Due to the close proximity of the prostate gland to the rectum, tumor growth may interfere with defecation. The client may experience changes in his stool and have pain on defecation.

Sociocultural Aspects, Lifestyle and Habits

The frequency of prostate cancer varies throughout the world. Japanese men experience a lower incidence than Caucasians. However, American-born Japanese men and Japanese immigrants to the United States show an increased incidence. Diet etiology has been proposed as an explanation for this epidemiologic finding. African-American men are at greater risk than white men. The risk for prostatic carcinoma increases with age and rarely occurs before the age of 50. Exposure to occupational carcinogens may be a factor in cancer of the prostate; therefore, an occupational history is important. Gonorrhea and exposure to a virus also are associated with an increased incidence of prostatic cancer.

Physical Assessment

As with any form of cancer, the potential for metastasis exists. With prostatic carcinoma, the most frequent site of metastasis is to the vertebral column. The two physiologic systems most affected are the genitourinary and musculoskeletal. An annual rectal examination is recommended for all men age 40 and older. It is the most inexpensive, quick, and easy method for early detection of prostatic cancer. To defer this examination is an unethical act from a humanitarian viewpoint. A 6-month rectal examination should be performed on any male client with continuing urinary symptoms and with a family history of a blood relative who had prostate cancer. During the physical examination, note any signs of vertebral compression, paresthesias, and pain. Carefully palpate the posterior lateral surfaces of the lobes of the prostate gland during the digital rectal examination. A mass may be detected or the midline furrow of the prostate gland may be obscured.

Testicular Carcinoma

Testicular carcinoma is the most common cancer of young men. An early childhood incidence peak is seen, with a far greater peak occurring around the 16- to 35-year age group. It seldom occurs after the age of 40. It is frequently detected in screenings of aggregates of young men, such as in the military, athletic teams, and in preschool and pre-employment physicals in university cities where there is an increased population of young men.

Reason for Seeking Health Evaluation

Detection of testicular masses usually occurs during a routine physical examination. The most common symptom of testicular carcinoma is an asymptomatic nodule or swelling, or a feeling of heaviness in the involved testicular area. These symptoms may not be enough to prompt a client to seek health evaluation. The knowledge of cancer of the testicles and of the process of performing self testicular examination are educational goals to encourage men to seek medical attention in the presence of an enlargement or heavy feeling in the testes. Testicular carcinoma is not always painless, but less than 50% of the cases experience testicular pain. Symptoms due to metastasis can range from weight loss to dyspnea, anorexia, nausea, vomiting, abdominal pain, back pain, and urinary obstruction. Early detection is essential to survival, and all testicular lesions should be considered malignant until proven otherwise.

Sociocultural Aspects, Lifestyle and Habits

Another deterrent in seeking nursing and medical advice stems from cultural teaching that it is taboo to talk about one's genitals. Feelings of embarrassment and guilt often accompany afflictions of the genitalia. Teenagers and young adults especially are facing strong physiologic sexual feelings and social mores that are causing conflict and confusion. As a result, it is quite difficult for young men to reveal or want to discover abnormalities within their genitals, and this difficulty could prove to be deadly, because testicular cancer is a disease of young men.

When investigating health habits, it is very important to check whether the young to middle-aged male client knows about testicular cancer and performs a self testicular examination monthly. Including risk factors for testicular carcinoma in history taking is to ascertain if the client has a medical history of cryptorchid (undescended testicles), an inguinal hernia in childhood, mumps, and orchitis; the latter may have been associated with strenuous exercise or a sexually transmitted disease.

Physical Assessment

Massive pulmonary metastasis in testicular cancer may manifest in dyspnea and supraclavicular adenopathy, along with excessive use of the respiratory accessory muscles of the neck and chest. Cyanosis may be evident. Other symptoms may include abnormal fremitus findings, dull percussion notes within the lung fields, respiratory asymmetry, or adventitious lung sounds. Unequal diaphragmatic excursions may exist. Examination of the breasts may reveal gynecomastia. Vague abdominal pain may be found. Abdominal or back pain may result from metastasis with retroperitoneal adenopathy. Palpation of the testes of all young and middle-aged men is a "must" in every physical examination. Clients should be instructed to seek immediate health evaluation for any change in previously normal testes. Swelling in the testicular area may be secondary to a mass or a hydrocele. Any swelling should be subject to the technique of transillumination. A hydrocele (collection of edema) will transilluminate, whereas a testicular lesion will not. Examination of the urinary system includes attention to any signs of urinary obstruction, such as urinary retention with overflow, dysuria, frequency, and change in the size or force of stream.

Sexual Dysfunction

Common types of sexual dysfunction may encompass penile erection difficulties, loss of libido, ejaculatory problems, and inability to achieve orgasm. The occurrence of one or more symptoms within these patterns that denote sexual dysfunction is commonly termed *impotence.* This term conveys the image of weakness, powerlessness, and worthlessness. Use of the term may prove to be detrimental to the client and may only reinforce or lead to poor self-esteem. This can only add to the psychological stress that often accompanies any sexual problem. Even as a health professional, there is most likely the unrecognized but biased impression of the client who is impotent as being a poor, weak, dejected, "less than a man" individual. Society has fostered the concept that "power" lies in the genitals and male sexual prowess (Farrell 1986). For this reason, it is suggested that the use of the term *impotence* should be avoided in the nurse-client interactions and those among health care providers.

Most clients do not readily talk about sexual problems and concerns unless questioned or unless discussion is initiated by the nurse. Sexual shortcomings are generally devastating to a client's self-esteem and confidence. If sexual difficulties are anticipated because of specific therapies and certain medical conditions, you have a professional obligation to discuss this with the client. Even if the client displays signs of embarrassment, a matter-of-fact and caring approach will help ease the discomfort and will be truly appreciated by the client. Furthermore, the client will perceive you as a knowledgeable and competent nurse.

The following are mythical sexual beliefs commonly held by American men and identified by Zilbergeld (Roberts 1990, p. 259):

1. Men should not have, or at least not express, certain feelings.
2. In sex, as elsewhere, it's performance that counts.
3. The man must take charge of and orchestrate sex.
4. A man always wants and is always ready to have sex.
5. All physical contact must lead to sex.
6. Sex equals intercourse.
7. Sex requires an erection.
8. Good sex is a linear progression of increasing excitement terminated only by orgasm.

9. Sex should be natural and spontaneous.
10. In this enlightened age, the preceding myths no longer have any influence on us.

Etiologies of Sexual Dysfunction

There are many possible causes of sexual difficulties, and often a single factor cannot be identified; the most common etiology is an anxiety or depressive state. Other than psychic causes, sexual dysfunction can result from organic causes and from the effects of certain drugs. The primary diagnostic goal is to determine whether the etiology is psychologically induced or is secondary to organic factors.

The inability to achieve orgasm is generally a result of psychogenic causes. Surrounding circumstances may be marital problems, disinterest in sexual partner, and stresses of work, play, family, and finances. Fear of rejection or sexual inadequacy, along with concern of pleasing a partner, contribute to the added pressure to perform. Other cognitive interferences may take the form of intense emotions (e.g., anger, chronic worry, anxiety, uncertainty of masculinity, self-consciousness, achievement-consciousness). A decrease in libido may result from stress as well. Other interacting factors that constitute a psychological cause of sexual difficulties include religious orthodoxy and homosexuality. Surprisingly, nocturnal erections occur more frequently and are of a longer duration in men who have psychogenic sexual dysfunctions compared with sexually healthy men. Erections that occur during REM sleep begin in early childhood and continue through the eighth decade. If the neurologic and cardiovascular systems that mediate erection are intact, nocturnal penile tumescence (NPT) will be experienced, and the etiology is probably psychogenic in nature.

Penile erection difficulties and ejaculatory problems, particularly premature ejaculation, may be related to psychosocial factors as well as to organic causes. Fatigue also may impact on sexual performance. Because organic causes of sexual dysfunction can arise from a large number of diseases and types of trauma, only the more common ones are mentioned.

Hypogonadism (chromosomal, pituitary, or testicular) displays itself as the nondevelopment or the regression of secondary sexual characteristics, decreased libido, the inability to obtain or maintain an erection, and absence of emission. The latter sign can be due also to retrograde ejaculation. Sexual dysfunction commonly occurs in such endocrine disorders as Klinefelter syndrome, hemochromatosis (an inherited disease characterized by iron deposits in the pituitary gland), pituitary gigantism, acromegaly, hypothyroidism, Addison's disease, Cushing's syndrome, and diabetes mellitus. Within the first 6 years of the onset of diabetes mellitus, 50% of the male clients develop sexual difficulties. The manifestation of *unexplained* erectile difficulties should prompt testing for *latent diabetes mellitus.* Signs of sexual dysfunction may be the first clinical signs of diabetic neuropathy.

The inability to obtain or maintain the erect state also might be secondary to insufficient blood flow to the penis, which could be caused by a penile thrombus. Severe arteriosclerosis also could be an etiology, and in addition, arteriosclerosis may hamper cognitive functioning and decrease sensation which could interfere with libido or thought process in planning and executing the sexual act. Mental retardation may influence the degree of understanding of sexual behavior and activities. Some clients with an abdominal aortic aneurysm may experience erectile difficulties as well. Other cardiovascular problems that may interfere with erection are sickle cell disease, Leriche syndrome, and leukemia.

Peyronie's disease, in which hard nodules develop beneath the skin on the dorsum and occasionally on the sides of the penis, causes a painful, arching distortion of the penile shaft; the deformity makes it virtually impossible to perform coitus. Another penile disease that interferes with sexual functioning is priapism (a painful, persistent erection that may often be unrelated to sexual activity). Additionally, penile trauma may result in sexual problems. Trauma from accidents and surgery can impact on sexual functioning.

With head injury, there is the possibility of the client's developing sexual dysfunction as long as several years following the accident. The incidence most often follows blows to the back of the head like those that are frequently experienced in boxing matches. Erectile problems and loss of sexual sensation may occur with spinal cord injuries and tumors with sacral and cauda equina destruction. In cord injuries of a higher level, some degree of reflex erections can occur. A transection above the sacral level results in the loss of sexual sensation; however, in some cases, tactile stimulation of the penis, cremasteric region, perineum, and anus can produce a reflexogenic erection. Problems with sexual functioning also can occur with injuries such as herniated disks and "crushed" pelvic fractures.

Yeager and Van Heerden (1980) stated that 15% of men under age 50 and 100% of men older than 70 experienced sexual dysfunction symptoms following abdominoperineal resection and proctocolectomy. Lower gastrointestinal track surgery and prostate surgery carry the risk of sexual dysfunction secondary to nerve damage and disrupted blood flow. With such surgeries as colostomy, ileostomy, and suprapubic prostatectomy, the potential neurologic and cardiovascular damage is commonly combined with psychic trauma; this makes it difficult to separate the cause and effect on sexual dysfunction as being due solely to the surgical trauma or resulting from the psychological responses to the illness (depression, anxiety) and associated poor self-image.

Krane (1988) pointed out that sexual dysfunction can occur from testicular atrophy if the testicular arteries are ligated during the surgical repair of a hernia. He also noted that radiation and chemotherapy could cause sexual dysfunction if destruction of the testes, hypothalamus, and pituitary gland occurred. In addition, he cited that a lumbar sympathectomy performed on older men yielded a 50% incidence of erectile problems. Ejaculatory capacity also may be disrupted following a sympathectomy and rhizotomies. A sympathectomy is sometimes performed to treat hypertension. Krane also stated that a 50% incidence of sexual dysfunction occurred in clients that had a pudendal neurectomy for neurogenic bladder.

Sociocultural Aspects, Lifestyle and Habits

Sexuality is a cultural phenomenon. Our beliefs and attitudes are socially learned and impact on our sexual behaviors. How a client views sexuality, sexual roles, and sexual practices has roots in his culture and his life experiences. Assessment of cultural variables may provide a crucial piece of information in diagnosing sexual dysfunction. Other areas that require exploration are occupational, exercise, and leisure activities; drug use (including alcohol); diet; family history; and medical history.

Listen carefully to the client's conversation; the content and specific words used will be clues to his attitudes and beliefs. Discussion of masculine and feminine roles and current events related to sexuality issues will aid in assessment of individual, culturally-influenced beliefs regarding sexual expectations and behavior. What does "being a man" mean to a client? How were incidents and discussions regarding sexual matters handled by his parents? What type of early sexual experiences did the client have? What style of parenting did the client experience as a child?

More explicit to sexual functioning would be to ascertain if the client is sexually active. At this point, you need to be aware of slang terms that the client may use in his conversation with you. If you are unsure of a term used by the client, ask him to explain what he means. Is he able to have sex? Is sex an important part of his life? Do any physical defects or illnesses interfere with his sexual experiences? Does he have any difficulty having or maintaining an erection (hard-on)? Is there any problem with ejaculation (coming)? Has drugs or drunkenness ever seemed to have interfered with his sexual performance? What role or actions does he believe a man (and a woman) should assume in the sex act?

Because extreme fatigue may impinge on sexual functioning, it is important to assess extent and stress of occupational activity and responsibility, amount and regularity of exercise regimens, and leisure activities. Regular sleep pattern and whether there have been changes in sleep pattern are investigated. Does the client use any medications or practices to induce sleep?

The number of drugs that interfere with male sexual functioning keeps growing. Smoking habits need to be assessed, as nicotine has been associated with erectile failure. Long-term use of marijuana is thought to have an impact on erectile function, secondary to its effect on diminishing serum testosterone levels. Medications commonly associated with male sexual dysfunction are listed in Table 22-1.

Sexual dysfunction may be caused by anxiety, or it could be the side effect of a psychotropic medication that has been prescribed to treat anxiety. The antihypertensives Regitine and Dibenzyline are known to have specifically caused inhibitory ejaculation. The drug Reglan can cause hyperprolactinemia, which frequently is associated with hypogonadism and decreased serum testosterone levels. The result is the absence of emission.

Table 22-1 **Drugs Associated With Male Sexual Dysfunction**

Antabuse
Anticholinergics (Norpace, Probanthine, Tagamet, Xantac)
Antihistamines
Amphetamines
Antihypertensives
Sympatholytics (Aldomet, Calapres, Serpasil, Sandril, Ismelin)
Alpha-adrenergic blocking agents (Minipress, Dibenzylene, Regitine)
Beta-adrenergic blocking agents (Inderal, Propranolol, Visken, Tenormen, Lopressor, Trandate, Normodyne)
Vasodilators (Apresoline, Loniten)
Diuretics (Diuril, Hydrodiuril, Hygroton, Aldactone)
Chemotherapy drugs
Corticosteroids
Digoxin
Estrogen
Lioresol (Rx of MS)
Psychotropic agents
Minor tranquilizers (Valium, Librium, Milltown, Sexax, Tranxene, Tybatron)
Major tranquilizers (Mellaril, Serentil, Thorazine)
Antidepressants (Tofranil, Elavil, Asenden, Desyrel, Norpramine, Vivactile, Eskalith, MAO inhibitors)
Psychedelics

Data from Braunwald et al (1987) and Krane (1988).

Chronic use of drugs of habituation tend to be associated with erectile failure (e.g., cocaine, heroin, methadone, codeine, merperidine, marijuana, nicotine, and alcohol). Acute alcoholic episodes also may affect erectile function. Alcoholism affects diet, and the secondary malnutritional vitamin deficiency of poor diet in alcoholism (thiamine, niacin, vitamin B12) can compound sexual dysfunction via pelvic neuropathy.

Lastly, data on family history (diabetes mellitus, peripheral vascular disease, hypertension) and the client's medical history (endocrine problems, genital disease, trauma and surgery, neurologic damage, lower gastrointestinal surgery, cardiovascular system problems, severe depression, anxiety, nervous breakdown) need to be collected and analyzed.

Clients with multiple sclerosis may experience absence of emission, a "dry" orgasm, due to retrograde ejaculation (secretions flow backward into the bladder). Retrograde ejaculation may be an early sign of diabetes mellitus—as much as a year prior to diagnosis. It also may occur following surgery on the neck of the bladder. Surgery involving the penis, prostate gland, rectum, or testicles could result in neurologic damage and sexual functioning problems. Genital trauma from accidents or cystoscopy and vasectomy procedures could give rise to sexual functioning problems as well. Furthermore, temporal lobe lesions and temporal lobe epilepsy have been associated with erectile problems and inability to achieve orgasm. Injury with neurogenic bladder dysfunction or that associated with diabetes mellitus could contribute to sexual functioning problems. Whether vascular problems such as priapism and intermittent claudication exist needs to be identified, as these may suggest an insufficient penile blood flow which will impede attainment and maintenance of the erect state of the penis. Krane (1988) stated that 60% of men on chronic hemodialysis experience erectile problems. This is thought to be due to azotemic effects on the neurologic system, and from hyperprolactinemia and decreased serum testosterone due to endocrine alterations. Additionally, the psychological response to the chronicity of the illness adds to the stress.

Mental Status Assessment

Because many sexual difficulties are caused by psychological factors, it is necessary to assess mental status. For instance, premature ejaculation is primarily related to a psychological state; it could be due to unreasonable performance expectations, to an emotional disorder, or to extreme anxiety or excitation in the sexual situation.

The client's self-concept is assessed. What is his perception of his sexual abilities? Has he had successful and unsuccessful sexual experiences? What are his usual sexual practices? Investigate his values of "right and wrong" surrounding sexual issues and activities in his cultural and societal realms and for himself. Does he have anxieties regarding sexual activity or ability? Does he practice safe sex? Explore relationships with his partner(s). How does he describe his ideal sexual partner? How does this ideal compare with his actual sexual partner(s)? Is there any evidence of marital discord? What turns him on? What turns him off? Is he under extreme pressure to perform sexually? Does he express any signs of feeling rejected or inadequate? How would he describe himself as a sexual partner? Does he express fear of sexual encounters and incompetence? Does he display any signs of chronic anxiety, guilt, or depression?

Physical Assessment

Examination of the skin may reveal abnormal body hair distribution and sparseness of hair, which may be a sign of hypogonadism. With vascular etiology, the examination of the eyegrounds may reveal changes consistent with vascular insufficiency and diabetes mellitus (e.g., narrowed arteries, hemorrhages, and exudates). If gynecomastia is observed, ask if the client is taking digoxin. Digoxin's chemical structure is similar to the sex steroids, and some clients have exhibited increased estrogen and decreased testosterone levels as side effects to its use. When assessing the cardiovascular system, note weakness and absence of pulses. To check the penile pulse, palpate the penile body between your thumb and forefinger on either side of the midline. A doppler check may be warranted. On examination of the genitourinary system, note any signs of dribbling, weakness of urinary stream, urgency, or frequency. Question the client about the existence of a "dry" orgasm and milky postcoital urine that would indicate retrograde ejaculation. When sexual dysfunction is associated with neurologic deficits, you may detect poor anal sphincter tone, loss of perineal sensation, and weakness or absence of the bulbocavernosus reflex; this reflex, when present, is the anal sphincter constriction that is elicited by squeezing the glans penis (tip). Also with neurologic alterations you may find distal muscle weakness, absent deep tendon reflexes in the lower extremities (particularly the Achilles' deep tendon reflex), diminished or absent vibratory and position sense, and decreased or absent tactile and pain sensation.

SUMMARY

This chapter explored the cultural impact on male identity and associated interactional practices. The traditional perception of masculinity in Western society was discussed in light of its impact on men interacting with health professionals, and on men in health professional roles. The issues of masculinity and gender surrounding morbidity and mortality rates included the lack of preventive health practices, longevity being less than that of women, and specific health problems and types of accidents that have a greater incidence in men. The selected health problems of men presented were cardiovascular disease, lung cancer, benign prostatic hyperplasia and prostatic carcinoma, testicular cancer, and sexual dysfunction. The associated symptomatology of these selected health problems that is inherent in sociocultural aspects, lifestyle and habits, mental status, and physical assessment was identified. Special health needs of men were highlighted, and a holistic view of the male client was emphasized.

DISCUSSION QUESTIONS/ ACTIVITIES

1. Identify sexual values and beliefs learned from your cultural background.
2. Share your impression of society's prevailing views of masculinity.
3. Discuss the issues of masculinity associated with male morbidity and mortality rates.
4. Identify nursing prescriptions (approaches, interventions) to improve men's health.

5. Discuss (or role-play) the data collection phase with a client experiencing sexual dysfunction.
6. List the variables pertinent to data collection in each of the following selected health problems of men: cardiovascular disease, lung cancer, benign prostatic hyperplasia and prostatic carcinoma, testicular cancer.

REFERENCES

Allen, D. G., and Whatley, M. 1986. Nursing and men's health—some critical considerations. *The Nursing Clinics of North America* 21(1):3–13.

Bozett, F. W., and Forrester, D. A. 1989. A proposal for a men's health nurse practitioner. *IMAGE: Journal of Nursing Scholarship* 21(3):158–164.

Braunwald, E.; Isselbacher, K.; Petersdorf, R.; Wilson, J.; Martin, J.; and Fauci, A. 1987. *Harrison's principles of internal medicine.* 11th ed. New York: McGraw-Hill.

Dean, Kathryn 1989. Self-care components of lifestyles: the importance of gender, attitudes, and the social situation. *Social Science Medicine* 29(2):137–152.

Doll, R., and Peto, R. 1981. The causes of cancer: quantitative estimates of avoidable risks of cancer in the United States today. *Journal of the National Cancer Institute* 66:1193–1308.

Farrell, W. 1986. *Why men are the way they are.* New York: McGraw Hill.

Foreman, M. D. 1986. Cardiovascular disease: a men's health hazard. *The Nursing Clinics of North America* 21(1):65–73.

Forrester, D. A. 1986. Myths of masculinity: impact upon men's health. *The Nursing Clinics of North America* 21(1):15–23.

Jourard, S. 1971. *The transparent self.* New York: Jossey Bass.

Krane, R. J. Impotence. *Semin Urol* 4(4):207–208.

Roberts, A. 1990. *Crisis intervention handbook: assessment, treatment, and research.* Belmont, Calif.: Wadsworth Publishing Company.

Waldron, I. 1982. An analysis of causes of sex differences in mortality and morbidity. In *The fundamental connection between nature and nurture,* ed. W. Gove and G. R. Carpenter, p. 69. Lexington, Mass.: Lexington Books.

Yeager, E. B., and Van Heerden, J. A. 1980. Sexual dysfunction following proctocolectomy and abdominoperineal resection. *Annuals of Surgery* 191:169.

Diagnostic criteria	Medical therapy	Complications and prognosis	Nursing management
Diagnosis by inspection and histologic examination	Treatment primarily symptomatic, with antihistamines, cool baths or compresses, topical steroids; clear nail polish may provide immediate relief by asphyxiating the mite. If secondary infection, antibiotics used Insect repellants or toxicants (benzyl benzoate) used to prevent bites.	Pruritus may persist for months. Secondary infection may occur.	Discuss with child and family methods for avoiding bites (not walking in grassy or bushy areas without proper clothing and repellant). Reinforce physician's instructions for symptomatic relief.
Diagnosis based on history of bites and microscopic examination	Antipruritics, topical calamine lotion, or corticosteroids used for symptomatic relief. Prevention involves spraying household, especially baseboards, basements, bedframes, and upholstery, and spraying affected pets.	May develop secondary infection from scratching; otherwise prognosis is very good.	Discuss with family the need for spraying house and pets. Advise avoiding unsprayed animals, especially if a child is susceptible to alteration.
Diagnosis based on inspection of lice and nits in hair and clothing, as well as microscopic examination; Wood's lamp may be used (lice appear fluorescent).	Most popular and effective treatment is 1.0% gamma benzene hexachloride (Kwell) lotion or shampoo. Proper hygiene and laundering are promoted, as lice live mainly in clothing.	Possible drug toxicity; prognosis is very good if treated.	Assess children for presence of lice and nits. Observe for behaviors of toxicity. Advise family to wash clothing and bedding. Advise against child sharing hats or combs with friends. Advise family to remove all dead nits after Kwell; some larvae may lie dormant. Allow family to air concerns about social embarrassment; state that lice have no respect for social class or income level.
Diagnosis based on history of itching, distribution of lesions, microscopic examination; burrows are very diagnostic.	Topical application of 1.0% gamma benzene hexachloride (Kwell) used most often; 10% Crotamiton, sulfur in petrolatum, 12.5–25% benzyl benzoate also used. Ointment is applied for 12 hr, then washed off to avoid toxic level of absorption; may be repeated 1 week later if more larvae are detected. Antipruritics and antibiotics used as needed	Possible drug toxicity Secondary infection from streptococci may lead to nephritis.	Instruct child and family on proper use of medications. Observe for behaviors of toxicity (eczema, urticaria, aplastic anemia, alopecia, irritability, nausea, vomiting, amblyopia, headache, dizziness, convulsions); these usually occur if medication ingested or overused. Discuss with family the need to launder clothing, bedding, curtains.

Continued

Table C-3 **Continued**

Alteration/parasite	Epidemiology and etiology	Pathophysiology	Behavioral assessment
Scabies, continued			*Sites:* Burrows on palms (90%), wrists, penis, nipples, axillae, natal cleft (between buttocks, above anus); vesicles on sides of fingers; nodules on scrotum, penis, buttocks, groin, axillary folds, upper back, abdomen, thighs
Ticks (hard and soft); large, globular arachnids with short legs and hard leathery skin	Live in grass, shrubs, vines, bushes, animals Female tick attaches self to skin and sucks blood from superficial blood vessels.	Toxin secreted by tick may cause pyrexia. Neurotoxin injected during several days of tick engorging itself on blood may cause paralysis; may cause Rocky Mountain spotted fever.	Initial bite usually painless but develops into infiltrated lesion with surrounding erythematous halo; persists 1–2 weeks. Tick mouth parts in the wound cause small, pruritic nodules. *Pyrexia:* Fever, chills, headache, vomiting, abdominal pain. Improvement 12–36 hr after tick removed *Paralysis:* Flaccid, ascending motor paralysis; death may result from respiratory paralysis.

Source: From J. Servonsky and S. Opas. *Nursing Management of Children.* Boston: Little, Brown, pp. 1198–1201.

Diagnostic criteria	Medical therapy	Complications and prognosis	Nursing management
			Overbathing may cause skin irritation. Pets may carry scabies; advise family to consult veterinarian.
Diagnosis based on history of tick bite or observation of tick on skin	Tick removed by heat, nail polish, mineral oil, petrolatum, ether, chloroform, or liquid nitrogen; removal of mouth parts must be ensured (may need punch biopsy). Paralysis disappears spontaneously 24 hr after tick removed. Prevent with repellants.	Respiratory paralysis may cause death if tick not removed; Rocky Mountain spotted fever can be a serious complication; otherwise, prognosis is good.	Advise child and family to avoid tick-infested areas, or to use effective repellants. If child has progressive paralysis of unknown origin, examine entire body for hidden tick.

Table C-4 **Animal and Insect Inflicted Injuries**

Injury	Behavioral assessment	Complications	Nursing management
Human bite	Localized redness and edema, teeth marks, potential break of the skin and bleeding	Secondary infection from streptococci or staphylococci	Culture wound, cleanse wound with high-pressure flow of normal saline, administer ordered antibiotics, culture the mouth and throat of the identified assailant, teach wound care and behaviors of secondary infection.
Dog bite	Localized redness and edema, teeth marks, potential break or tearing of the skin and bleeding, absence of tissue	Secondary infection from *Pasturella multocida*	Remove clothing and cleanse wound with high-pressure flow of normal saline; administer ordered analgesics, antibiotics, and tetanus vaccine; teach wound care and behaviors of secondary infection; teach children to stay away from dogs who are unknown, eating, or irritable.
Wild animal bite	Same as for dog bites	Rabies (rare), secondary infection from *Streptobaccilus moniliformis* or *Spirillum minus*	Cleanse wound with high-pressure flow of normal saline; administer ordered analgesics, antibiotics, and antitoxins; teach wound care and behaviors of secondary infection; teach children to keep a distance between themselves and all wild animals.
Cat scratch	Localized redness and edema, claw marks, potential break of the skin and bleeding	Secondary infection from *Pasturella multocida, Staphylococcus epidermidis, Streptococcus viridans* and diptheroides	Cleanse wound with normal saline or soap and water, teach wound care and behaviors of secondary infection.

Continued

Table C-4 **Continued**

Injury	Behavioral assessment	Complications	Nursing management
Venomous snake bite	Localized edema, presence of fang marks, progressive edema, paresthesia, and paralysis	Paralysis, respiratory insufficiency, disseminated intravascular coagulation, cardiac arrest	Know the endemic venomous snakes for the area, observe the site for fang marks, observe every 15 minutes for progression of neurologic behaviors, administer ordered antivenin, keep area immobilized and child quiet, release tourniquet every 15 minutes, check nailbeds for capillary refill, do not apply ice, have resuscitation equipment available, teach children precautions for hiking in deserts.
Venomous spider bite	Localized redness, nausea, sweating and fever, headache, muscle cramps, apprehension, paresthesias or hyperesthesias	Ulceration and necrosis of the bite area, coma	Observe the site for an inoculation (puncture), assess every 15 minutes for progression of neurologic behaviors and induration, administer ordered antivenin (if available), teach care of ulceration, administration of ordered antibiotics for prophylaxis of secondary infection, and precautions for children's play areas.
Nonvenomous spider bite	Localized redness and itching	Localized infection from skin abrasion	Observe site for an inoculation, observe for unexpected systemic behaviors, teach children precautions for play in basements, sheds, and wood piles.
Jellyfish sting	Painful stinging sensation, localized redness and itching, chills and fever, nausea and vomiting, weakness	Respiratory failure and death	Cleanse area with water; to cause diffusion of the venom through the skin, apply seaweed, wet teabags, or lime juice; teach children to observe for sealife when walking on beaches and in the ocean.
Bee sting	Localized itching, appearance of a stinger, histamine response	Anaphylaxis, respiratory failure and death	Remove stinger, apply a paste of baking soda to draw out the stinger, administer ordered antihistamines, observe for behaviors of anaphylaxis, apply topical antihistamines (such as calamine lotion) for localized itching and irritation.
Mosquito bite	Localized itching, histamine response	Localized infection from skin abrasion	Teach prophylactic use of mosquito repellants, apply topical antihistamines for localized itching and irritation.
Flea bite	Localized itching, histamine response	Localized infection from skin abrasion	Teach family to keep home and pets free of fleas and to change clothes and bedding when fleas are uncontrolled, apply topical antihistamines for localized itching and irritation, cut fingernails to prevent secondary infections from skin abrasion, teach children good health habits.

Source: J. Servonsky and S. Opas. *Nursing Management of Children.* Boston: Little, Brown, 1987, p. 1002.

APPENDIX

D

Common Laboratory Values

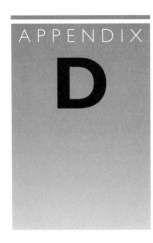

Table D-1 Normal Leukocyte Differential Count in Peripheral Blood

	Segmented neutrophils		Band* neutrophils		Eosinophils		Basophils		Lymphocytes		Monocytes	
Age	%	No./µL	%	No./µL	%	No./µL	%	No./µL	%	No./µL	%	No./µL
At birth	47 ± 15	8400	14.1 ± 4	2540	2.2	400	0.6	100	31 ± 5	5500	5.8	1050
12 hr	53	12,100	15.2	3460	2.0	450	0.4	100	24	5500	5.3	1200
24 hr	47	8870	14.2	2680	2.4	450	0.5	100	31	5800	5.8	1100
1 wk	34	4100	11.8	1420	4.1	500	0.4	50	41	5000	9.1	1100
2 wk	29	3320	10.5	1200	3.1	350	0.4	50	48	5500	8.8	1000
4 wk	25 ± 10	2750	9.5 ± 3	1150	2.8	300	0.5	50	56 ± 15	6000	6.5	700
2 mo	25	2750	8.4	1100	2.7	300	0.5	50	57	6300	5.9	650
4 mo	24	2730	8.9	1000	2.6	300	0.4	50	59	6800	5.2	600
6 mo	23	2710	8.8	1000	2.5	300	0.4	50	61	7300	4.8	580
8 mo	22	2680	8.3	1000	2.5	300	0.4	50	62	7600	4.7	580
10 mo	22	2600	8.3	1000	2.5	300	0.4	50	63	7500	4.6	550
12 mo	23	2680	8.1	990	2.6	300	0.4	50	61	7000	4.8	550
2 yr	25	2660	8.0	850	2.6	280	0.5	50	59	6300	5.0	530
4 yr	34 ± 11	3040	8.0 ± 3	710	2.8	250	0.6	50	50 ± 15	4500	5.0	450
6 yr	43	3600	8.0	670	2.7	230	0.6	50	42	3500	4.7	400
8 yr	45	3700	8.0	660	2.4	200	0.6	50	39	3300	4.2	350
10 yr	46 ± 15	3700	8.0 ± 3	645	2.4	200	0.5	40	38 ± 10	3100	4.3	350
12 yr	47	3700	8.0	640	2.5	200	0.5	40	38	3000	4.4	350
14 yr	48	3700	8.0	640	2.5	200	0.5	40	37	2900	4.7	380
16 yr	49 ± 15	3800	8.0 ± 3	620	2.6	200	0.5	40	35 ± 10	2800	5.1	400
18 yr	49	3800	8.0	620	2.6	200	0.5	40	35	2700	5.2	400
20 yr	51	3800	8.0	620	2.7	200	0.5	40	33	2500	5.0	380
21 yr	51 ± 15	3800	8.0 ± 3	620	2.7	200	0.5	40	34 ± 10	2500	4.0	300

*Note that these values are higher than those found in other references. They have been obtained by using strict criteria in differentiating segmented from band forms. Dr. Wallach does not classify a neutrophil as a segmented form unless a typical threadlike filament is visible.

Source: Wallach J. *Interpretation of Diagnostic Tests: A Synopsis of Laboratory Medicine* (5th ed). Boston: Little, Brown, 1992, pp. 4–5.

Table D-2 **Blood Chemistries—Reference Values (alphabetic)**

These values will vary, depending on the individual laboratory as well as the methods used. Each clinician should compare the transferability of these data to their own situation.

Acetone Aldolase		0.3–2.0 mg/dL
0–3 years		<16.3 units/L
4–16 years		<8.3 units/L
Adults (≥17 years)		<7.4 units/L
Ammonia		12–55 μg/dL
Amylase (total)		
<18 years		0–260 units/L
adults (≥18 years)		35–115 units/L
Base, excess		
Newborns		−10 to −2 mEq/L
Infants		−7 to −1 mEq/L
Children		−4 to +2 mEq/L
Adults		−2 to +3 mEq/L
Bicarbonate		
Age (years)		
Males	Females	
1–2	1–3	17–25 mEq/L
3–4	4–5	18–26 mEq/L
4–5	6–7	19–27 mEq/L
6–7	8–9	20–28 mEq/L
≥8*	≥10*	21–29 mEq/L
Bilirubin		
Total		<1.6 mg/dL
Direct		
1 month–adult		<0.5 mg/dL
Calcium		
Age (years)		
Males	Females	
Total		
1–14	1–11	9.6–10.6 mg/dL
15–16		9.5–10.5 mg/dL
17–18	12–14	9.5–10.5 mg/dL
19–21		9.3–10.3 mg/dL
>21*	>18*	8.9–10.1 mg/dL
Ionized		
1–19	1–17	4.9–5.5 mg/dL
≥20*	>18*	4.75–5.3 mg/dL
Carbon dioxide		
Total (content)		
Arterial		19–24 mEq/L
Venous		22–26 mEq/L
PCO_2 arterial or capillary		
Infants		27–40 mm Hg
Male adults		35–48 mm Hg
Female adults		32–45 mm Hg
PCO_2 venous		6–7 mm Hg > arterial blood
Ceruloplasmin		23–43 mg/dL
Chloride		
1–17 years		102–112 mEq/L
≥18 years		100–108 mEq/L
Cholesterol (see Lipid Fractionation)		

Cholinesterase		
Plasma		7–25 units/mL
RBC		0.65–1.3 pH units
Copper		70–150 μg/dL
Creatinine kinase (CK) (Ektachem)		
1–3 years		60–305 units/L
4–6 years		75–230 units/L
7–9 years		60–365 units/L
Males		
10–11 years		55–215 units/L
12–13 years		60–330 units/L
14–15 years		60–335 units/L
16–19 years		55–370 units/L
Females		
10–11 years		80–230 units/L
12–13 years		50–295 units/L
14–15 years		50–240 units/L
16–19 years		45–230 units/L
Creatinine kinase isoenzymes		MB < 5%
Creatinine		
Age (years)		
Males	Females	
1–2	1–3	0.2–0.6 mg/dL
3–4	4–5	0.3–0.7 mg/dL
5–9	6–8	0.5–0.8 mg/dL
10–11	≥9*	0.6–0.9 mg/dL
12–13		0.6–1.0 mg/dL
14–15		0.7–1.1 mg/dL
≥16*		0.8–1.2 mg/dL
Cryoglobulins		0
Fibrinogen		150–350 mg/dL
Gamma-glutamyl transpeptidase (GGT) (Ektachem)		
1–3 years		6–19 units/L
4–6 years		10–22 units/L
7–9 years		13–25 units/L
Males		
10–11 years		17–30 units/L
12–13 years		17–44 units/L
14–15 years		12–33 units/L
16–19 years		11–34 units/L
Females		
10–11 years		17–28 units/L
12–13 years		14–25 units/L
14–15 years		14–26 units/L
16–19 years		11–28 units/L
Glucose (fasting)		60–100 mg/dL (depends on method)
Iron, serum		
0–30 days		95–225 μg/dL
1–48 months		60–116 μg/dL
5–17 years		50–200 μg/dL
Adult males		75–175 μg/dL
Adult females		65–165 μg/dL

Table D-2 Continued

Iron-binding capacity	250–450 μg/dL
% saturation	20–50%
Isocitric dehydrogenase (ICD)	3–85 units/L
Lactic acid	
Venous	4.5–23 mg/dL
Arterial	4.5–14 mg/dL
Lactic dehydrogenase (LDH) (Ektachem)	
1–3 years	500–920 units/L
4–6 years	470–900 units/L
7–9 years	420–750 units/L
Males	
10–11 years	432–700 units/L
12–13 years	470–750 units/L
14–15 years	360–730 units/L
16–19 years	340–670 units/L
Females	
10–11 years	380–770 units/L
12–13 years	380–640 units/L
14–15 years	390–580 units/L
16–19 years	340–670 units/L
Lactic dehydrogenase isoenzymes	
I	17–28%
II	30–36%
III	19–25%
IV	10–16%
V	6–13%
Lead	<20 μg/dL
Leucine aminopeptidase (LAP)	Depends on method
Lipase	<1.5 units/mL
Lipid fractionation	
Cholesterol esters	60–75% of total
Phospholipids	180–320 mg/dL
Magnesium	1.7–2.1 mg/dL
Myoglobin, serum	≤90 ng/ml
Osmolality	275–295 mOsm/kg
Oxygen	
Saturation, arterial	96–100% of capacity
Tension, PO_2 arterial	
While breathing room air	
Newborns	60–75 mm Hg
<60 years	>85 mm Hg
60 years	>80 mm Hg
70 years	>70 mm Hg
80 years	>60 mm Hg
90 years	>50 mm Hg
While breathing 100% oxygen	>500 mm Hg
pH, arterial	7.35–7.45
Phenylalanine	
≤1 week	0.69–2.05 mg/dL
<1 month	0–2 mg/dL
<16 years	0.43–1.42 mg/dL
≥16 years	0.68–1.12 mg/dL
Tyrosine	
≤1 week	0.60–2.20 mg/dL
<16 years	0.47–1.34 mg/dL
≥16 years	0.82–1.99 mg/dL
Prostate specific antigen	
>40 years	≤4.0 ng/mL
≤40 years	≤2.7 ng/mL
Prostatic acid phosphatase (PAP), serum	<3.7 ng/mL

*Adult values.

Source: From J. Wallach. *Interpretation of Diagnostic Tests: A Synopsis of Laboratory Medicine* (5th ed.). Boston: Little, Brown, 1992. pp. 10–13.

Table D-3 Color Variations in Urine

Color	Cause
Straw-colored (dilute urine)	Nervous conditions, diabetes insipidus, granular kidney, large fluid intake
Dark yellow or amber (concentrated urine)	Acute febrile diseases, small fluid intake, vomiting, diarrhea
Turbid or smoky	Blood, chyle, spermatozoa, prostatic fluid, fat droplets
Red or red-brown	Porphyrin, hemoglobin, myoglobin, erythrocytes, transfusion reaction, hemorrhage, bleeding in urogenital tract, pyrvinium pamoate (Povan)
Orange-red or orange-brown	Drugs such as phenozyopyridine (Pyridium), urobilin
Yellow-brown or green-brown	Jaundice, obstruction of bile duct, phenol poisoning
Dark brown or black	Methylene blue medication, chorea, typhus
Cloudy	Pus, blood, epithelial cells, fat, phosphate bacteria, colloidal particles, urates, all-vegetable diet

Table D-4 **Normal Urine Values***

Constituent	24-hour excretion or as noted
Aldosterone	2–10 µg
Ammonia nitrogen	20–70 mEq
Amylase	35–260 Somogyi units/L
Calcium	
20 mg diet	<7.5 mEq
Catecholamines	
Free, epinephrine and norepinephrine	<100 µg
Metanephrine	<1.3 mg
VMA	<8 mg
Chloride	110–250 mEq
Coproporphyrin	100–300 µg
Cortisol	2–10 mg
Free cortisol	7–25 mg male 4–15 mg female
Creatine	
Adult male	<50 mg
Adult female	<100 mg
Higher in children and pregnancy	
Creatinine	1–1.6 g (15–25 mg kg)

Constituent	24-hour excretion or as noted
5-HIAA	2–9 mg
Lead	<120 mcg
Phosphorus	0.9–1.3 Gm
Porphobilinogen	<2 mg
Potassium	25–100 mEq
Protein	<50 mg
Sodium	100–260 mEq
Urea nitrogen	6–15 Gm
Uric acid	0.2–0.6 Gm
Urobilinogen	1–3.5 mg

	Estrone	Estradiol in µ	Estriol
Estrogens			
Female postpubertal	5–20	2–10	5–30
Female postmenopausal	0.3–2.4	0–14	2.2–7.5
Male } Female prepubertal }	0–15	0–5	0–10

*Specific gravity: 1.015–1.025; pH: 4.8–8.5; volume: 600–2500 mL/24 hr.

Source: Adapted from: *Harrison's Textbook of Medicine*, 8th edition, McGraw-Hill, 1977; *Textbook of Medicine*, Besson P., McDermott, W., 14th edition. W. B. Saunders Company, 1975.

Table D-5 **Pulmonary Function Tests**

Test	Age 20–39	40–59	60+
VC (liters)			
Men	3.35–5.90	2.72–5.30	2.42–4.70
Women	2.45–4.38	2.09–4.02	1.9–3.66
FEV_1 (liters)			
Men	3.11–4.64	2.45–3.98	2.09–3.32
Women	2.16–3.65	1.60–3.09	1.30–2.53
FEV% (FEV_1/VC%)			
Men	77	70	60
Women	82	77	74
Residual volume (liters)			
Men	1.13–2.32	1.45–2.62	1.77–2.77
Women	1.00–2.00	1.16–2.20	1.32–2.40
Total lung capacity (liters)			
Men	4.80–7.92	4.50–7.62	4.35–7.32
Women	3.61–6.18	3.41–6.02	3.31–5.86

FEV, forced expiratory volume; VC, vital capacity.

Source: From S. M. Tilkian, M. B. Conover, and A. G. Tilkian. *Clinical Implications of Laboratory Tests* (4th ed.). St. Louis: Mosby, 1987, p. 221.

Table D-6 Normal Values for Gastric Analysis

	Conventional units	Factor	S.I. units
Basal gastric secretion (1 hour)			
Concentration	(Mean ± 1 S.D.)		(Mean ± 1 S.D.)
Males	25.8 ± 1.8 mEq/L	1.0	25.8 ± 1.8 mmol/L
Females	20.3 ± 3.0 mEq/L		20.3 ± 3.0 mmol/L
Output	(Mean ± 1 S.D.)		(Mean ± 1 S.D.)
Males	2.57 ± 0.16 mEq/hr	1.0	2.57 ± 0.16 mmol/hr
Females	1.61 ± 0.18 mEq/hr		1.61 ± 0.18 mmol/hr
After histamine stimulation			
Normal	Mean output 11.8 mEq/hr	1.0	Mean output 11.8 mmol/hr
Duodenal ulcer	Mean output 15.2 mEq/hr		Mean output 15.2 mmol/hr
After maximal histamine stimulation			
Normal	Mean output 22.6 mEq/hr	1.0	Mean output 22.6 mmol/hr
Duodenal ulcer	Mean output 44.6 mEq/hr		Mean output 44.6 mmol/hr
Diagnex blue (Squibb):		1.0	
Anacidity	0–0.3 mg in 2 hrs		0–0.3 mg in 2 hr
Doubtful	0.3–0.6 mg in 2 hrs		0.3–0.6 mg in 2 hr
Normal	Greater than 0.6 mg in 2 hrs		Greater than 0.6 mg in 2 hr
Volume, fasting stomach content	50–100 mL	—	0.05–0.1 L
Emptying time	3–6 hrs	—	3–6 hr
Color	Opalescent or colorless	—	Opalescent or colorless
Specific gravity	1.006–1.009	—	1.006–1.009
pH (adults)	0.9–1.5	—	0.9–1.5

Source: From R. B. Conn, Jr. Laboratory reference values of clinical importance. In H. F. Conn, *Current Therapy 1981.* Philadelphia, W. B. Saunders Company, 1981.

Table D-7 Gastrointestinal Absorption Tests

Test	Conventional units	Factor	S.I. units
d-Xylose absorption test	After an 8-hour fast, 10 mL/kg body weight of a 0.05 solution of d-xylose is given by mouth. Nothing further by mouth is given until the test has been completed. All urine voided during the following 5 hours is pooled, and blood samples are taken at 0, 60, and 120 minutes. Normally 0.26 (range 0.16–0.33) of ingested xylose is excreted within 5 hours, and the serum xylose reaches a level between 25 and 40 mg/100 mL after 1 hour and is maintained at this level for another 60 minutes.		No change
Vitamin A absorption	A fasting blood specimen is obtained and 200,000 units of vitamin A in oil is given by mouth. Serum vitamin A level should rise to twice fasting level in 3 to 5 hours.		No change

Source: From R. B. Conn, Jr. Laboratory reference values of clinical importance. In H. F. Conn. *Current Therapy 1981.* Philadelphia, W. B. Saunders Company, 1981.

Table D-8 Liver Function Tests

Generalizations on liver function test interpretation

Patterns of abnormalities rather than single test changes are particularly useful despite sensitivities of only 65% in some cases.

Tests may be abnormal in many conditions that are not primarily hepatic (e.g., heart failure, sepsis, infections such as brucellosis, subacute bacterial endocarditis), and individual tests may be positive in other conditions than liver disease. Individual tests are normal in high proportions of patients with proven specific liver diseases, and normal values may not rule out liver disease.

Table D-8 Continued

Some common patterns (test combinations) of liver function changes	
Serum bilirubin (direct-total ratio)	
<20%	Constitutional hyperbilirubinemias (e.g., Gilbert's disease, Crigler Najjar syndrome)
	Hemolytic states
20–40%	Favors hepatocellular disease rather than extrahepatic obstruction
40–60%	Occurs in either hepatocellular or extrahepatic type
>50%	Favors extrahepatic obstruction rather than hepatocellular disease

Total serum bilirubin must exceed 2.5 mg/dL to produce clinical jaundice.

Total serum bilirubin > 5 mg/dL seldom occurs in uncomplicated hemolysis unless hepatobiliary disease is also present.

Total serum bilirubin level is generally less markedly elevated in hepatocellular jaundice (≤10 mg/dL) than in periampullary carcinomas (≤20 mg/dL) or intrahepatic cholestasis. In extrahepatic biliary obstruction, bilirubin may rise progressively to a plateau of 30–40 mg/dL (due in part to balance between renal excretion and diversion of bilirubin to other metabolites). Such a plateau tends not to occur in hepatocellular jaundice, and bilirubin may exceed 50 mg/dL (partly due to concomitant renal insufficiency and hemolysis).

Serum bilirubin levels are generally higher in obstruction due to carcinoma than due to stones.

Increased serum bilirubin with normal alkaline phosphatase suggests constitutional hyperbilirubinemias or hemolytic states.

Normal serum bilirubin with increased alkaline phosphatase (of liver origin) suggests obstruction of one hepatic duct or metastatic or infiltrative disease of liver. Metastatic and granulomatous lesions of liver cause 1.5–3.0 times increase of serum alkaline phosphatase.

Mild increase of serum glutamic-oxaloacetic (SGOT) and glutamic-pyruvic transaminases (SGPT) (usually <500 IU/L) with alkaline phosphatase increased >3 times normal indicates cholestatic jaundice, but more marked increase of SGOT and SGPT (especially >1000 IU/L) with alkaline phosphatase increased <3 times normal indicates hepatocellular jaundice.

SGOT and SGPT are most markedly increased in viral hepatitis, drug injury, carbon tetrachloride poisoning (100–2000 IU/L). SGOT >10 times normal indicates acute hepatocellular injury, but lesser increases are nonspecific and may occur with virtually any other form of liver injury. Levels are usually <200 IU/L in posthepatic jaundice and intrahepatic cholestasis. Levels are usually <50 IU/L in fatty liver, <100 IU/L in alcoholic cirrhosis, <150 IU/L in alcoholic hepatitis (may be higher if patient has delirium tremens), <200 IU/L in 65% of patients with cirrhosis, <200 IU/L in 50% of patients with metastatic liver disease, lymphoma, and leukemia.

SGOT-SGPT ratio > 1 with SGOT < 300 IU/L favors alcoholic hepatitis in cases of liver disease. Increased SGOT > SGPT also occurs in cirrhosis and metastatic liver disease. Increased SGOT < SGPT favors viral hepatitis, posthepatic jaundice, intrahepatic cholestasis. *SGOT is increased in acute myocardial infarction and in muscle diseases, but SGPT is normal. SGPT is more specific for liver disease than SGOT.*

SGOT soaring to peak of 1000–9000 IU/L, declining by 50% within 3 days and to <100 IU/L within a week suggests shock liver with centrolobular necrosis (e.g., due to congestive heart failure, arrhythmia, sepsis, GI hemorrhage); serum bilirubin and alkaline phosphatase reflect underlying disease. Rapid rise of SGOT and SGPT to very high levels (e.g., >600 IU/L and often >2000 IU/L) followed by a sharp fall in 12–72 hours is said to be typical of acute biliary duct obstruction. Abrupt SGOT rise may also be seen in acute fulminant viral hepatitis (rarely >4000 IU and decline more slowly; positive serologic tests) and acute chemical injury.

Gamma-glutamyl transpeptidase (GGT)–alkaline phosphatase ratio > 5 favors alcoholic liver disease.

Isolated elevation of GGT is a sensitive screening and monitoring test for alcoholism.

Serum 5′-nucleotidase and leucine aminopeptidase (LAP) parallel the increase in alkaline phosphatase in obstructive type of hepatobiliary disease, but the 5′-nucleotidase is increased only in the latter and is normal in pregnancy and bone disease, whereas the LAP is increased in pregnancy but usually normal in bone disease. GGT is normal in bone disease and pregnancy. Therefore, these enzymes are useful in determining the source of increased serum alkaline phosphatase.

Continued

Table D-8 **Continued**

Serum Enzyme	Biliary Obstruction	Pregnancy	Bone Disease
Alkaline phosphatase	I	I	I
5′-Nucleotidase	I	N	N
LAP	I	I	N
GGT	I	N	N

(I = increased; N = normal)

Serum alkaline phosphatase is the best indicator of biliary obstruction but does not differentiate intrahepatic cholestasis from extrahepatic obstruction. High values (>5 times normal) favor obstruction, and normal levels virtually exclude this diagnosis. Is markedly increased in infants with congenital intrahepatic bile duct atresia but is much lower in extrahepatic atresia.

Bilirubin ("bile") in urine implies increased serum direct bilirubin and excludes hemolysis as the cause. Often precedes clinical icterus. May occur without jaundice in anicteric or early hepatitis, early obstruction, or liver metastases. (Tablets detect 0.05–0.1 mg/dL; dipsticks are less sensitive; test is negative in normal persons.)

Complete absence of urine urobilinogen strongly suggests complete bile duct obstruction; normal in incomplete obstruction. Decreased in some phases of hepatic jaundice. Increased in hemolytic jaundice and subsiding hepatitis. Increase may evidence hepatic damage even without clinical jaundice (e.g., some patients with cirrhosis, metastatic liver disease, congestive heart failure). Presence in viral hepatitis depends on phase of disease. (Normal is <1 mg or 1 Ehrlich unit/2-hour specimen.)

Serum cholesterol

- May be normal or slightly decreased in hepatitis
- Markedly decreased in severe hepatitis or cirrhosis
- Increased in posthepatitic jaundice or intrahepatic cholestasis
- Markedly increased in primary biliary cirrhosis

Prothrombin time (PT) may be prolonged due to lack of vitamin K absorption in obstruction or lack of synthesis in hepatocellular disease. Corrected by parenteral administration of vitamin K (10 mg/day for 3 days) in obstructive but not in hepatocellular disease. Markedly prolonged PT is a good index of severe liver cell damage in hepatitis and cirrhosis; not useful when only slightly prolonged.

Serum gamma globulin tends to increase with most forms of chronic liver disease; marked increases (e.g., >3 gm/dL) are suggestive of chronic active hepatitis. Serum albumin is slow to reflect liver damage. Is usually normal in hepatitis and cholestasis.

Unusual patterns:

- Some patients do not present the usual pattern: SGOT and SGPT are <200 units in 20% of acute viral hepatitis. Serum alkaline phosphatase is increased >3 times in 5% of acute hepatitis.
- Normal values may not rule out liver disease: SGPT is normal in 50% and SGOT is normal in 25% of patients with alcoholic cirrhosis.
- Liver function test abnormalities may occur in systemic diseases, e.g., systemic lupus erythematosus (SLE), sarcoidosis, tuberculosis, subacute bacterial endocarditis, brucellosis, sickle cell disease.
- A confusing pattern may occur in mixed forms of jaundice, e.g., sickle cell disease producing hemolysis and complicated by pigment stones causing duct obstruction.

Serologic tests for viral hepatitis A (HAV)

Anti-HAV-IgM appears at the same time as symptoms and is detectable for 3–12 weeks after symptoms subside. Presence confirms the diagnosis of recent acute infection.

Anti-HAV-IgG appears after the acute period and is usually detectable for life; found in 45% of adult population. Indicates previous exposure to HAV, recovery, and immunity to type A hepatitis. Usually order anti-HAV-total and anti-HAV-IgM tests simultaneously; positive anti-HAV-total and negative anti-HAV-IgM indicates anti-HAV-IgG and immunity.

Serial testing is usually not indicated.

Serologic tests for viral hepatitis B (HBV)

Hepatitis B Surface Antigen (HB_sAg)

Table D-8 Continued

Earliest indicator of HBV infection. Usually appears in 27–41 days (as early as 14 days). Appears 7–26 days before biochemical abnormalities. Persists during the acute illness. Usually disappears 1–13 weeks after onset of laboratory abnormalities. Is the most reliable serologic marker of HBV infection. May also be found in chronic infection. HB vaccination does not cause a positive HB_sAg. Titers are not of clinical value. Present sensitive assays detect <1.0 ng/mL of circulating antigen, which is the level needed to find 10–15% of reactive blood donors who carry antigen but express only low levels.

Source: From J. Wallach. *Interpretation of Diagnostic Tests: A Synopsis of Laboratory Medicine.* (5th ed.). Boston: Little, Brown, 1992, pp. 170–172.

Table D-9 Laboratory Examination of Stool

Normal Values

Bulk:	100–200 g
Water:	up to 75%
Total osmolality:	200–250 mOsm
pH:	7.0–7.5 (may be acid with high lactose intake)
Nitrogen:	<2.5 g/d
Coproporphyrin:	400–1000 mg/24 h
Trypsin:	20–950 units/g

Color

Brown: normal
Clay color (gray-white): biliary obstruction
Tarry: if >100 mL of blood in upper GI tract
Red: blood in large intestine or undigested beets or tomatoes
Black: blood or iron or bismuth medication
Various colors: depending on diet

Source: From J. Wallach. *Interpretation of Diagnostic Tests: A Synopsis of Laboratory Medicine* (5th ed.). Boston: Little, Brown, 1992, p. 153.

Table D-10 Renal Function Tests

Urine concentration test
Restrict water intake for 14–16 hours; then collect three urine specimens at 1-, 2-, and 4-hour intervals, and measure specific gravity.

Normal: Urine specific gravity is ≥1.025.

With decreased renal function, specific gravity is <1.020. As renal impairment is more severe, specific gravity approaches 1.010.

The test is sensitive for early loss of renal function, but a normal finding does not necessarily rule out active kidney disease.

The test is unreliable in the presence of any severe water and electrolyte imbalance (e.g., adrenal cortical insufficiency, edema formation), low-protein or low-salt diet, chronic liver disease, pregnancy, lack of patient cooperation.

Fluid deprivation may be contraindicated in heart disease or early renal failure.

Vasopressin (pitressin) concentration test
The bladder is emptied, and urine is collected 1 and 2 hours after subcutaneous injection of 10 units of vasopressin. Water intake is not restricted, but no diuretics should be administered.

Normal: The specific gravity should reach ≥1.020.

Interpretation is the same as in the urine concentration test.

In diabetes insipidus, urine specific gravity becomes normal after vasopressin administration but not after fluid restriction.

The test may be used in the presence of edema or ascites. It is contraindicated in coronary artery disease and pregnancy.

Urine osmolality
Measurement of urine osmolality during water restriction is an accurate, sensitive test of decreased renal function.

The patient is on a high-protein diet for 3 days; has a dry supper and no fluids on the evening before the test; empties the bladder at 6 A.M., discards urine, and returns to bed. Test urine specimen is collected at 8 A.M.

Continued

Table D-10 Continued

Normal: concentration of >800 mOsm/kg

Minimal impairment of renal concentrating ability: 600–800 mOsm/kg

Moderate impairment: 400–600 mOsm/kg

Severe impairment: <400 mOsm/kg

Urine osmolality may be impaired when other tests are normal (Fishberg concentration test, serum urea nitrogen [BUN], phenolsulfonphthalein [PSP] excretion, creatinine clearance, IV pyelogram); may be especially useful in diabetes mellitus, essential hypertension, silent pyelonephritis.

It may be well also to measure serum osmolality and calculate urine-serum ratio (normal >3).

Urine dilution test

No breakfast is allowed; 1500 mL of water is taken within 30–45 minutes, and urine is collected every hour for 4 hours.

Normal: Urine volume is >80% of ingested amount (1200 mL).

Specific gravity is 1.003 in at least one specimen.

With decreased renal function there is a smaller volume of urine.

Specific gravity may not fall below 1.010.

Loss of dilution ability occurs later than loss of concentrating ability.

Water loading may be contraindicated in kidney and heart disease.

Phenolsulfonphthalein (PSP) excretion test

Administer an IV injection of 1 mg/kg body weight or usually 6 mg in 1-mL volume. Collect urine and (sometimes) blood samples at 15-, 30-, and 60-minute intervals.

Normal > 25% in urine in 15 minutes; 55–75% in 2 hours

The test is useful to detect slight to moderate decrease in renal function. It is not useful in chronic azotemia with fixed specific gravity (serum creatinine and creatinine clearance are more useful then).

It is hazardous in severe renal insufficiency or heart failure because adequate prior hydration is required to obtain sufficient urine volume. Using small urine volume magnifies errors.

The test is distorted by residual bladder urine, abnormal drainage sites (e.g., fistulas), and interfering substances (e.g., hematuria).

Hepatic disease may give falsely elevated values (because 20% of the dye is normally removed by the liver). False results may also occur in multiple myeloma (because of excessive protein binding) and in hypoalbuminemia. Certain drugs may interfere with PSP excretion (e.g., salicylates, penicillin, some diuretic and uricosuric drugs, and some x-ray contrast media).

The 15-minute PSP excretion correlates with the glomerular filtration rate (GFR); a normal 15-minute value indicates normal GFR. Progressive decrease of 15-minute value is proportional to decreased GFR (e.g., 15% PSP excretion in 15 minutes approximates a 45% GFR). If the GFR is normal, the PSP test indicates renal blood flow or tubular function; there are better tests available for measuring these two functions, and the PSP test is now rarely used.

Increased dye excretion in later time periods compared to the initial 15-minute period suggests increased residual urine due to obstructive uropathy or incomplete bladder emptying; the latter can be ruled out by indwelling catheterization during the test.

PSP that is normal with increased BUN and serum creatinine and decreased GFR suggests acute glomerulonephritis. PSP parallels these parameters in most chronic renal diseases.

Glomerular filtration rate

(See standard laboratory texts for information on the technical performance of clearance tests.)

Elderly patients with a normal serum creatinine and diminished muscle mass may have a 30% decrease in GFR.

GFR is measured with urea clearance, creatinine clearance, or inulin clearance.

Source: From J. Wallach. *Interpretation of Diagnostic Tests: A Synopsis of Laboratory Medicine* (5th ed.). Boston: Little, Brown, 1992, pp. 555–556.

Index